Fungal Infections of the Central Nervous System

Mehmet Turgut • Sundaram Challa
Ali Akhaddar
Editors

Fungal Infections of the Central Nervous System

Pathogens, Diagnosis, and Management

Springer

Editors
Mehmet Turgut
Department of Neurosurgery
Aydın Adnan Menderes University
School of Medicine
Aydın
Turkey

Ali Akhaddar
Department of Neurosurgery
Avicenne Military Hospital
Mohammed V University in Rabat
Marrakech
Morocco

Sundaram Challa
Department of Pathology
Basavatarakam Indo-American Hospital
& Research Institute
Hyderabad
Telangana
India

ISBN 978-3-030-06087-9 ISBN 978-3-030-06088-6 (eBook)
https://doi.org/10.1007/978-3-030-06088-6

This Springer imprint is published by the registered company Springer Nature Switzerland AG
The registered company address is: Gewerbestrasse 11, 6330 Cham, Switzerland

Preface I

Fungal infections of the central nervous system, once considered rare, have become more frequent and pose a diagnostic and therapeutic challenge in the day-to-day practice. Better awareness of the epidemiological features and elucidation of the risk factors along with advancements in technology in imaging and molecular diagnostics contributed to better understanding of the disease mechanisms and diagnosis. However, geographic variations due to environmental factors, emerging fungi in different clinical scenarios, and genetic factors influence the incidence of fungal infections. Though there is a wealth of information on fungal infections of the central nervous system, textbook like this provides a comprehensive and rapid access to the various aspects of these diseases and serves as a ready reference for the trainee and practicing neuroscientists.

The book has six sections with each section dedicated to one aspect of the disease. The authors were chosen from various parts of the world, based on their contributions and special interest in that subspecialty. Each chapter was edited by an expert in the field to provide concise and up-to-date information on the subject. The chapters were well-illustrated with tables and figures and provided with extensive references to guide further reading for residents, neurologists, internists, and neurological surgeons.

We are grateful to all the authors for their contributions and support to complete this book project in time. We especially wish to thank Springer Nature for their support in ensuring quality publication of the book. We are truly humbled by this experience. We hope this book will be a unique and important addition to the existing books on this subject.

Aydın, Turkey	Mehmet Turgut
Hyderabad, India	Sundaram Challa
Marrakech, Morocco	Ali Akhaddar

Preface II

Fungi are ubiquitous organisms found in the soil, water, and environment. Infections of humans are uncommon with only a few species being pathogenic. However, with changes in the environmental factors and immune status of individuals, fungal infections are on the rise. The incidence of fungal infections of the central nervous system (CNS) parallels that of the systemic fungal infections. Fungal infections of the CNS are being increasingly diagnosed in the past few decades due to steady increase in the number of immunosuppressed individuals, better awareness, and improved diagnostic modalities. Infections of the CNS are associated with high morbidity and mortality, but the diagnosis and treatment remain a challenge. Understanding the pathogenesis and host pathogen interactions helps in devising new diagnostic modalities and therapeutic interventions.

The etiologic agents include yeasts, filamentous fungi, and dimorphic fungi. The common yeast fungi include *Cryptococcus* and *Candida*, whereas filamentous fungi with hyaline septate hyphae include *Aspergillus*, *Fusarium*, and *Mucorales* and the pigmented fungi include dematiaceous fungi. The dimorphic fungi include *Blastomyces*, *Histoplasma*, *Coccidioides*, and *Paracoccidioides*. *Aspergillus* and *Mucorales* are usually opportunistic, but *Aspergillus* can cause infections in immunocompetent hosts in certain geographical regions. Dematiaceous fungi are neurotropic and cause infection in immunocompetent hosts, and dimorphic fungi cause infections which are geographically restricted.

The portal of entry is usually by inhalation and subsequent hematogenous dissemination to the CNS. The infection may spread from contiguous structures like paranasal sinuses, orbit, mastoid, or skull bone and by direct inoculation from surgery or trauma.

The size of the conidia or yeast, the virulence factors, and angioinvasiveness of the fungus are important in the pathogenesis. The interplay between host defenses and the strategy of the pathogen to evade immune attack, acquire nutrients, degrade extracellular matrix, and disseminate are not yet completely understood.

The immune status, portal of entry, type of the fungus, and virulence of the organism determine the pathology which in turn manifests as the clinical syndrome. The clinical syndromes include meningitis, intracranial space-occupying lesion, stroke-like manifestation, or spinal syndrome. The pathology includes abscess, granuloma, meningitis, infarct with or without hemorrhage, or subarachnoid hemorrhage. Imaging provides important clues to diagnosis in appropriate clinical setting.

Diagnosis is established by cerebrospinal fluid examination or tissue obtained at surgery along with culture. Histopathology is useful for delineation of fungal morphology, but species confirmation by culture is needed. Molecular tests, especially in disseminated disease, are warranted. Serum galactomannan is widely used but has several limitations. High index of clinical suspicion in appropriate clinical setting, along with epidemiological consideration, is important for early diagnosis. Management includes neurosurgical intervention, especially for intracranial space-occupying lesions, administration of antifungal treatment, and correction of immune impairment or risk factors.

In this textbook, in several chapters contributed by experts in the field, the epidemiological, clinical, diagnostic, and management aspects of various fungal infections of the CNS are addressed.

Aydın, Turkey Mehmet Turgut
Hyderabad, India Sundaram Challa
Marrakech, Morocco Ali Akhaddar

Contents

Part I

General Considerations

Historical Aspects of Fungal Infections

1

Nikolaos Ch. Syrmos, Vaitsa Giannouli, and Mehmet Turgut

Abbreviations

CNS Central nervous system
CSF Cerebrospinal fluid
USA United States of America

1.1 Introduction

Scientific research documented in the particular field of fungal infections should be explored through the perspectives of continuously changing biological, medical, and public profiles. In this chapter, a brief review of ancient to modern approaches to manage the central nervous system (CNS) infections caused by fungal pathogens will be given according to the historical references in the following subheadings of the history of medicine: "Ancient Greece," "Mid Modern Period," and "Contemporary Period."

N. C. Syrmos (✉) · V. Giannouli
Medical School, Aristotle University of Thessaloniki, Thessaloniki, Macedonia, Greece

M. Turgut
Department of Neurosurgery, Aydın Adnan Menderes University School of Medicine, Aydın, Turkey

1.2 Ancient Greece

The description and the scientific study of fungal infections remains an interesting and attractive topic since the antiquity. The father of the documented medicine, Hellenic Hippocrates of Kos, was the first physician who observed (Ancient Greek word παρατήρισις) and described the candidiasis phenomenon with white patches into the oral cavity in a weak and infirm patient. His main contribution initiated the human society's development of medicine through a well-documented and delicate blending of the art of healing and scientific observations and studies (Fig. 1.1) (Syrmos et al. 2010; Giannouli and Syrmos 2011; Syrmos 2011).

1.3 Mid Modern Period

Pier Antonio Micheli (1679–1737 AD) (Fig. 1.2), a catholic priest from Pisa, Central Italy, in his observations and studies, described *Aspergillus* (Schaechter 2011). Initially, his aim was to study the nine different fungal species that resembled aspergillum (Sumbali and Johri 2005). This was very often used, perforated, to sprinkle the holy water during Christian ceremonies (Schaechter 2000). Antonio also became a well-known academic botanist, a ranking professor, and also a curator of the Orto Botanico di Firenze, in Central Italy (Giardino dei Semplici). He made various

M. Turgut et al. (eds.), *Fungal Infections of the Central Nervous System*,
https://doi.org/10.1007/978-3-030-06088-6_1

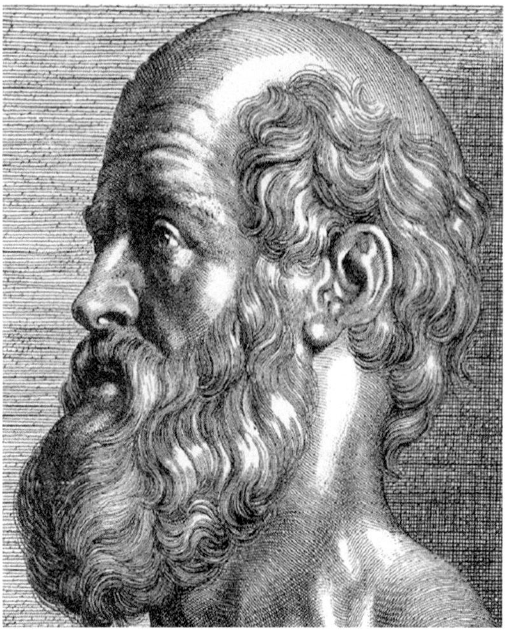

Fig. 1.1 A photograph of Hippocrates of Kos

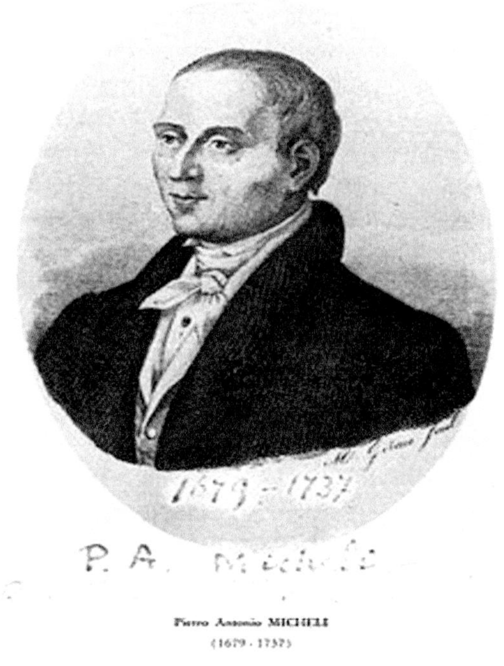

Fig. 1.2 A photograph of Pier Antonio Micheli (1679–1737 AD)

well-documented projects and wrote a paper entitled "Nova plantarum genera: iuxta Tournefortii methodum disposita" (Geronimus 2007). Over the years, he performed profound research about

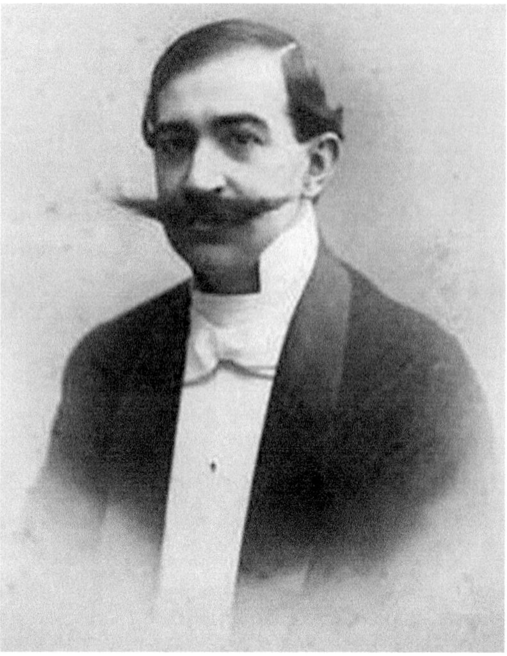

Fig. 1.3 A photograph of Alejandro Posadas (1870–1902 AD)

mushroom spores, managed to become an undisguised authority on cryptogams, and became a widely recognized figure in the scientific community of his era (Geronimus 2007). His main achievement was the connection between generations of microfungi such as *Aspergillus*, *Botrytis*, and others (Schaechter 2000; Geronimus 2007).

Later, around 1840, the fungal etiology of these manifestations was documented, thanks to the Berg-Bennett studies (Gholami-Shabani et al. 2018). Kurchenmeister in 1855 was the first who described human zygomycetes after isolation of nonseptate hyphae from a cancerous lung (Guého et al. 1992). Twenty one years later in 1861, Zenkar described the first case of human intracerebral candidiasis (McPartland and Goff 1991).

In 1892, Alejandro Posadas (1870–1902 AD) (Fig. 1.3), an Argentinian surgeon specializing in the general and pediatric surgery, started his scientific collaboration with Carl Wernicke (1848–1905 AD). Wernicke was at the same time an anatomist and a psychiatrist, from Germany (Fig. 1.4) (Sharpton et al. 2009; Miranda 2015). Together, they performed a series of well-documented neurological, biological, and specific pathological studies about human coccidioidomycosis.

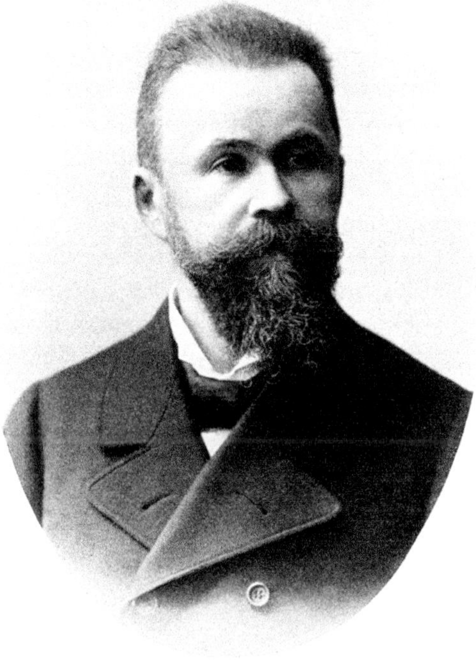

Fig. 1.4 A photograph of Carl Wernicke (1848–1905 AD)

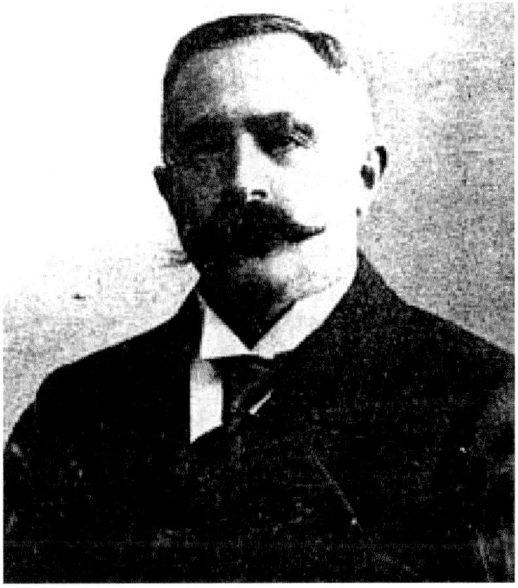

Fig. 1.5 A photograph of Abraham Buschke (1868–1943 AD)

Invaluable studies were performed by Abraham Buschke (1868–1943 AD) from Nakel, Posen, Germany (Fig. 1.5) (Sharpton et al. 2009). He was actually a dermatologist (Miranda 2015). In 1894, in collaboration with Otto Busse (1867–1922 AD), they described the "Busse-Buschke disease," an infectious pathological situation caused by the fungus *Cryptococcus neoformans*.

Around 1897, Oppe presented in the scientific community the first case of cerebral aspergillosis extending from sphenoid sinusitis (Antoniades et al. 2008). In 1905, Von Hansemann demonstrated *Cryptococcus* in cerebrospinal fluid (CSF) (Genkal et al. 2011). The name *Cryptococcus* was derived from the Greek word *kryptus* meaning "hidden." It was used to describe a specific group of yeasts that lacked the ability to produce endospores by Friedrich Traugott Kützing (1807–1893 AD), a German pharmacist, botanist, and phycologist (Fig. 1.6) (McPartland and Goff 1991; Sharpton et al. 2009).

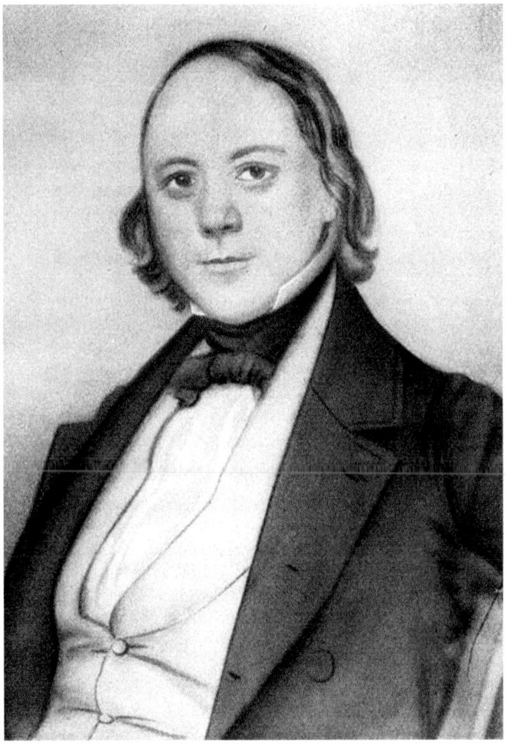

Fig. 1.6 A photograph of Friedrich Traugott Kützing (1807–1893 AD)

In the same time period, cerebral *Cryptococcus* and the blast mycosis were described, and the organism was successfully grown in culture (Miranda 2015). The triple scientific collaboration between Smith, Sano, and Miale reported the instances of meningeal implication caused by

Candida albicans (Antoniades et al. 2008; Genkal et al. 2011). They also described *Candida* meningitis for the first time (Gavito-Higuera et al. 2016; Pappas et al. 2016; Correia and Campos 2003).

1.4 Contemporary Period

Ophuls made the first human report of a coccidioidal brain lesion during his studies around 1905 (Huntington 1976, 1985). The next huge step in understanding the disease was made by William Ophuls (Patrick Ophuls) (1871–1933 AD) (Fig. 1.7), an academic pathologist in 1921, in Stanford Medical School, USA. Ophuls managed to clearly identify the fungal nature of this organism with mice transmission (Huntington Jr. 1986). He performed clinical studies of the disease in a documented series of cases of coccidioidomycosis in a patient who died because of disseminated coccidioidomycosis, the first documented case of the disease in the history (Hirschmann 2007). After decades of studies and many efforts, the researchers made the clear definition and manifestation of coccidioidomycosis in scientific publications. Further description of the disease was reported by Evans in 1909. The first case with both coccidioidal meningitis and hydrocephalus was described by Ryfkogel. He managed also to perform an accurate description of coccidioidal meningitis (Veterans Affairs Armed Forces, 1955–1958) (Correia and Campos 2003).

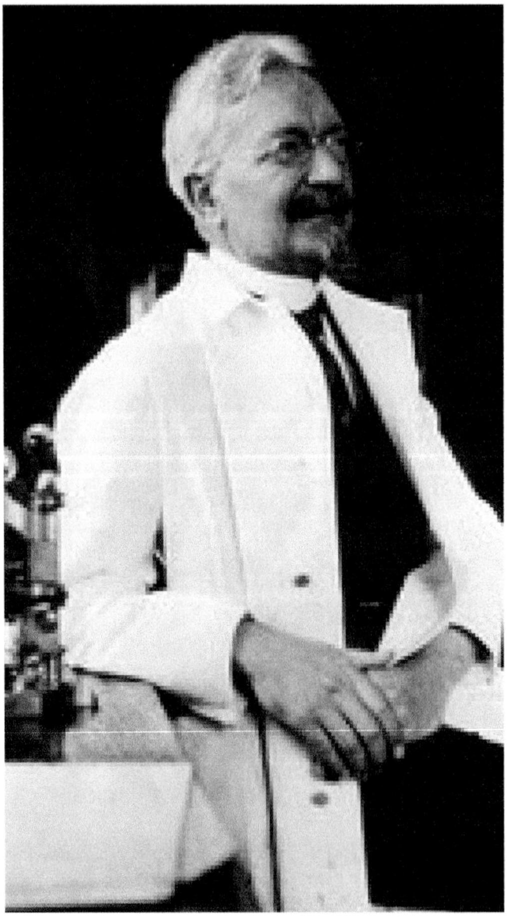

Fig. 1.7 A photograph of William Ophuls (1871–1933 AD)

Adolfo Lutz (1855–1940 AD), a Brazilian physician and pioneer tropical medical doctor, was the first to describe paracoccidioidomycosis in 1908 (Fig. 1.8). He performed zoological studies, epidemiological investigations, and infectious diseases research (Correia and Campos 2003).

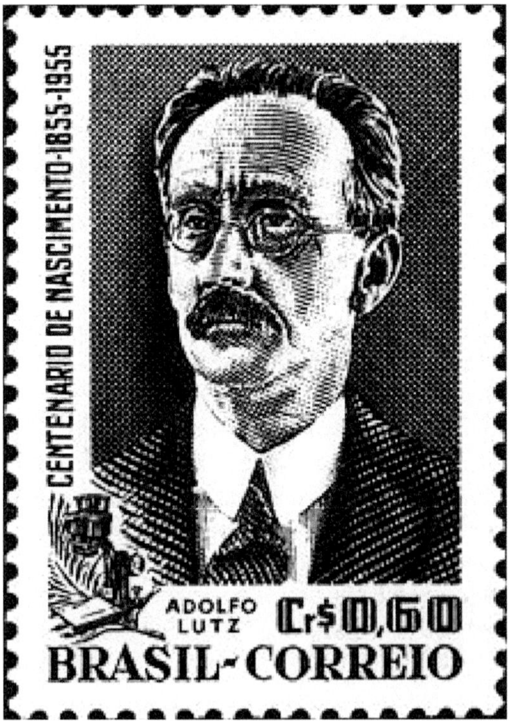

Fig. 1.8 A photograph of Adolfo Lutz (1855–1940 AD)

Morris was the first to report coccidioidomycosis as the only site of dissemination outside of the pulmonary area in 1924 (Morris 1924). Abbott and Cutler made review studies regarding 14 cases in 1936 with description of the typical CSF findings (Correia and Campos 2003). Subsequent pathological reports were very important in order to clarify the association between meningeal involvement and CNS coccidioidal infection (Spellberg et al. 2005).

Edmond Isidore Etienne Nocard (1850–1903 AD) performed studies in Provins (Seine-et-Marne, France) (Fig. 1.9) (Haas 2000). He was the first scientist who managed to describe the acid-fast aerobic cattle actinomycetes (Mathijsen 2003). Trevisan called them by the name *Nocardia farcinica* in 1889 (Pospischil 2002). An essential step was performed in 1891 by Eppinger with the first documented report of metastatic human cerebral nocardiosis from the lung (Pospischil 2002).

Histoplasmosis was described by Darling around 1906: the report was about a documented disseminated granulomatous infection in a patient (Beolens et al. 2011). About 18 years later in 1924, Morris reported a unique case of coccidioidomycosis outside the pulmonary function as a result of dissemination (Smit et al. 2003). Then, a total of 14 cases of typical CSF findings were reviewed by Abbott and Cutler in 1936 (Abbott and Cutler 1936). The association of meningeal involvements with coccidioidal infections of the CNS was documented in an accurate pathological report.

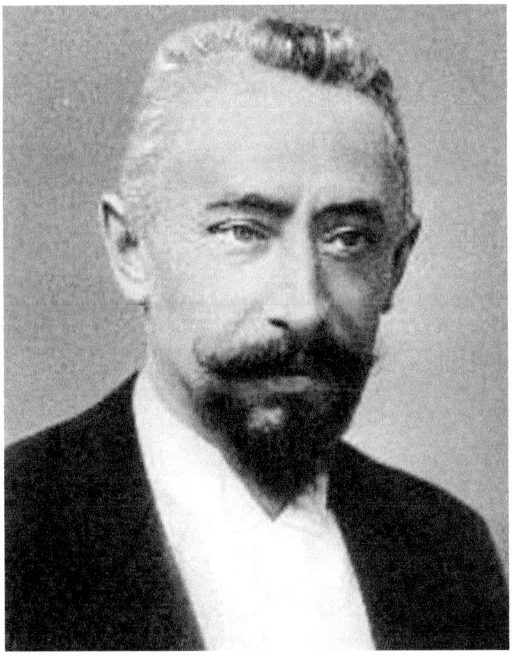

Fig. 1.9 A photograph of Edmond Isidore Etienne Nocard (1850–1903 AD)

In general, histiocytes were studied with *Histoplasma capsulatum*. On the other hand, rhinocerebral zygomycosis was accurately described and presented in a series of three cases by Gregory Binford in Maryland, USA, in 1943 (Chiller 2016). In 1952, he published a case report of brain abscess attributed to *Cladosporium* (Chiller 2016).

Moreover, we have to mention that before the use of the antifungal drugs, such cases with combination of fungal infections of the CNS and later improvement following surgical removal of cerebral abscess and evacuation of granulomatous lesion were rarely published in the current literature. In 1903, antifungal chemotherapy started successfully using potassium iodide in cases of cutaneous or subcutaneous sporotrichosis (Chiller 2016). The next decades involved with the introduction of mucosal and systemic mycoses: in 1953, nystatin, the first useful polyene drug, and in 1956, amphotericin B, the second useful polyene drug. Amphotericin B remains till today the best option about these infection types (Moen et al. 2013). Although these infections have been recognized for over a century, until the use of amphotericin B, fungal infections of the CNS remained a pathological situation with difficult effective treatment.

During the next few years, in 1964, flucytosine (5-fluorocytosine); in 1970, azole drugs; in 1978, miconazole; in 1981, ketoconazole; in 1990, fluconazole; in 1992, itraconazole; and in 2000–2010, other drugs against the fungal infections of the CNS were developed (Chiller 2016; Moen et al. 2013). In order to avoid the toxicity of amphotericin B, the following were introduced: liposomal amphotericin B with/without lipids, triazoles like voriconazole and posaconazole, and echinocandins like anidulafungin, caspofungin, and micafungin (Chiller 2016). The use of these combinations in situations such as cases of patients with severe invasive mycoses provided good results and in this way improved the outcome and ameliorated the health-related quality of life of these patients (Moen et al. 2013).

Finally, Fragoyannis, van Wyk, and de Beer reported of North American blastomycosis in South Africa (Fragoyannis et al. 1977). Gonyea (1978) reported a three-patient series with blastomycosis meningitis without extracranial infection (Schlech et al. 1985; Hurwitz et al. 1986).

1.5 Conclusion

Fungal infections have been known since early times, in particular since the nineteenth century. Although many fungal infections of the CNS are rare, there is no doubt further research is still needed in order to describe their formation in detail. Microbiologically, there are some morphologic similarities in various fungi, and therefore there is a difficulty in differential diagnosis of these complex forms but also the functional deficits that may cause.

References

Abbott KH, Cutler OI. Chronic coccidioidal meningitis: review of the literature and report of seven cases. Arch Pathol. 1936;21:320–30.

Antoniades D, Hamilton PB, Douglas MSV, Smol JP. Diatoms of North America: the freshwater floras of Prince Patrick, Ellef Ringnes and northern Ellesmere Islands from the Canadian Arctic Archipelago. Iconogr Diatomol. 2008;17:1–64.

Beolens B, Watkins M, Grayson M. The eponym dictionary of reptiles. Baltimore, MD: Johns Hopkins University Press; 2011.

Chiller TM. Histoplasmosis. CDC yellow book: CDC Health Information for International Travel. 2016.

Correia MI, Campos AC. Prevalence of hospital malnutrition in Latin America: the multicenter ELAN study. Nutrition. 2003;19:823–5.

Fragoyannis S, van Wyk G, de Beer M. North American blastomycosis in South Africa: a case report. S Afr Med J. 1977;51:169–71.

Gavito-Higuera J, Mullins CB, Ramos-Duran L, Olivas Chacon C, Hakim N, Enrique Palacios E. Fungal infections of the central nervous system: a pictorial review. J Clin Imaging Sci. 2016;6:24.

Genkal SI, Bondarenko NA, Schur LA. Diatoms in the lakes of the Southern and Northern Eastern Siberia. Rybinsk: Rybinsky Dom Pechati; 2011. p. 71.

Geronimus D. Piero di Cosimo: visions beautiful and strange. New Haven, CT: Yale University Press; 2007.

Gholami-Shabani M, Zamani S, Moosa H, Ghahfarokhi M, Jamzivar F, Mehdi Razzaghi-Abyaneh M. Recent advances in fungal infections of the central nervous system: from etiology to diagnosis and management. In: Kon K, Rai M, editors. The microbiology of central nervous system infections. Volume 3 in clinical microbiology: diagnosis, treatments and prophylaxis of infections. Cambridge, MA: Academic Press; 2018. p. 215–59.

Giannouli V, Syrmos N. Information about Macedonian medicine in ancient Greece. Hell J Nucl Med. 2011;14:324–5.

Guého E, de Hoog GS, Smith MT. Neotypification of the genus Trichosporon. Antonie Van Leeuwenhoek. 1992;61:285–8.

Haas L. Edmond Isidore Etienne Nocard (1850–1903). J Neurol Neurosurg Psychiatry. 2000;69:1.

Hirschmann JV. The early history of coccidioidomycosis: 1892–1945. Clin Infect Dis. 2007;44:1202–7.

Huntington RW. William Ophuls, pioneer coccidioidomycologist. Sabouraudia. 1976;14:231–5.

Huntington RW. Four great coccidioidomycologists: William Ophuls (1871–1933), Myrnie Gifford (1892–1966), and Charles Edward Smith (1904–1967) and William A. Winn (1903–1967). Sabouraudia. 1985;23:361–70.

Huntington RW Jr. Coccidioidomycosis—a great imitator disease. Arch Pathol Lab Med. 1986;110:182.

Hurwitz MD, Kallenbach JM, Behr A, Chun R, Baynes RD. Blastomycosis: a case report. S Afr Med J. 1986;70:622–4.

Mathijsen AH. Predecessors: veterinarians from earlier times (51). Edmond Isidore Etienne Nocard (1850–1903). Tijdschr Diergeneeskd. 2003;128:488–9.

McPartland JM, Goff JP. Neotypification of Trichosporon beigelii: morphological, pathological and taxonomic considerations. Mycotaxon. 1991;41:173–8.

Miranda E. Coccidioides posadasii. The encyclopedia of life (EOL) the earliest account of human cryptococcosis (Busse-Buschke disease) in a woman with chronic osteomyelitis of the tibia. Pediatr Infect Dis J. 2015;34:1278.

Moen MD, Lyseng-Williamson KA, Scott LJ. Liposomal amphotericin B. Drugs. 2013;69:361–92.

Morris M. Coccidioides of the central nervous system. California West Med. 1924;22:483–5.

Pappas PG, Kauffman CA, Andes DR, Clancy CJ, Marr KA, Ostrosky-Zeichner L, Reboli AC, Schuster MG, Vazquez JA, Walsh TJ, Zaoutis TE, Sobel JD, Kauffman CA, Andes DR. Clinical practice guideline for the management of Candidiasis: 2016 update by the Infectious Diseases Society of America. Clin Infect Dis. 2016;62(4):e1–50.

Pospischil A. Chlamydia, if it exists, is everywhere. Edmond Nocard (1850–1903). Schweiz Arch Tierheilkd. 2002;144(9):461.

Schaechter M. Pier Antonio Micheli, the father of modern mycology: a paean. In: McIlvainea. Official organ of the NAMA, vol. 14 2000.

Schaechter M. Eukaryotic microbes. Amsterdam: Academic Press; 2011. p. 19.

Schlech WF, Ward JI, Band JD, Hightower A, Fraser DW, Broome CV. Bacterial meningitis in the United States, 1978 through 1981. The national bacterial meningitis surveillance study. JAMA. 1985;253:1749–54.

Sharpton TJ, Stajich JE, Rounsley SD, Gardner MJ, Wortman JR, Jordar VS, Maiti R, Kodira CD, Neafsey DE, Zeng Q, Hung CY, McMahan C, Muszewska A, Grynberg M, Mandel MA, Kellner EM, Barker BM, Galgiani JN, Orbach MJ, Kirkland TN, Cole GT, Henn MR, Birren BW, Taylor JW. Comparative genomic analyses of the human fungal pathogens Coccidioides and their relatives. Genome Res. 2009;19:1722–31.

Smit LHM, Leemans R, Overbeek BP. Nocardia farcinica as the causative agent in a primary psoas abscess in a previously healthy cattle inspector. Clin Microbiol Infect. 2003;9:445–8.

Spellberg B, Edwards J Jr, Ibrahim A. Novel perspectives on mucormycosis: pathophysiology, presentation, and management. Clin Microbiol Rev. 2005;18:556–69.

Sumbali G, Johri BM. The fungi. Oxford: Alpha Science International Limited; 2005. p. 11.

Syrmos N. Microcephaly in ancient Greece—the Minoan Microcephalus of Zakros. Childs Nerv Syst. 2011;27:685–6.

Syrmos N, Ampatzidis G, Fachantidou A, Mouratidis A, Syrmos C. Historical back training in most important points of neurosurgery. Ann General Psychiatry. 2010;9(Suppl 1):S89.

Epidemiology of Central Nervous System Fungal Infections

2

Sanjeet Singh Dadwal

Abbreviations

CARD9	Caspase recruitment domain-containing protein 9 deficiency
CGD	Chronic granulomatous disease
CNS	Central nervous system
GvHD	Graft-versus-host disease
HCT	Hematopoietic cell transplantation
HIV/AIDS	Human immunodeficiency virus/acquired immunodeficiency syndrome
ICU	Intensive care unit
IFI	Invasive fungal infection
SOT	Solid organ transplantation
TNF-α	Tumor necrosis factor-alpha

2.1 Introduction

The burden of invasive fungal infection (IFI) has been increasing in both immunocompetent and the immunocompromised hosts (Vallabhaneni et al. 2016). This phenomenon is due to multiple factors that include increased awareness of fungal infections leading to an increased diagnostic testing, improvements in the diagnostic capabilities, and an ever-increasing pool of at-risk population: cancer, hematopoietic cell transplantation (HCT), solid organ transplantation (SOT), newer immunosuppressive therapies, and neonatal and elderly patients (Powers-Fletcher and Hanson 2016; Vallabhaneni et al. 2016). The spectrum includes fungi that are opportunistic pathogens and true pathogens (latter can lead to fungal infection without any apparent immunodeficiency). This chapter will discuss general considerations of central nervous system (CNS) IFI epidemiology and epidemiology of specific class of fungi: yeasts and molds that are most commonly associated with CNS infection.

2.2 General Considerations of Epidemiology of CNS Fungal Infection

In the absence of an immunocompromising condition, fungal infection of the CNS is uncommon as the host defense and the anatomy of the CNS (functional and structural) help prevent invasion of their CNS (Chakrabarti 2007; Marra et al. 2014). Although this protects vast majority of mankind, exposures related to diverse environmental/ecological niches of various fungal pathogens can lead to IFI in the context of their endemic distribution: *Coccidioides* (Brown et al. 2013), *Cryptococcus gattii* (Chen et al. 2014; Datta et al. 2009), *Histoplasma* (Chu et al. 2006; Hammerman et al. 1974), and *Blastomyces*

S. S. Dadwal (✉)
Division of Infectious Disease, City of Hope National Medical Center, Duarte, CA, USA
e-mail: sdadwal@coh.org

M. Turgut et al. (eds.), *Fungal Infections of the Central Nervous System*,
https://doi.org/10.1007/978-3-030-06088-6_2

(Baumgardner et al. 1992; Dworkin et al. 2005). The sinonasal fungal infection when invasive in nature can extend beyond the extracranial compartment into the brain (Kourkoumpetis et al. 2012; McCarthy et al. 2014) and may manifest as meningitis or space-occupying lesions/abscess. Certain epidemiologic exposures such as drowning have led to infection of the CNS with *Scedosporium apiospermum* (Kantarcioglu et al. 2008) and *Aspergillus* spp. (Kowacs et al. 2004). Diabetic ketoacidosis, steroid use, and iron overload are known risk factors for mucormycosis (Spellberg et al. 2005). Furthermore, iatrogenic fungal infections have occurred in the setting of outbreaks such as with *Exserohilum rostratum* due to contaminated compounded methylprednisolone for spinal injections in 2013 (Chiller et al. 2013), *Exophiala* infection from contaminated injectable steroids (From the Centers for Disease Control and Prevention 2003), and *Aspergillus* meningitis after spinal anesthesia in pregnant women (Gunaratne et al. 2007).

Perhaps, the most significant group that contributes to the burden of IFI is the immunocompromised patient. The high-risk group include, neutropenia in patients undergoing cytotoxic chemotherapy for hematologic malignancy, those who have undergone allogeneic HCT (Kontoyiannis et al. 2010), especially those with graft-versus-host disease (GVHD) requiring immunosuppressive therapy, SOT (Pappas et al. 2010; Singh 2003; Singh and Paterson 2005), use of biologic agents such as TNF-α (Warris et al. 2001), use of Bruton tyrosine kinase inhibitor, ibrutinib (Bercusson et al. 2018; Peri et al. 2018), congenital immunodeficiency such as chronic granulomatous disease (CGD) (Alsultan et al. 2006; Dotis et al. 2007; Henriet et al. 2013), and caspase recruitment domain-containing protein 9 deficiency (CARD9) (Gavino et al. 2014; Lanternier et al. 2015; Rieber et al. 2016). Within the SOT recipients, the type of organ transplant has an impact on the risk of IFI (Munoz et al. 2016). ICU patients are also at high risk for IFI: mainly candida and aspergillus (Denning 2004; Pittet et al. 1994). Patients with human immunodeficiency virus/acquired immunodeficiency syndrome (HIV/AIDS) are at high risk for cryptococcal infection (Rajasingham et al. 2017), and the risk correlates with the status of the cell-mediated immunity.

The CNS IFI can manifest as meningitis, which is the inflammation of the meninges. The symptoms are often protean and can vary from acute onset to subacute and chronic in nature. Patients often present with headaches that are subacute to chronic and may have visual changes, cranial nerve abnormalities, and other symptoms of elevated intracranial pressure. Nuchal rigidity may or may not exist. At times, patients may present with the symptoms/signs of cerebritis suggesting parenchymal involvement. The inflammatory component can result in endarteritis that may result in stroke manifesting with focal neurologic defects. In patients with immunocompromised state, symptoms and signs may be minimal or atypical that often result in delayed diagnosis. Intracranial abscess-/mass-like lesions are mostly encountered with invasive mold infections. Mold infections of the CNS are mostly encountered in the immunocompromised patients and typically present with space-occupying parenchymal lesions/abscesses and less likely to be associated with meningitis.

This chapter will provide an outline of the epidemiology for CNS infections related to common fungal pathogens (true and opportunistic), and the description will be centric to the specific organism.

2.3 Yeast Infections of the CNS

2.3.1 *Cryptococcus neoformans*

This pathogen belongs to basidiomycetous fungi and is the leading cause of CNS fungal infection manifesting as meningitis and may be accompanied by brain abscesses "cryptococcomas." Its distribution is worldwide and is ubiquitously found in soil, bird droppings, and animals. Humans can be colonized with it as well. There are eight genotypes, with the most common being *C. neoformans* var. *neoformans* in the USA and Europe. *C. neoformans* var. *grubii* is most common in the rest of the world. The most significant burden from this pathogen is in the

HIV/AIDS patient population, and the risk of developing this infection is directly correlated with the cell-mediated immunity that increases with the declining CD4 count (most cases occur when CD4 is <100 cells/μl) (Rajasingham et al. 2017). With the availability of HAART, the incidence of cryptococcal CNS infection has decreased in the USA, although it is still a major cause for morbidity and mortality in the developing world (Rajasingham et al. 2017). After HIV/AIDS, SOT recipients have the highest rate of CNS infection (Pappas et al. 2010), but it is rare in recipients of HCT (with more cases observed in autologous than allogeneic) (Kontoyiannis et al. 2010). In the SOT, *Cryptococcus* contributed to 8% of all IFI in a large prospective study (Pappas et al. 2010), and the CNS is the most common extrapulmonary site of infection. Increased risk for CNS involvement was correlated with abnormal mental status, late-onset disease, and high serum cryptococcal antigen titer (Osawa et al. 2010).

C. gattii is an emerging pathogen worldwide that was previously described primarily in tropical and subtropical areas such as Australia, New Guinea, Hawaii, Southern California, Central Africa, and Southeast Asia (Maziarz and Perfect 2016). Originally described with eucalyptus trees, the recent outbreaks noted association with trees such as oaks and firs. There has been an evolving epidemic in the Vancouver Island and Pacific Northwest, USA, and cases have been described in multiple states across the USA (Harris et al. 2011). This pathogen primarily affects the healthy individuals although there is an association with anti-GM-CSF antibodies and *C. gattii* infection (Rosen et al. 2013; Saijo et al. 2014). The disease process is frequently severe with meningitis and cryptococcomas in the immunocompetent patients (Chen et al. 2014).

2.3.2 *Candida*

Candida species are an important cause of healthcare-associated infection presenting as disseminated infection (candidemia). They are found in soil, on inanimate objects, and on hospital surfaces and colonize the respiratory/GI tract of normal and immunocompromised hosts. The risk factors for candidemia include critically ill neonates associated with prematurity, low APGAR score, shock, intubation and congenital malformations, neutropenic host, HCT recipients with mucositis or graft-versus-host disease (GVHD) of the gut, SOT, use of broad-spectrum antibiotics, central venous catheter, intravenous drug use, total parenteral nutrition, gastrointestinal surgery, diabetes, sepsis, pancreatitis, ICU stay, and dialysis (Blumberg et al. 2001). *C. albicans* is the most frequent cause of infection in the USA followed by *C. glabrata* (Matsumoto et al. 2014), and there is variability in the distribution of species based on geography and patient population (Pfaller et al. 2012); *C. glabrata* is more frequently isolated from SOT and elderly patients. Additionally, there has been emergence of drug-resistant *Candida* spp. such as triazole and echinocandin resistance in *C. glabrata* (Pfaller et al. 2010; Pfaller et al. 2011). *Candida auris*, a multidrug-resistant candida species, has gained notoriety in recent years as a cause of outbreaks associated with high morbidity and mortality (Sarma and Upadhyay 2017).

Candida used to be the most common cause of fungal meningitis, but that has been replaced by *C. neoformans*. *Candida* meningitis/brain abscesses occur in the context of disseminated candida infection in premature infants and neonates (Faix 1984; Fernandez et al. 2000) and patients with AIDS (Casado et al. 1997), neutropenia from chemotherapy (Flynn et al. 1993), CGD (Cohen et al. 1981), and SCID (Smego Jr et al. 1984). Direct inoculation may occur with traumatic injuries (Brenier-Pinchart et al. 1999), CNS ventricular shunts (Baradkar et al. 2009; Shapiro et al. 1989) and polymer wafers used in local chemotherapy are additional risk factors (Glick et al. 2010).

2.3.3 *Coccidioides*

The disease caused by *Coccidioides* is commonly referred to as coccidioidomycosis or "valley fever," named after the common occurrence of this endemic fungal infection in the San Joaquin Valley in California. *C. immitis* and *C. posadasii* are the two species that cause disease in humans. It is a dimorphic fungus that is able to survive in dry and arid environment. It is highly infectious and inhalation of even a few arthroconidia can lead to infection (Kong et al. 1964). Endemic areas include California, with particularly high rates in Kern and Fresno counties, Arizona, New Mexico, Nevada, Utah, Washington, Texas, Mexico, Central America, Honduras and Guatemala, and South America: Brazil, Venezuela, Argentina, and Paraguay (Stevens 1995). Changing environmental and human factors in the endemic area, changes in surveillance and definitions, diagnostic methods, and increasing pool of immunocompromised patients may be affecting the increase of rates in California and Arizona (Stockamp and Thompson 3rd 2016). Certain natural disasters such as major earthquakes (Schneider et al. 1997), digging/excavation activities, and dust storms may lead to local epidemics. Coccidioidal meningitis is a dreaded complication that is associated with significant morbidity and mortality. Basilar meningitis with its inflammatory exudate is commonly complicated with obstructive hydrocephalus that requires ventricular shunt. Patients with coccidioidomycosis with headache, visual changes, or any CNS symptom or sign should undergo spinal tap.

In a study of allogeneic HCT recipients living in endemic areas with prior history of exposure/infection, 11/426 (2.6%) were noted to develop active coccidioidomycosis post-HCT (Mendoza et al. 2015). In a study with SOT recipients with prior history of coccidioidomycosis, reactivation was observed in 5% despite antifungal prophylaxis (Keckich et al. 2011). Mortality rates of up to 55% have been reported in allogeneic HCT (Mendoza et al. 2015) and 28% in SOT (Mendoza and Blair 2013). Other risk factors include the use of TNF-α blockers (Bergstrom et al. 2004) and HIV/AIDS (CD4 less than 250) (Masannat and Ampel 2010), pregnant women, and race. It is more frequently observed in African Americans and Filipinos with the propensity to develop CNS involvement.

2.3.4 *Blastomyces*

Blastomyces dermatitidis is a dimorphic fungus that is endemic in the Midwestern states of the USA, Canadian provinces along the great lakes, and the Mississippi and Ohio river valleys (Castillo et al. 2016). Cases have been reported from other states and countries too. Even though surveys from Wisconsin show high rates of endemicity, the true prevalence is unknown, secondary to a lack of mandatory reporting. The infection has been associated with exposure to decaying wood or disturbing the soil. The most common site of infection is the skin and lungs with the propensity to develop disseminated disease. CNS involvement occurs in about a third of all infected patients. In a pediatric study that reviewed 114 children with *Blastomyces* infection, 21% had extrapulmonary disease, and only 2 had CNS involvement. The majority of the infections were due to *B. gilchristii* followed by *B dermatitidis*, and the latter was associated with more extrapulmonary disease (Frost et al. 2017). In a study of 22 patients with CNS involvement, 22.7% had isolated involvement of the CNS (Bariola et al. 2010). Presentation varies from symptoms/signs of acute meningitis to chronic meningitis and brain abscess. AIDS patients have high burden from CNS disease developing in 40% of patients (Grim et al. 2012), while it is of rare occurrence in SOT and HCT recipients (Kauffman et al. 2014). Furthermore, the use of corticosteroids and TNF-α blockers also increases the risk (Pappas et al. 1993; Smith and Kauffman 2009).

Blastomyces helicus is an emerging fungus that has been reported to be associated with disseminated disease with CNS involvement in 20% of the infected patients. The primary route of acquisition is inhalational and skin involvement is rare. In a case series of ten patients, six had underlying immunocompromising condition, and 50% had fungemia which is extremely uncommon with *B. dermatitidis* (Schwartz et al. 2018).

2.3.5 *Histoplasma*

Histoplasma capsulatum leads among the other causes for endemic mycoses (Chu et al. 2006; Hammerman et al. 1974). In the USA, it is most prevalent in the Ohio and Mississippi river valleys. Outside of the USA, it has been reported from Mexico, South American countries, parts of Asia, and Southeast Asia. Exposure to soil rich in bird or bat guano is a risk factor for the acquisition of *Histoplasma* (Wheat et al. 2016). The activities that are mostly reported to be significant exposures include farming, cave exploration, remodeling of old buildings, clearing brushes, or cutting trees at sites that had supported blackbird roosting. The highest numbers were seen in the context of HIV/AIDS epidemic (Assi et al. 2007; Kaur and Myers 1983) and, subsequently, exposure in the immunocompromised patients with T cell dysfunction, exposure to TNF-α blockers, SOT, and HCT (Wheat et al. 2016). It is encountered more commonly in the SOT group, while a lower incidence is observed in HCT recipients (Kauffman et al. 2014). Dissemination to the CNS is infrequent and is mostly observed in the immunocompromised patient with development of meningitis or focal lesions in 5–10% of the cases (Chen et al. 2014). A recent retrospective study reviewing 77 cases noted male predominance with most frequent underlying diagnosis of HIV/AIDS in 44% followed by transplantation in 13%, and 14% had other immunocompromising conditions (Wheat et al. 2018). Morbidity and mortality are high in patients with CNS involvement.

2.3.6 *Sporothrix schenckii*

S. schenckii is a dimorphic fungus that is most commonly found in the tropical and subtropical areas. It has been reported mostly from Japan, India, Mexico, Brazil, Uruguay, and Peru. In the USA, outbreaks related to pine seedlings and manipulation of the moss have been reported from the Mississippi Valley (Barros et al. 2011). The activities associated with risk for acquisition of *Sporothrix* are agriculture, floriculture, wood exploration, mining, and exposure to cats that are infected with this fungus (veterinarians, owners, and caretakers of cats) (Barros et al. 2004; Vilela et al. 2007). The most common site of infection is the skin although it can be acquired via inhalation and has the propensity to disseminate in the immunocompromised patients (Barros et al. 2011). CNS involvement has been reported in patients with underlying immunodeficiency (Gullberg et al. 1987; Hardman et al. 2005) and mostly manifests as meningitis.

2.4 Mold Infections of CNS

2.4.1 *Aspergillus*

The increase in the number of at-risk patients undergoing transplantation, chemotherapy for hematologic malignancies, and use of novel immunosuppressive medications has led to a spurt in invasive aspergillosis. *Aspergillus* spp. have a ubiquitous distribution in the nature and are commonly found in soil, decaying vegetation, and food material. The primary route of acquisition is inhalational, although infection related to skin patch dressing and trauma has been observed.

Risk factors for invasive aspergillosis include neutropenia in patients undergoing induction chemotherapy for hematologic malignancy and HCT especially in the context of GVHD that requires treatment with steroids or agents such as infliximab, and ibrutinib (bruton tyrosine kinase inhibitor) and in SOT (Bercusson et al. 2018; Kourkoumpetis et al. 2012; McCarthy et al. 2014; Pappas et al. 2010; Peri et al. 2018; Singh and Paterson 2005). Inherited conditions such as CGD and CARD9 deficiency are also associated with increased risk of *Aspergillus* infection (Alsultan et al. 2006; Dotis et al. 2007; Henriet et al. 2013; Rieber et al. 2016). Patients with diabetes, recent CNS surgery, lumbar puncture, paranasal sinusitis, chronic steroid use, intravenous drug use, pulmonary tuberculosis, and alcoholic liver disease are also at risk.

Aspergillus is now the most common cause of IFI in the allogeneic HCT patients having surpassed *Candida* as reported in a large prospective database (Kontoyiannis et al. 2010). In SOT, the highest incidence is noted in lung, lung-heart transplant (about 6%), and liver and kidney transplants (Pappas et al. 2010). CNS involvement occurred in 15.4% of cases in the context of disseminated disease from a large study in Europe

(Gavalda et al. 2005). *A. fumigatus*, *A. terreus*, *and A. flavus* are the most common species associated with CNS disease. CNS aspergillosis can manifest as meningitis, infarction, or a brain abscess with the latter two presentations being more common.

2.4.2 Non-*Aspergillus* Mold Infections

2.4.2.1 *Mucormycosis*

Mucormycosis is an infection caused by fungi from the *Mucorales* order (Mendoza et al. 2014), with *Rhizopus* spp. the most common offending agent. The organism is found in the decaying organic matter such as vegetables, seeds, fruits, manure, and compost. It releases spores that when airborne can be inhaled.

The incidence of this devastating illness has been increasing over the last decade, in the HCT and SOT, patients with hematologic malignancy (HM) undergoing cytotoxic chemotherapy, uncontrolled diabetes mellitus with acidosis, burns, and trauma (Roden et al. 2005; Walsh et al. 2012). Voriconazole and echinocandin prophylaxis has been associated with increased risk of mucormycosis, while tacrolimus is protective (Singh et al. 2009).

The spread to CNS is primarily via the hematogenous route, although direct extension from the sinuses to the intracranial compartment is well known. In a large retrospective study of 929 patients, CNS involvement was described in one-third of the patients, and of that 69% were related to sinonasal source (Roden et al. 2005). Injection drug users manifest predominantly with cerebral involvement—abscesses or infarcts (Fong et al. 1990; Stave et al. 1989).

2.4.2.2 *Phaeohyphomycoses (Dematiaceous Fungi)*

This is a diverse group of pigmented fungi that are emerging as a cause of CNS fungal infections. Many of the fungi in this group are neurotropic, such as *Cladophialophora bantiana*, *Exophiala dermatitidis*, and *Rhinodadeiella mackenziei* (Chakrabarti 2007).

Although *Cladophialophora* infections are reported worldwide, the majority are in areas that have a warm and humid climate (Kantarcioglu et al. 2017). A systematic review of *C. bantiana* cases reported that the majority of cases are from India, the USA, Brazil, Canada, France, Spain, South Africa, and Italy, with sporadic cases from various other countries. The majority of patients were immunocompetent (58.3%) and 97% had brain abscess. Regardless of the immune status, mortality was high at 65% (Kantarcioglu et al. 2017).

Exophiala dermatitidis notoriously causes brain abscesses and is mostly reported from the Asian countries. CARD9 deficiency has been identified as a risk factor (Lanternier et al. 2015). Other molds such as *Lomentospora prolificans*, *Alternaria* spp., *Exserohilum rostratum*, *Scopulariopsis* spp., *Curvularia* spp., *Bipolaris* spp., *Chaetomium*, and *Ochroconis gallopava* are more often encountered in immunocompromised hosts (Kontoyiannis et al. 2010; Pappas et al. 2010). In a review of 72 cases of phaeohyphomycosis (Revankar et al. 2002), the majority of patients (76%) had underlying immunodeficiency, and CNS involvement was identified in 22/72 (30.5%). Only three of the patients with CNS infection did not have an underlying immunologic deficit (two caused by *Curvularia* spp. and one by *Wangiella dermatitidis*). A case series of 12 SOT patients with *Ochroconis gallopava* infection described high mortality rate in those with CNS involvement that reached 80% (Shoham et al. 2008).

From an iatrogenic standpoint, a large outbreak of fungal meningitis due to *Exserohilum rostratum* in the USA resulted in patients who had received contaminated compounded methylprednisolone used for spinal/epidural injections (Chiller et al. 2013).

2.5 Miscellaneous Fungi

Scedosporium apiospermum is ubiquitously found in the environment, especially polluted environment of high human activity, agricultural soil, and polluted water (Ramirez-Garcia et al. 2018). *Scedosporium* and *Lomentospora* accounted for the majority of non-*Aspergillus* mold infections in both HCT and SOT, 71% and 29%, respectively (Husain et al. 2005).

Paracoccidioides brasiliensis is the main cause for paracoccidioidomycosis that is endemic in South America, and chronic disease is a risk factor for CNS involvement (Shikanai-Yasuda et al. 2017). *Fusarium* spp., *Acremonium* spp., and *Paecilomyces* spp. have also been associated with CNS involvement in patients with disseminated disease. Dermatophytes such as *Trichophyton* and *Microsporum* have also been described in immunocompromised patients leading to CNS infection. *Emmonsia* is another emerging fungus that has the ability to cause disseminated disease.

2.6 Conclusion

Fungi are ubiquitous in the environment and exposure to them is inevitable. The epidemiologic trends of CNS yeast and mold infections demonstrate varying risk based on the host immune status and environmental exposures especially in the context of endemic fungi, as well as non-endemic fungi. With the advancement in the care of very ill patients and neurosurgical interventions, these infections may occur more frequently. Increased awareness coupled with diagnostic advances over time should result in the timely establishment of diagnosis and intervention with a potential improvement in outcomes. The CNS IFI carries high morbidity and mortality and is a challenging medical/surgical condition.

References

Alsultan A, Williams MS, Lubner S, Goldman FD. Chronic granulomatous disease presenting with disseminated intracranial aspergillosis. Pediatr Blood Cancer. 2006;47:107–10.

Assi MA, Sandid MS, Baddour LM, Roberts GD, Walker RC. Systemic histoplasmosis: a 15-year retrospective institutional review of 111 patients. Medicine (Baltimore). 2007;86:162–9.

Baradkar VP, Mathur M, Sonavane A, Kumar S. Candidal infections of ventriculoperitoneal shunts. J Pediatr Neurosci. 2009;4:73–5.

Bariola JR, Perry P, Pappas PG, Proia L, Shealey W, Wright PW, Sizemore JM, Robinson M, Bradsher RW Jr. Blastomycosis of the central nervous system: a multicenter review of diagnosis and treatment in the modern era. Clin Infect Dis. 2010;50:797–804.

Barros MB, Schubach Ade O, do Valle AC, Gutierrez Galhardo MC, Conceicao-Silva F, Schubach TM, Reis RS, Wanke B, Marzochi KB, Conceicao MJ. Cat-transmitted sporotrichosis epidemic in Rio de Janeiro, Brazil: description of a series of cases. Clin Infect Dis. 2004;38:529–35.

Barros MB, de Almeida Paes R, Schubach AO. Sporothrix schenckii and Sporotrichosis. Clin Microbiol Rev. 2011;24:633–54.

Baumgardner DJ, Buggy BP, Mattson BJ, Burdick JS, Ludwig D. Epidemiology of blastomycosis in a region of high endemicity in north central Wisconsin. Clin Infect Dis. 1992;15:629–35.

Bercusson A, Colley T, Shah A, Warris A, Armstrong-James D. Ibrutinib blocks Btk-dependent NF-kB and NFAT responses in human macrophages during Aspergillus fumigatus phagocytosis. Blood. 2018;132(18):1985–8.

Bergstrom L, Yocum DE, Ampel NM, Villanueva I, Lisse J, Gluck O, Tesser J, Posever J, Miller M, Araujo J, Kageyama DM, Berry M, Karl L, Yung CM. Increased risk of coccidioidomycosis in patients treated with tumor necrosis factor alpha antagonists. Arthritis Rheum. 2004;50:1959–66.

Blumberg HM, Jarvis WR, Soucie JM, Edwards JE, Patterson JE, Pfaller MA, Rangel-Frausto MS, Rinaldi MG, Saiman L, Wiblin RT, Wenzel RP. Risk factors for candidal bloodstream infections in surgical intensive care unit patients: the NEMIS prospective multicenter study. The National Epidemiology of Mycosis Survey. Clin Infect Dis. 2001;33:177–86.

Brenier-Pinchart MP, Leclercq P, Mallie M, Bettega G. Candida meningitis possibly resulting from a harpoon injury. Eur J Clin Microbiol Infect Dis. 1999;18:454–5.

Brown J, Benedict K, Park BJ, Thompson GR 3rd. Coccidioidomycosis: epidemiology. Clin Epidemiol. 2013;5:185–97.

Casado JL, Quereda C, Oliva J, Navas E, Moreno A, Pintado V, Cobo J, Corral I. Candidal meningitis in HIV-infected patients: analysis of 14 cases. Clin Infect Dis. 1997;25:673–6.

Castillo CG, Kauffman CA, Miceli MH. Blastomycosis. Infect Dis Clin North Am. 2016;30:247–64.

Chakrabarti A. Epidemiology of central nervous system mycoses. Neurol India. 2007;55:191–7.

Chen SC, Meyer W, Sorrell TC. Cryptococcus gattii infections. Clin Microbiol Rev. 2014;27:980–1024.

Chiller TM, Roy M, Nguyen D, Guh A, Malani AN, Latham R, Peglow S, Kerkering T, Kaufman D, McFadden J, Collins J, Kainer M, Duwve J, Trump D, Blackmore C, Tan C, Cleveland AA, MacCannell T, Muehlenbachs A, Zaki SR, Brandt ME, Jernigan JA. Clinical findings for fungal infections caused by methylprednisolone injections. N Engl J Med. 2013;369:1610–9.

Chu JH, Feudtner C, Heydon K, Walsh TJ, Zaoutis TE. Hospitalizations for endemic mycoses: a population-based national study. Clin Infect Dis. 2006;42:822–5.

Cohen MS, Isturiz RE, Malech HL, Root RK, Wilfert CM, Gutman L, Buckley RH. Fungal infection in chronic granulomatous disease. The importance of the phagocyte in defense against fungi. Am J Med. 1981;71:59–66.

Datta K, Bartlett KH, Baer R, Byrnes E, Galanis E, Heitman J, Hoang L, Leslie MJ, MacDougall L, Magill SS, Morshed MG, Marr KA. Spread of Cryptococcus gattii into Pacific Northwest region of the United States. Emerg Infect Dis. 2009;15:1185–91.

Denning DW. Aspergillosis in "nonimmunocompromised" critically ill patients. Am J Respir Crit Care Med. 2004;170:580–1.

Dotis J, Iosifidis E, Roilides E. Central nervous system aspergillosis in children: a systematic review of reported cases. Int J Infect Dis. 2007;11:381–93.

Dworkin MS, Duckro AN, Proia L, Semel JD, Huhn G. The epidemiology of blastomycosis in Illinois and factors associated with death. Clin Infect Dis. 2005;41:e107–11.

Faix RG. Systemic Candida infections in infants in intensive care nurseries: high incidence of central nervous system involvement. J Pediatr. 1984;105:616–22.

Fernandez M, Moylett EH, Noyola DE, Baker CJ. Candidal meningitis in neonates: a 10-year review. Clin Infect Dis. 2000;31:458–63.

Flynn PM, Marina NM, Rivera GK, Hughes WT. Candida tropicalis infections in children with leukemia. Leuk Lymphoma. 1993;10:369–76.

Fong KM, Seneviratne EM, McCormack JG. Mucor cerebral abscess associated with intravenous drug abuse. Aust N Z J Med. 1990;20:74–7.

From the Centers for Disease Control and Prevention. Exophiala infection from contaminated injectable steroids prepared by a compounding pharmacy—United States, July–November 2002. JAMA. 2003;289:291–3.

Frost HM, Anderson J, Ivacic L, Meece J. Blastomycosis in children: an analysis of clinical, epidemiologic, and genetic features. J Pediatric Infect Dis Soc. 2017;6:49–56.

Gavalda J, Len O, San Juan R, Aguado JM, Fortun J, Lumbreras C, Moreno A, Munoz P, Blanes M, Ramos A, Rufi G, Gurgui M, Torre-Cisneros J, Montejo M, Cuenca-Estrella M, Rodriguez-Tudela JL, Pahissa A. Risk factors for invasive aspergillosis in solid-organ transplant recipients: a case-control study. Clin Infect Dis. 2005;41:52–9.

Gavino C, Cotter A, Lichtenstein D, Lejtenyi D, Fortin C, Legault C, Alirezaie N, Majewski J, Sheppard DC, Behr MA, Foulkes WD, Vinh DC. CARD9 deficiency and spontaneous central nervous system candidiasis: complete clinical remission with GM-CSF therapy. Clin Infect Dis. 2014;59:81–4.

Glick JA, Graham RS, Voils SA. Candida meningitis post Gliadel wafer placement successfully treated with intrathecal and intravenous amphotericin B. Ann Pharmacother. 2010;44:215–8.

Grim SA, Proia L, Miller R, Alhyraba M, Costas-Chavarri A, Oberholzer J, Clark NM. A multicenter study of histoplasmosis and blastomycosis after solid organ transplantation. Transpl Infect Dis. 2012;14:17–23.

Gullberg RM, Quintanilla A, Levin ML, Williams J, Phair JP. Sporotrichosis: recurrent cutaneous, articular, and central nervous system infection in a renal transplant recipient. Rev Infect Dis. 1987;9:369–75.

Gunaratne PS, Wijeyaratne CN, Seneviratne HR. Aspergillus meningitis in Sri Lanka—a post-tsunami effect? N Engl J Med. 2007;356:754–6.

Hammerman KJ, Powell KE, Tosh FE. The incidence of hospitalized cases of systemic mycotic infections. Sabouraudia. 1974;12:33–45.

Hardman S, Stephenson I, Jenkins DR, Wiselka MJ, Johnson EM. Disseminated Sporothrix schenckii in a patient with AIDS. J Infect. 2005;51:e73–7.

Harris JR, Lockhart SR, Debess E, Marsden-Haug N, Goldoft M, Wohrle R, Lee S, Smelser C, Park B, Chiller T. Cryptococcus gattii in the United States: clinical aspects of infection with an emerging pathogen. Clin Infect Dis. 2011;53:1188–95.

Henriet S, Verweij PE, Holland SM, Warris A. Invasive fungal infections in patients with chronic granulomatous disease. Adv Exp Med Biol. 2013;764:27–55.

Husain S, Munoz P, Forrest G, Alexander BD, Somani J, Brennan K, Wagener MM, Singh N. Infections due to Scedosporium apiospermum and Scedosporium prolificans in transplant recipients: clinical characteristics and impact of antifungal agent therapy on outcome. Clin Infect Dis. 2005;40:89–99.

Kantarcioglu AS, Guarro J, de Hoog GS. Central nervous system infections by members of the Pseudallescheria boydii species complex in healthy and immunocompromised hosts: epidemiology, clinical characteristics and outcome. Mycoses. 2008;51:275–90.

Kantarcioglu AS, Guarro J, De Hoog S, Apaydin H, Kiraz N. An updated comprehensive systematic review of Cladophialophora bantiana and analysis of epidemiology, clinical characteristics, and outcome of cerebral cases. Med Mycol. 2017;55:579–604.

Kauffman CA, Freifeld AG, Andes DR, Baddley JW, Herwaldt L, Walker RC, Alexander BD, Anaissie EJ, Benedict K, Ito JI, Knapp KM, Lyon GM, Marr KA, Morrison VA, Park BJ, Patterson TF, Schuster MG, Chiller TM, Pappas PG. Endemic fungal infections in solid organ and hematopoietic cell transplant recipients enrolled in the Transplant-Associated Infection Surveillance Network (TRANSNET). Transpl Infect Dis. 2014;16:213–24.

Kaur J, Myers AM. Homosexuality, steroid therapy, and histoplasmosis. Ann Intern Med. 1983;99:567.

Keckich DW, Blair JE, Vikram HR, Seville MT, Kusne S. Reactivation of coccidioidomycosis despite antifungal prophylaxis in solid organ transplant recipients. Transplantation. 2011;92:88–93.

Kong YC, Levine HB, Madin SH, Smith CE. Fungal multiplication and histopathologic changes in vaccinated mice infected with coccidioides immitis. J Immunol. 1964;92:779–90.

Kontoyiannis DP, Marr KA, Park BJ, Alexander BD, Anaissie EJ, Walsh TJ, Ito J, Andes DR, Baddley JW, Brown JM, Brumble LM, Freifeld AG, Hadley S, Herwaldt LA, Kauffman CA, Knapp K, Lyon GM, Morrison VA, Papanicolaou G, Patterson TF, Perl TM, Schuster MG, Walker R, Wannemuehler KA, Wingard JR, Chiller TM, Pappas PG. Prospective surveillance for invasive fungal infections in hematopoietic stem cell transplant recipients, 2001–2006: overview of the Transplant-Associated Infection Surveillance Network (TRANSNET) Database. Clin Infect Dis. 2010;50:1091–100.

Kourkoumpetis TK, Desalermos A, Muhammed M, Mylonakis E. Central nervous system aspergillosis: a series of 14 cases from a general hospital and review of 123 cases from the literature. Medicine (Baltimore). 2012;91:328–36.

Kowacs PA, Monteiro de Almeida S, Pinheiro RL, Fameli H, Piovesan EJ, Correia A, Werneck LC. Central nervous system Aspergillus fumigatus infection after near drowning. J Clin Pathol. 2004;57:202–4.

Lanternier F, Barbati E, Meinzer U, Liu L, Pedergnana V, Migaud M, Heritier S, Chomton M, Fremond ML, Gonzales E, Galeotti C, Romana S, Jacquemin E, Angoulvant A, Bidault V, Canioni D, Lachenaud J, Mansouri D, Mahdaviani SA, Adimi P, Mansouri N, Jamshidi M, Bougnoux ME, Abel L, Lortholary O, Blanche S, Casanova JL, Picard C, Puel A. Inherited CARD9 deficiency in 2 unrelated patients with invasive Exophiala infection. J Infect Dis. 2015;211:1241–50.

Marra CM, Whitley RJ, Scheld WM. Approach to the patient with central nervous system infection. In: Infections of the central nervous system. Philadelphia: Wolters Kluwer Health; 2014.

Masannat FY, Ampel NM. Coccidioidomycosis in patients with HIV-1 infection in the era of potent antiretroviral therapy. Clin Infect Dis. 2010;50:1–7.

Matsumoto E, Boyken L, Tendolkar S, McDanel J, Castanheira M, Pfaller M, Diekema D. Candidemia surveillance in Iowa: emergence of echinocandin resistance. Diagn Microbiol Infect Dis. 2014;79:205–8.

Maziarz EK, Perfect JR. Cryptococcosis. Infect Dis Clin North Am. 2016;30:179–206.

McCarthy M, Rosengart A, Schuetz AN, Kontoyiannis DP, Walsh TJ. Mold infections of the central nervous system. N Engl J Med. 2014;371:150–60.

Mendoza N, Blair JE. The utility of diagnostic testing for active coccidioidomycosis in solid organ transplant recipients. Am J Transplant. 2013;13:1034–9.

Mendoza L, Vilela R, Voelz K, Ibrahim AS, Voigt K, Lee SC. Human fungal pathogens of Mucorales and Entomophthorales. Cold Spring Harb Perspect Med. 2014;5 https://doi.org/10.1101/cshperspect.a019562.

Mendoza N, Noel P, Blair JE. Diagnosis, treatment, and outcomes of coccidioidomycosis in allogeneic stem cell transplantation. Transpl Infect Dis. 2015;17:380–8.

Munoz P, Giannella M, Vena A. Mold infections in solid transplant recipients. In: Transplant infections. Switzerland: Springer; 2016.

Osawa R, Alexander BD, Lortholary O, Dromer F, Forrest GN, Lyon GM, Somani J, Gupta KL, Del Busto R, Pruett TL, Sifri CD, Limaye AP, John GT, Klintmalm GB, Pursell K, Stosor V, Morris MI, Dowdy LA, Munoz P, Kalil AC, Garcia-Diaz J, Orloff S, House AA, Houston S, Wray D, Huprikar S, Johnson LB, Humar A, Razonable RR, Fisher RA, Husain S, Wagener MM, Singh N. Identifying predictors of central nervous system disease in solid organ transplant recipients with cryptococcosis. Transplantation. 2010;89:69–74.

Pappas PG, Threlkeld MG, Bedsole GD, Cleveland KO, Gelfand MS, Dismukes WE. Blastomycosis in immunocompromised patients. Medicine (Baltimore). 1993;72:311–25.

Pappas PG, Alexander BD, Andes DR, Hadley S, Kauffman CA, Freifeld A, Anaissie EJ, Brumble LM, Herwaldt L, Ito J, Kontoyiannis DP, Lyon GM, Marr KA, Morrison VA, Park BJ, Patterson TF, Perl TM, Oster RA, Schuster MG, Walker R, Walsh TJ, Wannemuehler KA, Chiller TM. Invasive fungal infections among organ transplant recipients: results of the Transplant-Associated Infection Surveillance Network (TRANSNET). Clin Infect Dis. 2010;50:1101–11.

Peri AM, Bisi L, Cappelletti A, Colella E, Verga L, Borella C, Foresti S, Migliorino GM, Gori A, Bandera A. Invasive aspergillosis with pulmonary and central nervous system involvement during ibrutinib therapy for relapsed chronic lymphocytic leukaemia: case report. Clin Microbiol Infect. 2018;24:785–6.

Pfaller MA, Castanheira M, Messer SA, Moet GJ, Jones RN. Variation in Candida spp. distribution and antifungal resistance rates among bloodstream infection isolates by patient age: report from the SENTRY Antimicrobial Surveillance Program (2008–2009). Diagn Microbiol Infect Dis. 2010;68:278–83.

Pfaller MA, Moet GJ, Messer SA, Jones RN, Castanheira M. Geographic variations in species distribution and echinocandin and azole antifungal resistance rates among Candida bloodstream infection isolates: report from the SENTRY Antimicrobial Surveillance Program (2008 to 2009). J Clin Microbiol. 2011;49:396–9.

Pfaller M, Neofytos D, Diekema D, Azie N, Meier-Kriesche HU, Quan SP, Horn D. Epidemiology and outcomes of candidemia in 3648 patients: data from the Prospective Antifungal Therapy (PATH Alliance(R)) registry, 2004–2008. Diagn Microbiol Infect Dis. 2012;74:323–31.

Pittet D, Monod M, Suter PM, Frenk E, Auckenthaler R. Candida colonization and subsequent infections in critically ill surgical patients. Ann Surg. 1994;220:751–8.

Powers-Fletcher MV, Hanson KE. Nonculture diagnostics in fungal disease. Infect Dis Clin North Am. 2016;30:37–49.

Rajasingham R, Smith RM, Park BJ, Jarvis JN, Govender NP, Chiller TM, Denning DW, Loyse A, Boulware DR. Global burden of disease of HIV-associated cryptococcal meningitis: an updated analysis. Lancet Infect Dis. 2017;17:873–81.

Ramirez-Garcia A, Pellon A, Rementeria A, Buldain I, Barreto-Bergter E, Rollin-Pinheiro R, de Meirelles JV, Xisto M, Ranque S, Havlicek V, Vandeputte P, Govic YL, Bouchara JP, Giraud S, Chen S, Rainer J, Alastruey-Izquierdo A, Martin-Gomez MT, Lopez-Soria LM, Peman J, Schwarz C, Bernhardt A, Tintelnot K, Capilla J, Martin-Vicente A, Cano-Lira J, Nagl M, Lackner M, Irinyi L, Meyer W, de Hoog S, Hernando FL. Scedosporium and Lomentospora: an updated overview of underrated opportunists. Med Mycol. 2018;56:102–25.

Revankar SG, Patterson JE, Sutton DA, Pullen R, Rinaldi MG. Disseminated phaeohyphomycosis: review of an emerging mycosis. Clin Infect Dis. 2002;34:467–76.

Rieber N, Gazendam RP, Freeman AF, Hsu AP, Collar AL, Sugui JA, Drummond RA, Rongkavilit C, Hoffman K, Henderson C, Clark L, Mezger M, Swamydas M, Engeholm M, Schule R, Neumayer B, Ebel F, Mikelis CM, Pittaluga S, Prasad VK, Singh A, Milner JD, Williams KW, Lim JK, Kwon-Chung KJ, Holland SM, Hartl D, Kuijpers TW, Lionakis MS. Extrapulmonary Aspergillus infection in patients with CARD9 deficiency. JCI Insight. 2016;1:e89890.

Roden MM, Zaoutis TE, Buchanan WL, Knudsen TA, Sarkisova TA, Schaufele RL, Sein M, Sein T, Chiou CC, Chu JH, Kontoyiannis DP, Walsh TJ. Epidemiology and outcome of zygomycosis: a review of 929 reported cases. Clin Infect Dis. 2005;41:634–53.

Rosen LB, Freeman AF, Yang LM, Jutivorakool K, Olivier KN, Angkasekwinai N, Suputtamongkol Y, Bennett JE, Pyrgos V, Williamson PR, Ding L, Holland SM, Browne SK. Anti-GM-CSF autoantibodies in patients with cryptococcal meningitis. J Immunol. 2013;190:3959–66.

Saijo T, Chen J, Chen SC, Rosen LB, Yi J, Sorrell TC, Bennett JE, Holland SM, Browne SK, Kwon-Chung KJ. Anti-granulocyte-macrophage colony-stimulating factor autoantibodies are a risk factor for central nervous system infection by Cryptococcus gattii in otherwise immunocompetent patients. MBio. 2014;5:e00912–4.

Sarma S, Upadhyay S. Current perspective on emergence, diagnosis and drug resistance in Candida auris. Infect Drug Resist. 2017;10:155–65.

Schneider E, Hajjeh RA, Spiegel RA, Jibson RW, Harp EL, Marshall GA, Gunn RA, McNeil MM, Pinner RW, Baron RC, Burger RC, Hutwagner LC, Crump C, Kaufman L, Reef SE, Feldman GM, Pappagianis D, Werner SB. A coccidioidomycosis outbreak following the Northridge, Calif, earthquake. JAMA. 1997;277:904–8.

Schwartz IS, Wiederhold NP, Hanson KE, Patterson TF, Sigler L. Blastomyces helicus, a new dimorphic fungus causing fatal pulmonary and systemic disease in humans and animals in Western Canada and United States. Clin Infect Dis. 2018; https://doi.org/10.1093/cid/ciy483.

Shapiro S, Javed T, Mealey J Jr. Candida albicans shunt infection. Pediatr Neurosci. 1989;15:125–30.

Shikanai-Yasuda MA, Mendes RP, Colombo AL, Queiroz-Telles F, Kono ASG, Paniago AMM, Nathan A, Valle A, Bagagli E, Benard G, Ferreira MS, Teixeira MM, Silva-Vergara ML, Pereira RM, Cavalcante RS, Hahn R, Durlacher RR, Khoury Z, Camargo ZP, Moretti ML, Martinez R. Brazilian guidelines for the clinical management of paracoccidioidomycosis. Rev Soc Bras Med Trop. 2017;50:715–40.

Shoham S, Pic-Aluas L, Taylor J, Cortez K, Rinaldi MG, Shea Y, Walsh TJ. Transplant-associated Ochroconis gallopava infections. Transpl Infect Dis. 2008;10:442–8.

Singh N. Fungal infections in the recipients of solid organ transplantation. Infect Dis Clin North Am. 2003;17:113–34., viii.

Singh N, Paterson DL. Aspergillus infections in transplant recipients. Clin Microbiol Rev. 2005;18:44–69.

Singh N, Aguado JM, Bonatti H, Forrest G, Gupta KL, Safdar N, John GT, Pursell KJ, Munoz P, Patel R, Fortun J, Martin-Davila P, Philippe B, Philit F, Tabah A, Terzi N, Chatelet V, Kusne S, Clark N, Blumberg E, Julia MB, Humar A, Houston S, Lass-Florl C, Johnson L, Dubberke ER, Barron MA, Lortholary O. Zygomycosis in solid organ transplant recipients: a prospective, matched case-control study to assess risks for disease and outcome. J Infect Dis. 2009;200:1002–11.

Smego RA Jr, Devoe PW, Sampson HA, Perfect JR, Wilfert CM, Buckley RH. Candida meningitis in two children with severe combined immunodeficiency. J Pediatr. 1984;104:902–4.

Smith JA, Kauffman CA. Endemic fungal infections in patients receiving tumour necrosis factor-alpha inhibitor therapy. Drugs. 2009;69:1403–15.

Spellberg B, Edwards J Jr, Ibrahim A. Novel perspectives on mucormycosis: pathophysiology, presentation, and management. Clin Microbiol Rev. 2005;18:556–69.

Stave GM, Heimberger T, Kerkering TM. Zygomycosis of the basal ganglia in intravenous drug users. Am J Med. 1989;86:115–7.

Stevens DA. Coccidioidomycosis. N Engl J Med. 1995;332:1077–82.

Stockamp NW, Thompson GR 3rd. Coccidioidomycosis. Infect Dis Clin North Am. 2016;30:229–46.

Vallabhaneni S, Mody RK, Walker T, Chiller T. The global burden of fungal diseases. Infect Dis Clin North Am. 2016;30:1–11.

Vilela R, Souza GF, Fernandes Cota G, Mendoza L. Cutaneous and meningeal sporotrichosis in a HIV patient. Rev Iberoam Micol. 2007;24:161–3.

Walsh TJ, Gamaletsou MN, McGinnis MR, Hayden RT, Kontoyiannis DP. Early clinical and laboratory diagnosis of invasive pulmonary, extrapulmonary, and disseminated mucormycosis (zygomycosis). Clin Infect Dis. 2012;54(Suppl 1):S55–60.

Warris A, Bjorneklett A, Gaustad P. Invasive pulmonary aspergillosis associated with infliximab therapy. N Engl J Med. 2001;344:1099–100.

Wheat LJ, Azar MM, Bahr NC, Spec A, Relich RF, Hage C. Histoplasmosis. Infect Dis Clin North Am. 2016;30:207–27.

Wheat J, Myint T, Guo Y, Kemmer P, Hage C, Terry C, Azar MM, Riddell J, Ender P, Chen S, Shehab K, Cleveland K, Esguerra E, Johnson J, Wright P, Douglas V, Vergidis P, Ooi W, Baddley J, Bamberger D, Khairy R, Vikram HR, Jenny-Avital E, Sivasubramanian G, Bowlware K, Pahud B, Sarria J, Tsai T, Assi M, Mocherla S, Prakash V, Allen D, Passaretti C, Huprikar S, Anderson A. Central nervous system histoplasmosis: multicenter retrospective study on clinical features, diagnostic approach and outcome of treatment. Medicine (Baltimore). 2018;97:e0245.

Morphological Classification of Fungal Infections (Yeasts, Mold, Dimorphic)

3

Lakshmi Vemu Gorthi

Abbreviation

TLM Transmitted light microscope

3.1 Introduction

Medical mycology is often referred to as an "exercise of contemplative observation" as it essentially relies on the time honoured observation of the morphology of the fungus to establish a definitive diagnosis (Rippon 1988). When a fungus is recovered from a clinical specimen, it is important to identify the fungus so as to determine whether it is a common pathogen or one of the opportunistic pathogens for a definitive diagnosis and an early management of the infection (Bennett 1992). The morphological studies of the major groups of medically important fungi and the relationships between them are based on colonial morphology and light microscopic examinations. All the observed features of a fungal isolate are accumulated and combined for an accurate identification and also to determine the taxonomy of the fungus (Rippon 1988; Lehmann 2009).

The three principal characteristics of the colonial morphology to be evaluated when fungi grow on standardized culture media are texture, growth rate and pigmentation (Chander 2018; Bennett 1992).

Most of the microscopic features of a fungus can be comfortably observed using a transmitted light microscope (TLM). However, in some cases, phase contrast microscopy and high-resolution digital photograph are required (Roberts and Goodman 2009). Though fungi are essentially unicellular organisms, in some fungal species the cells show varying degrees of specialization in the form of fruiting structures unique to a genus or species of the fungus. Thus, the major microscopic features used in morphological classification of fungi include not only the basic shape of the fungal thallus, presence or absence of septa in hyphae and pigmentation but also the structure of the fruiting bodies, especially formation and release mechanisms of reproductive propagules (Rippon 1988; Bennett 1992).

Based on the gross morphological characteristics, pathogenic fungi infecting humans are conveniently separated into two basic groups, *yeasts* and *molds*. The simplest morphological form of a fungus is the unicellular budding yeast cell. A number of pathogenic fungi alternate between a yeast phase (at 37 °C or in tissues) and a hyphal phase (at 28 °C) and are termed as *dimorphic fungi* (Chander 2018; Lehmann 2009).

L. V. Gorthi (✉)
Department of Microbiology, Kamineni Academy of Medical Sciences and Research Centre, Hyderabad, Telangana, India

M. Turgut et al. (eds.), *Fungal Infections of the Central Nervous System*, https://doi.org/10.1007/978-3-030-06088-6_3

3.2 Yeasts

3.2.1 The Yeast Cell (Chander 2018; Lehmann 2009)

Defined morphologically, a yeast is a single-celled fungus (spherical to ellipsoid forms with a diameter of 3–15 μm) that reproduces by simple budding. The size and shape of cells within a strain are the same when the yeast is propagated under identical conditions and may change with the nutrient and the environment. The yeast cell may elongate to form pseudo-hyphae and pseudo-mycelium under certain conditions (Chander 2018; Rippon 1988).

The morphological features essential in the classification and identification of yeasts include:

- The shape, size and internal structure of the yeast cells.
- The method of asexual reproduction by the vegetative cells and the position of the newly formed cells to their parent.
- The macroscopical appearance of a yeast growth visible to the naked eye.

It should be understood that the term *yeasts* is of no taxonomic significance. Instead, they are growth forms shown by a range of unrelated fungi. In the dimorphic fungi, the yeasts are a phase of growth in the life cycle of the filamentous fungus (Chander 2018).

3.2.2 Yeast Colonies (Roberts and Goodman 2009; Bennett 1992)

Yeast colonies on solid media resemble bacterial colonies, soft, dry, opaque, 1–3 mm in size and cream coloured. However, colony morphology is not a definitive differentiating feature among the yeasts (Lehmann 2009).

3.2.3 True/Budding Yeasts (Bennett 1992; Lehmann 2009)

These fungi predominantly are one-cell forms with round or oval bodies which reproduce by an asexual process called budding in which the cell develops a protuberance with a narrow base. This blastospore enlarges and eventually separates from the parent cell by cleavage of the cross wall to further develop and propagate the yeast colony. Some yeasts may produce buds simultaneously at several points (Lehmann 2009). In the true yeast, *Cryptococcus neoformans*, the daughter cells are attached to the parent cell by a narrow base, while in *Blastomyces dermatitidis*, the budding is broad based (Chander 2018).

3.2.4 Yeast-Like Fungi

In some of the medically important yeasts, the bud remains attached to the mother cell and continuously grows without separation to form chains of elongated cells called *pseudo-hyphae*, which form a pseudo-mycelium (e.g. *Candida* species) (Lehmann 2009). The short oval cells formed by budding at the ends of the long pseudomycelial cells are the "blasto-spores" and those developed on the sides of pseudomycelia are the "blastoconidia." The pseudo-hyphae are vegetative with no reproductive value. During adverse conditions, some of the hyphae become enriched with nutritive material and enlarge to form a thick wall called *chlamydospore*. These resting forms of the yeast-like fungi are usually larger than the other cells and develop at intercalary, terminal or sessile positions on the pseudo-hyphae (Chander 2018).

3.2.5 Fission Yeasts (Bennett 1992; Lehmann 2009)

A second form of cell division in the yeasts is by fission. The parental yeast cell elongates and separates from the progeny by a septum, resulting in several shapes (e.g. *Talaromyces (Penicillium) marneffei*).

3.3 Molds or Filamentous Fungi (Chander 2018; Rippon 1988; Bennett 1992; Lehmann 2009)

The filamentous fungi are popularly known as molds. They form true mycelium and reproduce by formation of different types of reproductive propagules. Example: dermatophytes and *Aspergillus*.

3.3.1 Key Morphological Features of Molds (Chander 2018; Rippon 1988; Lehmann 2009)

The standard method for identifying molds is by observing their colonial and microscopic morphology and following taxonomic keys to make a definite identification. The colony of a mold developed from a single reproductive propagule is called "thallus" (*TW*). The unit of a mold is called a *hypha* and is the actively growing assimilative phase. Branching and intertwining of hypha leads to the formation of a *mycelium*. Hyphae are usually 1.5–3.5 μm. in diameter in all molds except *Zygomycetes*. As the hypha develops, it gets divided into compartments or cells by the formation of cross walls called *septa*, which may be partial, complete or perforated. In general, all mycelial fungi, other than the *Zygomycetes*, have perforated (single or multiple) septa (Chander 2018).

3.3.2 Macroscopic Morphology of Molds

In general, molds grow as pigmented or white cottony to woolly colonies with or without aerial hyphae. Older colonies exhibit different colours based on the pigmentation of the conidiophores and conidia (Rippon 1988).

3.3.3 Microscopic Morphology of Molds

Using TLM with a 40× magnification, the important structures to be examined for a mold are the width of the hyphal filaments, presence or absence of pigmentation, septation and nature of branching of the hyphae especially the reproductive hyphae and the spores/conidia they bear, formation and size, shape and arrangement of spores/conidia and their surface (smooth or rough) and pigmentation (Roberts and Goodman 2009). These are the basis for identification of the molds to genus and species levels (Rippon 1988). The vegetative hyphae tend to be simple and exhibit few characteristic differentiating features between the genera and species. Grossly, all the molds have thin septate profusely branching hyphae except the *Mucormycotina* (Chander 2018).

3.4 Dimorphic Fungi (Kidd et al. 2016)

(Di: both; morphism: morphological form). Many medically important fungal pathogens, that cause endemic, systemic or subcutaneous infections, e.g. *Histoplasma*, *Sporothrix*, *Blastomyces*, *Paracoccidioides*, and *Penicillium*, transform from hyphal growth at body temperature (35–37 °C) to yeast cells, at ambient temperature (25–30 °C), in response to host stimuli. These dimorphic fungi exist as molds in the environment and as yeasts (or other structures, e.g. spherules in the case of *Coccidioides immitis*) in human tissues (a reversible phenomenon) (Chander 2018). These dimorphic fungal pathogens can overcome the physiological and cellular defences of the normal human host by changing their morphological form. *Coccidioides* and *Pneumocystis* species produce spherules and cysts, respectively, which allow for the production of offspring in a protected environment (Kidd et al. 2016).

For a definitive diagnosis of the dimorphic fungal infections, the two phases of the dimorphic fungus have to be reproduced in the clinical laboratory by growing these fungi both at 25 °C and 37 °C in appropriate culture media (Roberts and Goodman 2009; Kidd et al. 2016).

The term dimorphism is applied loosely to denote morphological changes in certain yeasts, with both yeast and mycelial phases. However, this feature should not be mistaken for dimorphism, as the phases are not temperature dependent. Both phases can be seen at 25 °C and 37 °C (Chander 2018; Köhler et al. 2015; Kidd et al. 2016).

3.5 General Morphological Features of Fungi (Chander 2018; Rippon 1988; Brandt et al. 2011; Lehmann 2009)

3.5.1 Mycelium

Characteristic of a filamentous fungus is derived from a single reproductive unit and is delineated into three general types that differ in function:

- *Vegetative mycelium*: Masses of hyphae within a colony adjacent to and growing into the substrate.
- *Submerged hyphae*: They are concerned with the digestion and assimilation of food materials from the substrate.
- *Reproductive/fertile hyphae*: Usually extend into the air to form an aerial mycelium. They give rise to various types of reproductive units.

3.5.1.1 Vegetative Hyphal Structures

Even though the vegetative hyphae have no reproductive significance, the different structures formed are of considerable value in the differentiation, especially among the dermatophytes (Rippon 1988).

- *Spirals or coiled hyphae*: They are bedspring-like, helical coils found at the ends of peridial hyphae surrounding an ascocarp or by themselves. They are very prominent in *Trichophyton mentagrophytes*.
- *Nodular organs*: Are enlargements in the mycelium, which consist of closely twisted hyphae as a knot, e.g. *Trichophyton mentagrophytes* and *Microsporum canis*.
- *Racquet mycelium*: These hyphae are larger than others with a regular enlargement of one end of each segment. Large and small ends are in opposition.
- *Pectinate body*: Is a unilateral, short, irregular projection formed on one side of a hypha, giving it a broken comb-like appearance, e.g. *Microsporum audouinii*.
- *Favic chandelier* (antler hyphae) formed by numerous multiple branches appearing at the end of a hypha. These resemble a reindeer antler or a chandelier. Occurs primarily in *Trichophyton schoenleinii* and *Trichophyton violaceum*.
- *Peridial hypha*: Is a wide, indented, multiseptated hypha which may terminate in a spiral. They are numerous in *Trichophyton mentagrophytes*.

3.6 Reproduction in Fungi

Majority of the medically important fungi have two reproductive states, sexual and asexual—the perfect or teleomorph or imperfect or anamorph state (Chander 2018; Rippon 1988; Köhler et al. 2015; Lehmann 2009).

3.6.1 Teleomorphs (Perfect State)

The sporulating structures that are associated with sexual spores produced after meiosis has occurred are called *teleomorphs (perfect state)*.

3.6.2 Anamorphs (Imperfect State)

Sporulating colonies that bear conidia or spores produced in an asexual process, wherein there is no prior fusion of nucleus nor subsequent meiosis, are known as *anamorphs (imperfect state)*. The asexual propagules arise following mitosis of the parent nucleus.

- *Asexual spores* are commonly formed by consecutive cleavage within a structure called sporangium, as seen in *Mucormycotina* (Brandt et al. 2011).
- *Conidia* are asexual, deciduous propagules produced exclusively by the filamentous fungi. Conidia arise by de novo budding of a conidiogenous hypha or by differentiation of preformed hyphae (Rippon 1988).

Both these reproductive states in fungi are separately classified and named for a genus and species. In general, medically important fungi are mainly described and identified based on the morphology of the asexual state (anamorph) which is the usual type of reproduction seen in the laboratory cultures while the sexual state is rarely manifested. The only exception is *Pseudoallescheria boydii*, an ascomycete, which is seen in its sexual state in the clinical specimen. Its asexual state, *Scedosporium apiospermum* may also be seen (Chander 2018).

3.6.3 Classification of Fungi into Phyla Based on Sexual Reproduction (Rippon 1988; Brandt et al. 2011)

The large numbers of morphological specifications associated with sexual sporulation in fungi is an important classification feature. And based on these features, medically important fungi are classified into three major phyla: the *Glomeromycota*, *Ascomycota* and *Basidiomycota*.

- Glomeromycota—fertilized cell becomes a zygote.
- Ascomycota—sexual spores are contained in an ascus or sac.
- Basidiomycota—sexual spores are produced at the end of the basidium.

3.6.3.1 Phylum *Glomeromycota* (Formerly *Zygomycota*) (Rippon 1988; Brandt et al. 2011)

Further classified as the subphylum *Mucormycotina* which accommodates the order *Mucorales*, which consists of the medically important genera, *Absidia*, *Mucor*, *Rhizomucor* and *Rhizopus*. The subphylum *Entomophthoromycotina* includes the genera *Basidiobolus* and *Conidiobolus* which are agents of subcutaneous infections.

Macroscopic Morphology/Colony Characteristics on Culture

Grow rapidly on agar in grey-white brown cottony or woolly colonies without distinct margins.

Microscopic Morphology

This group of lower fungi is characterized by an aseptate thallus. They typically develop coenocytic hyphae that are sparsely septate, broad (10–15 μm), colourless and ribbon like, branching irregularly. *Zygomycetes* rarely have septa, but if present, the septa are complete and at the site of formation of a zygospore.

Mucoromycotina

The characteristics of the asexual spore-bearing structures are distinct and help in differentiating the several genera. The important features that have to be examined include height and branching of sporangiophore, arrangement of sporangiospores and sporangiophores, size of sporangiospore, sporangium shape and size, presence or absence of columella (a sterile column of hyphae within a spore-bearing structure, extending as a supporting stalk), shape and size of columella and apophyses and presence or absence of rhizoids and their location (nodal or internodal) (a root-like structure, a filamentous branch-like extension for feeding rather than reproduction) (Brandt et al. 2011).

The distinct morphological features of the main genera of subphylum *Mucoromycotina* are:

- *Mucor*: Rhizoids are absent and the sporangiophores tend to branch and often bear large round sporangia.
- *Rhizopus*: Rhizoids are large and originate immediately on the stolon adjacent to sporangiophore (nodal). The latter are usually unbranched, long and terminate in a columella and a dark round sporangium with oval colourless to brown spores.
- *Absidia*: Rhizoids arise on the stolon between two sporangiophores (internodal). *Rhizomucor*: Is a variant of *Mucor*, but has poorly developed rhizoids and can grow at 60 °C (Chander 2018; Rippon 1988).

Entomophthoromycota (Formerly Subphylum Entomophthoromycotina)

Species in the *Entomophthoromycota* generally share several characteristics. Their vegetative cells are coenocytic; sporulation occurs by production of forcibly discharged dispersive or infective conidia; and their zygospores (which also function as resting spores) are homothallic (Rippon 1988; Brandt et al. 2011).

3.6.3.2 Phylum *Ascomycota* (Rippon 1988; Brandt et al. 2011)

These fungi have a septate thallus. Asexual reproduction consists of the production of conidia from a conidiogenous cell. In some species conidiogenous cell directly arises from mycelium while in some species it is contained in the conidiophore. Sexual reproduction results in ascospores produced in a saclike structure called ascocarp.

This phylum consists of the genus *Ajellomyces*, the main teleomorph of dimorphic systemic fungal pathogens. Anamorphic genera are *Blastomyces*, *Histoplasma*, *Pseudoallescheria*, teleomorph of the anamorph *Scedosporium*.

3.6.3.3 Phylum *Basidiomycota* (Rippon 1988; Brandt et al. 2011)

Most members of this phylum are septate, filamentous fungi, but some are typical yeasts. Asexual reproduction is variable with some species producing conidia. But many others do not produce conidia at all. Sexual reproduction results in production of basidiospores on the outside of the generative cell, called basidium. The spores are often forcibly discharged. The most prominent fungi in this phylum are the basidiomycetous yeasts with anamorphic stage belonging to the genera *Cryptococcus*, *Malassezia* and *Trichosporon*.

3.6.4 Anamorphic Fungi (Fungi Imperfecti, Deuteromycota) (Chander 2018; Rippon 1988; Brandt et al. 2011)

In majority of the medically important fungi, asexual reproduction has proved so successful that the sexual stage has disappeared. The members in this group of anamorphic fungi are classified into *Blastomycetes*, *Coelomycetes* and *Hyphomycetes*—based on their form of growth and asexual reproduction.

- *Blastomycetes* contain yeasts that reproduce by budding.
- *Coelemycetes* septate molds that produce conidia within a cavity of fungal tissue referred to as pycnidium.
- *Hyphomycetes* septate molds that produce conidia directly on the hyphae or on conidiophores. Important genera are included in this group, e.g. *Aspergillus*, *Blastomyces*, *Cladophialophora*, *Fusarium*, *Microsporum*, *Penicillium*, *Phialophora*, *Scedosporium*, *Histoplasma* and *Trichophyton*. The conidiogenesis in *Hyphomycetes* is either blastic or thallic. The *Hyphomycetes* are further divided as being either *dematiaceous* (darkly pigmented conidiophore and conidia) or *halohyphomycetes* (non-pigmented conidiophore and conidia) (Rippon 1988; Brandt et al. 2011).

3.7 Asexual Reproduction in Molds (Bennett 1992; Brandt et al. 2011)

Many reproductive propagules (conidia) are produced in an asexual reproductive phase of a mold. Conidia are produced free either by segmentation or by budding of the tips of the reproductive hyphae. The hyphae that bear the conidia are called conidiophores on conidiogenous cells. Smaller and unicellular conidia are called microconidia while large and multicellular conidia are termed as macroconidia. The conidial forms, shape, septation and colour together form the basis for identification of the fungi and was earlier known as the Saccardoan scheme after PA Saccardo.

3.7.1 Position of Conidium (Chander 2018)

- *Terminal*: On the end of the reproductive hypha.
- *Synchronous*: Several conidia develop at the same time from a botryose conidiogenous cell.
- *Basipetal*: The youngest conidium is at the bottom of a chain as in the phialidic *Aspergillus* or annellidic *Scopulariopsis*.
- *Acropetal*: The youngest conidium is at the top of the chain.

3.7.2 Conidiophore (Rippon 1988; Brandt et al. 2011)

Conidiophore is a simple or branched hypha (a fertile hypha) bearing conidiogenous cells. Important morphologic features are point of origin of the conidiophore on the mycelium, single or multiple, with or without branching presence or absence of foot cell, length of the conidiophore and pigmentation.

3.7.3 Conidiogenous Cell (Rippon 1988; Brandt et al. 2011)

Conidiogenous cells directly produce conidia. They may be *determinant* (no growth of the conidiophore after the formation of conidia) or *sympodial* (a mode of growth which results in the development of conidia on a geniculate or zig-zag rachis). Conidiogenous cell may be non-specialized or specialized into a phialide or an annellide.

3.7.3.1 Phialide (Brandt et al. 2011)

Phialide is a typically a flask-shaped cell that develops an open end from which conidia are produced in basipetal succession. Phialides are a characteristic of *Penicillium* and *Aspergillus* spp.

3.7.3.2 Annellide (Brandt et al. 2011)

Annellide is a specialized conidiogenous cell producing conidia in basipetal succession by a series of short percurrent proliferations (annellations). The tip of an annellide increases in length and becomes narrower as each subsequent conidium is formed. It is a complex phialide with a collar developing for each conidium produced (Rippon 1988).

Other types of conidiogenesis include blastoconidium, aleuroconidium and poroconidium (Chander 2018).

3.8 Conidium (Chander 2018; Rippon 1988)

Conidium is an asexually formed spore; a relatively thin-walled spore that is terminal on the conidiophore and deciduous at maturity.

3.8.1 Conidial Characteristics

The features include shape, size and colour of the conidia, septation, wall texture (rough, spiny or smooth), number of conidial types present and arrangement of conidia borne on the conidiogenous cells: whether solitary, catenulate (in chains), acropetal or basipetal.

3.8.2 Arthrospore

Arthrospore is a conidium formed from restructuring the walls of a septate hypha, so that it breaks into separate segments (hyphal fragmentation), e.g. *Geotrichum* (Brandt et al. 2011).

3.9 Fruiting Structures (Brandt et al. 2011)

These are due to certain modifications of the hyphal structures.

- *Synnemata*—A group of erect conidiophores that are cemented together producing conidia at the apex and/or along the sides of upper portion.
- *Sporodochium*—A cushion-shaped stroma covered with conidiophores.
- *Pycnidium*—It is globose to flask-shaped fruiting body with an inner lining of conidiogenous cell containing conidia. It is large up to several millimeters in diameter and may have a hard wall surrounded by peridial hyphae. Some strains of *Trichophyton mentagrophytes* produce pycnidia, especially when grown on soil—hair agar (Chander 2018; Rippon 1988).

3.10 Significance of Fungal Morphology (Webster and Weber 2007; Köhler et al. 2015)

Mycologists are interested in the structure of the reproductive bodies and the manner in which they are produced as these features constitute the most important basis for classification and taxonomy of the fungi.

On the other hand, morphogenesis is an important virulence factor related to pathogenic fungi (Li and Nielsen 2017). Although fungal hyphae can pierce tissue barriers owing to the turgor pressure at their tips, yeast can readily disseminate to distant sites in the host. Fungi that infect healthy humans do so almost exclusively in their yeast form. But for most fungi, the ability to assume various shapes is critical for infecting humans, because many enter the body in the form of small, round airborne dispersal propagules, sporangiospores or conidia, which are produced from hyphal cells. Thus, the array of morphological changes in the fungal pathogens are closely associated with virulence (Webster and Weber 2007; Köhler et al. 2015).

3.11 Conclusion

Although future taxonomic systems obviously will rely more on molecular characteristics, the present classification of fungi is mainly built on their morphology. Given the importance of morphological transitions in the pathogenesis of the human fungal pathogens, more extensive and more detailed studies are needed to gain deeper insights into the commonalities between the morphologies and their function during infection. Ultimately, future studies addressing how human fungal pathogens control morphology and virulence in response to host environmental cues will provide information that could lead to the development of novel treatment strategies, which are aimed at blocking these important morphological changes (Webster and Weber 2007; Köhler et al. 2015).

References

Brandt ME, Lockhart SR, Warnock DW. Laboratory aspects of medical mycology. In: Kauffmann CA, Pappas PG, Sobel JD, Dismukes WE, editors. Essentials of clinical mycology. 2nd ed. New York. ISBN: 978-1-4419-6639-1: Springer; 2011. p. 3–26. https://doi.org/10.1007/978-1-4419-6640-7.

Chander J. Fungal morphology. In: Text book of medical mycology. 4th ed. New Delhi: Jaypee Brothers Medical Publishers; 2018. p. 24–38.

Kidd S, Halliday C, Alexiou H, Ellis D. Dimorphic fungi in descriptions of medical fungi. 3rd ed. Adelaide, South Australia: Authors; 2016. ISBN: 9780646951294.

Köhler JR, Casadevall A, Perfect J. The spectrum of fungi that infects humans. Cold Spring Harb Perspect Med. 2015;5:a019273.

Kwon-Chung KJ, Bennett JE. Medical mycology. 2nd ed. Philadelphia: Lea & Febiger; 1992.

Lehmann PF. Fungal structure and morphology. In: Merz WG, Hay RJ, editors. Topley & Wilson's medical mycology. 10th ed. USA: John Wiley & Sons; 2009. p. 69–81.

Li Z, Nielsen K. Morphology changes in human fungal pathogens upon interaction with the host. J Fungi (Basel). 2017;3:66. https://doi.org/10.3390/jof3040066.

Rippon JW. Characteristics of fungi. In: Medical mycology. The pathogenic fungi and the pathogenic actinomycetes. 3rd ed. Philadelphia–London–Toronto–Montreal–Sydney–Tokyo: WB Saunders Company, Harcourt Brace Jovanovich, Inc.; 1988. p. 119–20.

Roberts GD, Goodman NL. Laboratory diagnosis. In: Merz WG, Hay RJ, editors. Topley & Wilson's medical mycology. 10th ed. USA: John Wiley & Sons; 2009. p. 82–96.

Webster J, Weber RWS. Introduction to fungi. 3rd ed. Cambridge: Cambridge University Press; 2007.

4 Pathogenesis of Fungal Infections

Chandrasekhar Srinivasamurthy Banushree and Neriyana Sannappa Madhusudhan

Abbreviations

ALS proteins	Agglutinin-like sequence proteins
CARD 9	Caspase recruitment domain-containing protein 9
CD	Cluster of differentiation
CLR	C-type lectin receptors
CNS	Central nervous system
CR	Complement receptor
CTLA-4	Cytotoxic T lymphocyte-associated protein 4
DC	Dendritic cell
DNA	Deoxyribonucleic acid
EC	Epithelial cell
EPA	Epithelial adhesin gene
HIV	Human immunodeficiency virus
Hsp	Heat shock protein
HYR	Hyphally regulated protein gene
IFN	Interferons
IL	Interleukin
IRIS	Immune reconstitution inflammatory syndrome
MR	Mannose receptors
NK	Natural killer
PAMP	Pathogen-associated molecular patterns
PD-1	Programmed cell death protein-1
PRR	Pattern recognition receptors
ROI	Reactive oxygen intermediates
Saps	Secreted aspartyl proteinases
Th	Thymus helper
TLO	Telomere-associated gene
TLR	Toll-like receptor
TNF-α	Tumor necrosis factor α
Treg cells	Regulatory T cells
YWP	Yeast-form wall protein

C. S. Banushree (✉)
Department of Pathology, Indira Gandhi Medical college and Research Institute, Puducherry, India

N. S. Madhusudhan
Department of Microbiology, Indira Gandhi Medical College and Research Institute, Puducherry, India

4.1 Introduction

Fungi are ubiquitous in nature such that they are present in soil, water both seawater and freshwater, plants, animals, food, woodworks like flooring, air conditioning in hospitals, schools, child day care centers, public transports, railway stations and even electronic devices (crevices of CD-ROM). Modern lifestyle has expanded range of exposure to fungi (Khan and Karuppayil 2012; Simoes et al. 2011). Fungal infections in humans are one of the most difficult diseases to manage. Fungal infections can occur in healthy as well as in seriously ill persons. Among 1.5 million fungal species, only three hundred cause the disease in humans and very few affect healthy individu-

M. Turgut et al. (eds.), *Fungal Infections of the Central Nervous System*,
https://doi.org/10.1007/978-3-030-06088-6_4

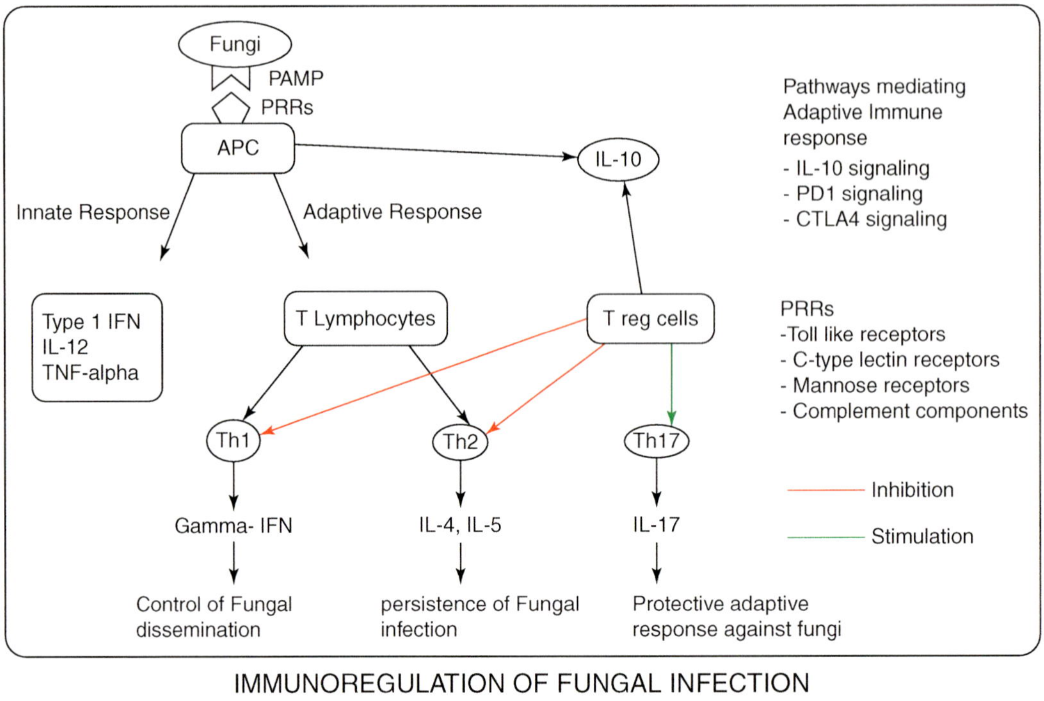

Fig. 4.1 Flow diagram depicting immunoregulation of fungal infection

Antibodies confer protection against fungal infections by multiple mechanisms that include direct neutralization of fungi and their antigens, inhibition of growth of fungi, modification of gene expression and signaling, lipid metabolism, causing iron starvation, inhibition of polysaccharide release, and biofilm formation. Antibodies promote opsonization of fungi and their phagocytosis, complement activation, and antibody-dependent cell toxicity (Elluru et al. 2014).

In CNS, immunological reactions comprise of both an innate response and an adaptive response. An innate response is initiated by microglia, and adaptive response depends upon the presentation of antigen by antigen-presenting cells such as macrophage and dendritic cells present in the leptomeningeal and perivascular region which has the potential to elicit T-cell response (Engelhardt et al. 2016). Microglia and perivascular macrophages release chemokines that regulate the neuroinflammatory response by increased recruiting of dendritic cells, neutrophils, and lymphocytes from peripheral tissue. The interaction of microglia and perivascular macrophages may be necessary to bridge the immunological communication between cells in the CNS and cells in the peripheral tissues (Li et al. 2015; Prinz and Priller 2014).

4.5 Evolution of Fungi

4.5.1 Role of Genes in Pathogenesis: Lessons Learnt from Comparative Genomic Studies (CGA)

The novel genes are acquired at the telomeric proximal regions of the pathogenic fungi which are nonexistent in their nonpathogenic relative species (Moran et al. 2011). This phenomenon is particularly well noticed in *Aspergillus* spp. Coordinated epigenetic regulation of expression of genes for virulence is facilitated by clustering. In a mouse infection model, about 30% of clustered genes were induced during initiation of invasive aspergillosis (McDonagh et al. 2008). Though horizontal gene transfer is seen

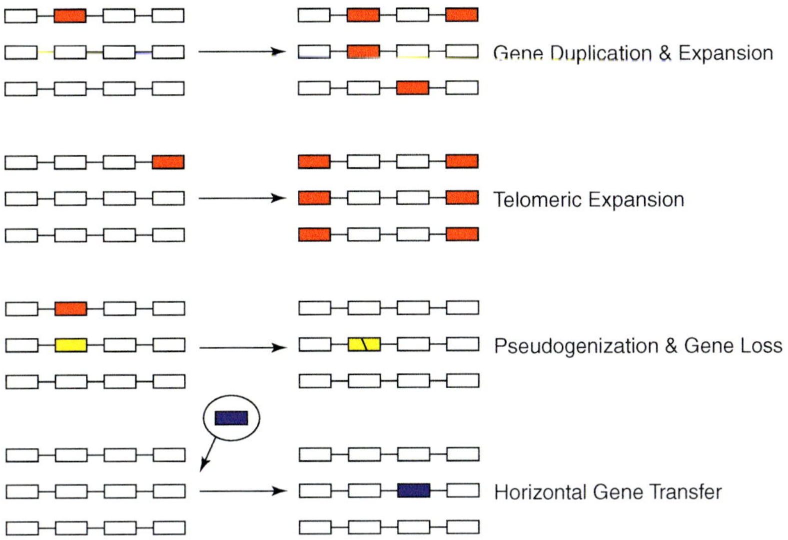

Fig. 4.2 Schematic diagram depicting genetic evolution of human fungal pathogens

in some fungi, their role in virulence of human pathogenic fungi is not clear (Moran et al. 2011). *Coccidioides* spp. which are regarded as pathogenic fungi have lost genes required to survive on plants as in *Aspergillus*. This supports that loss of gene during evolution has helped to create habitat specificity (Sharpton et al. 2009). Not only acquisition of genes but functional expression of these is crucial in virulence of the fungi. This has been studied in *Candida* spp. by transcript profiling and chromatin immunoprecipitation-microarray (ChIP-chip) analysis of the transcriptional networks (Tuch et al. 2008).

4.5.2 Genetic Basis for Evolution of Pathogenic Fungi (Moran et al. 2011)

- Gene duplication and expansion—genes for metalloproteases in *Coccidioides*, Saps, and ALS gene in Candida.
- Gene loss and pseudo-genetization—HYR1 in *Candida dubliniensis*, galactose metabolism in *C. glabrata.*
- Telomeric expansion—TLO genes in *Candida albicans*, EPA genes in *Candida glabrata*, secondary metabolite clusters in *Aspergillus.*
- Rarely horizontal transfer—proline racemase in *Candida parapsilosis. The genetic basis for evolution is summarized in Fig. 4.2.*

4.5.3 Secretory Factors

Enzymes produced by fungi, viz., protease, phospholipase, and elastase, cause tissue damage and impairment of host defenses (Romani 2004). Fungi produce enzymes like catalase, substrates like mannitol, and melanin that act as scavengers of oxidative killing, thereby countering the effects of reactive oxygen intermediates (ROI). Thus, innate immune response against fungi is hampered (Hamilton and Holdon 1999).

4.6 Mechanism of Pathogenesis

Cutaneous and mucosal physical barriers resist fungi infection. However, fungi often develop both virulence mechanisms and morphologic changes that facilitate their multiplication within the host. The development and severity of disease by fungal organisms depends upon the size of the inoculum, magnitude of tissue destruction, the ability of the fungi to multiply in tissues, as well as the immunologic status of the host (Kobayashi

Table 4.1 Prevalence of common systemic fungal infections involving CNS

Systemic fungal infection	Prevalence of CNS involvement
Candidiasis	50% (Pendelbury et al. 1989)
Aspergillosis	14–40% (Jantunen et al. 2003)
Blastomycosis	5–40% (Friedman et al. 2000)
Histoplasmosis	10–20% (Wheat et al. 1990)

1996). The prevalence of common systemic fungal infections involving CNS is represented in Table 4.1. The mechanism includes entry and adherence, invasion, colonization and dissemination in the host tissue, and damage to the host tissue by evasion of immune system (Khan et al. 2010).

4.6.1 Portal of Entry and Adherence

Fungal species are widely found in soil, plant debris, and other organic substrates and are eukaryotic species present on earth, although only a limited number of species are human pathogens (Dadiee and Hashemizadeh 2014). The incidence of invasive fungal infections is much lower than superficial fungal infections, but the high mortality rate associated with invasive fungal infections is of great concern (Brown et al. 2012). Invasive fungal infections can be due to dimorphic(endemic) mycoses that are caused by true pathogenic fungi or the opportunistic mold and yeast infections that are saprophytes which only infect an immunocompromised host. Histoplasmosis, coccidioidomycosis, blastomycosis, and paracoccidioidomycosis cause dimorphic mycoses. The most common opportunistic fungi are *Candida* and *Aspergillus* (de Pauw 2011). In dimorphic mycoses, conversion to pathogenic yeast form occurs after inhalation of microconidia and small mycelial fragments by the host. Histoplasmosis is caused by *Histoplasma capsulatum*, a dimorphic intracellular fungal pathogen. The cell surface heat shock protein (hsp)60 mediates binding and internalization of yeasts and conidia by macrophages, via the CD18 family integrin receptor (Tronchin et al. 2008; Long et al. 2003). Coccidioidomycosis is caused by *Coccidioides immitis* which converts from a mold form in the environment to a unicellular spherule containing sporangia in infected tissue (de Pauw 2011). Blastomycosis is caused by *Blastomyces dermatitidis* by inhalation of microconidia from soil. Blastomyces adhesin-1 present only on yeast form mediate binding of yeast cells to human macrophages through their CD14 and CR3 (CD11b/CD18) receptors (Long et al. 2003; Newman et al. 1995). Paracoccidioidomycosis is caused by thermally dimorphic fungi, *Paracoccidioides brasiliensis.* Inhalation of microconidia causes a primary lung infection and is followed by the morphological transition into the pathogenic yeast form. Glycoprotein 43 of cell wall helps in binding the macrophage (Tronchin et al. 2008; Lupi et al. 2005). Candida species are normal commensals of humans and are frequently isolated from the skin, gastrointestinal tract, and urine. The most common species that cause invasive infections are *C. albicans*, *C. glabrata*, *C. parapsilosis*, *C. tropicalis*, and *C. krusei* (Garcia-Vidal et al. 2013). *Candida albicans* is the predominant cause of invasive fungal infections from yeasts. *Candida albicans* as a commensal organism exists in a unicellular yeast-like morphology, but when it invades tissues, it becomes filamentous (de Pauw 2011). *Candida albicans* ability for mucosal adherence and biofilm formation is an important virulence factor. Aspergillus species are found in soil, air, food, and common decaying organic material. Among 200 recognized species, *A. fumigatus* is the most common cause of invasive fungal infection, followed by *A. flavus*, *A. terreus*, *A. niger*, and *A. nidulans*. The conidia produced by aspergillus disperse into the air, and when inhaled by an immunosuppressed patient, they germinate and become hyphae causing the invasive aspergillosis (Garcia-Vidal et al. 2013).

In CNS, fungal infections may develop via hematogenous dissemination from a distant focus such as lung, through direct implantation after trauma or secondary to the local extension from sino-nasal, orbital, or spinal infections (Mohan et al. 2012). Fungi enter from the bloodstream and possess surface components that allow them to traverse the capillary tight junctions and cause the infection (Sundaram et al. 2011).

One of the key factors contributing to pathogenesis of these organisms is morphogenetic variation like formation of yeasts, hyphae, and spherules that facilitate their multiplication within the host at higher temperature. *Candida albicans* switches between the growth forms like round yeast, elongated pseudohyphae and filamentous hyphae in the host. Yeast cells of many *Candida* species form filamentous pseudohyphae and hyphae in tissues, whereas *Cryptococcus neoformans* yeasts become coated with a capsule. *Coccidioides immitis* develops swollen, septated spherules in the host, and other fungi like *Histoplasma capsulatum*, *Blastomyces dermatitidis*, and *Penicillium marneffei* form filamentous mycelia in the environment but convert to yeast morphology upon contact with the human host (Rappleye and Goldman 2006).

Temperature plays a key role in the morphogenetic transition of *C. albicans* from yeast to filamentous growth. The heat shock transcription factor Hsf1 and the molecular chaperones Hsp70 and Hsp90 regulate the heat shock response in *Candida albicans* (Leach and Cowen 2013). *C. albicans* expresses adhesin agglutinin-like sequence (AIs) proteins. Among at least eight AIs, Als1p, Als3p, and Als5p play a major role in adherence of *C. albicans* to the host cells. Als1p and Als3p help in binding to endothelial and epithelial cells, whereas Als5p binds to extracellular matrix (ECM) proteins. The hyphal wall protein 1 (Hwp1p) adhesin present at the germ tube surface mediates tight binding to buccal epithelial cells and is required for biofilm formation (Tronchin et al. 2008; Loza et al. 2004).

C. albicans hyphae are hydrophobic and adhere to various biomaterials, such as catheters, prostheses, or medical implants, and form biofilms which contribute to tissue colonization. Biofilms are complex three-dimensional surface-associated communities of yeast and hyphal cells within an extracellular matrix (Hawser and Douglas 1994; Kojic and Darouiche 2004). The destruction of host tissues by *Candida* in the local environment may be facilitated by the release of hydrolytic enzymes such as secreted aspartyl proteinases (Saps), phospholipases, lipases, and hemolysins (Garcia-Vidal et al. 2013). Saps aids in nutrient uptake, tissue invasion, adherence, and dissemination (Khan et al. 2010).

Glucuronoxylomannan is the major constituent of the capsule produced by *Cryptococcus neoformans*. Glucuronoxylomannan causes immunosuppressive and immunodysregulatory effects on the host by partially activating TLR-dependent signal transduction pathways (Romani 2004).

Titan cells play a central role in *C. neoformans* pathogenicity. Titan cells can be of 100 μM and are formed from *C. neoformans* cell of 5–10 μM through various signaling pathways. They will have a thicker cell wall, denser capsule, and tetraploid or octaploid DNA content which prevents phagocytosis (Zaragoza et al. 2010; Zaragoza and Nielsen 2013). Melanization of *C. neoformans* occurs during infection, and overexpression of melanin results in decreased recognition by the host and modulation of host cell immune responses (Nosanchuk et al. 1999). Urease expression in *C. neoformans* is linked with increased invasion across the blood-brain barrier, and phospholipases A, B, C, and D help in tissue invasion and adherence (Khan et al. 2010; Olszewski et al. 2004).

H. capsulatum antigenic cell surface β glucans are hidden under a layer of α-(1,3)-glucan to avoid interaction with host phagocytes. After internalization through hsp60, interactions with CR3 do not result in a strong immune response allowing *H. capsulatum* to grow and survive within macrophages (Rappleye et al. 2007). Catalase present in *H. capsulatum* prevents from oxidative killing (Khan et al. 2010).

Coccidioides immitis develops swollen, septated spherules in the host which is required for dissemination; hyphal phase can tolerate pH 2–12. Elastase enzyme secreted causes destruction of lung interstitium and blood vessels, and estrogen-binding protein accelerates spherule maturation and endospore release (Kobayashi 1996; Khan et al. 2010).

Blastomyces adhesin-1 in *Blastomyces dermatitidis* acts as an adhesin and immunomodulator. α-1,3-Glucan in cell wall helps in adhesion and masking of cell surface receptors from being recognized by immune cells (Khan et al. 2010; Newman et al. 1995).

Mucormycosis is a serious life-threatening infection most commonly caused by *Rhizopus oryzae* that occurs in patients who are immunocompromised because of diabetic ketoacidosis, neutropenia, organ transplantation, and/or increased serum levels of available iron (Ibrahim et al. 2012). Fungi obtain iron from the host by using high-affinity iron permeases or low-molecular-weight iron chelators (siderophores) as iron is required for cell growth and development of fungi (Stearman et al. 1996). Moreover, glucose-regulated protein (GRP78) acts as a receptor that mediates binding and penetration of endothelial cells. The other virulence factors are aspartic proteinases and active ketone reductase system which accelerates the growth in the acidic and glucose-rich environment seen in ketoacidotic states (Farley and Sullivan 1998; Anand et al. 1992).

4.6.2 Invasion and Dissemination

The invasion of nonphagocytic host cells by fungi plays an important role in the pathogenesis of fungal infections. The invasion of natural cellular carriers such as vascular endothelium or pulmonary epithelium prevents phagocytosis by neutrophils and macrophages. The invaded host cell may serve as a source of nutrients like carbon and nitrogen for the fungus to sustain biosynthetic processes. Fungi have liking for certain carbon and nitrogen sources that are rapidly metabolized and therefore provide quick energy for growth and niche colonization (Sheppard and Filler 2015; Ries et al. 2018).

The yeast form of *C. albicans* is seen in commensal state while filamentous form in invasive disease. The hyphal form can escape from phagocytic cells. Sustained polarized hyphal growth prevents the entrapment of *C. albicans* intracellularly. Yeast cells also produce proteins like Ywp1 that weaken adherence and promote dissemination. This bidirectional morphotype conversion augments the ability of *C. albicans* to invade and disseminate. *C. albicans* invade epithelial cells by induced endocytosis and active penetration (Lin et al. 2015).

C. neoformans can cross brain endothelial cells by proteolytic degradation of tight junctions, induced endocytosis, and macrophage transport. Degradation of intercellular tight junction is facilitated by urease produced by *C. neoformans*. Binding of *C. neoformans* hyaluronic acid to CD44 present on brain endothelial cell activates the protein kinase C (PKC)-α signaling pathway resulting in rearrangement of endothelial cell actin microfilaments and the formation of pseudopods that engulf the organism and draw it into the endothelial cell. *C. neoformans* can invade the brain via a Trojan horse mechanism, whereby the organism is phagocytosed by a monocyte, which then diapedeses across the blood-brain barrier into the brain, carrying the fungus with it (Sheppard and Filler 2015).

In *A. fumigatus*, exposure of surface β-1,3-glucans of germinating conidia induces the activation of phospholipase D via a dectin-1-dependent mechanism which helps in endocytosis by epithelial cells (Han et al. 2011). Hyphae will penetrate more deeply into pulmonary tissues and invade pulmonary vascular endothelial cells from their abluminal side. Later, traverse the cell to gain access to the vascular compartment. From vascular compartment, hyphal fragments can disseminate to distal sites by invading vascular endothelial cells from the luminal side before penetrating further into other deep tissues such as the brain (Kamai et al. 2009; Filler and Sheppard 2006). Angiotropism is an important virulence factor, in particular among *Zygomycetes* leading to cavernous sinus thrombosis, ischemic infarction, and rupture of mycotic aneurysms (Rangel-Guerra et al. 1996). Dissemination to various organs occurs in some fungal infections due to bloodstream infection. Infection of bloodstream may occur through breaks in mucosal barrier as in systemic candidiasis (Eggimann et al. 2003; Pappas et al. 2009).

Animal studies in mice show hydroxamate-type siderophores are essential for proliferation inside the macrophages. *H. capsulatum* are known to produce hydroxamate-type siderophores for assimilation of iron from bloodstream for its growth (Hwang et al. 2008; Hilty et al. 2011). *Candida* and *Cryptococcus* are capable of utilizing the services of siderophores produced by other organisms. They do not produce their own siderophores (Tangen et al. 2007; Heymann et al. 2002).

Fungal infections present the greatest challenge to the immune system. Multiple mechanisms help the body to defend against the fungus. A profound adaptive response and genetic evolution by fungi to the changing microenvironment is seen. Some of them are well elucidated and some are poorly understood. An insight into the understanding of mechanism of pathogenesis helps in developing approach to combat fungal invasion and thereby preventing the fungal diseases. However, genetic profiling of fungi has unmasked many novel genes and many more to be studied in the light of emerging uncommon fungal infections.

4.7 Conclusion

Majority of the fungal infections of the CNS are opportunistic. The epidemiological and environmental factors, uncontrolled diabetes mellitus, immunosuppressive therapy for various diseases, trauma and intra venous drug abuse are some of the important predisposing factors. Host recognizes the fungal pathogens and activates immune response to inhibit/kill the pathogen and makes essential nutrients like iron unavailable to the fungus. The host defense depends on the immune status and type of the fungus. The fungal pathogen enters, adheres, adapts to the high body temperature of humans, evades immune attack by the host, elaborates various virulence factorsand enzymes by epigenetic regulation of gene expression to grow, replicate, invade and disseminate. The understanding of the host-pathogen interaction provides important therapeutic targets.

References

de Almeida SM. Central nervous system paracoccidioidomycosis: an overview. Braz J Infect Dis. 2005;9:126–33.

Anand VK, Alemar G, Griswold JA Jr. Intracranial complications of mucormycosis: an experimental model and clinical review. Laryngoscope. 1992;102:656–62.

Aristizabal BH, Clemons KV, Cock AM, Restrepo A, Stevens DA. Experimental Paracoccidioides brasiliensis infection in mice: influence of the hormonal status of the host on tissue responses. Med Mycol. 2002;40:169–78.

Bellocchio S, Montagnoli C, Bozza S, Gaziano R, Rossi G, Mambula SS, et al. The contribution of the Toll-like receptor superfamily to innate and adaptive immunity to fungal pathogens in vivo. J Immunol. 2004;172(5):3059–69.

Bhabhra R, Miley MD, Mylonakis E, Boettner D, Fortwendel J, Panepinto JC, et al. Disruption of the Aspergillus fumigatus gene encoding nucleolar protein CgrA impairs thermotolerant growth and reduces virulence. Infect Immun. 2004;72:4731–40.

Breneman E, Colford JM Jr. Aspergillosis of the CNS presenting as a aseptic meningitis. Clin Infect Dis. 1992;15:737–8.

Brown GD, Denning DW, Gow NA, Levitz SM, Netea MG, White TC. Hidden killers: human fungal infections. Sci Transl Med. 2012;4:165rv13.

Byrnes I, Edmond J, Bildfell RJ, Frank SA, Mitchell TG, Marr KA, et al. Molecular evidence that the range of the Vancouver Island outbreak of Cryptococcus gattii infection has expanded into the pacific northwest in the United States. J Infect Dis. 2009;199(7):1081–6.

Colombo AL, Tobón A, Restrepo A, Queiroz-Telles F, Nucci M. Epidemiology of endemic systemic fungal infections in Latin America. Med Mycol. 2011;49(8):785–98.

Dadiee P, Hashemizadeh Z. Opportunistic invasive fungal infections: diagnosis & clinical management. Indian J Med Res. 2014;139(2):195–204.

Davis LE. Fungal infections of the central nervous system. Neurol Clin. 1999;17:761–81.

van de Veerdonk FL, Netea MG. T-cell subsets and antifungal host defenses. Curr Fungal Infect Rep. 2010;4:238–43.

Drewniak A, Gazendam RP, Tool ATJ, van Houdt M, Jansen MH, van Hamme JL, et al. Invasive fungal infection and impaired neutrophil killing in human CARD9 deficiency. Blood. 2013;121(13):2385–92.

Drummond RA, Brown GD. The role of Dectin-1 in the host defence against fungal infections. Curr Opin Microbiol. 2011;14(4):392–9.

Drummond RA, Saijo S, Iwakura Y, Brown GD. The role of Syk/CARD9 coupled C-type lectins in antifungal immunity. Eur J Immunol. 2011;41(2):276–81.

Eggimann P, Garbino J, Pittet D. Epidemiology of Candida species infections in critically ill non-immunosuppressed patients. Lancet Infect Dis. 2003;3:685–702.

Elluru SR, Kaveri SV, Bayry J. The protective role of immunoglobulins in fungal infections and inflammation. Semin Immunopathol. 2014;37(2):187–97.

Engelhardt B, Carare RO, Bechmann I, Flügel A, Laman JD, Welle RO. Vascular, glial, and lymphatic immune gateways of the central nervous system. Acta Neuropathol. 2016;132:317.

Farley PC, Sullivan PA. The Rhizopus oryzae secreted aspartic proteinase gene family: an analysis of gene expression. Microbiology. 1998;144:2355–66.

Filler SG, Sheppard DC. Fungal invasion of normally non-phagocytic host cells. PLoS Pathog. 2006;e129:2.

Flaherman VJ, Hector R, Rutherford GW. Estimating severe coccidioidomycosis in California. Emerg Infect Dis. 2007;13(7):1087–90.

Freeman GJ, Long AJ, Iwai Y, Bourque K, Chernova T, Nishimura H, et al. Engagement of the PD-1 immunoinhibitory receptor by a novel B7 family member leads to negative regulation of lymphocyte activation. J Exp Med. 2000;192:1027–34.

Friedman JA, Wijdicks EF, Fulgham JR, Wright AJ. Meningoencephalitis due to *Blastomyces dermatitidis*: case report and literature review. Mayo Clin Proc. 2000;75:403–8.

Garcia-Solache MA, Casadevall A. Global warming will bring new fungal diseases for mammals. MBio. 2010;1(1):e00061–10.

Garcia-Vidal C, Viasus D, Carratala J. Pathogenesis of invasive fungal infections. Curr Opin Infect Dis. 2013;26:270–6.

Hamilton AJ, Holdon MD. Antioxidant systems in the pathogenic fungi of man and their role in virulence. Med Mycol. 1999;37:375–89.

Han X, Yu R, Zhen D, Tao S, Schmidt M, Han L. β-1,3-Glucan-induced host phospholipase D activation is involved in Aspergillus fumigatus internalization into type II human pneumocyte A549 cells. PLoS One. 2011;6:e21468.

Hardison SE, Brown GD. C type lectin receptors orchestrate antifungal immunity. Nat Immunol. 2012;13(9):817–22.

Hawser SP, Douglas LJ. Biofilm formation by Candida species on the surface of catheter materials in vitro. Infect Immun. 1994;62:915–21.

Heymann P, Gerads M, Schaller M, Dromer F, Winkelmann G, Ernst JF. The siderophore iron transporter of Candida albicans (Sit1p/Arn1p) mediates uptake of ferrichrome-type siderophores and is required for epithelial invasion. Infect Immun. 2002;70:5246–55.

Hilty J, George Smulian A, Newman SL. Histoplasma capsulatum utilizes siderophores for intracellular iron acquisition in macrophages. Med Mycol. 2011;49:633–42.

Hole CR, Wormley FL Jr. Vaccine and immunotherapeutic approaches for the prevention of cryptococcosis: lessons learned from animal models. Front Microbiol. 2012;3:291.

Hwang LH, Mayfield JA, Rine J, Sil A. Histoplasma requires SID1, a member of an iron-regulated siderophore gene cluster, for host colonization. PLoS Pathog. 2008;4:e1000044.

Ibrahim AS, Spellberg B, Walsh TJ, Kontoyiannis DP. Pathogenesis of mucormycosis. Clin Infect Dis. 2012;54:S16–22.

Jantunen E, Volin L, Salonen O, Piilonen A, Parkkali T, Anttila VJ, et al. Central nervous system aspergillosis in allogenic stem cell transplant recipients. Bone Marrow Transplant. 2003;31:191–6.

Juvvadi PR, Lee SC, Heitman J, Steinbach WJ. Calcineurin in fungal virulence and drug resistance: prospects for harnessing targeted inhibition of calcineurin for an antifungal therapeutic approach. Virulence. 2017;8:186–97.

Kamai Y, Lossinsky AS, Liu H, Sheppard DC, Filler SG. Polarized response of endothelial cells to invasion by Aspergillus fumigatus. Cell Microbiol. 2009;11:170–82.

Kauffman CA. Histoplasmosis: a clinical and laboratory update. Clin Microbiol Rev. 2007;20(1):115–32.

Khan AAH, Karuppayil SM. Fungal pollution of indoor environments and its management. Saudi J Biol Sci. 2012;19:405–26.

Khan MS, Ahmad I, Aqil F, Owais M, Shahid M, Musarrat J. Virulence and pathogenicity of fungal pathogens with special reference to Candida albicans. In: Ahmad I, Owais M, Shahid M, Aqil F, editors. Combating fungal infections: problems and remedy. Berlin, Heidelberg, Germany: Springer-Verlag; 2010. p. 21–45.

Khuu D, Shafir S, Bristow B, Sorvillo F. Blastomycosis mortality rates, United States, 1990–2010. Emerg Infect Dis. 2014;20(11):1789–94.

Kobayashi GS. Chapter 74: Disease mechanisms of fungi. In: Baron S, editor. Medical microbiology. 4th ed. Galveston, TX: University of Texas Medical Branch at Galveston; 1996.

Kohler JR, Casadevall A, Perfect J. The spectrum of fungi that infects humans. Cold Spring Harb Perspect Med. 2014;5:a019273.

Kojic EM, Darouiche RO. Candida infections of medical devices. Clin Microbiol Rev. 2004;17:255–67.

Kunadharaju R, Choe U, Harris JR, Lockhart SR, Greene JN. Cryptococcus gattii, Florida, USA, 2011 [Letter]. Emerg Infect Dis. 2013;19(3):519–21.

Leach MD, Cowen LE. Surviving the heat of the moment: a fungal pathogens perspective. PLoS Pathog. 2013;9:e1003163.

Lee PPW, Chan K-W, Lee T-L, Ho MH-K, Chen X-Y, Li C-H, et al. Penicilliosis in children without HIV infection—are they immunodeficient? Clin Infect Dis. 2012;54(2):e8–e19.

Li L, Eter N, Heiduschka P. The microglia in healthy and diseased retina. Exp Eye Res. 2015;136:116–30.

Lin H, Rathmell JC, Gray GS, Thompson CB, Leiden JM, Alegre ML. Cytotoxic T lymphocyte antigen 4 (CTLA4) blockade accelerates the acute rejection of cardiac allografts in CD28-deficient mice: CTLA4 can function independently of CD28. J Exp Med. 1998;188:199–204.

Lin XR, Alspaugh JA, Liu HP, Harris S. Fungal morphogenesis. Cold Spring Harb Perspect Med. 2015;5:a019679.

Long KH, Gomez FJ, Morris RE, Newman SL. Identification of heat shock protein 60 as the ligand on Histoplasma capsulatum that mediates binding to CD18 receptors on human macrophages. J Immunol. 2003;170:487–94.

Loza L, Fu Y, Ibrahim AS, Sheppard DC, Filler SG, Edwards JE Jr. Functional analysis of the *Candida albicans* ALS1 gene product. Yeast. 2004;21:473–82.

Lupi O, Tyring SK, McGinnis MR. Tropical dermatology: fungal tropical diseases. J Am Acad Dermatol. 2005;53:931–51.

McDonagh A, Fedorova ND, Crabtree J, Yu Y, Kim S, Chen D, et al. Sub-telomere directed gene expression during initiation of invasive aspergillosis. PLoS Pathog. 2008;4:e1000154.

Mendoza L, Vilela R, Voelz K, Ibrahim AS, Voigt K, Lee SC. Human fungal pathogens of Mucorales and Entomophthorales. Cold Spring Harb Perspect Med. 2015;5:1–33.

Mohan S, Jain KK, Arabi M, Shah GV. Imaging of meningitis and ventriculitis. Neuroimaging Clin N Am. 2012;22:557–83.

Moran GP, Coleman DC, Sullivan DJ. Comparative genomics and the evolution of pathogenicity in human pathogenic fungi. Eukaryot Cell. 2011;10(1):34–42.

Murdock BJ, Teitz-Tennenbaum S, Chen GH, Dils AJ, Malachowski AN, Curtis JL, et al. Early or late IL-10 blockade enhances Th1 and Th17 effector responses and promotes fungal clearance in mice with cryptococcal lung infection. J Immunol. 2014;193:4107–16.

Newman SL, Chaturvedi S, Klein BS. The WI-1 antigen of Blastomyces dermatitidis yeasts mediates binding to human macrophage CD11b/CD18 (CR3) and CD14. J Immunol. 1995;154:753–61.

Nosanchuk JD, Valadon P, Feldmesser M, Casadevall A. Melanization of Cryptococcus neoformans in murine infection. Mol Cell Biol. 1999;19:745–50.

Olszewski MA, Noverr MC, Chen GH, Toews GB, Cox GM, Perfect JR, et al. Urease expression by Cryptococcus neoformans promotes microvascular sequestration, thereby enhancing central nervous system invasion. Am J Pathol. 2004;164:1761–71.

Pandiyan P, Conti HR, Zheng L, Peterson AC, Mathern DR, Hernandez-Santos N, et al. CD4+CD25+Foxp3+ regulatory T cells promote Th17 cells in vitro and enhance host resistance in mouse Candida albicans Th17 cell infection model. Immunity. 2011;34:422–34.

Pappas PG, Kauffman CA, Andes D, Benjamin DK Jr, Calandra TF, Edwards JE Jr, et al. Infectious Diseases Society of a clinical practice guidelines for the management of candidiasis: 2009 update by the Infectious Diseases Society of America. Clin Infect Dis. 2009;48:503–35.

de Pauw BE. What are fungal infections? Mediterr J Hematol Infect Dis. 2011;3(1):e2011001.

Pendelbury WW, Perl DP, Munoz DG. Multiple microabscesses in the central nervous system: a clinicopathologic study. J Neuropathol Exp Neurol. 1989;48:290–300.

Pfaller MA, Diekema DJ. Epidemiology of invasive mycoses in North America. Crit Rev Microbiol. 2010;36:1–53.

Polvi EJ, Li X, O'Meara TR, Leach MD, Cowen LE. Opportunistic yeast pathogens: reservoirs, virulence mechanisms, and therapeutic strategies. Cell Mol Life Sci. 2015;72:2261–87.

Prinz M, Priller J. Microglia and brain macrophages in the molecular age: from origin to neuropsychiatric disease. Nat Rev Neurosci. 2014;15:300–12.

Rangel-Guerra RA, Martinezz HR, Saenz C, Bosques-Padilla F, Estrada-Bellmann I. Rhinocerebral and systemic mucormycosis. Clinical experience with 36 cases. J Neurol Surg. 1996;143:19–30.

Rappleye CA, Goldman WE. Defining virulence genes in the dimorphic fungi. Annu Rev Microbiol. 2006;60:281–303.

Rappleye CA, Eissenberg LG, Goldman WE. Histoplasma capsulatum a-(1,3)-glucan blocks innate immune recognition by the b-glucan receptor. Proc Natl Acad Sci U S A. 2007;104:1366–70.

Ries LNA, Beattie S, Cramer RA, Goldman GH. Overview of carbon and nitrogen catabolite metabolism in the virulence of human pathogenic fungi. Mol Microbiol. 2018;107:277–97.

Romani L. Immunity to fungal infections. Nat Rev Immunol. 2004;4:1–23.

Romani L, Puccetti P. Protective tolerance to fungi: the role of IL-10 and tryptophan catabolism. Trends Microbiol. 2006;14:183–9.

Roussey JA, Olszewski MA, Osterholzer JJ. Immunoregulation in fungal diseases. Microorganisms. 2016;4:47.

Roy M, Benedict K, Deak E, Kirby MA, McNiel JT, Sickler CJ, et al. A large community outbreak of blastomycosis in Wisconsin with geographic and ethnic clustering. Clin Infect Dis. 2013;57(5):655–62.

Rutz S, Ouyang W. Regulation of interleukin-10 expression. Adv Exp Med Biol. 2016;941:89–116.

Santelli AC, Blair JE, Roust LR. Coccidioidomycosis in patients with diabetes mellitus. Am J Med. 2006;119(11):964–9.

Sharma RR. Fungal infections of the nervous system: current perspective and controversies in management. Int J Surg. 2010;8:591–601.

Sharpton TJ, Stajich JE, Rounsley SD, Gardner MJ, Wortman JR, Jordar VS, et al. Comparative genomic analyses of the human fungal pathogens Coccidioides and their relatives. Genome Res. 2009;19:1722–31.

Shelburne SA 3rd, Hamill RJ, Rodriguez-Barradas MC, Greenberg SB, Atmar RL, Musher DW, et al. Immune reconstitution inflammatory syndrome: emergence of a unique syndrome during highly active antiretroviral therapy. Medicine. 2002;81:213–27.

Sheppard DC, Filler SG. Host cell invasion by medically important fungi. Cold Spring Harb Perspect Med. 2015;5:a019687.

Shih RY, Koeller KK. Bacterial, fungal, and parasitic infections of the central nervous system: radiologic-pathologic correlation and historical perspectives. Radiographics. 2015;35:1141–69.

Simoes SA, Leite DP Jr, Hahn RC. Fungal microbiota in air-conditioning installed in both adult and neonatal intensive treatment units and their impact in two university hospitals of the central western region, Mato Grosso, Brazil. Mycopathologia. 2011;172:109–16.

Stearman R, Yuan DS, Yamaguchi-Iwai Y, Klausner RD, Dancis A. A permease-oxidase complex involved in high-affinity iron uptake in yeast. Science. 1996;271:1552–7.

Sundaram C, Shankar SK, Thong WK, Pardo-Villamizar CA. Pathology and diagnosis of central nervous system infections. Pathol Res Int. 2011;2011:878263.

Tangen KL, Jung WH, Sham AP, Lian T, Kronstad JW. The iron- and cAMP-regulated gene SIT1 influences ferrioxamine B utilization, melanization and cell wall structure in Cryptococcus neoformans. Microbiology. 2007;153:29–41.

Taylor LH, Latham SM, Woolhouse ME. Risk factors for human disease emergence. Philos Trans R Soc Lond B Biol Sci. 2001;356:983–9.

Tronchin G, Pihet M, Lopes-Bezerra LM, Bouchara JP. Adherence mechanisms in human pathogenic fungi. Med Mycol. 2008;46:749–72.

Tuch BB, Galgoczy DJ, Hernday AD, Li H, Johnson AD. The evolution of combinatorial gene regulation in fungi. PLoS Biol. 2008;6:e38.

Verma A, Wuthrich M, Deepe G, Klein B. Adaptive immunity to fungi. Cold Spring Harb Perspect Med. 2015;5:a019612.

Wheat LJ, Batteiger BE, Sathapatayavongs B. Histoplasma capsulatum infections of the central nervous system. Medicine. 1990;69:244–60.

Whibley N, Maccallum DM, Vickers MA, Zafreen S, Waldmann H, Hori S, et al. Expansion of Foxp3+ T-cell populations by Candida albicans enhances both Th17-cell responses and fungal dissemination after intravenous challenge. Eur J Immunol. 2014;44:1069–83.

Zaragoza O, Nielsen K. Titan cells in Cryptococcus neoformans: cells with a giant impact. Curr Opin Microbiol. 2013;16:409–13.

Zaragoza O, Garcia-Rodas R, Nosanchuk JD, Cuenca-Estrella M, Rodriguez-Tudela JL, Casadevall A. Fungal cell gigantism during mammalian infection. PLoS Pathog. 2010;6:e1000945.

Predisposing Factors

5

Shruti Gupta and Sanjay Behari

Abbreviations

BWI	Burn wound infection
CNS	Central nervous system
CVID	Common variable immunodeficiency
HIV	Human immunodeficiency virus
HSCT	Haematopoietic stem cell transplant
IV	Intravenous
MDR	Multidrug-resistant
SCID	Severe combined immunodeficiency

5.1 Introduction

The central nervous system (CNS) is an uncommon site for fungal infections. A rise of infections in the immunocompromised patient population, along with an increase in their life expectancy due to improved medical care, has led to an increase in the prevalence of CNS mycotic infections. An early diagnosis and prompt management, both medical and surgical, are essential for improving the clinical outcome.

5.2 CNS Pathogens/Pathogenic Fungi

The fungi that commonly affect the CNS can be divided in to three types: *yeasts*, *filamentous fungi* and *dimorphic fungi* (Chakrabarti 2007). *Yeasts* are unicellular fungi, and those that commonly affect the CNS include *Candida* spp. and *Cryptococcus* spp. *Filamentous fungi* can be further subdivided into 'septate fungi' such as *Aspergillus* spp. and 'non-septate fungi' like *Rhizopus* and *Mucor* (Chakrabarti 2007; Scully et al. 2008). The *dimorphic* fungi are the endemic fungi which exist in two morphologic forms, spores at 35° and filamentous at 25 °C temperature. These include *Histoplasma*, *Blastomyces* and *Coccidioides* (Scully et al. 2008).

Other fungi that primarily infect the brain include the *true* 'neurotropic' fungi also known as the melanised fungi. These include *Exophiala dermatidis*, *Cladophialophora bantiana* and *Ramichloridium mackenzie* under the order Chaetothyriales (Chakrabarti 2007).

5.3 Mode of CNS Inoculation/ Mode of Spread

CNS contamination is usually via the hematogenous route. This is closely followed by contiguous spread from a para-meningeal focus such as the paranasal sinuses, orbit and ear. Direct inoculation of fungi/spores during surgery or at the

S. Gupta · S. Behari (✉)
Department of Neurosurgery, Sanjay Gandhi Postgraduate Institute of Medical Sciences, Lucknow, Uttar Pradesh, India

M. Turgut et al. (eds.), *Fungal Infections of the Central Nervous System*,
https://doi.org/10.1007/978-3-030-06088-6_5

time of trauma might also result in CNS disease (Sethi et al. 2012).

5.4 Pathogenesis of CNS Fungal Mycoses

A myriad of factors influence the ability of the fungus to infect the CNS. These include host factors as well as the virility of the fungi. The host susceptibility depends upon the immune system and its response to fungal inoculation. If a host fails to eliminate the fungi at a primary site, for example, the lungs, hematogenous dissemination to the brain occurs. Once the brain comes in contact with the fungus, the phagocytic cells such as microglia as well as astrocytes are activated. Both cellular and humoral immune responses are activated, and cytokine release occurs (Sethi et al. 2012).

The virility of the fungus depends on the mode and the size of inoculum, the ability of fungi to adapt to the body temperature of the host, the hypoxic state at the cellular level and its ability to overcome the host immune response.

5.5 Pathobiology of Fungal Lesions

The pathobiology of the fungal manifestations depends on the morphology of the fungus (Chakrabarti 2007; Sethi et al. 2012; Murthy 2007; Low and Rotstein 2011).

5.5.1 Yeasts

Yeasts or the unicellular fungi like *Candida* and *Cryptococcus* affect the capillaries and small arterioles and, hence, commonly cause meningitis and small subpial ischaemic lesions. In case of *Cryptococcus*, parenchymal infestation manifests as granulomas called cryptococcomas or cortical nodules. Medium-sized yeast fungi like *Candida* with pseudobranching may cause brain abscess formation (Sethi et al. 2012; Naik et al. 2015; Shankar et al. 2007).

5.5.2 Filamentous Fungi

The large filamentous fungi with septate or aseptate hyphae, like *Aspergillus* and *Zygomycetes*, can obstruct large- and intermediate-sized arteries. They result in the development of necrotizing angiitis, thrombosis, and large-sized infarcts. The haemorrhagic infarcts later convert to septic infarcts with abscesses and cerebritis. Skull base involvement and invasive infections can occur from the paranasal sinuses. Invasive infection, in its most severe forms, may spread to the orbit causing visual loss, to the palate causing necrosis, as well as to the brain leading to a high mortality. In addition to this, aspergillosis can result in the formation of an intracranial space occupying lesion and, often, can lead to the occurrence of chronic infection in the immune-competent host (Chakrabarti 2007; Sethi et al. 2012; Bozorgi et al. 2016).

5.5.3 Dimorphic Fungi

These fungi are commonly associated with self-limited pulmonary illness or mild systemic illness when their manifestations occur in the mildest forms. Dissemination to the CNS constitutes nearly one-third to half of the extra-pulmonary dissemination. Common manifestations include chronic basilar meningitis with or without hydrocephalus and the development of vasculitic infarcts (Drake and Adam 2009).

5.6 Clinical Spectrum

Fungal infections of the CNS more commonly affect males, with the male/female ratio being as high as 70:30 in some studies (Sethi et al. 2012). The CNS manifestations, as in the case of any other infection, vary depending upon the virulence of the affecting fungi as well as the host immune response. CNS fungal infections commonly occur in the immunocompromised host; infections in the immunocompetent hosts are known but are less prevalent. Fungi can infect the meninges, the brain or spinal cord parenchyma, intracranial vasculature, cerebrospinal fluid as well as the calvarium or the skull, most commonly the paranasal sinuses and the skull base (Scully et al. 2008; Murthy 2007; Naik et al. 2015). Consequently, the patient may present with a clinical syndrome related to any part of the cranio-spinal axis as fungal CNS infection may result in meningitis, encephalitis, abscess formation, intracranial fungal granuloma, vasculitis and subsequent infarcts (Scully et al. 2008; Murthy 2007; Naik et al. 2015; Shankar et al. 2007). Certain fungi have specific involvement patterns, such as the rhinocerebral involvement by the *Mucor* and *Rhizopus* and the skull base involvement by *Aspergillus*. Overall, the most common symptoms are headache, nausea and vomiting, fever, focal neurological deficits, seizures and cranial nerve palsies (Chakrabarti 2007; Sethi et al. 2012; Bozorgi et al. 2016).

5.7 Specific Predisposing Factors

Fungi are ubiquitous in distribution and are known to be opportunistic pathogens. A number of conditions decrease the immune response of the host and predispose them to fungal infections. These include both primary and secondary immunodeficiency states. Primary immunodeficiency states are those wherein there are hereditary immune defects. In contrast, secondary immunodeficiency states refer to a decrease in immunity due to acquired conditions like infection (human immunodeficiency virus [HIV], tuberculosis), malnutrition, immunosuppressive drugs, etc. Apart from this, environmental exposure also plays an important role in precipitating infection by fungi in human beings.

5.7.1 Primary Immunodeficiency State/Hereditary Immune Defects

Hereditary immune disorders are genetic disorders which affect the immune response of the host to the fungi. These immune defects may involve the *humoral immune system* which involves B-lymphocytes and antibody production or the *cellular immune system* which involves T-lymphocytes, or both (Low and Rotstein 2011). Phagocyte and complement function may also be impaired. Examples of defective humoral immunity include common variable immunodeficiency (CVID) and transient hypogammaglobulinemia of the infant; defective cellular immunity may occur in chronic mucocutaneous candidiasis and DiGeorge syndrome, whereas both cellular and humoral deficiencies occur in severe combined immunodeficiency (SCID). Apart from these, chronic granulomatous disease and cyclic neutropenia also favour the invasion by opportunistic infections owing to phagocyte dysfunction. Prophylaxis with both antifungal medications and antibiotics is recommended in these immunodeficiency states.

5.7.2 Secondary Immunodeficiency States

5.7.2.1 Human Immunodeficiency Virus (HIV) Seropositivity

HIV or the human immunodeficiency virus causes an impairment of host immune responses, leading to the 'acquired immunodeficiency syndrome'. This causes a variety of opportunistic infections, fungal infections being one of them. Several factors like the viral load, the cluster of differentiation (CD)4+ lymphocyte count and the cytokine level affect the manifestations of the disease as well as the propensity of opportunist pathogens to infect human beings. Invasion of the CNS occurs during the early course of the disease, and the virus targets the astrocytes and perivascular microglial cells; astrocytes act as reservoirs for the virus, and the macrophages form the typical multinucleated giant cells. Neurons are affected indirectly by the toxic effects of inflammatory cytokines and neurotoxins like the envelope glycoprotein (gp) 120, as well as by the oxidative stress. Apart from these primary effects on CNS, HIV also predisposes to various fungal brain infections, typically at a

CD4+ count <200 per μL of blood. Areas endemic for HIV/AIDS show a high prevalence of cryptococcal meningitis, and approximately 5–10% patients with HIV have this meningitis as an AIDS-defining illness (Shankar et al. 2007). Cryptococcal fungemia can follow inhalation of fungal spores, and *Cryptococcus neoformans* can then cross the blood-brain barrier by transcytosis. It leads to leptomeningeal and brain inflammation with CD8+ lymphocytes and macrophage-predominant infiltrates.

5.7.2.2 Intravenous (IV) Drug Abuse

Fungal infections may account for up to 5–50% of serious infections in IV drug abusers (Leen and Brettle 1991). The most common fungi isolated are *Candida* spp. and *Aspergillus* spp. Fungal infections in intravenous drug abusers are chiefly due to contaminated, unsterile needles and injections. Multiple injections and sharing of injecting needles also predispose this group of patients to a high risk of HIV infection, which is an independent risk factor for mycotic infections (Low and Rotstein 2011; Leen and Brettle 1991).

5.7.2.3 Chronic Renal Failure

It is stated that end-stage renal disease results in an impairment of both humoral and cellular immunity owing to the uremic milieu, and the degree of impairment is directly related to the duration of renal failure (Gandhi et al. 2005). Defects in humoral immunity lead to an impaired T-helper cell function and antibody production; defects in the cellular immunity cause defective lymphocytic response to antigen exposure and impaired phagocytosis. The use of chronic indwelling catheters, multiple antibiotic use, corticosteroid treatment, repeated dialysis, the use of iron chelating agents, endotracheal or nasogastric tube, hyperalimentation and metabolic acidosis are conditions that further increase the chances of mycoses in these patients (Gandhi et al. 2005).

5.7.2.4 Diabetes Mellitus

Diabetes mellitus, more commonly the diabetic ketoacidotic state, is a fertile ground for the multiplication of fungi. The carbohydrate-rich ketotic state helps in proliferation of the fungus, and the acidotic environment causes failure of phagocytosis, thus protecting the fungus from the host immune responses (Sethi et al. 2012; Bozorgi et al. 2016). This is especially true for the filamentous fungi belonging to the order Mucorales viz. *Rhizopus* and *Mucor*.

5.7.2.5 Immunosuppressive Medication and Solid Organ Transplant

The most commonly affected patient population belongs to the group that has undergone a small bowel transplantation; and the risk of fungal infection is relatively lower in those patients who have undergone a renal or liver transplantation (Low and Rotstein 2011). Both medical and surgical factors play an important role. Immunosuppressive medications used in these patients including various chemotherapeutic agents, high-dose steroids as well as anti-lymphocyte globulins directly inhibit cell-mediated immunity and place the afflicted individuals at an increased risk of local, systemic and CNS mycoses. Extrinsic factors, such as radiation, further aggravate this inhibition of host immune responses. Surgical factors include prolonged ischemia time, renal failure requiring multiple haemodialysis, fulminant hepatitis, re-transplantation, older age at transplantation and graft-versus-host disease (Low and Rotstein 2011).

5.7.2.6 Haematological Malignancies and Haematopoietic Stem Cell Transplant (HSCT)

Patients with haematological malignancies like acute leukaemia are at a risk of fungal infections, especially associated with their invasive and acutely fulminant forms. The risk of infection in these patients depends on the type of leukaemia, duration of leukaemia, degree of neutropenia and the type of chemotherapeutic agents used for treatment. Specific at-risk populations include those with de novo leukaemia; those in post-remission status; those afflicted with the hairy cell, acute myelogenous or acute lymphocytic leukaemic variants; those with relapsed leukaemia; and those with leukaemia refractory to medical treatment (Low and Rotstein 2011). In addition to these factors, those patients with a breach in the skin or mucosa, secondary to a central venous catheter placement or mycotoxin chemotherapy exposure, are at a higher risk for developing fungal infections.

Patients receiving HSCT are at an increased risk of fungal infections depending upon a variety of factors in the host, the graft as well as the treatment (immunosuppressive drugs) and procedures (invasive catheters) done during the conduction of HSCT. Host factors like an older age and human leukocyte antigen mismatch affect the patient early after the HSCT. Pre-transplant treatment with immunosuppressive drugs and post-transplant complications like graft-versus-host disease and *Cytomegalovirus* infection may lead to profound phagocytic defects, primarily affecting the alveolar macrophages. This leads to an increased propensity of these patients to develop invasive aspergillosis and candidiasis (Scully et al. 2008; Low and Rotstein 2011).

5.7.2.7 Tuberculosis

Tuberculosis is an important predisposing factor for the development of concomitant fungal infections. The disease almost reaches epidemic proportions in developing countries. Fungal infections, both pulmonary and extra-pulmonary, increase in the setting of tuberculosis. Fungi can cause both mono- and poly-microbial infections. The fungi that have been most frequently isolated include *Aspergillus* spp. viz. *A. niger*, *A. fumigatus* and *A. flavus* (Osman et al. 2013). A significant association has been noted in male patients, smokers, diabetics, patients with concomitant HIV infection, patients suffering from multidrug-resistant (MDR) tuberculosis and patients suffering from lung abscess and from other severe forms of pulmonary lesions. Fungemia and fungal seeding of CNS are also favoured in patients who have been treated with broad-spectrum antibiotics where all the bacterial pathogens have been eliminated. In addition, it is also proposed that in MDR tuberculosis, the mycobacterium affects the cell-mediated immunity as the condition decreases the production and effect of gamma interferon.

5.7.2.8 Surgery

A positive history of neurosurgical procedures per se is a risk factor for the development of fungal infections, although most postsurgical infections, both local and systemic, are pyogenic in nature. Pyogenic infections are frequently caused by Gram-positive cocci like *Staphylococcus epidermidis* and *Staphylococcus aureus* (O'Brien et al. 2011). These patients often receive prolonged broad-spectrum antibiotics and harbour indwelling catheters and hence are at risk of candedemia and CNS seeding. Surgery for aneurysmal subarachnoid haemorrhage, placement of an external ventricular drain and conduction of CSF diversion procedures like the ventriculo-peritoneal and the lumbo-peritoneal shunts are specific at-risk procedures. In a series of 18 patients, the rate of Candida inoculation at the time of surgery was as high as 72% and the time to infection from the insertion of indwelling catheter was 13–36 days (Scully et al. 2008; O'Brien et al. 2011). The concomitant presence of other risk factors such as HIV seropositivity, and extremes of age, favour CNS mycotic infections.

5.7.2.9 Burns

Burn wound infection (BWI) is an important health problem, and fungi can cause infection as a part of poly- or mono-microbial infection. They may cause fungemia, extensive soft tissue infection and opportunistic infections as well. In fact, fungi are the second most important cause of BWI after bacteria. The prevalence of *Candida albicans* in burn patients is up to 15–30%, and infections with moulds such as *Aspergillus* are also on a rise in burn patients (Capoor et al. 2010). The risk factors associated with fungal infections in patients with burns include an advanced age of the burns, the presence of deep burns, a high percentage of burn area, inhalational burns, a prolonged hospital stay, the presence of indwelling catheters and the prolonged use of antibiotics.

5.7.2.10 Iron Overload States

Patients undergoing frequent blood transfusions, haemodialysis and being treated with iron chelators like deferoxamine or those suffering from hereditary iron overload states such as hemochromatosis are at a higher risk of infections with fungi like *Aspergillus*, *Zygomycetes*, *Candida*, *Cryptococcus*, *Histoplasma* and *Paracoccidioides* (Alexander et al. 2006).

There are two mechanisms that have been proposed for fungal infections in iron overload states. It has been observed that a virtually iron-free environment is needed for the proper functioning of the immune responses, and hence, the presence of iron impairs the host immune response. The second mechanism proposed is that over the years, fungi have developed sophisticated mechanisms to utilize iron, which act as cofactors in several enzymatic reactions and hence favour the growth of fungi in an iron-rich environment.

5.7.2.11 Malnutrition

Nutritional deficiency is an important cause of secondary immunodeficiency state. When the body weight falls to 80% of the recommended level for the age and height, the immune system is impaired, and when it falls to 70% of the recommended level, the immune system impairment is severe. The deficiency of one or more essential micronutrients, such as calcium, zinc or selenium, also impairs the immune response of the host and hence predisposes to a multitude of infections including fungal infections.

5.7.2.12 Trauma

Trauma in both the civilian (motor vehicle accidents, agriculture-related and natural calamities) and the military (explosive devices) setting has been associated with fungal infections. Trauma leads to direct inoculation with fungi especially from the soil. Elasticised bandages of wounds have also been implicated in infection with fungi, e.g., *Zygomycetes*.

5.7.2.13 Neutropenia

Neutrophils are rapidly destructive for fungal hyphae and constitute an important defence mechanism against fungal infections. A reduction in the neutrophil count is termed as neutropenia. Neutropenia is defined as an absolute neutrophil count of <1500 per μL of blood (Scully et al. 2008; Sethi et al. 2012; Low and Rotstein 2011). Both the duration and the severity of neutropenia influence the extent and outcome of CNS mycotic infections. Neutropenia due to aplastic anaemia and bone marrow failure may be responsible for the highest level of risk. Filamentous fungi, like *Aspergillus* spp., commonly affect neutropenic patients.

5.7.3 Environmental Exposure to Fungal Spores

Fungi are ubiquitous in distribution and are abundant in the soil and in the decaying waste. Environmental exposure to fungal spores dispersed in the air as well as encountered in the farm and animal waste, like bat or pigeon droppings, has been implicated in CNS fungal infections. Specific fungi like *Cryptococcus* have also been associated with eucalyptus tree plantations and pigeon droppings; *Histoplasma* infections have been associated with bat droppings in caves (Sethi et al. 2012).

5.8 Clinical Outcome

Mortality rates as high as up to 80% have been reported in CNS mycoses (Bozorgi et al. 2016). The mortality rate in immunocompromised patients is higher than in the immunocompetent counterparts (Scully et al. 2008; Sethi et al. 2012; Low and Rotstein 2011). Apart from the immunocompromised state, the severity of neutropenia, the age at presentation, the neurologic status at presentation and the duration of hospital stay are independent risk factors associated with morbidity and mortality. With the advent of novel antifungal drugs, such as liposomal amphotericin B and voriconazole, and with extensive surgical debridement that is now possible with advances in surgical techniques, the mortality rates have been reduced to as low as 10–15% in the recent times (Bozorgi et al. 2016).

5.9 Conclusion

- Fungal infections of the CNS are on the rise. They affect the immunocompromised individuals more commonly but can also affect the immunocompetent hosts.
- The presence of predisposing conditions should be carefully assessed in arriving at the diagnosis.
- An early diagnosis and prompt introduction of treatment can help in decreasing the mortality.
- Treatment/correction of the predisposing factors is vital in reducing the morbidity and mortality associated with fungal infections of the central nervous system.

References

Alexander J, Limaye AP, Ko CW, Bronner MP, Kowdley KV. Association of hepatic iron overload with invasive fungal infection in liver transplant recipients. Liver Transpl. 2006;12:1799–804.

Bozorgi V, Talebitaher M, Shalbaf N, Radmanesh N, Nasri F, Ansari-Ramandi MM. Epidemiological aspects and clinical outcome of patients with Rhinocerebral zygomycosis: a survey in a referral hospital in Iran. Pan Afr Med J. 2016;13(24):232.

Capoor MR, Sarabahi S, Tiwari VK, Narayanan RP. Fungal infections in burns: diagnosis and management. Indian J Plast Surg. 2010;43(Suppl):S37–42.

Chakrabarti A. Epidemiology of central nervous system mycoses. Neurol India. 2007;55:191–7.

Drake KW, Adam RD. Coccidioidal meningitis and brain abscesses: analysis of 71 cases at a referral center. Neurology. 2009;73:1780–6.

Gandhi BV, Bahadur MM, Dodeja H, Aggrwal V, Thamba A, Mali M. Systemic fungal infections in renal diseases. J Postgrad Med. 2005;51(Suppl 1):S30–6.

Leen CL, Brettle RP. Fungal infections in drug users. J Antimicrob Chemother. 1991;28(Suppl A):83–96.

Low C-Y, Rotstein C. Emerging fungal infections in immunocompromised patients. F1000 Med Rep. 2011;3:14.

Murthy JM. Fungal infections of the central nervous system: the clinical syndromes. Neurol India. 2007;55:221–5.

Naik V, Ahmed FU, Gupta A, Garg A, Sarkar C, Sharma B, Mahapatra AK. Intracranial fungal granulomas:a single institutional clinicopathologic study of 66 patients and review of the literature. World Neurosurg. 2015;83:1166–72.

O'Brien D, Stevens NT, Lim CH, O'Brien DF, Smyth E, Fitzpatrick F, Humphreys H. Candida infection of the central nervous system following neurosurgery: a 12-year review. Acta Neurochir (Wien). 2011;153:1347–50.

Osman NM, Gomaa AA, Sayed NM, Abd el Aziz AA. Microarray detection of fungal infection in pulmonary tuberculosis. Egypt J Chest Dis Tuberc. 2013;62:151–7.

Scully EP, Baden LR, Katz JT. Fungal brain infections. Curr Opin Neurol. 2008;21:347–52.

Sethi PK, Khanna L, Batra A, Anand I, Sethi NK, Torgovnick J, Arsura E. Central nervous system fungal infections: observations from a large tertiary hospital in northern India. Clin Neurol Neurosurg. 2012;114:1232–7.

Shankar SK, Mahadevan A, Sundaram C, Sarkar C, Chacko G, Lanjewar DN, Santosh V, Yasha TC, Radhakrishnan VV. Pathobiology of fungal infections of the central nervous system with special reference to the Indian scenario. Neurol India. 2007;55:198–215.

Histopathology

6

Leonardo F. Jurado
and Rocío del Pilar López-Panqueva

Abbreviations

AIDS	Acquired immunodeficiency syndrome
BAL	Broncoalveolar lavage
CNS	Central nervous system
CSF	Cerebrospinal fluid
HIV	Human immunodeficiency virus
PAS	Periodic acid-Schiff

6.1 Introduction

As a result of advancements in transplantation and the concomitant use of immunosuppressive drugs, the human immunodeficiency virus (HIV) pandemic, the high prevalence of chronic diseases such as diabetes, the incidence of invasive fungal infections, and central nervous system (CNS)-involvement have increased during the last decades (Raman-Sharma 2010; Brumble et al. 2017). Nevertheless, CNS compromise remains uncommon, but its associated morbidity and mortality are quite high. Even for immunocompetent hosts, the cure rate for patients receiving antifungal therapy for cryptococcal meningitis is around 75% and is only 25% for aspergillosis and mucormycosis (Perdigao et al. 2004).

Fungal infections have been recognized historically, but CNS fungal infections have been recognized recently. The first description of a fungal infection is attributed with Hippocrates, in his book *Of the Epidemics* (400 B.C.E.) (The Library of Victoria University, Toronto n.d.), in which he described white patches in the oral cavity of a debilitated patient (candidiasis). Zenkar in 1861 described a fatal case of intracerebral candidiasis, and Smith and Sano were the first reporting a case of *Candida* meningitis in 1933 (Segal and Elad 2010).

CNS fungal infections can be classified as parenchymal (i.e., abscess, granulomas, cerebritis), extra-axial (meningitis), or vascular (vasculitis), or in some cases a combination of them (Mathur et al. 2012). Fungi are ubiquitous in the environment, and CNS compromise often occurs after a pulmonary infection. Delay in diagnosis and management is a major complicating factor. Symptoms are nonspecific, and even patients with disseminated infection and multi-organ involvement may not develop organ-specific changes or clinical signs (Liu et al. 2011).

L. F. Jurado (✉)
Pathology and Laboratories Department, Fundación Santa Fe de Bogotá University Hospital, Bogotá, Colombia
e-mail: lfjuradoz@unal.edu.co

R. d. P. López-Panqueva
Pathology and Laboratories Department, Fundación Santa Fe de Bogotá University Hospital, Bogotá, Colombia

School of Medicine, Los Andes University, Bogotá, Colombia

M. Turgut et al. (eds.), *Fungal Infections of the Central Nervous System*,
https://doi.org/10.1007/978-3-030-06088-6_6

An Indian study including 130 histopathologically confirmed CNS fungal infection cases (Sundaram et al. 2006) reported that the most frequent pattern was granulomatous inflammation in the majority of patients (74 cases), followed by angioinvasion with infarcts and abscesses in 31 cases and angioinvasion with infarcts in 9 cases. Macroscopically, mycotic aneurysm with rupture and subarachnoid hemorrhage were seen in two patients, chronic meningitis in two, abscess in eight (single in three, multiple in five), and encephalitis with vasculitis and infarcts in four patients.

Fungal infections of the CNS could be caused by a large group of organisms; in addition, they are not including in a mandatory report disease by the public health authorities, and therefore, robust epidemiological information on their global burden is not available (Schwartz et al. 2018). However, according to reports from reference centers (Schwartz et al. 2018; Naggie and Perfect 2009), and the review in the present book, the most important and frequent entities include candidiasis, aspergillosis, cryptococcosis, mucormycosis, histoplasmosis, coccidioidomycosis, and blastomycosis.

Fungi are ubiquitous environmental organisms that may be unicellular (yeast), filamentous (molds), or show a dimorphic morphology. More than one million known mycotic species exist in nature, and around 200 species are known to be pathogenic for the human being. However, only about 20 fungal species produce invasive systemic infections, including CNS invasion (Guarner and Brandt 2011).

According to its morphology, fungi can be classified as follows: pseudomycetes/yeasts (*Candida* spp., *Cryptococcus* spp., *Histoplasma* spp., *Blastomyces* spp., *Coccidioides* spp., *Paracoccidioides* spp., and *Sporotrichum* spp.), septate mycetes (*Aspergillus* spp., *Penicillium* spp., *Cephalosporium* spp., *Cladosporium* spp., *Diplorhinotrichum* spp., *Hormodendrum* spp., and *Paecilomyces* spp.), and nonseptate mycetes (*Mucor* spp., *Rhizopus* spp., *Absidia* spp., *Basidiobolus* spp., *Cunninghamella* spp., and *Mortierella* spp.).

Dimorphic fungi such as *Histoplasma* spp., *Coccidioides* spp., *Blastomyces* spp., *Sporotrichum* spp., and *Paracoccidioides* spp. display a mycelial form at 25 °C (filamentous in nature) and transform into yeast (spherules) at normal human body temperature (37 °C). Encapsulated yeast, *C. neoformans*, preserves its morphology in normal human tissues and in the environment, similar to some septate and nonseptate mycetes.

In general, fungal infections are becoming more frequent because of expansion of at-risk populations (transplanted patients, those receiving immunosuppressive and chemotherapeutic agents, HIV-infected patients, premature infants, the elderly, and patients undergoing major surgery) (Table 6.1) and also because availability of treatment schemas permit longer survival of these patients (Naggie and Perfect 2009). Certain variations in the geographical distribution of endemic fungal infections can be attributed to climate

Table 6.1 Fungal pathogens of the CNS associated with specific conditions

	Fungi
Disease-induced immunosuppression	
HIV infection	*Cryptococcus neoformans*
Diabetes and iron overload	Mucorales
Hematological malignancies (e.g., acute leukemia)	*Aspergillus* spp., and other molds
Neutropenia (e.g., aplastic anemia)	*Aspergillus* spp.
Prematurity	*Candida* spp.
Drug-induced immunosuppression	
Corticosteroids	*Aspergillus* spp., and other molds
Biological drugs (TNFα inhibitors)	Molds, dimorphic fungi, *Cryptococcus* spp.
Immunomodulatory agents (e.g., ibrutinib)	*Aspergillus* spp., *Cryptococcus* spp.
Hematopoietic stem cell transplantation	*Aspergillus* spp., non-*Aspergillus* molds
Solid organ transplantation	*Candida* spp., *Aspergillus* spp., non-*Aspergillus* molds
Medical interventions	
Neurosurgery, spinal anesthesia, injection	*Aspergillus* spp., other molds, *Candida* spp.
Intravascular or intracranial devices	*Candida* spp.
Other	
Intravenous drug use	*Candida* spp.

Adapted from: Lancet Neurol. 2018;17(4):362–72. https://doi.org/10.1016/S1474-4422(18)30030-9 (Schwartz et al. 2018)

changes, an extension of human habitats, ease of travel, and shifting populations. Therefore, during the last decades, a shift in the epidemiology of human mycoses has occurred (Guarner and Brandt 2011).

Before the twenty-first century, bloodstream infections were mostly caused by *Candida* spp., and the most frequent invasive pulmonary infections included primarily aspergillosis and endemic mycoses. Nowadays, fungi previously not considered pathogenic, including mucoraceous genera (formerly called zygomycetes), and many hyaline and dematiaceous molds are frequently seen affecting immunocompromised patients. Therefore, diagnosis of infection versus colonization with these fungi is a common issue that has important treatment implications (Guarner and Brandt 2011). Moreover, advances in diagnostic imaging and specific patient support have permitted the possibility of collecting biopsy specimens for histological examination from sites previously not reachable; nevertheless, these advantages come with challenges related to the limited amount of tissue obtained and the architectural distortion produced by the procedure (Gavito-Higuera et al. 2016).

In histological terms, evidence of damaging tissue is a sufficient diagnostic proof of a CNS infection, even in patients with negative results in cultures and other tests. However, this demonstration requires a brain biopsy, which is one of the most important limitations (De Pauw et al. 2008). Frequently, fungi when present in tissue are not easily visible using routine stains; thus, Gomori methenamine silver or periodic acid Schiff (PAS) staining can be used to improve their visibility and allow a better morphological identification (Schwartz et al. 2018; De Pauw et al. 2008). Some microscopic fungal characteristics can allow its identification to a genus level. For example, *Aspergillus* species can be differentiated from *Mucorales* by their septate, dichotomous branching hyphae, whereas *Mucorales* have an irregular shape of mostly uniseptate or pauciseptate hyphae. Some organisms show specific morphological characteristics, which can help in their identification. For example, *H. capsulatum* are small intracellular, budding yeasts; *B. dermatitidis* are thick-walled, broad-based budding yeasts; *P. brasiliensis* is big yeasts with small yeasts attached given a so-called pilot-wheel configuration; and *Coccidioides* species manifest themselves as large spherules that contain endospores (De Pauw et al. 2008; McCarthy et al. 2014).

Histopathological examination represents a rapid and cost-effective approach of providing a presumptive or definitive diagnosis of an invasive fungal infection. Nevertheless, microbiologists, pathologists, and clinicians need to be aware of the limitations of histological diagnosis, the pitfalls of morphological diagnosis, and the additional tests that can be performed (Guarner and Brandt 2011).

In this chapter, we review the most representative microscopic findings and interpretation pitfalls regarding the most frequently encountered fungi in CNS infections. We also present the complementary or alternative tests that can be performed in the biopsy specimen and other samples.

6.2 Disease Caused by *Aspergillus* spp.

The genus *Aspergillus* is represented by molds (Fig. 6.1a, c (Courtesy of D. Palacios M.D.), e (Courtesy of Z. DL Rosa R.M.)) that reproduce asexually producing conidia (Fig. 6.1b, d (Courtesy of Z. DL Rosa R.M.)) (Bennett 2009). These fungi are ubiquitous and have been used for centuries for industrial proposes. This genus is able to survive in a variety of habitats from leaf litter to human tissues. The most frequent species associated with human disease is *A. fumigatus*, and other species, such as *A. niger*, cause disease in immunosuppressed individuals. *Aspergillus* fungi produce three particular clinical entities: allergic bronchopulmonary aspergillosis, chronic pulmonary aspergillosis/aspergilloma, and invasive or systemic aspergillosis (Riscili and Wood 2009).

Invasive pulmonary aspergillosis generally occurs in critically immunosuppressed patients, including patients with prolonged neutropenia, organ transplant recipients, patients with AIDS, premature newborns, and patients with chronic granulomatous disease (Sherif and Segal 2010).

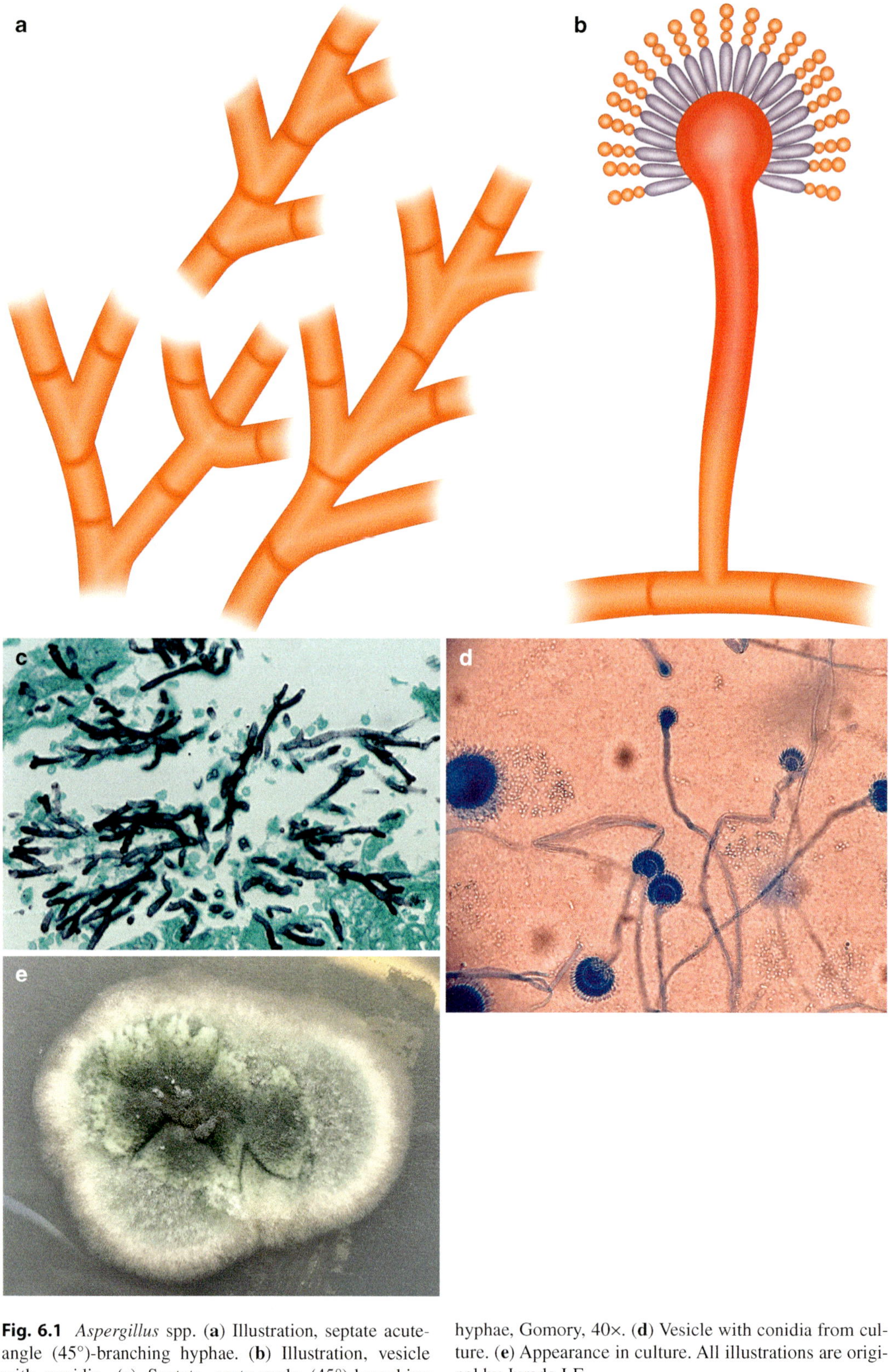

Fig. 6.1 *Aspergillus* spp. (**a**) Illustration, septate acute-angle (45°)-branching hyphae. (**b**) Illustration, vesicle with conidia. (**c**) Septate acute-angle (45°)-branching hyphae, Gomory, 40×. (**d**) Vesicle with conidia from culture. (**e**) Appearance in culture. All illustrations are original by Jurado LF

Apparition of neurological signs of stroke or seizures usually indicates that the fungus has reached the CNS.

Aspergillus spp. are one of the most frequent fungi isolated from neurological infections, most infections of the CNS are due to *A. fumigatus*, which gets into the CNS by hematogenous spread from the primary site of infection (lungs) or from contiguous anatomical sites, such as the paranasal sinuses (McCarthy et al. 2014). Focal lesions or a brain abscess are the predominant findings (Barrera-Herrera et al. 2015), while cerebral infarction caused by septic embolism, vascular thrombosis, or mycotic aneurysms are less frequent (McCarthy et al. 2014), and meningitis (without parenchymal involvement) is rarely reported (Antinori et al. 2013). Microscopically, *Aspergillus* spp. are thin (3–12 μm), septate, acute-angle (45°), or dichotomous branching hyphae (Fig. 6.1a, c), and when present in cavitary lesions, vesicles with conidia can be also identified (Fig. 6.1b, d).

In a retrospective study performed by Sundaram et al. (2006), 56% of the cases were caused by *Aspergillus* spp., 25% of them had a positive culture, and the majority of patients were immunocompetent. The most common source of spreading was continuity from sinuses, orbit or ear, followed by the hematogenous route; however, in eight cases, no source of infection was identified. Histologically, granulomas and dense fibrosis were the most frequent features. Eight cases presented isolated intracerebral granulomas; fibrosis was less marked in these lesions. The granulomas observed differed from tuberculous granulomas by the prominence of multinucleated giant cells, an abundance of neutrophils and plasma cells with lymphocytes and few epitheloid cells and marked fibrosis. Microscopic identification of the fungus was performed on GMS and PAS, and the culture positivity was 25%. The most common isolated organisms were *A. flavus*, *A. fumigatus*, *A. niger*, and *A. terreus*.

Lee et al. (2010) reported a series of 393 patients with evidence of fungal infection on histologic examination (a total of 231 (58.8%) were rhinocerebral infections); they analyzed the culture-histology concordance of filamentous fungi in 122 specimens; they showed concordance in 83% on cases with septated, acute-angle-branching hyphae and the presence of *Aspergillus* spp. in culture; *Fusarium* spp., *Trichophyton* spp., and others were recovered in culture from the discordant cases. Among the *Aspergillus* species isolated, *A. fumigatus*, *A. flavus*, *A. niger*, *A. nidulans*, and *A. terreus* were identified.

Cases of mixed infection, involving *Aspergillus* spp. and *Candida* or mucoraceous genera, have been described, posing an important dilemma. To be able to identify mixed infections, it is crucial to use alternative diagnostic testing (Hofman et al. 2010). In cases of invasive pulmonary aspergillosis, cultures are positive in only 50% of bronchoalveolar lavage (BAL) fluid specimens, and organisms recovered from BAL fluid samples could reflect colonization rather than the actual infection. In cases of invasive disease, isolation of *Aspergillus* spp. in blood cultures is approximately 5% (Sherif and Segal 2010).

Regarding the complementary test that can be performed when a case of aspergillosis is suspected, galactomannan and (1 → 3)-β-D-glucan, which are components of the fungi cell wall, can be measured in body liquids using commercially available kits (Sherif and Segal 2010). However, this analysis presents false-positive results in approximately 50% of individuals taking antibiotics (piperacillin, amoxicillin) and all patients receiving substances that contain products of *A. niger* fermentation (plasmalyte). This test also presents cross-reaction with other fungi, such as *Penicillium* spp. and *Histoplasma* spp. (Guarner and Brandt 2011). A study (Chong et al. 2016) that evaluated galactomannan testing in CSF from 17 patients with CNS *Aspergillus* infection and 27 controls reported a sensitivity of 88% and a specificity of 96%, which indicates a high diagnostic performance.

The (1 → 3)-β-D-glucan is present in a broad range of fungi (Alexander et al. 2010). There are commercially available assays for testing circulating (1 → 3)-β-D-glucan; it has been detected in patients with systemic fungal infections (invasive aspergillosis, candidemia, and *Pneumocystis* pneumonia) (Persat et al. 2008). The evidence on CNS infection is scarce; recently a study showed that its measurement in CSF represents a good approach for diagnosing and therapeutic monitoring of CNS fungal infection in children (Salvatore et al. 2016).

6.3 Disease Caused by *Candida* spp.

Candida spp. are small (4–6 μm), oval, thin-walled yeast-like fungi, which reproduce by budding or fission (Fig. 6.2a–c (Courtesy of Z. DL Rosa R.M.)). On culture media, *Candida* spp. form smooth, creamy white, glistening colonies (Fig. 6.2d (Courtesy of Z. DL Rosa R.M.)). The genus *Candida* is represented by over 2000 species, but only a few cause diseases in humans. Although more than 17 different *Candida* species have been reported as pathogens, the majority of invasive infections are attributed to 5 species: *Candida albicans*, *Candida glabrata*, *Candida parapsilosis*, *Candida tropicalis*, and *Candida krusei* (Vazquez and Sobel 2011).

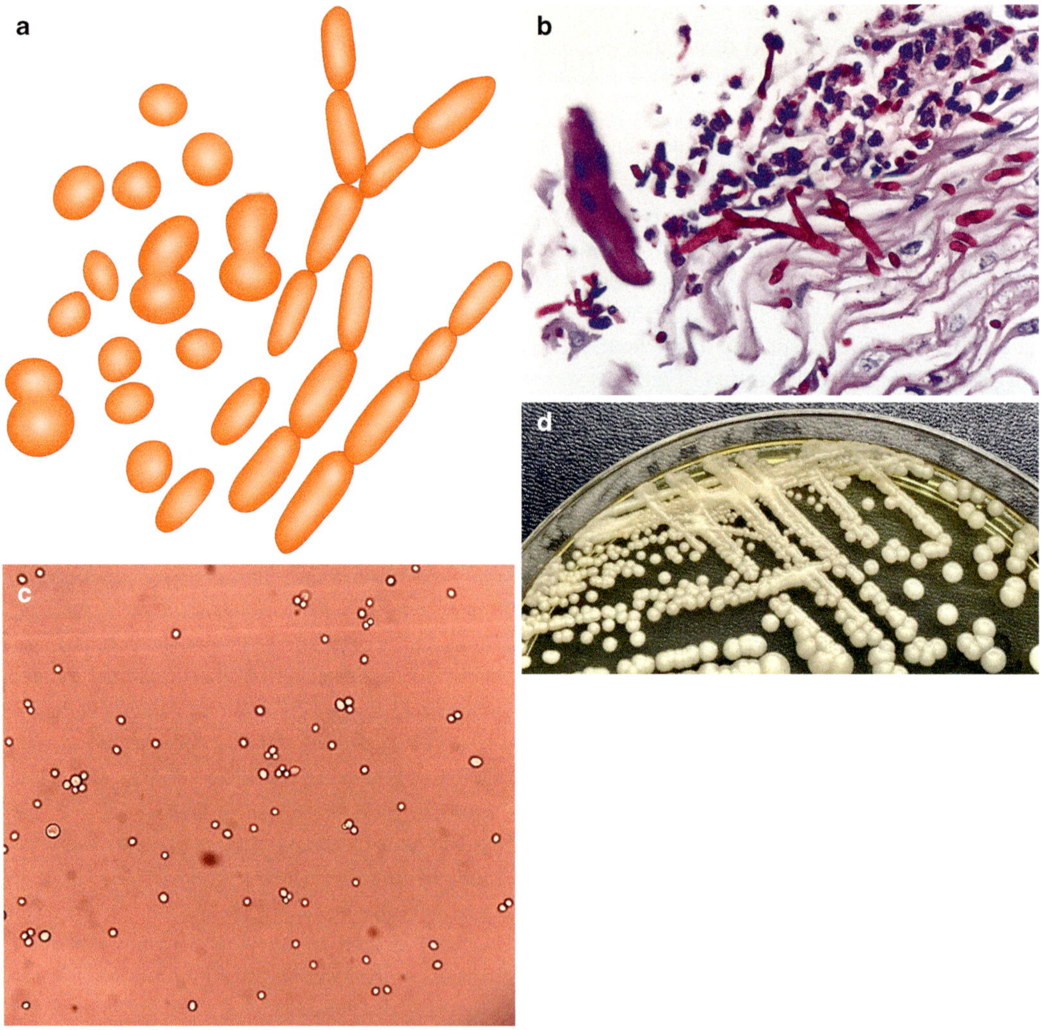

Fig. 6.2 *Candida* spp. (**a**) Illustration, budding yeasts and thin branching, pseudohyphae or filaments showing periodic constrictions. (**b**) Pseudohyphae over tissular inflammatory reaction H&E, 100×. (**c**) Budding yeasts from culture. (**d**) Appearance in culture. All illustrations are original by Jurado LF

During the last decades, *Candida* species have evolved from infrequent to relevant and common human pathogens causing a wide spectrum of clinical syndromes. *Candida albicans* usually colonizes the oropharynx and vagina, and viable organisms can be cultured from these surfaces (Southern et al. 2008). When there are microbial imbalances caused by antibiotic use, hormonal deregulations, and immunosuppression (HIV infection, diabetes), superficial infections in the gastrointestinal or genitourinary tract can occur (Concia et al. 2009). Invasive candidiasis occurs frequently as a healthcare-associated infection, and patients at risk include those under broad-spectrum antibiotic treatment, immunosuppressant drugs, those with vascular access devices, cancer diagnosis, and neutropenia (Darouiche 2009).

CNS infections caused by *Candida* species usually arise from hematogenous spread, and most of these are caused by *Candida albicans* (Kullberg and Arendrup 2015). Epidemiological data on the *Candida* species distribution in CNS infections is not available; in the published series, *Candida* spp. usually appears in the second or third place of frequency (Brumble et al. 2017; Sundaram et al. 2006). Meningitis is the most common clinical form of CNS involvement due to *Candida* spp., but chronic meningitis, brain abscess formation, ventriculitis, mycotic aneurysms, and vasculitis have also been reported (Zimmermann et al. 2016; Merwick et al. 2015; Fennelly et al. 2013).

Candida organisms can form mats of budding yeasts and thin branching pseudohyphae, also called filaments, that may show periodic constrictions (Fig. 6.2a). The organisms can be seen with H&E (Fig. 6.2b), GMS, and PAS stains, but *C. glabrata* does not produce filaments. During histopathologic examination, it is very important to identify invasion of tissues and vessels, considering that isolation from the skin, lungs, and the gastrointestinal or genitourinary tract may be indicative of colonization (Southern et al. 2008; Darouiche 2009).

The usual tissue reaction, both in superficial and invasive disease, consists of neutrophilic inflammation with few lymphocytes and macrophages, fibrin, and coagulative necrosis (van de Veerdonk et al. 2010); sparse giant cells and granulomas can also be found. Due to the bloodstream nature of the infection, mycotic aneurysms or thrombophlebitis can develop. In candidemia cases, necrotizing vasculitis has been described; interestingly, organisms are not observed in affected vessels, supporting the idea that *Candida* soluble fractions are responsible for this pathogenic pattern (Sargent et al. 2010). In neutropenic patients, the necrosis is frequently accompanied by hemorrhage, and few lymphocytes and macrophages can be seen (Schuetz and Walsh 2015).

Candida spp. are yeasts that produce pseudohyphae (Fig. 6.2a, b), thus requiring differentiation from other yeasts and molds that produce hyphae in tissues, such as *Aspergillus* spp. and *Trichosporon* spp. Elongated *Candida* pseudohyphae can appear to be branching but can be differentiated because pseudohyphae are thin and do not have septations (Fig. 6.2b). Another pitfall is the germinating blastospores that appear to be branching but can be distinguished due to the absence of a constriction between the base of the blastospore and the germ tube (Guarner and Brandt 2011; Schuetz and Walsh 2015).

When the invasive disease is suspected, blood cultures are the most important tool for diagnosis; after all, blood culture positivity is around 50–70% of tested cases. Additionally, the peptide nucleic acid fluorescent *in situ* hybridization assay (PNA FISH) can be used to identify the most common *Candida* species in smears made from positive blood culture bottles (Posch et al. 2017).

Another diagnostic option for invasive infection is the multiplex-tandem PCR, which can be performed in whole blood, serum, or plasma and has yielded better and faster results compared with blood culturing; nevertheless, this methodology is still for research use only and needs to be validated for diagnostic purposes (Lau et al. 2010).

6.4 Disease Caused by *Rhizopus* spp. and *Mucor* spp.

Since the 1800s, researchers have investigated a group of entities caused by ribbon-like, pauciseptate, hyaline molds (Fig. 6.3a–e (Courtesy of A. Agudelo M.D.)); however, the nomenclature of these fungi has not been completely defined (Ribes et al. 2000). Historically, these molds have been called *Zygomycota* (not used anymore) and *Mucorales*; therefore, the disease is known as mucormycosis or zygomycosis. Currently, it is accepted that the subphylum *Mucoromycotina* has two orders, the *Mucorales* and the

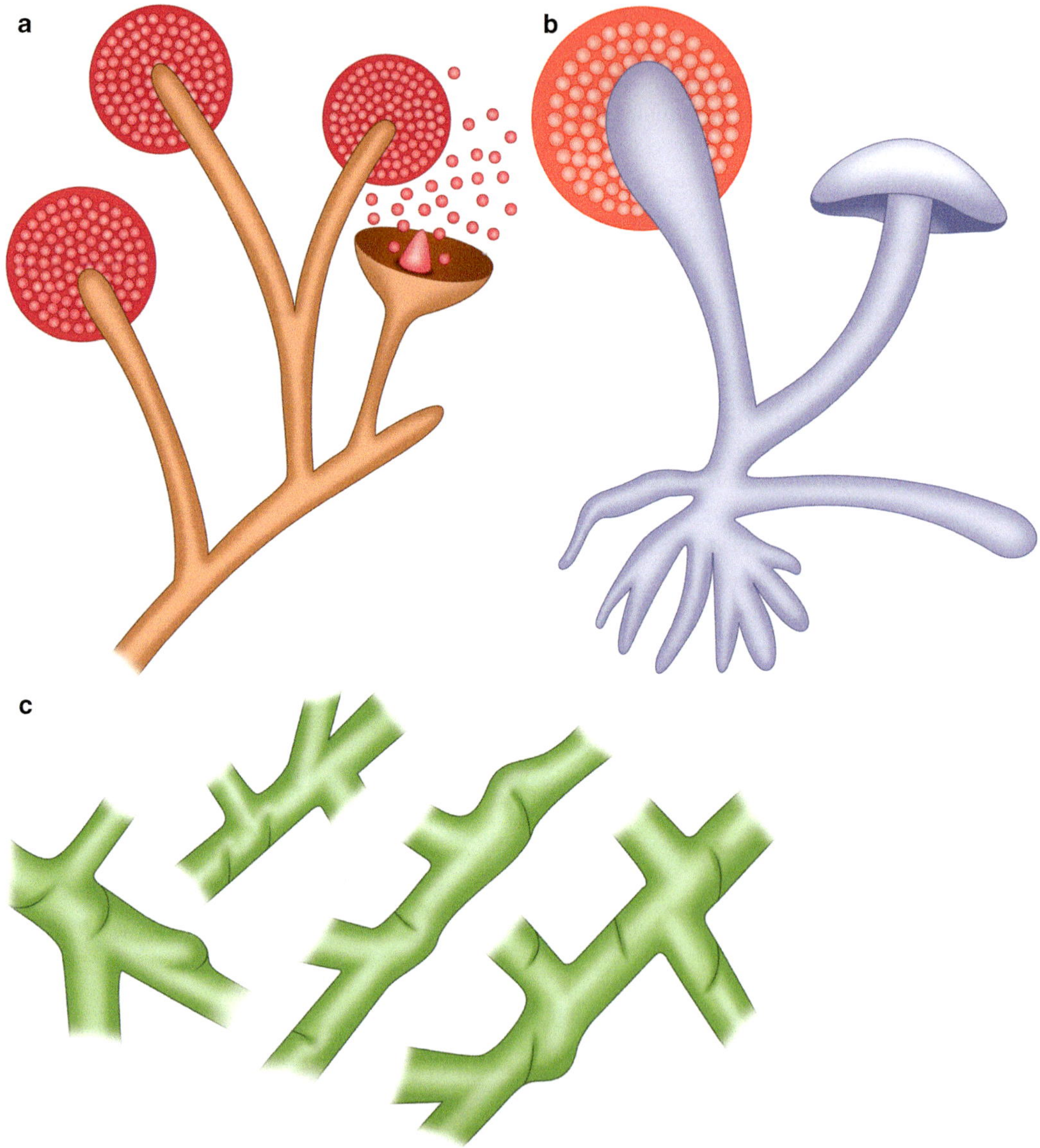

Fig. 6.3 Mucorales. (**a**) Illustration, usual appearance of *Mucor* spp. (**b**) Illustration, usual appearance of *Rhizopus* spp. (**c**) Illustration, hyphae with some septations (pauciseptate) and a 90° angle branching. (**d**) *Rhizopus* spp. from culture

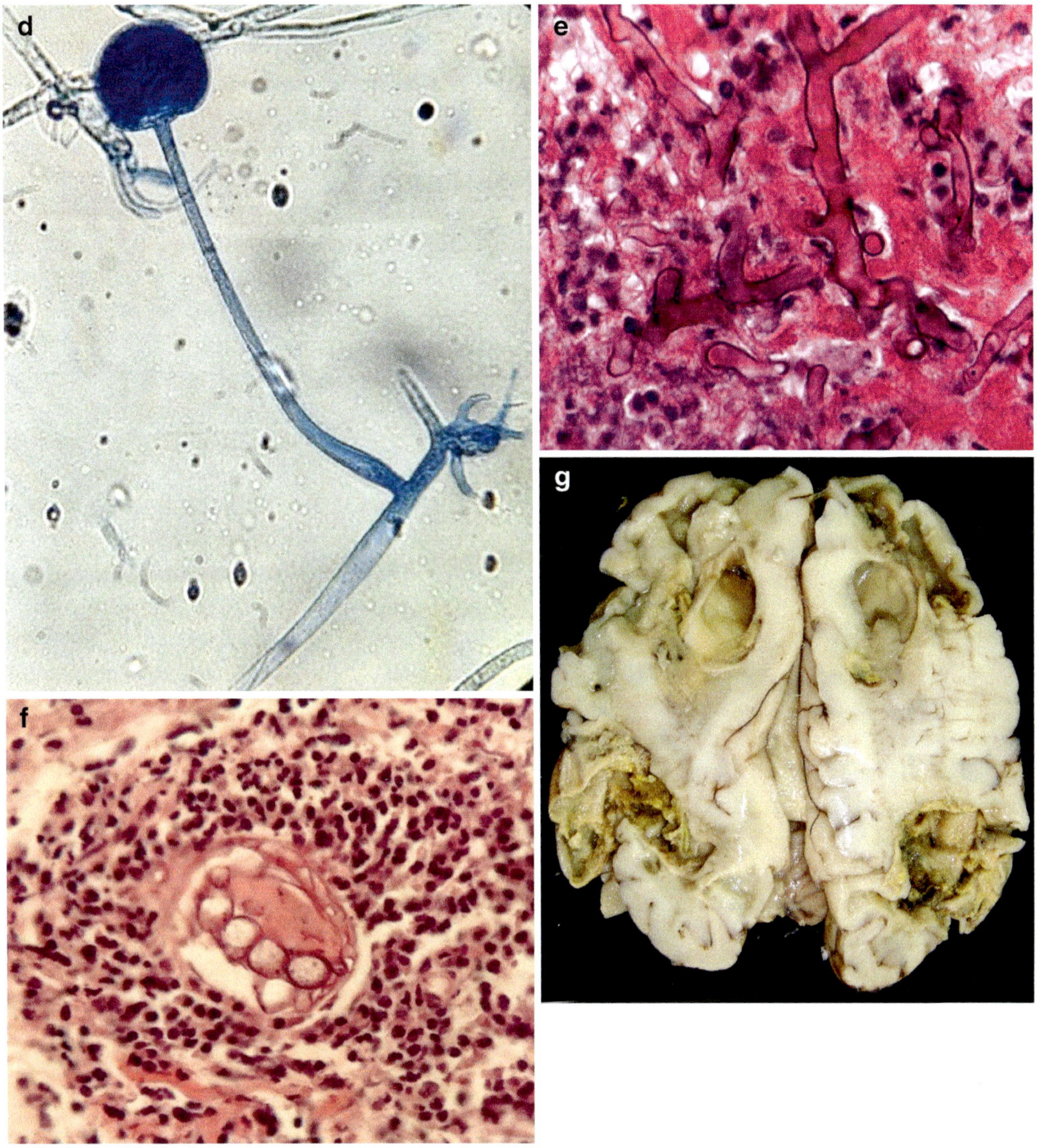

Fig. 6.3 (continued)

Entomophthorales. The former was originally identified as affecting insects and causing mucocutaneous disease in immunocompetent human hosts, while the *Mucorales* cause a spectrum of predominantly angioinvasive disease in immunosuppressed patients (Fig. 6.3f (Courtesy of A. Agudelo M.D.)). Among the *Mucorales*, *Rhizopus* is the most frequent genus that causes human disease; conversely, *Mucor* spp. produce disease in less than 20% of cases (Naggie and Perfect 2009).

Mucorales are ubiquitous in the environment and are usually found in soil and decomposing organic matter (Ribes et al. 2000). Their spores are easily airborne, frequently causing contamination in the laboratory; considering this, isolation of these molds must be correlated with the clinical history, in order to define their clinical significance. Inhaled spores can produce respiratory disease in immunosuppressed individuals, and the spores can also invade the skin and subcutaneous tissue by traumatic inoculation, contaminated needles, and even insect bites; less commonly, spores can be swallowed and cause gastrointestinal disease (Prabhu and Patel 2004).

When the immune response is not able to control the initial infection, the spores germinate and invade the surrounding tissue. Initially, there is an edematous reaction, and by the time the hyphae invade blood vessels, (Fig. 6.3f) the tissue becomes necrotic and acquires a characteristic black color. By contrast, immunocompetent individuals develop an intense inflammatory response and can present with a mass in the skin, respiratory sinuses, or the gastrointestinal tract (Roilides et al. 2014).

In general terms, mucormycosis presents itself in three main clinical ways, which are rhinocerebral (Fig. 6.3g (Courtesy of A. Rueda M.D.)), pulmonary, and cutaneous. Mortality due to disseminated disease is extremely high, and it is influenced by the predisposing factors and the clinical presentation (Roden et al. 2005). Early identification of the initial infection site is imperative to start a proper surgical and antifungal treatment. Additionally, for diagnosis, tissue specimens should be both cultured and histopathologically analyzed.

Identification of these molds in tissues is very important since it allows distinguishing the presence of the fungi as a pathogen from a culture contaminant and also is indispensable to define the presence of blood vessel affectation (Fig. 6.3f). Mucorales genera are characterized by nonpigmented, wide (5–20 μm), thin-walled, ribbon-like hyphae with some septations (pauciseptate) and a 90° angle branching (Ribes et al. 2000) (Fig. 6.3c, e). The hyphae may vary in width, appear folded or crinkled, and be sparse or fragmented. In lesions exposed to air and in culture media, thick-walled spherical structures can form at the ends of the hyphae (Fig. 6.3a, b, d). Routine H&E stains may show only the cell wall without structure inside (Fig. 6.3e, f); in cytologic specimens, the hyphae can be identified using Papanicolaou and calcofluor white stains; and GMS and PAS can also help highlight the fungal wall (Naggie and Perfect 2009).

In some situations, the hyphae may look degenerated, and many of the characteristics may not be appreciated in the specimen. In these cases, the pathologist must describe the degenerate hyphal elements observed in the specimen. This identifies the tissue where the fungus is found, ruling out the common possibility of culture contamination.

In immunosuppressed patients, the hyphal elements are usually found immersed in abundant necrosis, hemorrhage, and blood vessel thrombosis (Ben-Ami et al. 2009). Another important diagnostic feature is the identification of fungal elements invading the blood vessel wall or inside the lumen (Fig. 6.3f). Neutrophilic inflammation could also be identified surrounding the lesion.

It is important to be careful in differentiating *Mucorales* from other fungi that produce nonpigmented hyphae in tissue (*Aspergillus* spp.), other hyaline septate molds (*Fusarium* and *Scedosporium*), and *Candida* spp. (Ribes et al. 2000). An important morphological pitfall is the presence of many septations and acute-angle branching, which suggest *Aspergillus* spp. or another hyaline septate mold, while the identification of yeasts and pseudohyphae formation should suggest *Candida* spp. When using GMS, poorly stained hyphae are observed, which should suggest mucormycosis. Therefore, specifically identifying *Mucorales* in tissues or detecting dual infections by *Mucorales* genera and other fungi, immunohistochemistry, in situ hybridization, or PCR can be very useful (Hofman et al. 2010).

Like in most mycotic infections, culture is indispensable for organism-specific diagnosis. Furthermore, during sample-processing, is important to handle the specimens carefully, since aggressive grinding of the tissue may render the fragile fungal elements nonviable (Ribes et al. 2000). Mucorales genera are fast-growing fungi, but unfortunately, the yield of cultures is low. Also, although serologic tests have been attempted, they are not recommended (Guarner and Brandt 2011).

The retrospective Indian study performed by Sundaram et al. (2006) included a total of 130 CNS fungal infection cases during a 17-year period; in the study, 30% of the cases (39 patients) were mucormycosis, and of these patients, 37 developed the rhinocerebral form. In three patients, the disease was limited to the CNS, and their clinical presentation was stroke-like and diffuse encephalopathy. The most frequent histologic pattern was hemorrhagic infarction with angioinvasion and neutrophilic infiltrates. And the identified fungal elements were hyaline hyphae, pale and nonseptate with irregular or right-angle branching (Fig. 6.3c, e). Cultures were performed in 15 (38%) patients and were positive in 33% (5 cases), and *Rhizopus oryzae* was the most frequently isolated organism.

6.5 Disease Caused by *Histoplasma* spp.

Histoplasma capsulatum is a cosmopolitan fungus that can be found in old buildings, caves, and soil rich in bird and bat droppings; nevertheless, there are areas of high concentration where the disease is endemic; these areas include the Ohio and Mississippi River valleys in the United States, some countries in Central and South America, southern Europe, areas in Africa, and southeastern Asia (Wheat et al. 2016; Colombo et al. 2011). In most areas of the world, human histoplasmosis is due to *H. capsulatum* var. *capsulatum*; nevertheless, in western and central regions of sub-Saharan Africa, the African clade of *Histoplasma capsulatum*, formerly named *H. capsulatum* var. *duboisii*, can be found as the etiological agent of the disease. Frequently, histoplasmosis occurs in outbreaks related with old buildings renovation/demolition, or when tourists visit caves, but most of these cases are sporadic (Loulergue et al. 2007).

As with most fungi that cause systemic disease, the infection spreads by airborne route. In other words, the human being gets infected of histoplasmosis by inhaling the microconidia, and the immediate clinical response depends on the amount of fungus inhaled and the immune response; individuals may show no symptoms, may have acute or chronic pulmonary disease, or may have a disseminated presentation (Bueno-Fischer et al. 2009; Kauffman 2009). After the conidia are inhaled, they are phagocytized by alveolar macrophages and change to the yeast phase (Fig. 6.4b, c). The organisms are able to survive inside macrophages for weeks, and the migration of macrophages to the lymph nodes facilitates its dissemination. The disseminated form can occur both after initial infection and as reactivation of latent infection in immunocompromised individuals (HIV-AIDS, hematologic cancer patients, solid organ transplanted individuals, corticosteroids, and tumor necrosis factor antagonists users) (Hage et al. 2010).

Patients with high exposure loads or those who are immunosuppressed are at high risk of developing acute pneumonia or ARDS (Wheat et al. 2016; Bueno-Fischer et al. 2009). The migration of macrophages to mediastinal lymph nodes can make patients present with mediastinitis, and as macrophages travel through the body, the fungi spread to other organs, such as the skin, gastrointestinal tract, liver, spleen, and bone marrow; further, although infrequent, central nervous system compromise can occur (Wheat et al. 2016).

Histoplasma capsulatum var. *capsulatum* in tissue is an oval 2–4 μm yeast and may show narrow-based buds (Wheat et al. 2016) (Fig. 6.4b, c). With H&E staining, the basophilic yeast cytoplasm looks separated from the surrounding tissue by a clear zone corresponding to the cell wall, and using GMS and PAS stains, it is possible to highlight the cell wall. Due to the initial immune response, the yeasts are phagocytized by histiocytes, so they appear to be clustered; therefore, some authors suggest this as an important diagnostic clue (Fig. 6.4b, c). Further, this yeast aggregation inside macrophages and occasionally neutrophils is the usual presentation of *Histoplasma* in fluids stained with Papanicolaou or blood smears stained with Giemsa (Gupta et al. 2009).

There is scarce information regarding the histologic presentation of acute pulmonary histoplasmosis; some authors have described nodular areas of parenchymal and vascular necrosis associated with lymphohistiocytic vasculitis (Mukhopadhyay and Katzenstein 2010). This histopathologic pattern simulates the lymphoma-a

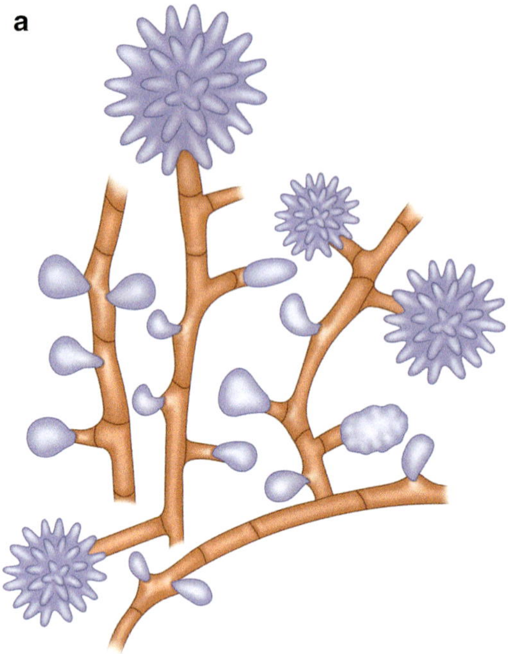

b

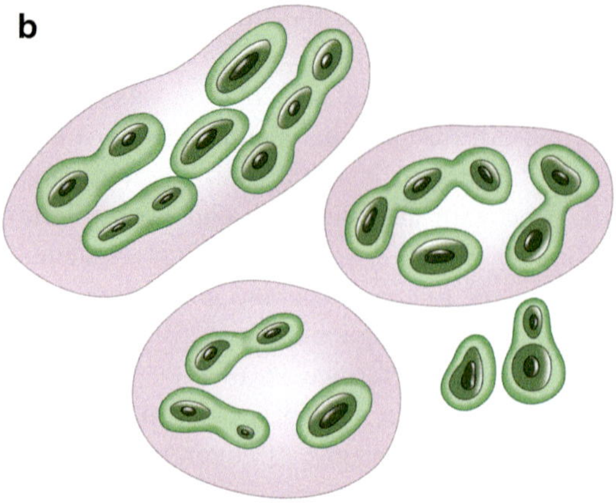

c

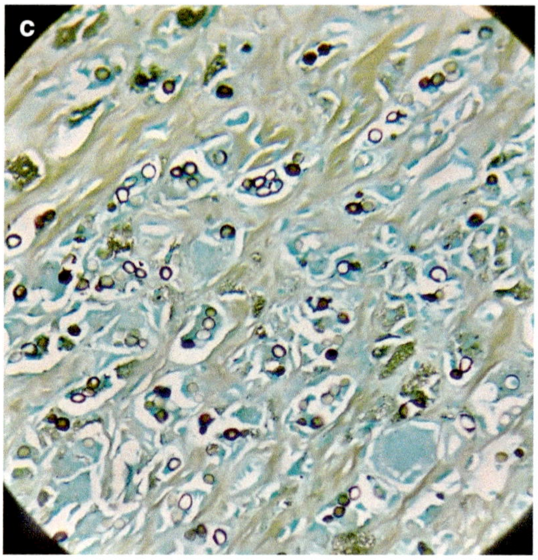

Fig. 6.4 *Histoplasma* spp. (**a**) Illustration, saprophytic form. (**b**) Illustration, parasitic form, yeast inside macrophages. (**c**) Multiple yeast infecting cells, Gomory, 40×. All illustrations are original by Jurado LF. (**d**) Nonpigmented, thin-walled, ribbon-like pauciseptate hyphae over necrotic tissue, H&E, 40×. (**e**) Fungal elements invading a blood vessel, H&E, 40×. (**f**) Macroscopic appearance of encephalic Mucormicosis, frontal lobes affected by hemorrhagic necrosis causing cavitary lesions. All illustrations are original by Jurado LF

toid granulomatosis but scattered small granulomas and the presence of yeasts must suggest the diagnosis of histoplasmosis.

The chronic pulmonary cases that radiographically appear as coin lesions show a granulomatous inflammation with the necrotic and calcified material, and it is common to find yeasts within the necrotic-calcified material (Wheat et al. 2016). When immunosuppressed patients develop disseminated disease, it is usual to observe sheets of macrophages filled with yeasts (Fig. 6.4b, c). The abundance of macrophages distorts the organ architecture and produces necrotic areas. Considering that the morphology of *H. capsulatum* is not specific, it is important to always perform clinical-epidemiologic correlation (Kauffman 2008).

Many fungi can be morphologically confused with *H. capsulatum* var. *capsulatum* when observed in tissue sections (Bueno-Fischer et al. 2009); for example, in the case of capsule-deficient cryptococci, size variation and weakly positive mucicarmine-stained yeasts may help to differentiate cryptococcosis from histoplasmosis.

Another case could be the small variant of *B. dermatitidis*, where it is useful to look for the presence of broad-based budding and larger forms, which can help in making the diagnosis of *B. dermatitidis* infection. The endospores of *Coccidioides* spp. can also be a challenging case, where looking for rest of a ruptured spherule or an intact spherule is paramount for its differentiation. Another important example involves *Pneumocystis jirovecii*, as when distinguishing this organism, it is important to know that it lacks budding and has an intracystic focus. For the cases of *Candida glabrata*, this organism may show more size variability than histoplasmosis, and the inflammation is mostly neutrophilic. Finally, in *Penicillium marneffei* infection, it is important to keep in mind that this organism forms a transverse septum rather than a budding pattern.

In addition to the mentioned fungi, some parasites can also appear morphologically similar to *Histoplasma* spp., agents of leishmaniasis, toxoplasmosis, and Chagas' disease, which also show intracellular organisms (Gupta et al. 2009). One of the most relevant histopathologic differences between these protozoans and *Histoplasma* is that H&E stains the entire organism, and none of them show the halo produced by the fungal cell wall. Kinetoplasts (a distinct hematoxylin-stained bar located to the side of the nucleus that represents a mass of mitochondrial DNA) should be observed in the cases of *Leishmania* or *Trypanosoma* infections. Finally, it is important to remember when toxoplasmosis and Chagas' disease are suspected, that the infected cells are somatic (cardiomyocytes or neurons) rather than macrophages. In summary, to perform a definitive diagnosis of histoplasmosis from tissue sections is challenging, and if cultures were not requested, alternative testing must be demanded.

The culture of blood samples can help in diagnosing disseminated disease, but since *Histoplasma* spp. are an intracellular organism, lysis-centrifugation methods must be used to liberate the yeasts from infected cells. Additionally, this fungus has a long generation period, so cultures must be incubated for 4–6 weeks before being reported as negative (Wheat et al. 2016; Kauffman 2008). On the other hand, there are immune-based methods, where testing for antibodies can be performed using complement fixation or immunodiffusion; however, in immunodeficient patients, production of antibodies may not even occur (Kauffman 2009). In addition, false-positive serology results can occur in individuals with lymphoma, tuberculosis, and other fungal infections, especially in cases of blastomycosis (Wheat et al. 2016).

Through enzyme immunoassay, it is possible to detect certain antigens in urine and serum; after all, the antigen is concentrated in the urine, making *Histoplasma* antigen detection more reliable (Wheat et al. 2016). In the same way to antibody testing, there are false-positive results with antigen testing; particularly, the cross-reactivity with blastomycosis is problematic because histoplasmosis and blastomycosis have overlapping endemicity and histopathologically can have a striking resemblance. Furthermore, in patients with localized disease (nondisseminated), the antigen burden is lower, and thus sensitivity is lower. With those limitations, combining the results of detection of antigen in urine and serum may increase the sensitivity in patients with localized histoplasmosis (Swartzentruber et al. 2009).

6.6 Disease Caused by *Coccidioides* spp.

Coccidioidomycosis is a disease of the Western hemisphere caused by a dimorphic soil-dwelling fungus of the genus *Coccidioides*. It was first recognized as a clinical condition in Argentina in 1882, and, soon after, another case in the San Joaquin Valley in California (USA) was reported (Rixford and Gilchrist 1896).

There are two primary species that cause the disease. *Coccidioides immitis* is endemic in some parts of the United States, particularly in the California desertic areas (Adam et al. 2009); additionally, *Coccidioides posadasii* is present in desertic regions of the United States (Arizona, Utah, New Mexico, and West Texas), northwest

Mexico, and desertic zones in Argentina, Paraguay, and areas of Central America (Colombo et al. 2011; Ampel 2009). Nevertheless, differences in morphology or clinical presentation have been found between the entities produced by each species. An interesting correlation between the incidence of the disease and specific environmental factors is commonly reported; for example, coccidioidomycosis incidence increases when there are rainy summers followed by dry winters, after earthquakes, or when humans establish themselves on the previously recognized endemic areas. Thus, when any of these situations take place, *Coccidioides* arthrospores are released in higher concentrations compared with the usual baseline (Parish and Blair 2008).

When susceptible individuals inhale the arthroconidia (Fig. 6.5a), this fungus reaches the alveoli and transforms into multinucleated spherical structures that contain hundreds of endospores (Fig. 6.5b, c (Courtesy of D. Palacios M.D.)) (Parish and Blair 2008). It is estimated that approximately 60% of infected people have no symptoms, while the remainder may present a clinical condition that simulates an acute community-acquired pneumonia, also known as "valley fever" (Adam et al. 2009; Ampel 2009). The chest X-rays may show lobar opacities and hilar adenopathy, and in some patients, cutaneous manifestations (erythematous rashes) are developed as reflections of the immune response to the acute infection (Gavito-Higuera et al. 2016).

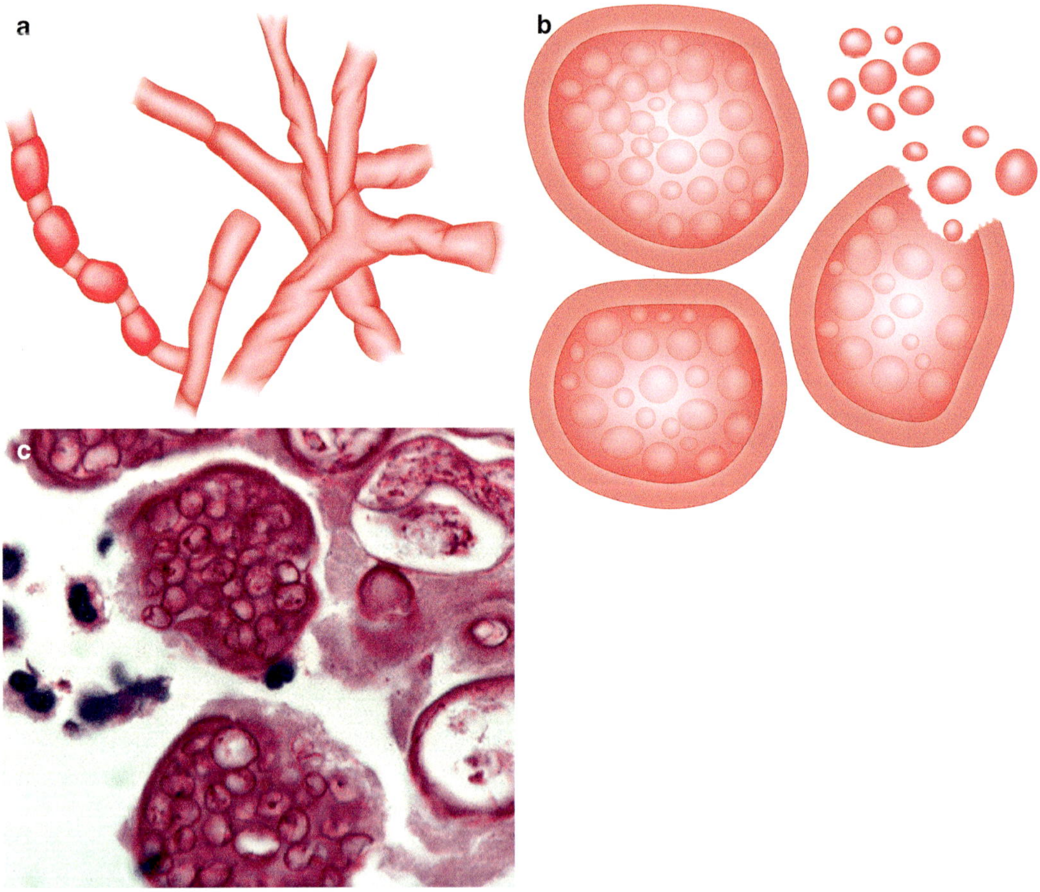

Fig. 6.5 *Coccidioides* spp. (**a**) Illustration, saprophytic form, showing arthroconidia development. (**b**) Illustration, spherules with multiple endospores inside. (**c**) Spherules with multiple endospores inside. H&E, 40×. All illustrations are original by Jurado LF

Most of acute infections resolve with no complications; however, in a minority of patients, the infection may progress to a chronic condition, developing either a cavity or a nodule (Wheat et al. 2016). It is recognized that specific risk groups (African Americans, Asians, pregnant women, patients with diabetes, patients receiving corticosteroids) are more likely to develop disseminated disease (Adam et al. 2009). The most common sites of extrapulmonary involvement are the skin, lymph nodes, bones, and joints; nevertheless, the most feared is the extension to the CNS (Kauffman 2008). In those cases, the most frequent presentation is meningitis. Therefore, the usual imaging findings are meningeal enhancement and hydrocephalus, but focal brain lesions, infarcts, or areas of cerebritis or cerebellitis can also be observed (Lammering et al. 2013).

The most characteristic morphological feature of *Coccidioides* is the presence of spherules of diverse sizes (10–100 μm) with multiple endospores (2–5 μm); those can be identified with H&E staining (Fig. 6.5c) (Saubolle 2007). Sometimes, the walls of the spherules are ruptured, and the endospores can appear spilled over the surrounding tissue. It is usual that active lesions contain multiple organisms, while lesions in resolution show a lower number of fungal structures (Guarner and Brandt 2011).

Using GMS, it is possible to highlight spherule and endospore walls. In contrast, PAS stain affinity varies with age of the structures; therefore, immature endospores and spherules stain strongly, while mature structures appear less stained (Saubolle 2007). Occasionally, in the cavitary lung or cutaneous lesions, mycelia can be observed (Saubolle 2007). The sensitivity of histopathology for *Coccidioides* identification is 84% and 75% for cytology (Adam et al. 2009).

The predominant inflammatory response to endospores is neutrophilic, whereas the reaction to spherules is mostly granulomatous. Thus, early in the infection process, the histologic pattern tends to look mixed (pyogranulomatous) because the concentration of both fungal structures is high. In addition, lymphocytic clusters of B and T cells next to well-constituted granulomas with necrosis have been described and appear to be an important hallmark of coccidioidomycosis (Li et al. 2005). Eosinophil infiltrates can also be abundant, which produces eosinophilic major basic protein, creating the Splendore-Höeppli phenomenon (an intense cover of eosinophilic material around the fungal elements) (Read et al. 2005).

The microorganism to consider for differential diagnosis, is *Rhinosporidium seeberi*, a parasite that causes polyps in the upper respiratory tract, produces big sporangia (some can be seen with the naked eye) with multiple internal endospores. This parasite has very similar morphology to *Coccidioides*; however, its sporangia and endospores are bigger than the fungal spherules, and its internal sporangial wall stains with mucicarmine (Malo et al. 2014).

Considering that one important characteristic of *Coccidioides* is the presence of spherules, it is important to remember that endospores outside spherules or immature spherules without endospores can be confused with yeasts such as *Blastomyces*, *Histoplasma*, *Candida*, or *Pneumocystis* (Saubolle 2007). It also needs to be remembered that in immunosuppressed patients, more than one organism may coexist; thus, in areas of endemicity, *Pneumocystis* and *Coccidioides* could be found in the same specimen.

Detection of antibodies can be a helpful diagnostic tool. Nowadays, IgM and IgG are generally measured using EIA or immunodiffusion; however, it is also possible to use tube precipitation to measure IgM and complement fixation for IgG antibodies. False-negative results have been reported in up to 38% of patients with hematogenous infection and 46% of fatal cases (Adam et al. 2009). Detection of antigens in the urine using EIA has shown positive results in 71% of patients with coccidioidomycosis but has a cross-reaction in 10% of patients with other endemic mycoses (Durkin et al. 2008).

6.7 Disease Caused by *Cryptococcus* spp.

Human cryptococcosis is a systemic mycosis caused by some species of the *Cryptococcus* genus. Up to 40 species have been described, but few are recognized as a human pathogen (May et al. 2016). The most relevant are *C. neoformans* and *C. gattii*, but two other species, *C. albidus* and *C. laurentii*, have been reported in rare cases, producing disease in humans (Johnson et al. 1998; Kordossis et al. 1998).

These organisms are found in soil and are related with pigeon droppings. Infection involves most frequently the lungs and the CNS and less frequently can compromise the skin and the skeletal system. Because its incidence is high in immunocompromised patients, especially individuals with AIDS and organ transplant recipients, cryptococcosis is considered an opportunistic disease (May et al. 2016).

Cryptococcal meningoencephalitis is a frequent and life-threatening complication in patients with HIV infection (Williamson et al. 2017) and is the most common fungal infection of the CNS worldwide (223,100 estimated cases in 2014) (Rajasingham et al. 2017) causing a substantial disease burden in countries with poor access to medical care and high numbers of people living with HIV.

C. neoformans is the causative agent for the majority of infections in immunocompromised individuals, while *C. gattii* causes disease in immunocompetent hosts (Huston and Mody 2009). Additionally, *C. neoformans* var. *grubii* (serotype A) and *C. neoformans* var. *neoformans* (serotype D) have a worldwide distribution and are primarily associated with pigeon guano. HIV infection is the most important risk factor for cryptococcal disease; however, other conditions associated with cryptococcosis include chronic lung, liver, and renal disease, autoimmune diseases, immunosuppressant use, and cancer (Galanis and MacDougall 2010).

Irrespective of the species, inhaling cryptococcal yeasts or basidiospores infects humans; therefore, the lung is always the first infected organ (Huston and Mody 2009). In contrast to other pathogenic fungi, few exposed individuals remain asymptomatic; most develop pneumonia, cryptococcomas, or pleural effusion. From the lungs, cryptococci can disseminate to the CNS, resulting in meningitis or cryptococcomas. Further, *C. gattii* more frequently causes solid lesions in the lungs and brain than *C. neoformans*. The occurrence of the disseminated disease depends on the host immune status; in immunocompetent patients the most frequent presentation is pulmonary, while immunosuppressed patients commonly develop CNS disease (Williamson et al. 2017).

Cryptococcus spp. is a spherical to oval encapsulated yeast, measuring approximately 5–10 μm in diameter in clinical specimens with a narrow-based budding and a capsule ranging in size from 1 to >30 μm (Fig. 6.6a, d). In specimens isolated from the outside environment, yeast tends to be smaller and with a thinner capsule (Neilson et al. 1997). The thick, polysaccharide capsule gives the yeasts a characteristic appearance of having a clear space around them (Fig. 6.6b, c (Courtesy of M. Tuñon M.D.), d).

When analyzing CSF, India ink is the ideal negative stain to highlight the capsule (Fig. 6.6d). Due to the capsule, the buds appear separate from the mother cell. The capsule can be stained with Alcian blue and Mayer's or Southgate's mucicarmine. As it happens with all other yeasts, the wall stains with GMS and PAS; moreover, for cryptococci, Fontana-Masson also results in a stain due to the presence of melanin (Williamson et al. 2017).

The histopathological reaction varies from well-formed granulomas, where the yeasts are found inside histiocytes and giant cells, to minimal inflammatory response with abundant extracellular organisms that distorts the tissue architecture (Gazzoni et al. 2009). When the granulomatous pattern is present, the granulomas show a spectrum from abundant necrosis to fibrosis (Fig. 6.6b, c). In some cases, the fibrosis is intense, with abundant stocky-spindle fibroblast cells in a storiform pattern accompanied by a background of lymphocytes and plasma cells, giving the appearance of an inflammatory pseudotumor (Sing and Ramdial 2007). Some authors have suggested that the histological reaction is related to the immune status of the patient and the presence or absence of capsule (Rajasingham et al. 2017).

In some cases, the yeast produces a thinner polysaccharide capsule; thus, these organisms may look similar to other yeasts, such as *Candida*

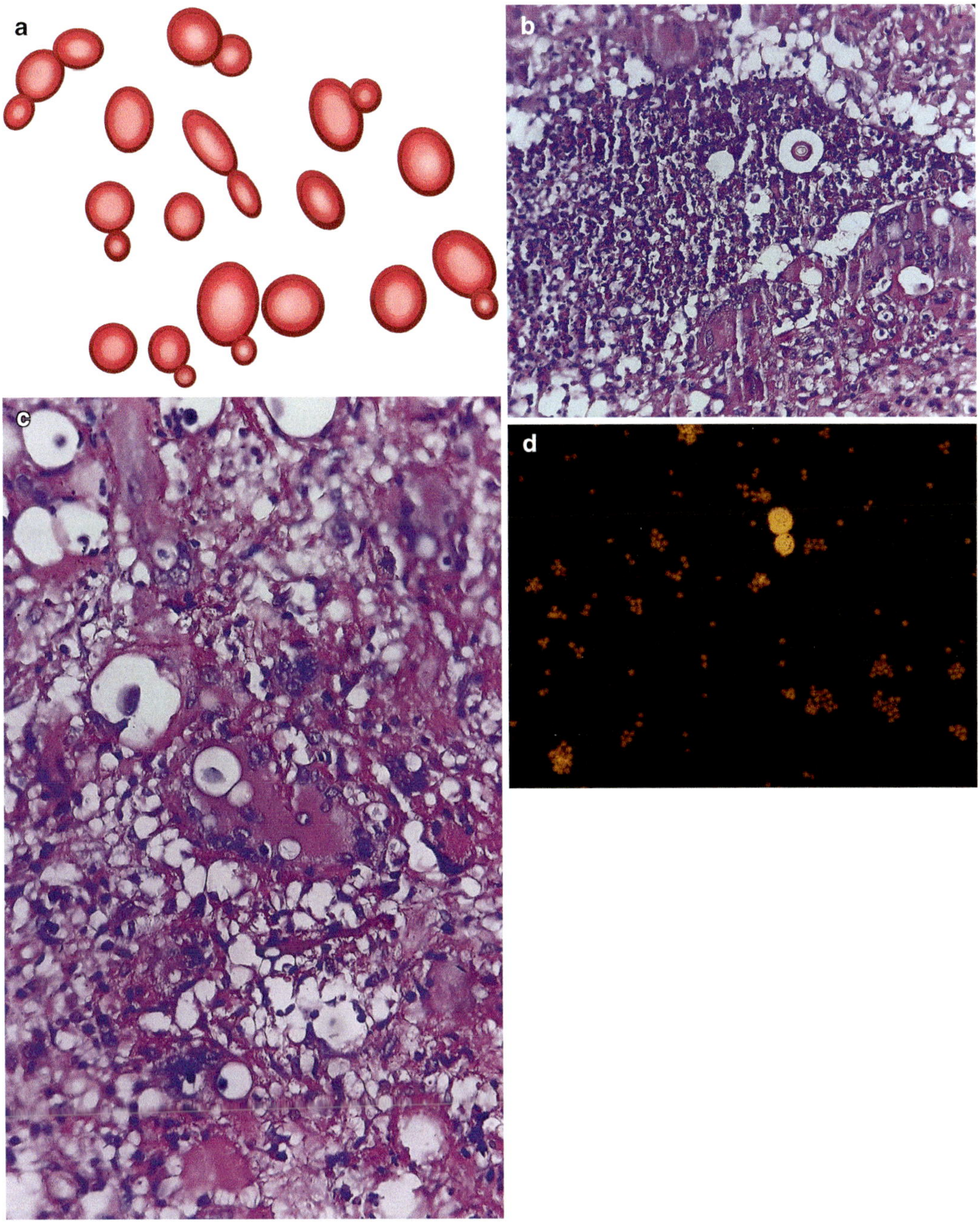

Fig. 6.6 *Cryptococcus* spp. (**a**) Illustration, narrow-based budding yeast. (**b**, **c**) Granulomatous reaction, multiple yeasts inside multinucleated giant cells, abundant lymphocytic infiltrate, H&E, 40×. (**d**) Yeast in CSF smear. Its thick polysaccharide capsule gives the yeasts a characteristic appearance of having a clear space around them. India ink, 40×. All illustrations are original by Jurado LF

spp. or *Histoplasma*. In this situation, staining these specimens with Fontana-Masson may show evidence of melanin, which is a hallmark of cryptococci. The use of cryptococcal antigen analysis in serum and CSF may not be useful in patients with poorly encapsulated cryptococci because most of the serologic tests detect capsular antigens (Gazzoni et al. 2009).

Cryptococcal antigen testing using latex agglutination or EIA can be performed in serum and CSF, showing a sensitivity and specificity of above 90%; nevertheless, false-negative results can occur due to a low fungal burden or a prozone phenomenon. Alternatively, false-positive results have been reported in infected individuals with *Trichosporon* spp. or *Klebsiella pneumoniae*, in those with a positive rheumatoid factor, or when the reagent was incubated with the specimen beyond the recommended time (Williamson et al. 2017). Cultures, using canavanine-glycine-bromothymol blue medium, that turn blue in the presence of *C. gattii* are helpful to identify the infective species and are indispensable for measuring antifungal susceptibility when indicated.

6.8 Disease Caused by *Blastomyces dermatitidis*

Gilchrist described blastomycosis in Baltimore (USA) during the 1890s as a skin infection caused by what he thought was a protozoan organism (Gilchrist 1894); thus, the disease was named as Gilchrist's disease. Initially, because skin manifestations of blastomycosis were very striking, it was considered a dermatologic condition (Gilchrist and Stokes 1898). The concept of airborne transmission was not recognized until pathologic descriptions allowed the pathophysiologic mechanisms to be elucidated (Sarosi and Davies 1979). There are infrequent cases of direct cutaneous inoculation in laboratory workers and veterinarians, but virtually all cases of blastomycosis are considered to originate primarily from lung disease (Sarosi and Davies 1979).

The etiological agent is the dimorphic fungus *Blastomyces dermatitidis*. The organism exists in nature in the mold or mycelial phase and converts to the yeast phase in tissues at body temperature (Fig. 6.7a, b). The mold is the infective form, producing conidia that can be aerosolized and subsequently inhaled. In culture, *B. dermatitidis* grows from 25 to 28 °C as a mold and at 37 °C as a yeast (Nemecek et al. 2006).

This fungus has been isolated from soil in the Mississippi and Ohio River valleys, around the Great Lakes and the Saint Lawrence River, which include multiple states in the United States (southeastern, south central, and upper Midwestern states); it has also been found in several Canadian provinces (McKinnell and Pappas 2009). Outbreaks of blastomycosis after a source exposure have been reported, but most cases occur sporadically in the endemic areas. Occasionally, cases are reported in areas where the disease is not endemic, such as Colorado, Texas, Kansas, and Nebraska in the United States, and from other countries around the world (Shukla et al. 2009).

Patients infected with *B. dermatitidis* can develop pneumonia, extrapulmonary disease, or both. Lung involvement often imitates an acute bacterial pneumonia, lung cancer, or tuberculosis. Cutaneous lesions, which can be present as verrucous or ulcerative lesions, are the most common extrapulmonary manifestation, followed by bone, prostate, and CNS disease.

In the yeast phase, the organism appears as spherical, budding, thick-walled yeast with a daughter cell forming a single bud with a broad base. Further, size varies from 5 to 15 μm, and most are spherical to oval and have a double cell wall appearance, which consists of the interior and exterior components of its thick cell surface (Fig. 6.7c). The yeast may be found inside or outside of macrophages in the pyogranulomatous tissue response (McKinnell and Pappas 2009).

After inhalation of the conidia, a variety of responses can occur in the lungs, from asymptomatic disease to acute and chronic pneumonia, and fatal acute respiratory distress syndrome (McKinnell and Pappas 2009; Patel et al. 2010). In up to 40% of cases, the disease has become systemic at the time of diagnosis, affecting the skin, soft tissue, bone, genitourinary tract, or the CNS (McKinnell and Pappas 2009). Blastomycosis in immunocompromised hosts appears to be more severe and frequently fatal. In patients with CNS involvement, diabetes mellitus is an important risk factor (Bariola et al. 2010).

B. dermatitidis in tissue appears as yeasts that measure 8–15 μm in diameter, have a thick refractile cell wall, and usually show a single,

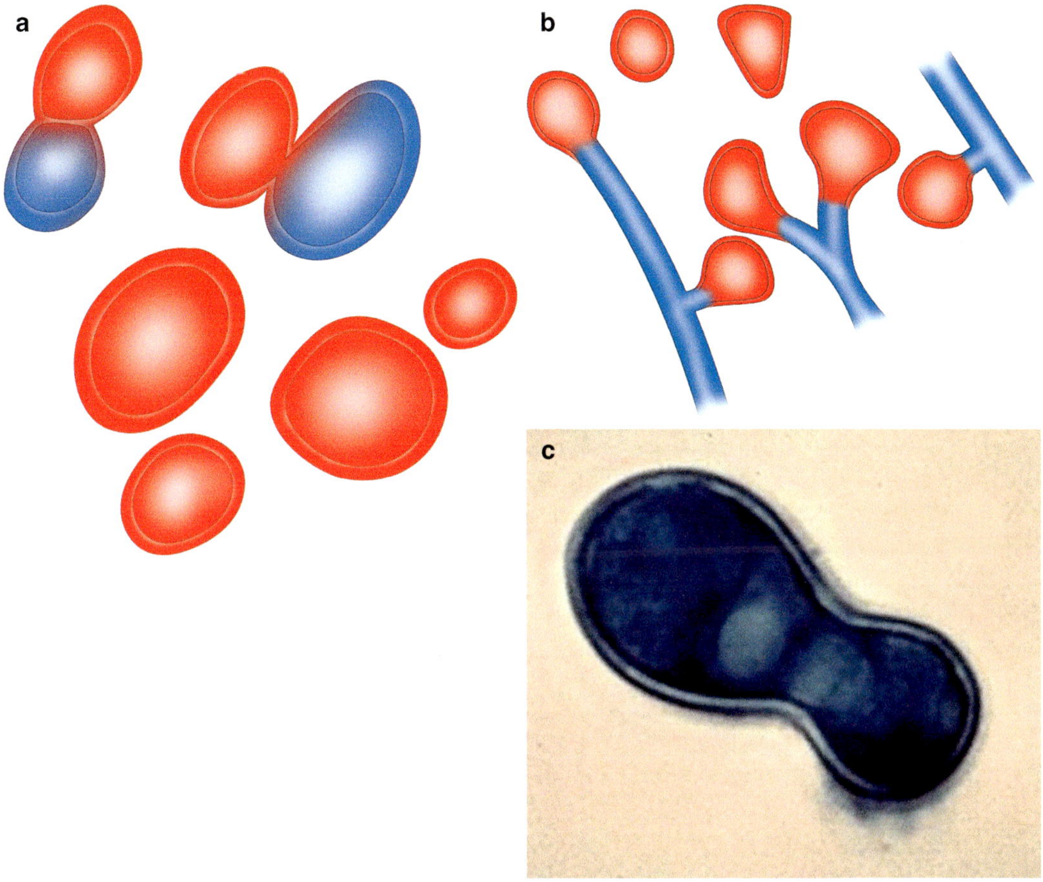

Fig. 6.7 *Blastomyces dermatitidis*. (**a**) Yeast form, with broad-based budding. (**b**) Mycelial or saprophytic form, forming single conidium showing its characteristic "lollipop" morphology. (**c**) Thick-walled yeast with broad-based budding, showing its "footprint" morphology. All illustrations are original by Jurado LF

broad-based bud (Fig. 6.7a, c). The yeasts can be identified in many samples, such as sputum, bronchoalveolar lavage, fine-needle aspirates, CSF, and biopsy specimens. When the H&E stain is used, the thick refractile cell wall gives the appearance of a space between the fungal cell contents and the surrounding tissue. The multiple nuclei of the yeast stain with hematoxylin. Sometimes, this fungus can show small yeast forms, called microforms. Additionally, *B. dermatitidis* can be identified with routinely used preparations such as Papanicolaou and KOH. The contour of the yeast is best appreciated with silver stains such as PAS or GMS (Patel et al. 2010; Lemos et al. 2000).

The histological reaction produced by the yeasts is mainly granulomatous with diverse degrees of neutrophilic infiltrate; therefore, as in the cases of coccidioidomycosis, it has been described as pyogranulomatous inflammation (Patel et al. 2010).

Few studies have compared the identification of broad-based budding yeasts in histopathologic or cytologic specimens with culture or other diagnostic methods that confirm the diagnosis of blastomycosis. Patel et al. (2010), in a retrospective study of 53 cases, reported that *Coccidioides immitis*, *Candida albicans*, and *Aspergillus* were recovered from 10% of the pathologic specimens, demonstrating broad-based budding yeasts in the direct histopathologic examination. A previous study by Lemos et al. (2000) of patients with blastomycosis showed that in a high percentage of the cultures,

Candida was isolated. These results suggest that not all broad-based budding yeasts in the 8–15 μm diameter range are *Blastomyces*.

Considering that histopathologic and cytologic studies can provide results before the culture, there is pressure to use these findings to guide treatment, particularly because *B. dermatitidis* can take up to 3 weeks to grow or may not grow. The sensitivity of culture varies depending on the specimen that was obtained and may range from 62% to 100% (Lemos et al. 2000; Martynowicz and Prakash 2002). The diagnostic yield of histopathology will depend on the expertise of the pathologist (McKinnell and Pappas 2009). Because of the possibility of false-positive results, pathologists must describe the yeast and budding pattern observed in the tissue and also should add a commentary in the report about the yeasts that can have similar morphology. In addition, alternative tests should be performed to determine if the patient truly has blastomycosis, especially in cases from areas where the disease is not endemic or when the clinical presentation is not usual.

B. dermatitidis antigens can be detected in the urine and serum by using an EIA. The sensitivity and specificity have been reported to be above 90%; nevertheless, cross-reactivity occurs in patients with histoplasmosis, paracoccidioidomycosis, and penicilliosis caused by *P. marneffei* (Durkin et al. 2004). Because of the cross-reactivity, it is useful to perform antigen tests for both blastomycosis and histoplasmosis. Detection of antibodies to *B. dermatitidis* in serum using traditional complement fixation and immunodifusion has poor specificity and sensitivity; however, as antigens have been better purified and used in radioimmunodiffusion and EIAs, the sensitivity and specificity of serology are significantly higher (McKinnell and Pappas 2009).

6.9 Conclusion

Due to the high morbidity and mortality rates associated with systemic fungal infections and particularly in cases of CNS involvement, a rapid and accurate diagnosis is always mandatory. The broad spectrum in clinical and pathogenic presentation makes its diagnosis a big challenge. When a tissue or liquid specimen is available, the pathological analysis is a very useful tool for rapid and accurate diagnosis. Usually, pathological studies can provide results before the culture or other analyses are available. Nevertheless, it is important to remember the limitations of this approach because many of the fungal structures among different species are very similar. Therefore, it could be really easy to misdiagnose a specific fungal infection, which would have a relevant impact on therapy. Thus, it is always important to consider the clinical information, as well as complementary analysis, in order to obtain a definitive ethological diagnosis.

References

Adam RD, Elliott SP, Taljanovicc MS. The spectrum and presentation of disseminated coccidioidomycosis. Am J Med. 2009;122:770–7.

Alexander B, Smith P, Davis R, Perfect J, Reller L. The (1, 3)-D glucan test as an aid to the early diagnosis of invasive fungal infections following lung transplantation. J Clin Microbiol. 2010;48(11):4083–8. https://doi.org/10.1128/JCM.01183-10.

Ampel NM. Coccidioidomycosis: a review of recent advances. Clin Chest Med. 2009;30:241–51.

Antinori S, Corbellino M, Meroni L, Resta F, Sollima S, Tonolini M, Tortorano AM, Milazzo L, Bello L, Furfaro E, Galli M, Viscoli C. Aspergillus meningitis: a rare clinical manifestation of central nervous system aspergillosis. Case report and review of 92 cases. J Infect. 2013;66:218–38.

Bariola J, Perry P, Pappas PG, Proia L, Shealey W, Wright PW, Sizemore JM, Matthew Robinson M, Bradsher RW. Blastomycosis of the central nervous system: a multicenter review of diagnosis and treatment in the modern era. Clin Infect Dis. 2010;50:797–804.

Barrera-Herrera LE, Vera A, Álvarez J, Lopez R. Necrotizing encephalitis caused by disseminated Aspergillus infection after orthotopic liver transplantation. Case Rep Gastroenterol. 2015;9(1):1–6. https://doi.org/10.1159/000371541.

Ben-Ami R, Luna M, Lewis RE, Walsh TJ, Kontoyiannis DP. A clinicopathological study of pulmonary mucormycosis in cancer patients: extensive angioinvasion but limited inflammatory response. J Infect. 2009;59:134–8.

Bennett JW. Aspergillus: a primer for the novice. Med Mycol. 2009;47:S5–S12.

Brumble LM, Reza MB, Dhakal LP, Cruz G, Saleh OMA. Fungal infections of the central nervous system: clinical, radiographic and laboratory manifestations. J Microbiol Exp. 2017;5(6):00167. https://doi.org/10.15406/jmcn.2017.05.00167.

Bueno-Fischer G, Mocelin H, Severo CB, Oliveira F d M, Xavier MO, Severo LC. Histoplasmosis in children. Paediatr Respir Rev. 2009;10:172–7.

Chong GM, Maertens JA, Lagrou K, Driessen GJ, Cornelissen JJ, Rijnders BJ. Diagnostic performance of galactomannan antigen testing in cerebrospinal fluid. J Clin Microbiol. 2016;54:428–31.

Colombo AL, Tobon A, Restrepo A, Queiroz-Telles F, Nucci M. Epidemiology of endemic systemic fungal infections in Latin America. Med Mycol. 2011;49:785–98.

Concia E, Azzini AM, Conti M. Epidemiology, incidence and risk factors for invasive candidiasis in high-risk patients. Drugs. 2009;69(Suppl 1):5–14.

Darouiche RO. Candida in the ICU. Clin Chest Med. 2009;30:287–93.

De Pauw B, Walsh TJ, Donnelly JP, Stevens DA, Edwards JE, Calandra T, Pappas PG, Maertens J, Lortholary O, Kauffman CA, Denning DW, Patterson TF, Maschmeyer G, Bille J, Dismukes WE, Herbrecht R, Hope WW, Kibbler CC, Kullberg BJ, Marr KA, Mu-oz P, Odds FC, Perfect JR, Restrepo A, Ruhnke M, Segal BH, Sobel JD, Sorrell TC, Viscoli C, Wingard JR, Zaoutis T, Bennett JE, European Organization for Research and Treatment of Cancer/Invasive Fungal Infections Cooperative Group; National Institute of Allergy and Infectious Diseases Mycoses Study Group (EORTC/MSG) Consensus Group. Revised definitions of invasive fungal disease from the European Organization for Research and Treatment of Cancer/Invasive Fungal Infections Cooperative Group and the National Institute of Allergy and Infectious Diseases Mycoses Study Group (EORTC/MSG) Consensus Group. Clin Infect Dis. 2008;46:1813–21. https://doi.org/10.1086/588660.

van de Veerdonk FL, Kullberg BJ, Mihai N. Pathogenesis of invasive candidiasis. Curr Opin Crit Care. 2010;16(5):453–45. https://doi.org/10.1097/MCC.0b013e32833e046e.

Durkin MJ, Witt A, LeMonte A, Wheat B, Connolly P. Antigen assay with the potential to aid in diagnosis of blastomycosis. J Clin Microbiol. 2004;42:4873–5.

Durkin M, Connolly P, Kuberski T, Myers R, Kubak BM, Bruckner D, Pegues D, Wheat LJ. Diagnosis of coccidioidomycosis with use of the *Coccidioides* antigen enzyme immunoassay. Clin Infect Dis. 2008;47:e69–73.

Fennelly AM, Slenker AK, Murphy LC, Moussouttas M, DeSimone JA. Candida cerebral abscesses: a case report and review of the literature. Med Mycol. 2013;51:779–84.

Galanis E, MacDougall L. Epidemiology of *Cryptococcus gattii*, British Columbia, Canada, 1999–2007. Emerg Infect Dis. 2010;16:251–7.

Gavito-Higuera J, Mullins CB, Ramos-Duran L, Olivas Chacon CI, Hakim N, Palacios E. Fungal infections of the central nervous system: a pictorial review. J Clin Imaging Sci. 2016;6:24. https://doi.org/10.4103/2156-7514.184244.

Gazzoni AF, Severo CB, Salles EF, Severo LC. Histopathology, serology and cultures in the diagnosis of cryptococcosis. Rev Inst Med Trop Sao Paulo. 2009;51:255–9.

Gilchrist TC. Protozoan dermatitis. J Cutan Genitourin Dis. 1894;12:496–9.

Gilchrist TC, Stokes WR. Case of pseudo-lupus vulgaris caused by *Blastomyces*. J Exp Med. 1898;3:53–78.

Guarner J, Brandt ME. Histopathologic diagnosis of fungal infections in the 21st century. Clin Microbiol Rev. 2011;24(2):247–80. https://doi.org/10.1128/CMR.00053-10.

Gupta N, Arora S, Rajwanshi A, Nijhawan R, Srinivasan R. Histoplasmosis: cytodiagnosis and review of literature with special emphasis on differential diagnosis on cytomorphology. Cytopathology. 2009; https://doi.org/10.1111/j.1365-2303.2009.00693.x.

Hage CA, Bowyer S, Tarvin SE, Helper D, Kleiman MB, Wheat LJ. Recognition, diagnosis, and treatment of histoplasmosis complicating tumor necrosis factor blocker herapy. Clin Infect Dis. 2010;50:85–92.

Hofman V, Dhouibi A, Butori C, Padovani B, Gari-Toussaint M, Garcia-Hermoso D, Baumann M, Vénissac N, Cathomas G, Hofman P. Usefulness of molecular biology performed with formaldehyde-fixed paraffin embedded tissue for the diagnosis of combined pulmonary invasive mucormycosis and aspergillosis in an immunocompromised patient. Diagn Pathol. 2010;5:1–7.

Huston SM, Mody CH. Cryptococcosis: an emerging respiratory mycosis. Clin Chest Med. 2009;30:253–64.

Johnson LB, Bradley SF, Kauffman CA. Fungaemia due to *Cryptococcus laurentii* and a review of non-neoformans cryptococcaemia. Mycoses. 1998;41:277–80.

Kauffman CA. Diagnosis of histoplasmosis in immunosuppressed patients. Curr Opin Infect Dis. 2008;21:421–5.

Kauffman CA. Histoplasmosis. Clin Chest Med. 2009;30:217–25.

Kordossis T, Avlami A, Velegraki A, Stefanou I, Georgakopoulos G, Papalambrou C, Legakis NJ. First report of Cryptococcus laurentii meningitis and a fatal case of Cryptococcus albidus cryptococcaemia in AIDS patients. Med Mycol. 1998;36:335–9.

Kullberg BJ, Arendrup MC. Invasive candidiasis. N Engl J Med. 2015;373:1445–56.

Lammering JC, Iv M, Gupta N, Pandit R, Patel MR. Imaging spectrum of CNS coccidioidomycosis: prevalence and significance of concurrent brain and spinal disease. AJR Am J Roentgenol. 2013;200:1334–46.

Lau A, Halliday C, Chen SC, Playford EG, Stanley K, Sorrell TC. Comparison of whole blood, serum, and plasma for early detection of candidemia by multiplex-tandem PCR. J Clin Microbiol. 2010;48:811–6.

Lee S, Yun NR, Kim KH, Jeon JH, Kim EC, Chung DH, Park WB, Oh MD. Discrepancy between histology and culture in filamentous fungal infections. Med Mycol. 2010;48:886–8.

Lemos LB, Guo M, Baliga M. Blastomycosis: organ involvement and etiologic diagnosis. A review of 123 patients from Mississippi. Ann Diagn Pathol. 2000;4:391–406.

Li L, Dial SM, Schmelz M, Rennels MA, Ampel NM. Cellular immune suppressor activity resides in lymphocyte cell clusters adjacent to granulomata in human coccidioidomycosis. Infect Immun. 2005;73:3923–8.

Liu X, Ling Z, Li L, Ruan B. Invasive fungal infections in liver transplantation. Int J Infect Dis. 2011;15(5):e298–304.

Loulergue P, Bastides F, Baudouin V, Chandenier J, Mariani-Kurkdjian P, Dupont B, Viard JP, Dromer F, Lortholary O. Literature review and case histories of *Histoplasma capsulatum* var. *duboisii* infections in HIV-infected patients. Emerg Infect Dis. 2007;13:1647–52.

Malo J, Luraschi-Monjagatta C, Wolk DM, Thompson R, Hage CA, Knox KS. Update on the diagnosis of pulmonary coccidioidomycosis. Ann Am Thorac Soc. 2014;11(2):243–53. https://doi.org/10.1513/AnnalsATS.201308-286FR.

Martynowicz M, Prakash UBS. Pulmonary blastomycosis: an appraisal of diagnostic techniques. Chest. 2002;121:768–73.

Mathur M, Johnson CE, Sze G. Fungal infections of the central nervous system. Neuroimaging Clin N Am. 2012;22(4):609–32.

May RC, Stone NR, Wiesner DL, Bicanic T, Nielsen K. Cryptococcus: from environmental saprophyte to global pathogen. Nat Rev Microbiol. 2016;14(2):106–17. https://doi.org/10.1038/nrmicro.2015.6.

McCarthy M, Rosengart A, Schuetz AN, Kontoyiannis DP, Walsh TJ. Mold infections of the central nervous system. N Engl J Med. 2014;371:150–60.

McKinnell JA, Pappas PG. Blastomycosis: new insights into diagnosis, prevention, and treatment. Clin Chest Med. 2009;30:227–39.

Merwick Á, Minhas Z, Curtis C, Thom M, Choi D, Mummery C. Intradural extramedullary spinal candida infection. Pract Neurol. 2015;15:400–4.

Mukhopadhyay S, Katzenstein ALA. Biopsy findings in acute pulmonary histoplasmosis: unusual histologic features in 4 cases mimicking lymphomatoid granulomatosis. Am J Surg Pathol. 2010;34:541–6.

Naggie S, Perfect JR. Molds: hyalohyphomycosis, phaeohyphomycosis, and zygomycosis. Clin Chest Med. 2009;30:337–53.

Neilson JB, Fromtling RA, Bulmer GS. *Cryptococcus neoformans*: size range of infectious particles from aerosolized soil. Infect Immun. 1997;17:634–8.

Nemecek JC, Wuthrich M, Klein BS. Global control of dimorphism and virulence in fungi. Science. 2006;312:583–8.

Parish JM, Blair JE. Coccidioidomycosis. Mayo Clin Proc. 2008;83:343–9.

Patel A, Gattuso JP, Reddy VB. Diagnosis of blastomycosis in surgical pathology and cytopathology: correlation with microbiologic culture. Am J Surg Pathol. 2010;34:256–61.

Perdigao J, Rojas R, Verzelli LF, Castillo M. Fungal infections of the central nervous system. Semin Roentgenol. 2004;39(4):505–18.

Persat F, Ranque S, Derouin F, Michel-Nguyen A, Picot S, Sulahian A. Contribution of the (1→3)-beta-D-glucan assay for diagnosis of invasive fungal infections. J Clin Microbiol. 2008;46:1009–13.

Posch W, Heimdörfer D, Wilflingseder D, Lass-Flörl C. Invasive candidiasis: future directions in non-culture based diagnosis. Expert Rev Anti Infect Ther. 2017;15(9):829–38. https://doi.org/10.1080/14787210.2017.1370373.

Prabhu RM, Patel R. Mucormycosis and entomophthoramycosis: a review of the clinical manifestations, diagnosis and treatment. Clin Microbiol Infect. 2004;10(Suppl 1):31–47. https://doi.org/10.1111/j.1470-9465.2004.00843.x.

Rajasingham R, Smith RM, Park BJ, Jarvis JN, Govender NP, Chiller TM, Denning DW, Loyse A, Boulware DR. Global burden of disease of HIV-associated cryptococcal meningitis: an updated analysis. Lancet Infect Dis. 2017;17:873–81.

Raman-Sharma R. Fungal infections of the nervous system: current perspective and controversies in management. Int J Surg. 2010;8(8):591–601.

Read RW, Zhang J, Albini T, Evans M, Rao NA. Splendore-Hoeppli phenomenon in the conjunctiva: immunohistochemical analysis. Am J Ophthalmol. 2005;140:262–6.

Ribes JA, Vanover-Sams CL, Baker DJ. *Zygomycetes* in human disease. Clin Microbiol Rev. 2000;13:236–301.

Riscili BP, Wood KL. Noninvasive pulmonary *Aspergillus* infections. Clin Chest Med. 2009;30:315–35.

Rixford E, Gilchrist TC. Two cases of protozoon (coccidioidal) infection of the skin and other organs. Johns Hopkins Hosp Rep. 1896;1:209–68.

Roden MM, Zaoutis TE, Buchanan WL, Knudsen TA, Sarkisova TA, Schaufele RL, Sein M, Sein T, Chiou CC, Chu JH, Kontoyiannis DP, Walsh TJ. Epidemiology and outcome of zygomycosis: a review of 929 reported cases. Clin Infect Dis. 2005;41:634–53.

Roilides E, Antachopoulos C, Simitsopoulou M. Pathogenesis and host defence against Mucorales: the role of cytokines and interaction with antifungal drugs. Mycoses. 2014;57(Suppl 3):40–7. https://doi.org/10.1111/myc.12236.

Salvatore CM, Chen TK, Toussi SS, De La Mora P, Petraitiene R, Finkelman MA, Walsh TJ. (1→3)-β-D-Glucan in cerebrospinal fluid as a biomarker for *Candida* and *Aspergillus* infections of the central nervous system in pediatric patients. J Pediatr Infect Dis Soc. 2016;5(3):277–86. https://doi.org/10.1093/jpids/piv014.

Sargent J, O'Marcaigh A, Smith O, Butler K, Gavin P, O'Sullivan M. *Candida albicans*-associated necrotizing vasculitis producing life-threatening gastrointestinal hemorrhage. Hum Pathol. 2010;41:602–4.

Sarosi GA, Davies SF. Blastomycosis. State of the art. Am Rev Respir Dis. 1979;120:911–38.

Saubolle MA. Laboratory aspects in the diagnosis of coccidioidomycosis. Ann N Y Acad Sci. 2007;1111:301–14.

Schuetz AN, Walsh TJ. Importance of fungal histopathology in immunocompromised pediatric patients: it's not just "Aspergillus" anymore. Am J Clin Pathol. 2015;144(2):185–7. https://doi.org/10.1309/AJCPE3NSJ2RYLENS.

Schwartz S, Kontoyiannis DP, Harrison T, Ruhnke M. Advances in the diagnosis and treatment of fungal infections of the CNS. Lancet Neurol. 2018;17(4):362–72. https://doi.org/10.1016/S1474-4422(18)30030-9.

Segal E, Elad D. Candidiasis. In: Mahy BW, Meulen Borriello VP, Murray PR, Funke G, Kaufmann SH, Steward HM, Merz WG, Hay RJ, Cox F, Wakelin D, Gillespie SH, Despommier DD, editors. Topley & Wilson's microbiology and microbial infections. New York: Wiley; 2010. https://doi.org/10.1002/9780470688618.taw0157.

Sherif R, Segal BH. Pulmonary aspergillosis: clinical presentation, diagnostic tests, management and complications. Curr Opin Pulm Med. 2010;16:242–50.

Shukla S, Singh S, Jain M, Kumar Singh S, Chander R, Kawatra N. Paediatric cutaneous blastomycosis: a rare case diagnosed on FNAC. Diagn Cytopathol. 2009;37:119–21.

Sing Y, Ramdial PK. Cryptococcal inflammatory pseudotumors. Am J Surg Pathol. 2007;31:1521–7.

Southern P, Horbul J, Maher D, Davis DA. *C. albicans* colonization of human mucosal surfaces. PLoS One. 2008;3:1–9.

Sundaram C, Umabala P, Laxmi V, Purohit AK, Prasad VSSV, Panigrahi M, Sahu BP, Sarathi MV, Kaul S, Borghain R, Meena AK, Jayalakshmi SS, Suvarna A, Mohandas S, Murthy JMK. Pathology of fungal infections of the central nervous system: 17 years' experience from Southern India. Histopathology. 2006;49:396–405. https://doi.org/10.1111/j.1365-2559.2006.02515.x.

Swartzentruber S, Rhodes L, Kurkjian K, Zahn M, Brandt ME, Connolly P, Wheat LJ. Diagnosis of acute pulmonary histoplasmosis by antigen detection. Clin Infect Dis. 2009;49:1878–82.

The Library of Victoria University, Toronto. Epidemics, hippocrates. Available at: https://archive.org/stream/L477HippocratesVII.EpidemicsLoebClassicalLibrary/L477-Hippocrates%20VII.%20Epidemics%20%28Loeb%20Classical%20Library%29_djvu.txt.

Vazquez J, Sobel J. Candidiasis. In: Kaufman C, Pappas P, Sobel J, Dismukes W, editors. Essentials of clinical mycology. 2nd ed. Oxford: Oxford University Press; 2011. p. 167–206.

Wheat LJ, Azar MM, Bahr NC, Spec A, Relich RF, Hage C. Histoplasmosis. Infect Dis Clin North Am. 2016;30:207–27. https://doi.org/10.1016/j.idc.2015.10.009.

Williamson PR, Jarvis JN, Panackal AA, Fisher MC, Molloy SF, Loyse A, Harrison TS. Cryptococcal meningitis: epidemiology, immunology, diagnosis and therapy. Nat Rev Neurol. 2017;13:13–24.

Zimmermann J, Guresir A, Nelles M, Guresir E. Rapid development and rupture of a cerebral mycotic aneurysm in Candida infective endocarditis. Intensive Care Med. 2016;42:275–6.

Molecular Genetics and Genomics of Fungal Infections

7

Shivaprakash M. Rudramurthy
and Arunaloke Chakrabarti

Abbreviations

AIDS	Acquired immunodeficiency syndrome
CDC	Centers for Disease Control and Prevention
CM	Cryptococcal meningitis
CNS	Central nervous system
CSF	Cerebrospinal fluid
CT	Computed tomography
EF	Elongation factor
HIV	Human immunodeficiency virus
HRCA	Hyperbranched rolling circle amplification
ISHAM	International Society for Human and Animal Mycology
ITS	Internal transcribed spacer
LAMP	Loop-mediated isothermal amplification
LFA	Lateral flow assay
ME	Meningitis/encephalitis
MIC	Minimal inhibitory concentration
MRI	Magnetic resonance imaging
PCR	Polymerase chain reaction
PLB	Phospholipase B

S. M. Rudramurthy
Department of Medical Microbiology, Postgraduate Institute of Medical Education and Research, Chandigarh, India

A. Chakrabarti (✉)
Department of Medical Microbiology, Postgraduate Institute of Medical Education and Research, Chandigarh, India

Center of Advance Research in Medical Mycology, WHO Collaborating Center for Reference and Research of Fungi of Medical Importance, National Culture Collection of Pathogenic Fungi, Chandigarh, India

7.1 Introduction

Central nervous system (CNS) is the second most common organ after lung where fungi invade during invasive fungal infections. Yeast (*Cryptococcus*, *Candida*), moulds (*Aspergillus*, *Mucorales*, non-*Aspergillus* hyaline molds, dematiaceous fungi) and dimorphic fungi can produce CNS infection. However, *Cryptococcus*, *Aspergillus*, *Mucorales* and neurotropic dematiaceous fungi (*Cladophialophora bantiana*, *Exophiala dermatitidis*, *Rhinocladiella mackenzie*, *Ochroconis gallopava* and *Chaetomium* spp.) are commonly isolated from CNS fungal infections. Molds, dimorphic fungi and *Cryptococcus* generally enter through respiratory tract in immunosuppressed hosts and subsequently infect CNS by haematogenous dissemination. *Cryptococcus* and neurotropic dematiaceous fungi may produce CNS infection even in immunocompetent host following the same route. Similarly any patient with candi-

M. Turgut et al. (eds.), *Fungal Infections of the Central Nervous System*,
https://doi.org/10.1007/978-3-030-06088-6_7

demia may lead to CNS infection. CNS fungal infections have also been reported after intravenous drug abuse. Other than haematogenous route, direct inoculation of CNS may occur by any fungus as a result of surgery, trauma and contaminated medical supplies. Direct extension from adjacent structure like paranasal sinuses, mastoid and orbit to CNS is also possible by fungus (McCarthy and Walsh 2017).

CNS fungal infection may manifest as meningitis, meningoencephalitis, hydrocephalus, space-occupying lesion, acute cerebrovascular events and spinal infections (Preuner and Lion 2009). The outcome of CNS fungal infections depends on early diagnosis and prompt management. But, the early diagnosis faces stiff challenges due to general considerations of rarity of CNS fungal infection, non-specific clinical symptoms and signs, difficulty in collection of samples for brain and absence of any standardized molecular tests. However, CNS fungal infection has drawn a lot of international attention after *Exserohilum rostratum* meningitis outbreak in the United States (Gade et al. 2013), though similar post-tsunami *Aspergillus* meningitis outbreak in Sri Lanka due to contaminated medical supplies occurred much earlier (Gunaratne et al. 2007).

Imaging including computerized tomography (CT) and magnetic resonance imaging (MRI) helps in suspecting CNS fungal infection. Any patient at risk of CNS fungal infection or documented fungal infection of lung or sinuses should be screened with neuroimaging. To confirm the diagnosis, invasive samples from CNS are required. Cerebrospinal fluid (CSF) sample helps in the diagnosis of meningitis or meningoencephalitis by direct demonstration of fungus on microscopy and/or culture, whereas biopsy sample is required for space-occupying lesion. The collection of biopsy sample may be a challenge in majority of the cases. In this difficult scenario, non-culture-based diagnostic tests of CSF may help in early detection of CNS mycosis. Among the non-culture-based diagnosis, molecular biomarkers and antigen detection in CSF have been developed as pan-fungal marker or pathogen-specific tests. Though promising results are reported for early diagnosis and monitoring therapy by those tests, none of those tests, except *Cryptococcus* antigen, has received United States Food and Drug Adminstration (US FDA) approval (Kami et al. 1999a; Buitrago et al. 2011; Binnicker et al. 2011; Vucicevic et al. 2010; Klingspor and Jalal 2006; Elsayed et al. 2001; Ralph and Hussain 1996). Researchers have also attempted the molecular genomic technology in diagnosis of fungal diseases, but the studies are few and far between. In the present chapter, we have reviewed the existing knowledge on molecular genomic tests for diagnosis and monitoring of CNS fungal diseases.

7.2 DNA-Based Molecular Diagnosis of CNS Fungal Infections

The currently available techniques such as conventional and biomarker tests have many limitations and often fail to provide a rational basis for institution of appropriate antifungal therapy. There is a need for the use of molecular techniques, which are rapid and sensitive and may detect the causative agent accurately that would help appropriate and prompt antifungal therapy. Molecular techniques are applied either for detection of nucleic acid in clinical samples or for the accurate identification of fungi isolated from the clinical specimen. Detection of nucleic acid in clinical sample faces the challenge of extraction of nucleic acid, inadequate amount nucleic acid in sample and contamination during test procedure. However, DNA-based molecular assays for the identification of majority of the fungi isolated from clinical specimen and for outbreak investigation are well established.

7.2.1 Molecular Test Formats

Polymerase chain reaction (PCR) is the commonly used test format for the molecular diagnosis of fungal infections. Either standard PCR or different modifications of the PCR including nested PCR, real-time PCR, multiplex PCR and

PCR-ELISA (enzyme-linked immunosorbent assay) are used to amplify the fungal nucleic acid from the specimen and simultaneous detection. The amplified products are identified by either DNA sequencing or use of DNA microarray chips or analysis by restricted fragment length polymorphism or use of specific hybridization probes captured to microbeads (Luminex technology) (Preuner and Lion 2009; Landlinger et al. 2009). Of all the PCR amplification formats available, real-time platforms are generally preferred due to (a) less chance of contamination in a closed system and without the requirement of post-PCR processing; (b) simultaneous quantification of the fungal load in the clinical sample; (c) simultaneous detection of the species either by use of specific probes or by melt curve analysis of amplified product; and (d) possible multiplex assay to detect multiple pathogen in single reaction (Khot and Fredricks 2009).

7.2.2 Targets for PCR Amplifications

The PCR-based assays allow the detection of either the broad range of fungus or specific species or genus. For the detection of presence of unknown fungi in the clinical specimen, pan-fungal primers that enable amplification of broad range of fungus are used. Many pan-fungal primers have been designed to amplify different regions of ribosomal genes such as internal transcribed spacer (ITS) regions 1 and 2, 18s region and 28s/26s region (Fig. 7.1).The multicopy of ribosomal genes also improves sensitivity of detection. The ITS region is specifically used, as this region has both the high conserved and variable areas. White et al. (1990) first time described the universal primers for the amplification of the ITS region, which is now widely used. Occasionally, this region may not be sufficient to discriminate the fungi to the species and subspecies level (Atkins and Clark 2004), and cross-reactivity with phylogenetically related fungi may be a problem for identification (Bialek et al. 2002). The diagnostic performance of ITS pan-fungal PCR has shown high concordance (>80%) with routine conventional methods including microscopy and isolation. The sensitivity and specificity were 57% and 97% even in cases with fungal infections having negative microscopy (Lass-Flörl et al. 2013). The other less frequently used targets include mitochondrial gene, beta tubulin gene, calmodulin gene, etc.

7.2.3 DNA Extraction

Extraction of the DNA from clinical sample may not be easy as the number of fungal cells present in the CSF is low in patients with space-occupying lesions. Hence, the extraction procedure should be of high quality without much damage to the DNA. Bialek et al. (2002) demonstrated that a simple freeze and boil procedure may be sufficient to free the *Cryptococcal* DNA from the brain tissue homogenates. Similarly, the DNA extracted from frozen neural tissue of patients with amyotrophic lateral sclerosis revealed multiple fungal genera including *Candida*, *Malassezia*, *Fusarium*, *Botrytis*, *Trichoderma* and *Cryptococcus*, which were responsible for the severity of the disease (Alonso et al. 2017). Different commercial kits are also being used for efficient DNA extraction from clinical specimen (DNeasy Blood & Tissue Kit, TaKaRa MiniBEST Universal Genomic DNA Extraction). The DNA from pure culture can be extracted using the physical methods such as boiling, grinding in liquid nitrogen, bead beating and use of cell-degrading enzymes or detergents such as sodium dodecyl sulphate followed by purification by phenol/chloroform isoamyl alcohol precipitation.

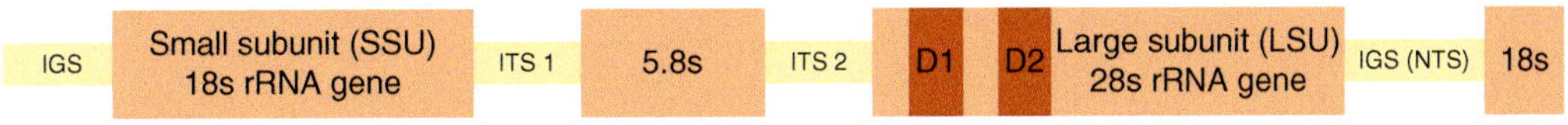

Fig. 7.1 Schematic diagram of ribosomal gene used as targets for molecular diagnosis of fungal infection or identification of fungi

7.3 Molecular Diagnosis of Cryptococcosis

Rapelli et al., for the first time, described PCR-based assay for the detection of the *Cryptococcus neoformans* from the CSF of the cryptococcal meningitis patients. They developed nested PCR-based assay using two nested primer pairs specific for ITS region of ribosomal DNA of *C. neoformans*. The assay identified all 21 proven cases of cryptococcal meningitis (CM) (sensitivity 100%) and was negative in the 19 control specimens tested (specificity 100%). As the cryptococcal antigen titre in the CSF persists and remains high even after 5 months of the adequate therapy, quantification of the DNA by PCR techniques may help to monitor the therapy. The quantity of fungal DNA decreases with response to therapy (Rappelli et al. 1998). The conventional single step PCR technique described by Paschoal et al. (2004) was of low sensitivity (76.8%) compared to culture possibly due to low copy number generated by the single-step PCR and failure to detect band on gel electrophoresis.

Bialek et al. compared and evaluated nested PCR and real-time PCR (LightCycler technology), targeting 18s rRNA in 100 brain homogenates of murine cryptococcal meningitis. Though both the protocols were successful in diagnosing cryptococcal meningitis in 86–87% of tissue samples, the real-time PCR was rapid and also offered the quantitative results (Bialek et al. 2002). Real-time PCR using TaqMan probes targeting ITS2-rDNA region has also been evaluated in CSF samples. The technique is highly sensitive and specific and could differentiate *C. neoformans* and *C. gattii* (Veron et al. 2009). Another real-time fluorescence quantitative PCR assay for cryptococcal meningitis that measures the Cryptococcus virulence-associated DEAD-box RNA helicase (VAD1) mRNA had sensitivity (96%) equal to cryptococcal antigen detection. Its level significantly correlated with the numbers of the *C. neoformans*, glucose concentration and intracranial pressure. The VAD1 mRNA level also decreased in the patients receiving antifungal therapy. Thus, the test may be useful to evaluate the antifungal therapy response (Qishui et al. 2012).

The loop-mediated isothermal amplification (LAMP) technology, an isothermal amplification, is considered as accurate, cost-effective and rapid and does not require sophisticated equipment like thermal cycler. The new LAMP assay was developed, targeting the intergenic spacer region of rRNA gene that could simultaneously identify and differentiate *C. neoformans* and *C. gattii* species complex. Recently, Chen et al. evaluated 85 CSF samples from 58 confirmed cryptococcal meningitis in non-HIV-infected patients by LAMP and qPCR and compared it with the lateral flow assay (LFA), India ink and culture (Chen et al. 2016). The LFA had the highest detection rate (97.6%) followed by the LAMP (87.1%), the qPCR (80.0%), India ink staining (70.6%) and culture (35.3%). The limit of detection of LAMP was 20 fg (approx. 30 genomic copies), and no cross-reaction was observed.

Martins et al. compared the utility of different primer sets CN4 and CN5 (those usually used for the molecular differentiation of the culture isolates) for the molecular diagnosis of cryptococcal meningitis from CSF. The test was successful in diagnosing 94.8% of the acquired immunodeficiency syndrome (AIDS) patients with cryptococcal meningitis. While the multiplex PCR was used to detect both the DNA of the *C. neoformans* (primer set CAN70s-CNA70A, amplify the coding sequence of putative aminotransferase gene on chromosome 3) and *C. gattii* (Cnb49S-CNb49A, coding sequence of putative polymerase on chromosome 2), it was positive in 64.6% of the samples. The positive samples gave the band size corresponding to the *C. neoformans* and none to *C. gattii*, indicating evaluation of patients with *C. neoformans* infections only in their series (Martins et al. 2015).

In the recent years, multiplex molecular panel tests have been developed to detect the pathogens based on clinical syndromic approach. The FilmArray Meningitis/Encephalitis (ME) panel (BioFire Diagnostics, Salt Lake City, UT) has been cleared by the FDA for the diagnosis of CNS infections directly from clinical samples. The FilmArray ME panel is rapid (~60 min) and syndromic-based for the diagnosis of select meningitis and encephalitis pathogens including *Cryptococcus* (Liesman et al. 2018). In addition to the common bacterial and viral pathogens, it also has the target for *C. neoformans*/*C. gattii*. Liesman et al. (2018) evaluated FilmArray ME panel on large number CSF samples (n = 291) and demonstrated an overall 52% (26/50) agreement for *Cryptococcus neoformans*/*Cryptococcus gattii* detection when compared with *Cryptococcus* antigen by LFA. However, when compared directly to the results of routine fungal smear or culture, overall agreement improved to 92.3% (12/13). In another study performed in human immunodeficiency virus (HIV)-infected patients, the multiplex panel could detect *Cryptococcus* culture-positive cases with 100% sensitivity and specificity and differentiate between relapse and paradoxical immune reconstitution inflammatory syndrome (Rhein et al. 2016). However, culture-positive cases may be missed occasionally by this panel (Chew et al. 2018). Therefore, this test should be used as an adjunct to other tests, such as culture, *Cryptococcus* antigen detection test and/or pathogen-specific PCR assay (Hanson 2016; Demogines et al. 2015).

7.4 Molecular Diagnosis of CNS Aspergillosis

CNS aspergillosis can present as meningitis, encephalitis, cerebral abscesses or strokes. Cerebral abscesses are common presentation. The disease may occur by direct extension from sinuses and ear or haematological dissemination. The major risk factors for CNS aspergillosis are prolonged neutropenia, corticosteroid therapy, haematopoietic and solid-organ transplant recipients and haematological malignancies on chemotherapy (Shamim et al. 2010). CNS aspergillosis is difficult to diagnose as the symptoms overlap with infections due to other disease aetiologies, leading to high mortality. Early definitive diagnosis is crucial to administer appropriate antifungal therapy. Though culture-based assays are considered the mainstay of microbiologic diagnosis, mere isolation from non-sterile clinical specimens may be suspicious due to ubiquity of this pathogen (Simoneau et al. 2005). Biomarker testing including galactomannan and glucans has good specificity but variable sensitivity (Barnes 2008; Leeflang et al. 2008). The test results do not identify the species of *Aspergillus* implicated with the disease, which may be important due to variability of antifungal susceptibility among the species. Thus, molecular methods are introduced, keeping in mind those inherent shortcomings in diagnosis. The rapidity of results, high sensitivity and ability to discriminate the species by molecular tests are useful for diagnosis and initiation of targeted antifungal therapy. However, only few studies compared PCR diagnosis to culture and serology. Valero et al. (2016) developed a real-time PCR assay using fluorescent-labelled sequence-specific probes. They validated their assays in 60 clinical samples, including five CSF samples, and recorded 100% sensitivity. Overall sensitivity was 83.3% and sequencing could be avoided in 67.7% of the samples. The test could identify the pathogen within 24 h of sample collection (Valero et al. 2016). Nested PCR testing was used in 113 CSF samples from 55 immunocompromised patients with proven/probable, possible or no CNS aspergillosis. CNS aspergillosis could be diagnosed with 100% sensitivity and 93% specificity in all the proven/probable cases. PCR was positive in 4 out of 22 possible cases and 2 negative CNS aspergillosis cases. Hummel et al. (2006) used PCR-based diagnosis on the 35 CSF samples from 6 patients with proven/probable and possible CNS aspergillosis; each patient had at least 1 positive sample by PCR. One of the earliest studies using molecular techniques for CNS aspergillosis diagnosis was from Japan. PCR was performed on CSF of five patients with pulmonary aspergillosis and focal neurological signs. PCR was positive in all five patients, but CSF cultures were negative in those patients, whereas serology was positive in four patients (80%) (Kami et al. 1999a). Other studies carried out with one or two patients have been included in Table 7.1 (Verweij et al. 1999; Kami et al. 1999b; Moling et al. 2002; Komatsu

Table 7.1 Review of genomic-based diagnosis of central nervous system fungal infections

Major fungal classes	Reference, country	No of samples/patients (controls)	Specimen	Positive culture/positive microscopy/histology/staining/smear or serology	Positive PCR	Sensitivity/specificity	Comments
Dimorphic fungi							
Histoplasmosis	Buitrago et al. (2011), Spain	1	CSF	NA	1/1	–	Possible case of histoplasmosis, real-time-PCR was used
Coccidioidomycosis	Binnicker et al. (2011), USA	2	CSF	Culture and serology negative	2/2	–	Real-time PCR
	Vucicevic et al. (2010), USA	5	CSF	1 CSF culture positive for *Coccidioides*	0/5	–	1 case of proven coccidioidomycosis, 1 probable, 3 unconfirmed
	Mitchell (2015), USA	82 pleural and spinal fluids	CSF	–	–	–	Real-time PCR using BD Max
Cryptococcosis	Saha (2009), India	46 diseased, 30 controls	CSF	Culture positive 44/46, India ink 43/46, LAT 46/46, EIA 46/46	46/46	100%/100%	Urine and serum were also tested by PCR, with 100% sensitivity and specificity
	Paschoal et al. (2004), Brazil	56 samples from acute cryptococcal meningitis, 16 samples from bacterial/viral meningitis	CSF	Culture positive 43/56, India ink positive 48/56	52/56	92.9%/100%	Proven and probable cases of cryptococcal meningitis
	Iyer (2002), India	17	CSF	Culture positive 13/17	13/17	–	18S rRNA was targeted
	Rappelli et al. (1998), Italy	21 samples from acute cryptococcal meningitis, 19 samples from bacterial/viral meningitis	CSF	Culture and India ink positive 21/21	21/21	–	Nested PCR
Candidiasis	Klingspor and Jalal (2006), Sweden	24	CSF	1/25	4/24	–	18S rRNA was targeted
	Elsayed et al. (2001), Canada	4	CSF	Culture positive 0/4, serology positive 2/4	2/4	–	Ribosomal DNA used as target

	Ralph and Hussain (1996), Canada	7 samples from 1 patient	CSF	Culture positive 1/7	4/6, 1 sample not tested	–	–
Non-Aspergillus moulds							
Mucormycosis	Bialek et al. (2005), Germany	2 brain biopsy samples	Brain biopsy tissue	Histopathology positive 2/2	2/2	–	Nested PCR of 18S rRNA
Exserohilum rostratum	Gade et al. (2015), USA	359 all case samples 729 all case specimens (461 case patients and 171 PCR positive for *E. rostratum*)	CSF	Cultures positive for *E. rostratum* (2), 2 for *E. nigrum*, 1 for *C. cladosporioides*	All case sample: 83 (23%) by conventional PCR and 138 (38%) by real-time PCR All case specimens: 91 (13%) by conventional PCR and 174 (24%) by real-time PCR	23%/38%	2 samples were not tested. All the culture-positive cases were also detected by both conventional and real-time PCR
Aspergillosis	Valero et al. (2016), Spain	5 CSF samples (60 clinical samples)	CSF	Microbiologic criteria positive in all cases	5/5	100%	Pan-fungal qPCR against ITS1, ITS2
	Reinwald et al. (2013), Germany	113 samples from 55 immunocompromised patients with suspected CNS aspergillosis	CSF	Microbiologic criteria positive in 8 cases (proven/probable CNS IA)	Positive for all proven/probable cases Positive for 4/22 possible cases Positive in 2/25 of no CNS IA cases	100%/93%	Nested PCR 18S rRNA followed by ETBr staining

(continued)

Table 7.1 (continued)

Major fungal classes	Reference, country	No of samples/patients (controls)	Specimen	Positive culture/ positive microscopy/ histology/staining/ smear or serology	Positive PCR	Sensitivity/ specificity	Comments
	Hummel et al. (2006), Germany	35 samples from 6 suspected patients of CNS aspergillosis	CSF	Microbiologic criteria positive in 4 cases (proven/ probable CNS IA) 2 cases of possible IA	Multiple samples tested per patient; each patient had one positive CSF sample	NA	Nested PCR 18S rRNA
	Bialek et al. (2005), Germany	2 brain biopsy samples	Brain biopsy tissue	Histopathology positive 2/2	2/2	–	Nested PCR of 18S rRNA
	Kami et al. (1999a, b), Japan	5	CSF	Culture positive 0/5, serology positive 4/5	5/5	100%/100%	–
	Verweij et al. (1999), Netherlands	26 samples from 1 patient	CSF	Culture positive 1/7	4/26	–	Genus-specific hot start PCR
	Komatsu et al. (2004), Japan	1	CSF	Culture and serology negative	1/1	–	18S rRNA
	Moling et al. (2002), Italy	2	CSF	Culture positive 2/2, serology 1/2	1/2	–	18S rRNA

et al. 2004). One study used nested PCR on paraffin wax-embedded brain biopsy samples (Bialek et al. 2005). They could detect *Aspergillus* in the brain biopsy samples, which correlated with histopathology findings (Bialek et al. 2005). Due to the promising results in patients with CNS aspergillosis, PCR testing could be used especially in patients who are not subjected to invasive procedures (Reinwald et al. 2013).

7.5 Non-*Cryptococcal* and Non-*Aspergillus* CNS Infections

Candida species may rarely cause meningoencephalitis in patients with haematological malignancy, post-neurosurgery and premature neonates (Pappas et al. 2004). The majority of the reported cases of *Candida* meningoencephalitis have been diagnosed by culture methods. Badiee et al. used the TaqMan probes designed from 18s region of rDNA, to detect the species-specific *Candida* in the CSF and serum of patients with suspected non-*Cryptococcal* fungal meningitis. Of 38 patients evaluated, they diagnosed 4 cases of Candidal meningitis, 3 due to *C. albicans* and 1 *C. glabrata* (Badiee and Alborzi 2011).

The large outbreak of fungal meningitis associated with the epidural injections of contaminated methylprednisolone acetate solution in the United States (Centers for Disease Control and Prevention (CDC) 2012) has helped in our understanding on the utility of the molecular tests for the diagnosis of the fungal meningitis. Though *A. fumigatus* was isolated from the index case, the vast majority of the laboratories confirmed the infections due to *Exserohilum rostratum*. For the development of the molecular diagnostic test to investigate this outbreak, two sets of primers, (1) broad spectrum primers (ITS3 and ITS4) that could amplify 350 bp fragment of any fungus and (2) *Exserohilum* specific primer that amplifies 250 bp variable region of ITS2, were used (Gade et al. 2013). The amplified products were identified by DNA sequencing. A total of 115/413 (28%) cases were positive for fungal DNA by PCR and sequencing. Broad-range PCR was positive in 96 cases; additionally 25 more cases were diagnosed by *Exserohilum*-specific PCR who were negative by broad-range PCR. Of CSF samples from 345 patients, 82 (24%) were positive for *E. rostratum*, and one CSF sample had *Cladosporium* DNA. The researchers later developed a validated TaqMan real-time PCR for the detection of *E. rostratum* in the body fluids (majority of samples were CSF) and identified 57 additional cases; 19%, 29% and 47% cases were positive by culture, conventional PCR and real-time PCR, respectively. They suggested that beta-D-glucan assay was more appropriate than the real-time PCR for monitoring the response to therapy, though cautioned about the possibility of contamination in both the test formats. Therefore, the results of the tests should be interpreted with clinical finding and epidemiological data (Gade et al. 2015). A highly sensitive species-specific molecular beacon real-time PCR assay that has the potential to detect and quantify *E. rostratum* in clinical sample has also been developed (Zhao et al. 2013).

PCR assay for the diagnosis of coccidioidomycosis was attempted by Vucicevic et al. They included 153 respiratory and 5 CSF samples (Vucicevic et al. 2010). The ITS2 LightCycler real-time PCR was positive in five respiratory samples, but the CSF samples were negative in all cases. Later using the same technique, two cases of meningeal coccidioidomycosis were diagnosed successfully, and the PCR results were positive 3 days before the serology and 3 weeks before the culture results (Binnicker et al. 2011). PCR test for meningeal coccidioidomycosis requires further evaluation. In case of histoplasmosis, though molecular PCR-based techniques are available for the detection and identification of *Histoplasma* from culture and animal model, application of molecular tests directly on clinical samples is very few and less successful (López et al. 2017).

7.6 Molecular Identification of the Fungal Isolates

Identification of the fungi to the species level is important for the initiation of appropriate antifungals. Conventional mode of identification of the fungal culture usually relies on morphological and physiological characters. It requires in-depth knowledge on the minute details of each species. In clinical laboratory this method of identification is usually difficult and takes time due to lack of expertise and slow-growing nature of many species. Accurate identification may be a problem even for experts in many cases due to morphological similarities of closely related species. Molecular techniques have been used successfully for identification of the fungi. Currently DNA sequencing is considered as the gold standard for the identification of the fungi. Different conserved and variable genes have been used, ITS region of the rDNA being the commonest. ITS2 region is commonly used as it contains both conserved and variable regions. The International Society for Human and Animal Mycology (ISHAM) has created the barcode database for identification of majority of the pathogenic fungi using ITS2 region.

Differentiation between *C. neoformans* and *C. gattii* is essential for epidemiology and management, as they differ in their distribution, ecology, clinical presentation, antifungal susceptibility and therapeutic outcomes (Trilles et al. 2012). Identification and differentiation of these two species by biochemical tests take time. Molecular technique has been developed to differentiate the two species from culture, but the technique was not successful for differentiating directly on clinical specimen. With the aim to develop the sensitive technique for the detection and differentiation of these two species directly from the clinical specimens, Trilles et al. (2012) developed hyper-branched rolling circle amplification (HRCA) technique to differentiate all seven major molecular types of *C. neoformans* (Trilles et al. 2014). Phospholipase B gene (PLB) was amplified by semi-nested PCR. They designed the species-specific padlock probes that produce minimum secondary structure at the 5′-end probe binding arm. For effective padlock probe binding, the annealing temperature was adjusted close to or above the ligation temperature. These probes were ligated to the amplified product, and HCRA reactions were performed in real-time PCR machine to amplify the probe signals. Using this technique, they could differentiate all major molecular types of *C. neoformans* and *C. gattii*. This technique is promising for the detection and differentiation of major *Cryptococcus* species directly from the clinical specimen. The semi-nested PCR used in this technique increased the detection limit to ~1 pg. HCRA had been developed earlier as well that targeted ITS regions of rDNA. The technique could only differentiate the known molecular types (Kaocharoen et al. 2008). Recently, real-time PCR assay, targeting intergenic spacer-1 region of rDNA locus, has been developed, which could differentiate the cultures of *C. neoformans* sensu lato and *C. gattii* sensu lato (Tavares et al. 2016). Though the detection limit of this technique is not better than the above-mentioned probe-based techniques, this method is affordable and has less chance of contamination, as it eliminates post-amplification processing.

Identification of *Aspergillus* to the species level is essential as few newly described species *A. lentulus*, *A. calidoustus*, *A. terreus* and *A. versicolor* have elevated MICs to several antifungal drugs (Balajee et al. 2005). The ITS sequences of *Aspergillus* do not have sufficient variation and fail to differentiate various *Aspergillus* species complexes. Other protein-coding loci, such as for beta-tubulin (BenA), calmodulin (CaM) and RNA polymerase 2 (RPB2), are used to differentiate *Aspergillus* species. Using the oligonucleotide probe and PCR-enzyme immunoassay, de Aguirre et al. (2004) successfully identified seven medically important *Aspergillus* species (*A. flavus*, *A. fumigatus*, *A. nidulans*, *A. niger*, *A. terreus*, *A. ustus* and *A. versicolor*). ISHAM working group recommends the use of ITS sequence for the identification up to *Aspergillus* species complex and BenA and CaM for identification of species within species complex. For *Candida* species ITS region and D1/D2 region of large subunit of rDNA (26s) are targeted. Robust techniques such as high-resolution melting curve analysis of ITS 1 and 2 region may also be applied to speciate *Candida* (Mandviwala et al. 2010). Nonamplified nucleic acid probes targeting the 26S rRNA region have been evaluated for the identification of fungi, employing peptide nucleic acid–FISH (flourescence in-situ hybridization) technology (Farina et al. 2012). But, the technique is expensive and tedious and may not be beneficial as sequencing is cheaper and more specific. For *Fusarium* species complex, other targets such as elongation factor 1 alpha (EF-1-α), β tubulin and RNA polymerase II subunit B are used to identify different species (O'Donnell et al. 2010). EF-1-α and β tubulin genes are employed for the identification of *Cladophialophora* species (de Hoog et al. 2007). Apart from ITS region, sequencing Hcp100 and $1281–1283_{(220)}$ molecular markers may be used for successful identification of *H. capsulatum* (Frías-De-León et al. 2017). Primers and fluorescence resonance energy transfer hybridization probes targeting glyceraldehyde-3-phosphate dehydrogenase genes have been utilized for molecular identification of *Histoplasma* species (Babady et al. 2011).

7.7 Molecular Diagnosis from Tissue

Though demonstration of fungal elements in tissue specimens by histopathology can prove invasive fungal infections, it may not help in differentiating the etiologic agent to the genus or species level. Therefore, results from histopathology are limited in guiding antifungal therapy. However, detection and identification of fungi from brain tissue specimens by employing molecular techniques are less well studied. The development of molecular-based identification of fungi in the paraffin-embedded tissue is an interesting approach, which may help in accurate identification of fungus and management. Bialek et al. developed a semi-nested PCR targeted against 18S rDNA of *Zygomycetes* and *Aspergillus* spp. The PCR assays were in concordance with histopathology results and could be used as a valuable tool for identification of fungus from tissue samples (Bialek et al. 2005).In another study, 18S rDNA regions were used to identify mucoralean fungi from fresh tissue samples (Zaman et al. 2017).

7.8 Conclusion

With the rise in number of fungal infection across the world, CNS fungal disease rate has also gone up. But, the success of ante-mortem diagnosis of CNS infection is never more than 50% due to low index of suspicion, difficulty in sample collection and low sensitivity of conventional techniques. Any patient who is at high risk of CNS fungal infection or already have documented fungal infection of lung or sinuses should be screened by neuroimaging. Every attempt should be made for collection of brain biopsy sample in suspected CNS fungal infection cases. The molecular genomic test may be used as an adjunct to conventional diagnostic procedures for early diagnosis, till an independent validated molecular genetic test is developed. The research should be directed for pan-fungal and pathogen-specific markers, good extraction procedure and use of a closed sensitive platform. The genomic test can be used for rapid identification of fungi and for outbreak investigation.

References

de Aguirre L, Hurst SF, Choi JS, Shin JH, Hinrikson HP, Morrison CJ. Rapid differentiation of Aspergillus species from other medically important opportunistic molds and yeasts by PCR-enzyme immunoassay. J Clin Microbiol. 2004;42:3495–504.

Alonso R, Pisa D, Fernández-Fernández AM, Rábano A, Carrasco L. Fungal infection in neural tissue of patients with amyotrophic lateral sclerosis. Neurobiol Dis. 2017;108:249–60.

Atkins SD, Clark IM. Fungal molecular diagnostics: a mini review. J Appl Genet. 2004;45:3–15.

Babady NE, Buckwalter SP, Hall L, Le Febre KM, Binnicker MJ, Wengenack NL. Detection of Blastomyces dermatitidis and Histoplasma capsulatum from culture isolates and clinical specimens by use of real-time PCR. J Clin Microbiol. 2011;49:3204–8.

Badiee P, Alborzi A. Assessment of a real-time PCR method to detect human non-cryptococcal fungal meningitis. Arch Iran Med. 2011;14:381–4.

Balajee SA, Gribskov JL, Hanley E, Nickle D, Marr KA. Aspergillus lentulus sp. nov., a new sibling species of A. fumigatus. Eukaryot Cell. 2005;4:625–32.

Barnes RA. Early diagnosis of fungal infection in immunocompromised patients. J Antimicrob Chemother. 2008;61(Suppl 1):i3–6.

Bialek R, Weiss M, Bekure-Nemariam K, Najvar LK, Alberdi MB, Graybill JR, et al. Detection of Cryptococcus neoformans DNA in tissue samples by nested and real-time PCR assays. Clin Diagn Lab Immunol. 2002;9:461–9.

Bialek R, Konrad F, Kern J, Aepinus C, Cecenas L, Gonzalez GM, et al. PCR based identification and discrimination of agents of mucormycosis and aspergillosis in paraffin wax embedded tissue. J Clin Pathol. 2005;58:1180–4.

Binnicker MJ, Popa AS, Catania J, Alexov M, Tsaras G, Lloyd F, et al. Meningeal coccidioidomycosis diagnosed by real-time polymerase chain reaction analysis of cerebrospinal fluid. Mycopathologia. 2011;171:285–9.

Buitrago MJ, Bernal-Martínez L, Castelli MV, Rodríguez-Tudela JL, Cuenca-Estrella M. Histoplasmosis and paracoccidioidomycosis in a non-endemic area: a review of cases and diagnosis. J Travel Med. 2011;18:26–33.

Centers for Disease Control and Prevention (CDC). Multistate fungal meningitis outbreak – interim guidance for treatment. MMWR Morb Mortal Wkly Rep. 2012;61:842.

Chew KL, Lee CK, Cross GB, Lum LHW, Yan B, Jureen R. Culture-confirmed cryptococcal meningitis not detected by Cryptococcus PCR on the Biofire meningitis/encephalitis panel®. Clin Microbiol Infect. 2018;24(7):791–2.

Demogines A, Fouch S, Everhart K, Leber A, Barney T, Daly JA, et al. Multi-center clinical evaluation of a multiplex meningitis/encephalitis PCR panel for simultaneous detection of bacteria, yeast, and viruses in cerebrospinal fluid specimens. J Clin Microbiol. 2015;54:2251–61.

Elsayed S, Fitzgerald V, Massey V, Hussain Z. Evaluation of the Candigen enzyme-linked immunosorbent assay for quantitative detection of Candida species antigen. Arch Pathol Lab Med. 2001;125:344–6.

Farina C, Perin S, Andreoni S, Conte M, Fazii P, Lombardi G, et al. Evaluation of the peptide nucleic acid fluorescence in situ hybridisation technology for yeast identification directly from positive blood cultures: an Italian experience. Mycoses. 2012;55:388–92.

Frías-De-León MG, Ramírez-Bárcenas JA, Rodríguez-Arellanes G, Velasco-Castrejón O, Taylor ML, Reyes-Montes M d R. Usefulness of molecular markers in the diagnosis of occupational and recreational histoplasmosis outbreaks. Folia Microbiol (Praha). 2017;62:111–6.

Gade L, Scheel CM, Pham CD, Lindsley MD, Iqbal N, Cleveland AA, et al. Detection of fungal DNA in human body fluids and tissues during a multistate outbreak of fungal meningitis and other infections. Eukaryot Cell. 2013;12:677–83.

Gade L, Grgurich DE, Kerkering TM, Brandt ME, Litvintseva AP. Utility of real-time PCR for detection of exserohilum rostratum in body and tissue fluids during the multistate outbreak of fungal meningitis and other infections. J Clin Microbiol. 2015;53:618–25.

Gunaratne PS, Wijeyaratne CN, Seneviratne HR. Aspergillus meningitis in Sri Lanka – a post-tsunami effect? N Engl J Med. 2007;356:754–6.

Hanson KE. The first fully automated molecular diagnostic panel for meningitis and encephalitis: how well does it perform, and when should it be used? J Clin Microbiol. 2016;54:2222–4.

de Hoog GS, Nishikaku AS, Fernandez-Zeppenfeldt G, Padín-González C, Burger E, Badali H, et al. Molecular analysis and pathogenicity of the Cladophialophora carrionii complex, with the description of a novel species. Stud Mycol. 2007;58:219–34.

Hummel M, Spiess B, Kentouche K, Niggemann S, Böhm C, Reuter S, et al. Detection of Aspergillus DNA in cerebrospinal fluid from patients with cerebral aspergillosis by a nested PCR assay. J Clin Microbiol. 2006;44:3989–93.

Kami M, Ogawa S, Kanda Y, Tanaka Y, Machida U, Matsumura T, et al. Early diagnosis of central nervous system aspergillosis using polymerase chain reaction, latex agglutination test, and enzyme-linked immunosorbent assay. Br J Haematol. 1999a;106:536–7.

Kami M, Shirouzu I, Mitani K, Ogawa S, Matsumura T, Kanda Y, et al. Early diagnosis of central nervous system aspergillosis with combination use of cerebral diffusion-weighted echo-planar magnetic resonance image and polymerase chain reaction of cerebrospinal fluid. Intern Med. 1999b;38:45–8.

Kaocharoen S, Wang B, Tsui KM, Trilles L, Kong F, Meyer W. Hyperbranched rolling circle amplification as a rapid and sensitive method for species identification within the Cryptococcus species complex. Electrophoresis. 2008;29:3183–91.

Khot PD, Fredricks DN. PCR-based diagnosis of human fungal infections. Expert Rev Anti Infect Ther. 2009;7:1201–21.

Klingspor L, Jalal S. Molecular detection and identification of Candida and Aspergillus spp. from clinical samples using real-time PCR. Clin Microbiol Infect. 2006;12:745–53.

Komatsu H, Fujisawa T, Inui A, Horiuchi K, Hashizume H, Sogo T, et al. Molecular diagnosis of cerebral aspergillosis by sequence analysis with panfungal polymerase chain reaction. J Pediatr Hematol Oncol. 2004;26:40–4.

Landlinger C, Preuner S, Willinger B, Haberpursch B, Racil Z, Mayer J, et al. Species-specific identification of a wide range of clinically relevant fungal pathogens by use of Luminex xMAP technology. J Clin Microbiol. 2009;47:1063–73.

Lass-Flörl C, Mutschlechner W, Aigner M, Grif K, Marth C, Girschikofsky M, et al. Utility of PCR in diagnosis of invasive fungal infections: real-life data from a multicenter study. J Clin Microbiol. 2013;51:863–8.

Leeflang MM, Debets-Ossenkopp YJ, Visser CE, Scholten RJ, Hooft L, Bijlmer HA, et al. Galactomannan detection for invasive aspergillosis in immunocompromised patients. Cochrane Database Syst Rev. 2008;(4):CD007394.

Liesman RM, Strasburg AP, Heitman AK, Theel ES, Patel R, Binnicker MJ. Evaluation of a commercial multiplex molecular panel for diagnosis of infectious meningitis and encephalitis. J Clin Microbiol. 2018;56:1–27.

López LF, Muñoz CO, Cáceres DH, Tobón ÁM, Loparev V, Clay O, et al. Standardization and validation of real time PCR assays for the diagnosis of histoplasmosis using three molecular targets in an animal model. PLoS One. 2017;12:e0190311.

Mandviwala T, Shinde R, Kalra A, Sobel JD, Akins RA. High-throughput identification and quantification of Candida species using high resolution derivative melt analysis of panfungal amplicons. J Mol Diagn. 2010;12:91–101.

Martins M d A, Brighente KBS, de Matos TA, Vidal JE, de Hipólito DDC, Pereira-Chioccola VL. Molecular diagnosis of cryptococcal meningitis in cerebrospinal fluid: comparison of primer sets for Cryptococcus neoformans and Cryptococcus gattii species complex. Braz J Infect Dis. 2015;19:62–7.

Mitchell M, Dizon D, Libke R, Peterson M, Slater D, Dhillon A. Development of a real-time PCR assay for identification of Coccidioides immitis by use of the BD Max system. J Clin Microbiol. 2015;53:926–9. https://doi.org/10.1128/JCM.02731-14.

McCarthy MW, Walsh TJ. Molecular diagnosis of invasive mycoses of the central nervous system. Expert Rev Mol Diagn. 2017;17:129–39.

Moling O, Lass-Floerl C, Verweij PE, Porte M, Boiron P, Prugger M, et al. Case reports. Chronic and acute Aspergillus meningitis – Falldarstellungen. Chronische und akute Aspergillus-Meningitis. Mycoses. 2002;45:504–11.

Chen M, Zhou J, Li J, Li M, Sun J, Fang WJ, Al-Hatmi AMS, Xu J, Boekhout T, Liao WQ, Pan WH. Evaluation of five conventional and molecular approaches for diagnosis of cryptococcal meningitis in non-HIV-infected patients. Mycoses. 2016;59(8):494–502. https://doi.org/10.1111/myc.12497.

O'Donnell K, Sutton DA, Rinaldi MG, Sarver BAJ, Balajee SA, Schroers H-J, et al. Internet-accessible DNA sequence database for identifying fusaria from human and animal infections. J Clin Microbiol. 2010;48:3708–18.

Pappas PG, Rex JH, Sobel JD, Filler SG, Dismukes WE, Walsh TJ, et al. Guidelines for treatment of candidiasis. Clin Infect Dis. 2004;38:161–89.

Paschoal RC, Hirata MH, Hirata RC, Melhem MDSC, Dias ALT, Paula CR. Neurocryptococcosis: diagnosis by PCR method. Rev Inst Med Trop Sao Paulo. 2004;46:203–7.

Preuner S, Lion T. Towards molecular diagnostics of invasive fungal infections. Expert Rev Mol Diagn. 2009;9:397–401.

Qishui O, Ling J, Ni L, Bin Y, Wen L. Comparison of real-time florescence quantitative PCR measurements of VAD1 mRNA with three conventional methods in diagnosis and follow-up treatment of Cryptococcus neoformans infection. Mycoses. 2012;55:326–32.

Ralph ED, Hussain Z. Chronic meningitis caused by Candida albicans in a liver transplant recipient: usefulness of the polymerase chain reaction for diagnosis and for monitoring treatment. Clin Infect Dis. 1996;23:191–2.

Rappelli P, Are R, Casu G, Fiori PL, Cappuccinelli P, Aceti A. Development of a nested PCR for detection of *Cryptococcus neoformans* cerebrospinal fluid. J Clin Microbiol. 1998;36:3438–40.

Reinwald M, Buchheidt D, Hummel M, Duerken M, Bertz H, Schwerdtfeger R, et al. Diagnostic performance of an Aspergillus-specific nested PCR assay in cerebrospinal fluid samples of immunocompromised patients for detection of central nervous system Aspergillosis. PLoS One. 2013;8:1–6.

Rhein J, Bahr NC, Hemmert AC, Cloud JL, Bellamkonda S, Oswald C, et al. Diagnostic performance of a multiplex PCR assay for meningitis in an HIV-infected population in Uganda. Diagn Microbiol Infect Dis. 2016;84:268–73.

Saha DC, Xess I, Biswas A, Bhowmik DM, Padma MV. Detection of Cryptococcus by conventional, serological and molecular methods. J Med Microbiol. 2009;58:1098–105. https://doi.org/10.1099/jmm.0.007328-0.

Shamim MS, Enam SA, Ali R, Anwar S. Craniocerebral aspergillosis: a review of advances in diagnosis and management. J Pak Med Assoc. 2010;60:573–9.

Simoneau E, Kelly M, Labbe AC, Roy J, Laverdière M. What is the clinical significance of positive blood cultures with Aspergillus sp in hematopoietic stem cell transplant recipients? A 23 year experience. Bone Marrow Transplant. 2005;35:303–6.

Tavares ER, Azevedo CS, Panagio LA, Pelisson M, Pinge-Filho P, Venancio EJ, et al. Accurate and sensitive real-time PCR assays using intergenic spacer 1 region to differentiate Cryptococcus gattii sensu lato and Cryptococcus neoformans sensu lato. Med Mycol. 2016;54:89–96.

Trilles L, Meyer W, Wanke B, Guarro J, Lazéra M. Correlation of antifungal susceptibility and molecular type within the Cryptococcus neoformans/C. gattii species complex. Med Mycol. 2012;50:328–32.

Trilles L, Wang B, Firacative C, Lazéra MDS, Wanke B, Meyer W. Identification of the major molecular types of Cryptococcus neoformans and C. gattii by Hyperbranched rolling circle amplification. PLoS One. 2014;9:e94648.

Valero C, De L, Cruz-Villar L, Zaragoza Ó, Buitrago MJ. New panfungal real-time PCR assay for diagnosis of invasive fungal infections. J Clin Microbiol. 2016;54:2910–8.

Veron V, Simon S, Blanchet D, Aznar C. Real-time polymerase chain reaction detection of Cryptococcus neoformans and Cryptococcus gattii in human samples. Diagn Microbiol Infect Dis. 2009;65:69–72.

Verweij PE, Brinkman K, Kremer HPH, Kullberg B, Meis JFGM. Aspergillus meningitis: diagnosis by non-culture-based microbiological methods and management Aspergillus meningitis: diagnosis by non-culture-based microbiological methods and management. J Clin Microbiol. 1999;37:1186–9.

Vucicevic D, Blair JE, Binnicker MJ, McCullough AE, Kusne S, Vikram HR, et al. The utility of Coccidioides polymerase chain reaction testing in the clinical setting. Mycopathologia. 2010;170:345–51.

White TJ, Bruns T, Lee S, Taylor J. Amplification and direct sequencing of fungal ribosomal RNA genes for phylogenetics. In: Innis MA, Gelfand DH, Shinsky JJ, White TJ, editors. PCR protocols: a guide to methods and applications. New York: Academic Press Inc.; 1990.

Zaman K, Rudramurthy SM, Das A, Panda N, Honnavar P, Kaur H, et al. Molecular diagnosis of rhino-orbito-cerebral mucormycosis from fresh tissue samples. J Med Microbiol. 2017;66:1124–9.

Zhao Y, Petraitiene R, Walsh TJ, Perlin DS. A real-time PCR assay for rapid detection and quantification of Exserohilum rostratum, a causative pathogen of fungal meningitis associated with injection of contaminated methylprednisolone. J Clin Microbiol. 2013;51:1034–6.

Part II

Fungal Pathogens: Pathogenesis, Pathology and Diagnosis

Aspergillosis

8

Sundaram Challa

Abbreviations

BAL	Broncoalveolar lavage
BBB	Blood-brain barrier
BG	B-D-glucan
CGD	Chronic granulomatous disease
CNS	Central nervous system
CR	Complement receptor
CSF	Cerebrospinal fluid
EM	Extracellular matrix
FFPE	Formalin-fixed parafin embedded
GAG	Galactosaminogalactan
GM	Galactomannan
GMS	Gomori's methenamine silver
H&E	Hematoxylin and eosin
HSCT	Hematopoietic stem cell transplant
IA	Invasive aspergillosis
ICSOL	Intracranial space occupying lesion
IHC	Immunohistochemistry
PAMP	Pathogen-associated molecular pattern
PCR	Polymerase chain reaction
PAS	Periodic acid-Schiff
PTX	Pentraxin
ROS	Reactive oxygen species
TLRs	Toll-like receptors
TNF	Tumor necrosis factor

S. Challa (✉)
Basavatarakam Indo-American Cancer Hospital & Research Institute, Hyderabad, Telangana, India

8.1 Introduction

Central nervous system (CNS) aspergillosis is a serious complication accounting for 10–20% of invasive aspergillosis (IA) (Denning 1998). It is the most common extra pulmonary site of involvement and is associated with high morbidity and mortality (Denning 1998; Walsh et al. 1985a; Chakrabarti et al. 2011; Dignani 2014). Once considered rare, CNS aspergillosis is diagnosed more frequently in the last few decades due to increase in at risk population and better diagnostic methods. It has protean clinical manifestations depending on the immune status of the host and mode of spread. Early diagnosis is important for timely treatment and improve outcome.

Most of the series from the west report CNS aspergillosis in immunosuppressed hosts only, whereas in countries like Saudi Arabia, Sudan, Pakistan, India, and some African countries, it is reported in both immunosuppressed and immunocompetent hosts (Denning 1998; Walsh et al. 1985a; Chakrabarti et al. 2011; Dignani 2014; Sundaram et al. 1989; Sharma et al. 1997; Murthy et al. 2000; Kleinschmidt-DeMasters 2002; Challa et al. 2004; Sundaram et al. 2006; Raja and Singh 2006; Murthy 2007; Shamim et al. 2007; Shankar et al. 2007; Uppin et al. 2011). Environmental factors, distribution of fungi, and socioeconomic factors are implicated in the geographical variations of IA (Chakrabarti et al. 2011; Murthy and Sundaram 2014; Patterson et al. 2016).

M. Turgut et al. (eds.), *Fungal Infections of the Central Nervous System*,
https://doi.org/10.1007/978-3-030-06088-6_8

Insights into the pathogenesis help to understand the host pathogen interactions better and facilitate development of immunotherapies (Posch et al. 2017). This review focuses on the pathogenesis, pathology, and diagnosis of CNS aspergillosis.

8.1.1 Risk Factors

Neutropenia and administration of corticosteroids are important risk factors for increasing the risk of IA and disseminated CNS aspergillosis. Hematopoietic stem cell transplantation (HSCT), hematological malignancies, solid organ transplantation, chronic granulomatous disease (CGD), acquired immunodeficiency syndrome, autoimmune diseases, certain drugs like anti CD-52 and tumor necrosis factor (TNF)-α inhibitors, coinfection with cytomegalovirus, and critical illness are some of the important risk factors (Mylonakis et al. 2000; Marr et al. 2002; Lundin et al. 2003; van Burik et al. 2007; Kontoyiannis et al. 2010; Neofytos et al. 2010; Pappas et al. 2010; Blot et al. 2012; Singh et al. 2013; Baddley et al. 2014; Spapen et al. 2014). The percentage proportion of each risk factor causing CNS aspergillosis varies, and all at-risk population does not develop disease. Environmental factors and genetic factors are also implicated as contributing factors (Chakrabarti et al. 2011; Sundaram et al. 2006; Murthy 2007; Kwon-Chung and Sugui 2013). Hot and humid climate with constant exposure to high inoculums of pathogen predisposes to infection in immunocompetent hosts (Chakrabarti et al. 2011; Murthy et al. 2000; Sundaram et al. 2006; Murthy 2007; Shamim et al. 2007; Murthy and Sundaram 2014; Patterson et al. 2016).

8.1.2 Pathogens

CNS aspergillosis is caused by various species of *Aspergillus*, and most infections are caused by *A. fumigatus*, *A. flavus*, *A. terreus*, and *A. niger*. Less common infection is caused by *A. nidulans*, especially in a setting of CGD (Perfect et al. 2001).

8.1.3 Mode of Spread

The conidia of *Aspergillus* are inhaled into the sinus/lung. CNS involvement may occur by (1) hematogenous spread, usually from the lung or heart; (2) contiguous spread from paranasal sinus (PNS), orbit, or ear; or (3) direct implantation during surgery or trauma. CNS may be the only or primary site of involvement rarely (Bokhari et al. 2014). *Aspergillus* species are ubiquitous in the environment and have a worldwide distribution. However, the risks of exposure vary both temporally and geographically and are dependent on precipitation patterns, humidity, temperature, and wind conditions (Panackal et al. 2010). The small size of the conidia of *A. fumigatus* facilitates its entry into pulmonary alveoli, whereas the larger conidial size of *A. flavus* gets it trapped in the sinuses. The conidia get directly implanted in the subarachnoid space or brain parenchyma due to trauma or surgery by mechanical disruption of blood-brain barrier (BBB).

A. fumigatus is the commonest cause of IA and dissemination to CNS in immunosuppressed hosts, due to the physical characteristics of the conidia and swift adaptability to the host environment (Kwon-Chung and Sugui 2013). *A. fumigatus* possesses a versatile metabolism that meets its nutritional requirements under different environmental conditions (Gibbons et al. 2012). Its angioinvasive nature facilitates dissemination to CNS.

A. flavus is the second leading cause of IA and is the commonest cause of sinocranial aspergillosis, especially in immunocompetent hosts (Sundaram et al. 2006; Murthy et al. 2001; Challa et al. 2010). The factors that contribute in its pathogenesis include (1) ability to grow in a wide range of temperatures, withstanding high temperatures up to 48 °C, (2) growth facilitated by humidity, (3) 100-fold more virulence than *A. fumigatus* (in experimental conditions) in terms of inoculum required, and (4) prevalence in the air in hospital wards and homes (Patterson et al. 2016; Hedayati et al. 2007). Extension from the sinuses via the orbital apex is the most common route. Invasion into CNS occurs by invasion of orbit, base of skull, parasellar area, and cribriform plate into anterior, middle, and posterior fossae (Shankar et al. 2007; Chimelli and Mahler-Araujo 1997).

8.1.4 Initiation of Disease at Peripheral Site

Normal host even when exposed to conidia does not develop disease due to adequate host defenses. In the lung or sinus, when the conidia begin to swell, the macrophages recognize the pattern-associated molecular patterns (PAMPs) on the surface of the conidia, phagocytose them, recruit neutrophils, and elaborate chemokines and cytokines to kill and eliminate the germinating conidia. However, immunosuppressed individuals, especially those with qualitative or quantitative defects in neutrophils, cannot prevent germination of conidia into hyphae. The hyphae enter the host epithelial cells, grow within them by preventing apoptosis, then invade blood vessels from abluminal surface, produce thrombosis, cause endothelial damage, and disseminate to extrapulmonary sites including CNS (Filler and Sheppard 2006; Hohl and Feldmesser 2007; Dagenais and Keller 2009).

Immunocompetent hosts exposed to constant exposure to high inocula of conidia, aided by hot and humid climate, also cannot prevent germination of conidia. The proteases secreted by the fungus degrade the extracellular matrix and provide nutrients as well as facilitate invasion (Hedayati et al. 2007; Krishnan et al. 2009; Raksha et al. 2017).

8.1.5 Pathogenesis of CNS Aspergillosis

This is poorly understood. The immune interactions between *A. fumigatus* and lung are well studied, but most of the understanding of CNS aspergillosis is drawn from animal studies. The brain is considered to be an immune privilege site. In a healthy host, CNS fungal infections are rare. The brain is protected from invasion of pathogens by BBB, blood-cerebrospinal fluid barrier, and intrinsic immune system (Dotis and Roilides 2007; Nau et al. 2014). The pathogenesis and pathology depend on the immune status of the host, route of entry, pathogen species, and its virulence (Fig. 8.1).

8.1.6 Innate Immune System in CNS

Microglia and perivascular, meningeal, and choroid plexus macrophages along with complement constitute the innate immune system in CNS (Nau et al. 2014). Microglia is the major immune surveillance cell of CNS and is similar to myeloid derived peripheral macrophages in its functions. The cerebrospinal fluid (CSF) also contains a trafficking population of mononuclear cells, comprising T cells, B cells, monocytes, and dendritic cells (Ransohoff and Engelhardt 2012). The microglia and the other immune cells continuously sample the brain microenvironment and subarachnoid space to identify any pathogen-related antigens (Dando et al. 2014). Microglia expresses germ line-encoded pattern recognition receptors (PRRs), on the surface or in the cytoplasm, which are crucial in the recognition of pathogens. These include Toll-like receptor-2/4 (TLRs), Dectin-1 and Dectin-2, complement receptor-3 (CR-3), CD45, CD86, and others. Complement aids in the recognition and killing

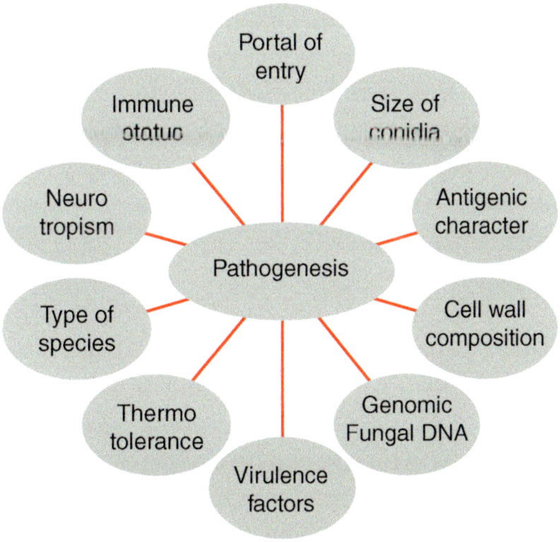

Fig. 8.1 Central nervous system aspergillosis: factors influencing pathogenesis

of the pathogen as well as bridging functions to other parts of the immune network (Ricklin et al. 2010). Neuronal and glial cells express TLRs as well as complement receptors (CR); however, production of complement in response to injury is controlled by fine-tuned regulatory mechanisms to protect the brain from injury (Veerhuis et al. 2011).

8.1.7 Host Defenses to *Aspergillus* Infection in CNS

The *Aspergillus* spp. hyphae on reaching the cerebral microvasculature interact with endothelial cells, microglia, and astrocytes. The microglial PRRs, TLR-4, CR-3, and Dectin-1, recognize the PAMPs, the β-glucan, and the mannose, on *Aspergillus* hyphae (Mogensen 2009; Hadas et al. 2010). This recognition and interaction trigger both humoral- and cell-mediated immune responses (Dotis and Roilides 2007).

The microglia and other resident immune cells express major histocompatibility complex Class I and Class II molecules. Microglia act as antigen-presenting cells and stimulate proliferation of T cells. Upon activation, the effector signal transduction pathways are initiated leading to NF-kB activation and production of cytokines and chemokines such as interferon-γ, TNF-α, interleukin-1β, IL-6, and IL-12. These enhance phagocytosis and kill the hyphae by the production of free radicals, nitric oxide, and superoxide anion. The chemokines recruit dendritic cells, neutrophils, CD4+ and CD8+ T cells, B lymphocytes, and macrophages from periphery and along with activated resident cells potentiate inflammation to kill the hyphae (Dotis and Roilides 2007).

On recognition *of Aspergillus* hyphae by PRRs, complement cascade gets activated and leads to the cleavage of C3 and formation of membrane attack complex. Astrocytes, oligodendroglia, neurons, and invading macrophages show increase in complement synthesis, whereas microglia show only minor amounts. Opsonization of conidia and hyphae with complement fragments like C3b and iC3b mediates phagocytosis, oxidative burst, and release of damaging compounds by binding to corresponding receptors on immune cells. *Aspergillus* also drives complement activation by interaction with the pattern recognition molecule pentraxin-3 (PTX-3). When *A. fumigatus* is opsonized with PTX-3, the complement cascade can be activated either by interaction between PTX-3 and C1q via the classical pathway or by interaction between PTX-3 and ficolin-2 via the lectin pathway (Ma et al. 2009; Moalli et al. 2010).

The host tries to inhibit the spread of fungus by forming abscess and sealing it off from adjacent brain parenchyma (Rambach et al. 2008; Speth and Rambach 2012). The cytokine IL-6 sequesters iron intracellularly, which is an important nutrient for *Aspergillus*, and restricts its growth (Erta et al. 2012).

8.1.8 Strategy of Pathogen

The virulence factors of *Aspergillus* help to evade immune attack and facilitate invasion (Rambach et al. 2005). The fungi hide from recognition, mask the receptors, acquire or produce complement regulatory molecules from the host, and secrete proteases to degrade complement factors (Rambach et al. 2008; Speth et al. 2008). *A. fumigatus* secretes alkaline protease which cleaves and destroys complement in the CSF and reduces the capacity to opsonize the hyphae (Rambach et al. 2010; Balenga et al. 2015). Fungal hyphae limit the surface deposition of C3 and thus interfere with complement-dependent phagocytosis. The level of complement deposition on different *Aspergillus* species correlates inversely with their pathogenicity: highly virulent species like *A. fumigatus* and *A. flavus* bind less C3 on their surface than nonpathogenic species like *A. glaucus* or *A. nidulans* (Henwick et al. 1993).

The melanin pigment blocks the C3 binding site and prevents phagocytosis and protects fungus against reactive oxygen species (ROS) to enable its survival in the host (Tsai et al. 1998; van de Veerdonk et al. 2017).

During its growth, *A. fumigatus* produces several enzymes and toxic substances. Mycotoxins, which include soluble galactosaminogalactan (GAG), gliotoxin, and fumagillin, inhibit phagocytosis, reduce ROS production by neutrophils, and inhibit T cell responses (Dagenais and Keller 2009; Tomee and Kauffman 2000). GAG induces neutrophil apoptosis and inhibits the IL-1-mediated inflammation and induces Th-17 T cells that protect the fungus (van de Veerdonk et al. 2017). Fumagillin inhibits the function of neutrophils. Gliotoxin can damage and kill microglial cells, astrocytes, and neurons via apoptosis and decreases macrophage function that is required for optimal phagocytosis and killing of the pathogens (Tomee and Kauffman 2000; Fallon et al. 2010; Schlam et al. 2016). Secretion of gliotoxin makes the fungal conidia less susceptible to opsonization, increasing the propensity of the fungus to invade the CNS through endothelial cell endocytosis (Rambach et al. 2008; Tomee and Kauffman 2000). *A. fumigatus* proteases damage and degrade the host tissue, facilitating the acquisition of essential nutrients, such as iron and zinc, which are required for its metabolism (van de Veerdonk et al. 2017). *A. fumigatus* has a remarkable adaptability to hypoxic conditions and changes its transcriptional profile and metabolism to survive and invade in the host (van de Veerdonk et al. 2017). *A. flavus* produces aflatoxin, and the strains that produce higher amounts of aflatoxin are pathogenic and exhibit increased host cell cytotoxicity (Qureshi et al. 2014).

8.1.9 Limitation of Host Defense

The protective action of microglia against infections critically depends on the cross talk with circulating granulocytes and monocytes, before circulating leukocytes enter the brain and CSF. Neutropenia, a common risk factor for disseminated aspergillosis, probably affects microglial function by impairing this cross-talk (Nau et al. 2014). Though microglia has a protective role, microglial activation and cytokine release disrupt BBB and increase the risk of CNS invasion (Streit 2002; Olson and Miller 2004). The cytokine/chemokine profile illustrates that CNS fungal infection is the result of an ineffective immune response, possibly due to an insufficient antifungal effector function of endogenous glial cells resulting from competing pro- and anti-inflammatory cytokines (Dotis and Roilides 2007; Licinio and Wong 1997). Specific T cell subsets which are activated as part of host response to *A. fumigatus* include both protective and disease-promoting T cells (van de Veerdonk et al. 2017).

The antifungal effect of complement depends on its concentration. CNS is a vulnerable organ as the complement levels are low in CSF and complement activation might be insufficient for an effective antifungal defense (Speth and Rambach 2012).

The formation of abscess to contain the spread hides the fungus from the attack of the complement and allows its growth (Rambach et al. 2008; Speth and Rambach 2012). The strategy of the pathogen versus the host defense is given in Fig. 8.2.

8.1.10 Pathology

Damage from *Aspergillus* spp. can result from fungal growth and tissue invasion or from inflammatory response (Hohl and Feldmesser 2007). The ineffective clearing of the organism and inability to down regulate the inflammatory response also contribute to the pathology. Neuropathologic features include hemorrhagic infarcts and/or necrosis, vascular thrombosis, meningitis, granuloma, and formation of solitary or multiple abscesses (Kleinschmidt-DeMasters 2002; Sundaram et al. 2006; Shankar et al. 2007; Walsh et al. 1985b; Hope et al. 2005; Ruhnke et al. 2007) (Fig. 8.3). The infarcts and abscess are usually due to *A. fumigatus* and are a result of hematogenous dissemination in immunosuppressed hosts, whereas granulomas are usually due to *A. flavus* resulting from contiguous spread from sinus, orbit, or ear in immunocompetent hosts. Spinal cord involvement is rare. It is reported as direct extension from lung or thoracic vertebrae and presents as epidural mass causing cord compression (Seres et al. 1972; Sheth et al. 1985).

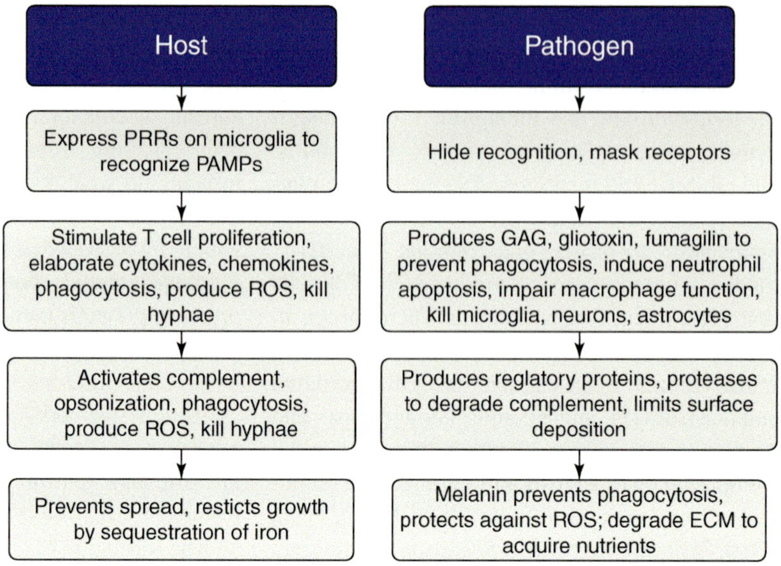

Fig. 8.2 Central nervous system aspergillosis: strategy of pathogen against host defense. Abbreviations: *PRR* pattern recognition receptor, *PAMP* pathogen-associated molecular pattern, *ROS* reactive oxygen species, *GAG* galactosaminogalactan, *ECM* extracellular matrix

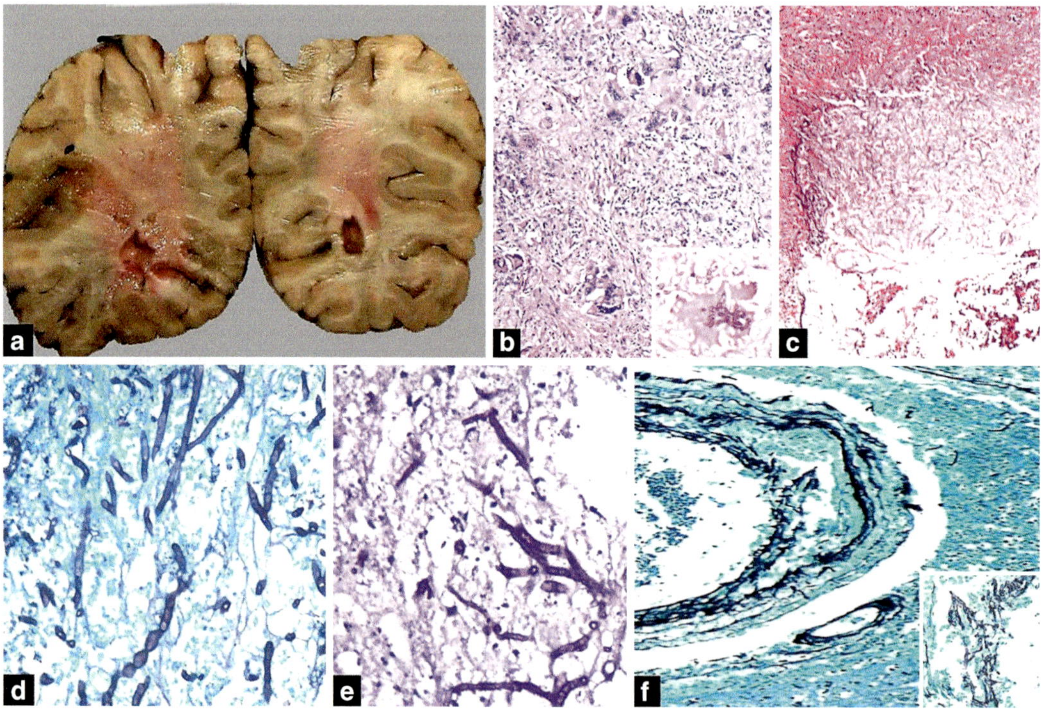

Fig. 8.3 (**a**) Coronal section of brain showing infarct (arrow). (**b**) Photomicrograph showing granulomas with predominance of multinucleated giant cells and extensive fibrosis (hematoxylin and eosin ×10); inset showing negative staining septate hyphae within giant cell (H&E ×40). (**c**) Photomicrograph showing abscess with necrotic material and numerous septate hyphae in the wall (H&E ×4). (**d**) Slender septate dichotomously branching hyphae (Gomori's methenamine silver ×40). (**e**) Slender septate hyphae (periodic acid-Schiff ×40). (**f**) Angioinvasion with destruction of elastic tissue (GMS ×10); inset showing septate hyphae of *Aspergillus* spp. in the vessel wall (GMS ×40)

8.1.11 Hemorrhagic Infarcts

These involve anterior and middle cerebral artery territories and are usually acute and necrotizing. These are due to direct invasion of vessel wall or secondary to septic embolus. In view of the angioinvasive nature of *Aspergillus*, the infarcts are usually hemorrhagic with areas of necrosis, which may convert into septic infarcts (Chimelli and Mahler-Araujo 1997). Arteritis with bland infarcts due to *Aspergillus* spp. is reported (Uppin et al. 2007). Histology shows vascular invasion with thrombosis and necrosis. The inflammatory infiltrate is usually sparse (Sundaram et al. 2006; Shankar et al. 2007; Chimelli and Mahler-Araujo 1997).

8.1.12 Mycotic Aneurysm

Mycotic aneurysms due to *Aspergillus* are rarely reported (Shankar et al. 2007; Chimelli and Mahler-Araujo 1997; Sundaram et al. 2007). These are fusiform and involve longer and proximal segments of vessels like basilar, middle, and posterior cerebral arteries. They result from direct invasion of the vessel wall by hyphae. The elastase elaborated by *Aspergillus* spp. digests the elastic lamina of artery leading to weakness of vessel wall with eventual rupture and subarachnoid hemorrhage. It is usually fatal (Sundaram et al. 2007).

8.1.13 Abscess

These may be solitary or multiple and are located at grey-white matter junction. They may be well circumscribed or poorly delineated from adjacent brain parenchyma depending on the immune status of the host. The abscess contains central necrotic material, surrounded by hemorrhagic necrosis and neutrophilic infiltrate with interspersed fungal hyphae (Shankar et al. 2007).

8.1.14 Granuloma

These are usually located in frontal or temporal regions. These may be extracerebral in continuity with sinus lesion, dural based with basal meningitis, or completely intraparenchymal (Sundaram et al. 2006; Shankar et al. 2007; Chimelli and Mahler-Araujo 1997; Sundaram and Murthy 2011). They are characterized by epitheloid cells, predominance of multinucleated giant cells, and infiltrates of neutrophils, lymphocytes, plasma cells, and eosinophils. The stroma is very dense and fibrous. Intraparenchymal granulomas with no obvious source of infection in the sinus, ear, or lung are reported (Sharma et al. 1997; Sundaram and Murthy 2011; Challa et al. 2007). They need to be differentiated from tuberculomas in countries endemic for tuberculosis, by the location, extensive fibrosis, minimal necrosis with prominence of foreign body giant cells, and nature of infiltrate along with appropriate fungal stains (Sundaram et al. 2006; Sundaram and Murthy 2011; Challa et al. 2007).

8.1.15 Meningitis

Meningitis is uncommon due to *Aspergillus* spp. However, meningitis is reported following surgical procedures or spinal anesthesia due to direct implantation of conidia. It is localized and may be an abscess or granuloma. Suboptimal hospital care practices and use of contaminated intravenous infusion sets or instruments in developing countries are implicated in this form of disease (Chakrabarti et al. 2011).

8.1.16 Diagnosis

Due to high morbidity and mortality of CNS aspergillosis, early and accurate diagnosis is essential for institution of appropriate treatment. The antifungal susceptibility varies among different spp. of *Aspergillus*. Hence it is important to diagnose *Aspergillus* and differentiate from other filamentous fungi with similar morphology and also get species identification for specific treatment.

The diagnostic tests include direct microscopy, culture, serology, and molecular tests. These tests are applied according to the clinical scenario and availability. Surgical excision and submission of tissue for histopathology and culture are done when there are mass lesions extending from sinus/

orbit/ear or intracranial space-occupying lesions (ICSOLs). In immunocompromised hosts with CNS involvement, biopsy from a peripheral site like lung may be obtained (Guarner and Brandt 2011). Serological and molecular tests are useful, in disseminated aspergillosis, subject to availability. The advantages and limitations of various diagnostic tests are given in Table 8.1.

8.1.17 Direct Microscopy

These include (1) wet mounts with or without potassium hydroxide, (2) fluorescent techniques applied to fresh fluid or tissue, and (3) frozen/formalin-fixed paraffin-embedded (FFPE) sections stained with hematoxylin and eosin (H&E), periodic acid-Schiff (PAS), and Gomori's methenamine silver (GMS) (Hope et al. 2005; Guarner and Brandt 2011; Barton 2013). The advantages include high sensitivity and rapid turnaround time, but the major disadvantage is its inability to differentiate *Aspergillus* from other filamentous fungi and species identification, compromising the diagnostic accuracy (Hope et al. 2005; Guarner and Brandt 2011; Barton 2013).

8.1.18 Wet Mounts

The wet mounts of the specimen delineate the hyphal morphology, and addition of 10% potassium hydroxide causes partial digestion of the proteinaceous material for better visualization. The fluorescent dye, Calcofluor-white, selectively binds to the polysaccharides in the fungal cell wall, but the stain is not specific to *Aspergillus* spp. (Chander et al. 1993).

8.1.19 Histopathology

Histopathology is very useful in the diagnosis, especially tissue obtained from sinus or ICSOL; however, it may not be possible to obtain tissue from lesions located in deep white matter of brain or vascular lesions. Routine histology with H&E stain helps in assessing tissue reaction, whereas special stains like PAS and GMS delineate the morphology of fungal hyphae much better. In the tissue, the *Aspergillus* spp. are seen as slender, septate, hyaline, nonpigmented, and dichotomously branching hyphae. Fungal hyphae may be seen as negative staining structures within the giant cells and in the stroma. PAS and GMS are complementary to each other with a concordance rate of 84% (Hope et al. 2005; Heaton et al. 2016). Frozen sections and squash smears are less sensitive (60%) but highly specific (98%) for the detection of fungal filaments; these, though useful in the rapid diagnosis, should not be used as a standalone method (Heaton et al. 2016; Sundaram 2003). In suspected cases of CNS aspergillosis, a combination of H&E, PAS, GMS, and Masson-Fontana stains helps in making a presumptive diagnosis (Hope et al. 2005; Guarner and Brandt 2011).

8.1.20 Limitations of Histopathology

Morphology cannot provide the fungal genus and species; speciation needs culturing and biochemical characterization (Shankar et al. 2007; Guarner and Brandt 2011). The septate hyaline dichotomously branching morphology alone cannot differentiate *Aspergillus* spp. from other hyaline molds like *Fusarium* spp. and *Scedosporium* spp. (Guarner and Brandt 2011). In addition, there may be difficulty in distinguishing *Aspergillus* spp. from *Mucorales*, which are pauci/aseptate, and dematiaceous fungi with less melanin in the cell walls, by using histopathology alone (Guarner and Brandt 2011; Tarrand et al. 2003; Sangoi et al. 2009; Lee et al. 2010; Sundaram et al. 2014; Challa et al. 2014). The concordance between morphologic diagnosis on histopathology and culture varies from 79% to 88% (Tarrand et al. 2003; Sangoi et al. 2009; Lee et al. 2010; Sundaram et al. 2014; Challa et al. 2014).Misdiagnosis and misclassification can occur in about 20% cases (Sundaram 2003; Tarrand et al. 2003; Sangoi et al. 2009; Lee et al. 2010; Sundaram et al. 2014). Tissue fungal infection burden of less than 10^3 CFU/gm of tissue usually proves to be

Table 8.1 Diagnostic tests for central nervous system aspergillosis: advantages and limitations

Test	Sample	Advantages	Limitations	Comment
Culture	Tissue Blood/BAL/CSF	Species identification Allows antifungal susceptibility/resistance	Yield less than 50%; long turnaround time; may fail to grow or sporulate	Yield on tissue better (79%); blood/BAL/CSF usually negative
Histopathology	Tissue from sinus/orbit/ICSOL Core biopsy from lung/skin in disseminated disease	Rapid, cost-effective presumptive diagnosis of invasive fungal disease; differentiates from contamination	Cannot identify genera/species; cannot differentiate from other hyaline septate fungi like *Fusarium* and *Scedosporium*; sometimes, difficult to differentiate from *Mucor*/*Candida*/dematiaceous fungi; architectural distortion; yield is 79%	Antifungal susceptibility differs among species/genera; misclassification up to 20%; use of IHC/in situ hybridization/PCR on FFPE tissue increases diagnostic accuracy; however, not yet validated
Galactomannan	Blood/BAL	Useful in disseminated disease in certain subpopulations like in HSCT/hematologic malignancy; rapid; early marker of invasive disease; sensitivity 40–100%; specificity 56–100%	False-positive results in patients (1) receiving antibiotics like piperacillin, amoxicillin, or ticarcillin; (2) receiving substances that contain products of fermentation of *A. niger*; (3) with infections with other fungi including *Penicillium*, *Paecilomyces*, *Alternaria*, and *Histoplasma* spp.; cutoff value controversial	Higher positive result than imaging and direct microscopy; low sensitivity in non-neutropenic patients
(1,3)-β-D Glucan	Serum	Rapid	Not specific for *Aspergillus*; false-positive results in patients receiving piperacillin/tazobactam	Marker of invasive disease in certain subpopulations like in HSCT/hematologic malignancy
PCR	Blood/BAL/FFPE/other fluids	Early marker of invasive disease; sensitivity 84%; specificity 86%	Yield on FFPE lower than in blood	Technique not yet recommended for routine use; combination of GM with validated PCR improves diagnosis of definite disease
Others	Fungal antibodies, metabolites		Not useful for diagnosis	

Abbreviations: *BAL* brochoalveolar lavage, *CSF* cerebrospinal fluid, *ICSOL* intracranial space-occupying lesion, *HSCT* hematopoietic stem cell transplant, *FFPE* formalin-fixed paraffin-embedded, *PCR* polymerase chain reaction, *GM* galactomannan histologically negative (Kahn et al. 1986). Tissue reaction depends on the immune status of the host and may be minimal in severely immunosuppressed host.

8.1.21 Ancillary Techniques to Histology

These include immunohistochemistry (IHC), immunofluorescence, in situ hybridization, and polymerase chain reaction (PCR). Immunohistochemical reagents that detect *Aspergillus* spp. in tissue are commercially available; however, the widespread presence of common antigens in fungi has resulted in cross-reactivity with other hyaline septated molds, *Mucorales*, and some yeasts (Phillips and Weiner 1987; Reed et al. 1993; Schuetz and Cohen 2009). In culture-proven aspergillosis, IHC positivity on FFPE tissues was reported to be 88–100% (Challa et al. 2015; Jung et al. 2015). IHC was found to be particularly useful to differentiate *Aspergillus* spp. from *Mucor* spp. when culture studies are not available (Challa et al. 2015; Jung et al. 2015).

The yield of fungal DNA from FFPE is low. These tests still need validation for routine diagnostic use (Patterson et al. 2016).

8.1.22 Culture Studies

Aspergillus spp. have the ability to grow at 37 °C and hence can be distinguished from other pathogenic fungi. It grows readily in blood agar, chocolate agar, and brain-heart infusion broth but better with Sabouraud dextrose agar, which is a fungal-specific medium (Hope et al. 2005). The recovery is improved by inhibiting growth of bacteria and environmental molds by the addition of chloramphenicol/gentamycin and cyclohexidine, respectively (Sutton 2003). The speciation is done by conidial morphology. In addition to diagnosis, culture enables susceptibility testing to antifungals as well as determines resistance. Certain species of *Aspergillus* like *A. terreus* and *A. nidulans* are resistant to amphotericin, and hence the culture studies help in therapeutic options (Walsh et al. 2003).

8.1.23 Limitations of Culture Studies

The turnaround time is long and may take a few days. The yield of organisms may be low; organisms may fail to grow or fail to sporulate, and sometimes the growth characteristics are atypical (Tarrand et al. 2003). Hence culture studies may be insensitive and nondiagnostic (Hope et al. 2005; Guarner and Brandt 2011).

8.1.24 Molecular Tests

In disseminated aspergillosis or IA involving CNS, when tissue cannot be obtained, molecular tests are useful. Blood cultures are usually negative. The molecular tests include (1,3)-β-D-glucan (BG) test, galactomannan (GM) antigenemia test, and PCR. Most of the tests are standardized and validated in serum or BAL fluid for *A. fumigatus* involving the lung. Galactomannan and validated PCR applied to blood can be used as screening tools to identify patients at high risk of developing IA (Jones and McLintock 2003). Detection of antibodies and metabolites of *Aspergillus* spp. was not found to be useful for diagnosis of IA (Hope et al. 2005).

8.1.25 BG Test

(1,3)-β-D-Glucan is a cell wall component of most fungi including *Aspergillus* spp. Serum assays are recommended for diagnosing IA in certain high-risk populations like hematologic malignancies and HSCT, but they are not specific for *Aspergillus* (Patterson et al. 2016). False-positive reactions are known to occur in some patients who are receiving piperacillin/tazobactam (Metan et al. 2010).

8.1.26 Galactomannan (GM) Test

GM is a polysaccharide antigen present on the cell wall of *Aspergillus*, and it is released into the blood during invasive infections. It can be detected in serum or brochoalveolar lavage

(BAL) fluid, CSF, or pleural fluid days before clinical symptoms appear and hence an effective method for early diagnosis of IA (Arvanitis et al. 2014; Feng 2015). It is a fairly sensitive and specific test, less time consuming and yields higher positive results compared to imaging and direct microscopy. The sensitivity and specificity range from 40% to 100% and 56% to 100%, respectively (Feng 2015). The positive cutoff value is controversial (Zhou et al. 2017). It gives a false-positive result in approximately 50% of patients receiving antibiotics like piperacillin, amoxicillin, or ticarcillin, 100% of patients receiving substances that contain products of *A. niger* fermentation (plasmalyte), and various percentages of patients with infections with other fungi, like *Penicillium*, *Paecilomyces*, *Alternaria*, and *Histoplasma* (Hachem et al. 2009). In non-neutropenic patients, the value of the detection of circulating GM is limited because of low sensitivity (Erjavec et al. 2009).

8.1.27 Polymerase Chain Reaction (PCR)

PCR amplifies target of rDNA and subsequent sequencing. Using real-time quantitative PCR allows fast and accurate diagnosis of IA and identification of species. PCR can be applied to blood, BAL, or FFPE on the extracted DNA (Feng 2015). *Aspergillus* DNA can be detected very early in patients with IA, much before onset of clinical signs and symptoms of invasive fungal infection (Cuenca-Estrella et al. 2009). Small studies of *Aspergillus* PCR on non-blood and extrapulmonary body fluids (pleural fluid, CSF, etc.) and paraffin-preserved and fresh tissues (lung, skin, sinus, lymph node) demonstrate sensitivity of 86% and specificity of 100% (Buitrago et al. 2013; Reinwald et al. 2013a, b). Concomitant use of GM and validated PCR applied to serum, other tissues, and fluids improves the sensitivity of diagnosis and enables a definite diagnosis of IA (Hope et al. 2005; Musher et al. 2004). However, the techniques still need standardization and validation for routine use.

Histopathology/cytology and culture are strongly recommended for the diagnosis of IA till molecular methods are available for routine use (Patterson et al. 2016). Despite the limitations, histopathology and culture remain gold standard for the diagnosis of CNS aspergillosis where tissue can be obtained. Molecular tests are useful in disseminated disease.

8.2 Conclusion

CNS aspergillosis occurs in both immunosuppressed and immunocompetent hosts with geographical variations. Ineffective defense mechanisms and strategy of pathogen to evade immune attack result in disease. The pathology and clinical manifestations depend on the immune status, risk factors, route of spread, and the species involved. Early diagnosis is important for institution of appropriate therapy as CNS aspergillosis is associated with high morbidity and mortality. Histopathology and culture remain gold standard where tissue can be obtained and molecular methods are important tools in disseminated disease.

Acknowledgment The author, who was former Dean and Senior Professor of Pathology at Nizam's Institute of Medical Sciences, Hyderabad, gratefully acknowledges all the colleagues, students, and technical staff for their contribution.

References

Arvanitis M, Ziakas PD, Zacharioudakis IM, Zervou FN, Caliendo AM, Mylonakis E. PCR in diagnosis of invasive aspergillosis: a meta-analysis of diagnostic performance. J Clin Microbiol. 2014;52(10):3731–42.

Baddley JW, Winthrop KL, Chen L, Liu L, Grijalva CG, Delzell E, et al. Non-viral opportunistic infections in new users of tumour necrosis factor inhibitor therapy: results of the SAfety Assessment of Biologic ThERapy (SABER) study. Ann Rheum Dis. 2014;73(11):1942–8.

Balenga NA, Klichinsky M, Xie Z, Chan EC, Zhao M, Jude J, et al. A fungal protease allergen provokes airway hyper-responsiveness in asthma. Nat Commun. 2015;6(1):6763.

Barton RC. Laboratory diagnosis of invasive aspergillosis: from diagnosis to prediction of out-

come. Scientifica. 2013;2013:459405. https://doi.org/10.1155/2013/459405.
Blot SI, Taccone FS, Van den Abeele A-M, Bulpa P, Meersseman W, Brusselaers N, et al. A clinical algorithm to diagnose invasive pulmonary aspergillosis in critically ill patients. Am J Respir Crit Care Med. 2012;186(1):56–64.
Bokhari R, Baeesa S, Al-Maghrabi J, Madani T. Isolated cerebral aspergillosis in immunocompetent patients. World Neurosurg. 2014;82(1–2):e325–33.
Buitrago MJ, Aguado JM, Ballen A, Bernal-Martinez L, Prieto M, Garcia-Reyne A, et al. Efficacy of DNA amplification in tissue biopsy samples to improve the detection of invasive fungal disease. Clin Microbiol Infect. 2013;19(6):E271–7.
van Burik J-AH, Carter SL, Freifeld AG, High KP, Godder KT, Papanicolaou GA, et al. Higher risk of cytomegalovirus and aspergillus infections in recipients of T cell-depleted unrelated bone marrow: analysis of infectious complications in patients treated with T cell depletion versus immunosuppressive therapy to prevent graft-versus-host disease. Biol Blood Marrow Transplant. 2007;13(12):1487–98.
Chakrabarti A, Chatterjee SS, Das A, Shivaprakash MR. Invasive aspergillosis in developing countries. Med Mycol. 2011;49(S1):S35–47.
Challa S, Prayaga AK, Vemu L, Sadasivan J, Jagarlapudi MKM, Digumarti R, et al. Fungal endocarditis: an autopsy study. Asian Cardiovasc Thorac Ann. 2004;12(2):95–8.
Challa S, Uppin SG, Purohit AK. Isolated cerebral Aspergillus granuloma with no obvious source of infection. Neurol India. 2007;55(3):289–91.
Challa S, Uppin SG, Hanumanthu S, Panigrahi MK, Purohit AK, Sattaluri S, et al. Fungal rhinosinusitis: a clinicopathological study from South India. Eur Arch Otorhinolaryngol. 2010;267(8):1239–45.
Challa S, Pamidi U, Uppin S, Uppin M, Vemu L. Diagnostic accuracy of morphologic identification of filamentous fungi in paraffin embedded tissue sections: correlation of histological and culture diagnosis. Indian J Pathol Microbiol. 2014;57(4):583.
Challa S, Uppin SG, Uppin MS, Pamidimukkala U, Vemu L. Diagnosis of filamentous fungi on tissue sections by immunohistochemistry using anti-aspergillus antibody. Med Mycol. 2015;53(5):470–6.
Chander J, Chakrabarti A, Sharma A, Saini JS, Panigarhi D. Evaluation of Calcofluor staining in the diagnosis of fungal corneal ulcer. Mycoses. 1993;36(7–8):243–5.
Chimelli L, Mahler-Araujo MB. Fungal infections. Brain Pathol. 1997;7(1):613–27.
Cuenca-Estrella M, Meije Y, Diaz-Pedroche C, Gomez-Lopez A, Buitrago MJ, Bernal-Martinez L, et al. Value of serial quantification of fungal DNA by a real-time PCR-based technique for early diagnosis of invasive aspergillosis in patients with febrile neutropenia. J Clin Microbiol. 2009;47(2):379–84.
Dagenais TRT, Keller NP. Pathogenesis of Aspergillus fumigatus in invasive aspergillosis. Clin Microbiol Rev. 2009;22(3):447–65.
Dando SJ, Mackay-Sim A, Norton R, Currie BJ, St. John JA, Ekberg JAK, et al. Pathogens penetrating the central nervous system: infection pathways and the cellular and molecular mechanisms of invasion. Clin Microbiol Rev. 2014;27(4):691–726.
van de Veerdonk FL, Gresnigt MS, Romani L, Netea MG, Latgé J-P. Aspergillus fumigatus morphology and dynamic host interactions. Nat Rev Microbiol. 2017;15(11):661–74.
Denning DW. Invasive aspergillosis. Clin Infect Dis. 1998;26(4):781–803.
Dignani MC. Epidemiology of invasive fungal diseases on the basis of autopsy reports. F1000Prime Rep. 2014;6:81.
Dotis J, Roilides E. Immunopathogenesis of central nervous system fungal infections. Neurol India. 2007;55(3):216–20.
Erjavec Z, Kluin-Nelemans H, Verweij PE. Trends in invasive fungal infections, with emphasis on invasive aspergillosis. Clin Microbiol Infect. 2009;15(7):625–33.
Erta M, Quintana A, Hidalgo J. Interleukin-6, a major cytokine in the central nervous system. Int J Biol Sci. 2012;8(9):1254–66.
Fallon JP, Reeves EP, Kavanagh K. Inhibition of neutrophil function following exposure to the Aspergillus fumigatus toxin fumagillin. J Med Microbiol. 2010;59(6):625–33.
Feng H. Research progress on diagnosis methods for fungal infection. Infect Int. 2015;4(4):102–7.
Filler SG, Sheppard DC. Fungal invasion of normally non-phagocytic host cells. PLoS Pathog. 2006;2(12):e129.
Gibbons JG, Beauvais A, Beau R, McGary KL, Latgé J-P, Rokas A. Global transcriptome changes underlying colony growth in the opportunistic human pathogen Aspergillus fumigatus. Eukaryot Cell. 2012;11(1):68–78.
Guarner J, Brandt ME. Histopathologic diagnosis of fungal infections in the 21st century. Clin Microbiol Rev. 2011;24(2):247–80.
Hachem RY, Kontoyiannis DP, Chemaly RF, Jiang Y, Reitzel R, Raad I. Utility of galactomannan enzyme immunoassay and (1,3) beta-D-glucan in diagnosis of invasive fungal infections: low sensitivity for Aspergillus fumigatus infection in hematologic malignancy patients. J Clin Microbiol. 2009;47(1):129–33.
Hadas S, Reichert F, Rotshenker S. Dissimilar and similar functional properties of complement receptor-3 in microglia and macrophages in combating yeast pathogens by phagocytosis. Glia. 2010;58(7):823–30.
Heaton SM, Weintrob AC, Downing K, Keenan B, Aggarwal D, Shaikh F, et al. Histopathological techniques for the diagnosis of combat-related invasive fungal wound infections. BMC Clin Pathol. 2016;16:11.
Hedayati MT, Pasqualotto AC, Warn PA, Bowyer P, Denning DW. Aspergillus flavus: human pathogen, allergen and mycotoxin producer. Microbiology. 2007;153(6):1677–92.
Henwick S, Hetherington SV, Patrick CC. Complement binding to Aspergillus conidia correlates with pathogenicity. J Lab Clin Med. 1993;122(1):27–35.

Hohl TM, Feldmesser M. Aspergillus fumigatus: principles of pathogenesis and host defense. Eukaryot Cell. 2007;6(11):1953–63.

Hope WW, Walsh TJ, Denning DW. Laboratory diagnosis of invasive aspergillosis. Lancet Infect Dis. 2005;5(10):609–22.

Jones BL, McLintock LA. Impact of diagnostic markers on early antifungal therapy. Curr Opin Infect Dis. 2003;16(6):521–6.

Jung J, Park YS, Sung H, Song JS, Lee S-O, Choi S-H, et al. Assessment of the accuracy of histomorphologic diagnosis of aspergillosis and mucormycosis by immunohistochemical tests. Clin Infect Dis. 2015;61(11):civ660.

Kahn FW, Jones JM, England DM. The role of bronchoalveolar lavage in the diagnosis of invasive pulmonary aspergillosis. Am J Clin Pathol. 1986;86(4):518–23.

Kleinschmidt-DeMasters BK. Central nervous system aspergillosis: a 20-year retrospective series. Hum Pathol. 2002;33(1):116–24.

Kontoyiannis DP, Marr KA, Park BJ, Alexander BD, Anaissie EJ, Walsh TJ, et al. Prospective surveillance for invasive fungal infections in hematopoietic stem cell transplant recipients, 2001–2006: overview of the transplant-associated infection surveillance network (TRANSNET) database. Clin Infect Dis. 2010;50(8):1091–100.

Krishnan S, Manavathu EK, Chandrasekar PH. *Aspergillus flavus*: an emerging non-*fumigatus Aspergillus* species of significance. Mycoses. 2009;52(3):206–22.

Kwon-Chung KJ, Sugui JA. Aspergillus fumigatus—what makes the species a ubiquitous human fungal pathogen? PLoS Pathog. 2013;9(12):e1003743.

Lee S, Yun NR, Kim K-H, Jeon JH, Kim E-C, Chung DH, et al. Discrepancy between histology and culture in filamentous fungal infections. Med Mycol. 2010;48(6):886–8.

Licinio J, Wong M-L. Pathways and mechanisms for cytokine signaling of the central nervous system. J Clin Invest. 1997;100(12):2941–7.

Lundin J, Hagberg H, Repp R, Cavallin-Ståhl E, Fredén S, Juliusson G, et al. Phase 2 study of alemtuzumab (anti-CD52 monoclonal antibody) in patients with advanced mycosis fungoides/Sezary syndrome. Blood. 2003;101(11):4267–72.

Ma YJ, Doni A, Hummelshøj T, Honoré C, Bastone A, Mantovani A, et al. Synergy between ficolin-2 and pentraxin 3 boosts innate immune recognition and complement deposition. J Biol Chem. 2009;284(41):28263–75.

Marr KA, Carter RA, Boeckh M, Martin P, Corey L. Invasive aspergillosis in allogeneic stem cell transplant recipients: changes in epidemiology and risk factors. Blood. 2002;100(13):4358–66.

Metan G, Ağkuş Ç, Buldu H, Koç AN. The interaction between piperacillin/tazobactam and assays for Aspergillus galactomannan and 1,3-beta-d-glucan in patients without risk factors for invasive fungal infections. Infection. 2010;38(3):217–21.

Moalli F, Doni A, Deban L, Zelante T, Zagarella S, Bottazzi B, et al. Role of complement and Fc receptors in the protective activity of the long pentraxin PTX3 against Aspergillus fumigatus. Blood. 2010;116(24):5170–80.

Mogensen TH. Pathogen recognition and inflammatory signaling in innate immune defenses. Clin Microbiol Rev. 2009;22(2):240–73.

Murthy JMK. Fungal infections of the central nervous system: the clinical syndromes. Neurol India. 2007;55(3):221–5.

Murthy JMK, Sundaram C. Fungal infections of the central nervous system. Hand book Clin Neurol. 2014;121:1383–401.

Murthy JM, Sundaram C, Prasad VS, Purohit AK, Rammurti S, Laxmi V. Aspergillosis of central nervous system: a study of 21 patients seen in a university hospital in South India. J Assoc Physicians India. 2000;48(7):677–81.

Murthy JM, Sundaram C, Prasad VS, Purohit AK, Rammurti S, Laxmi V. Sinocranial aspergillosis: a form of central nervous system aspergillosis in South India. Mycoses. 2001;44(5):141–5.

Musher B, Fredricks D, Leisenring W, Balajee SA, Smith C, Marr KA. Aspergillus galactomannan enzyme immunoassay and quantitative PCR for diagnosis of invasive aspergillosis with bronchoalveolar lavage fluid. J Clin Microbiol. 2004;42(12):5517–22.

Mylonakis E, Paliou M, Sax PE, Skolnik PR, Baron MJ, Rich JD. Central nervous system aspergillosis in patients with human immunodeficiency virus infection. Report of 6 cases and review. Medicine (Baltimore). 2000;79(4):269–80.

Nau R, Ribes S, Djukic M, Eiffert H. Strategies to increase the activity of microglia as efficient protectors of the brain against infections. Front Cell Neurosci. 2014;8:138.

Neofytos D, Fishman JA, Horn D, Anaissie E, Chang C-H, Olyaci A, et al. Epidemiology and outcome of invasive fungal infections in solid organ transplant recipients. Transpl Infect Dis. 2010;12(3):220–9.

Olson JK, Miller SD. Microglia initiate central nervous system innate and adaptive immune responses through multiple TLRs. J Immunol. 2004;173(6):3916–24.

Panackal AA, Li H, Kontoyiannis DP, Mori M, Perego CA, Boeckh M, et al. Geoclimatic influences on invasive aspergillosis after hematopoietic stem cell transplantation. Clin Infect Dis. 2010;50(12):1588–97.

Pappas PG, Alexander BD, Andes DR, Hadley S, Kauffman CA, Freifeld A, et al. Invasive fungal infections among organ transplant recipients: results of the transplant-associated infection surveillance network (TRANSNET). Clin Infect Dis. 2010;50(8):1101–11.

Patterson TF, Thompson GR, Denning DW, Fishman JA, Hadley S, Herbrecht R, et al. Practice guidelines for the diagnosis and management of aspergillosis: 2016 update by the Infectious Diseases Society of America. Clin Infect Dis. 2016;63(4):e1–60.

Perfect JR, Cox GM, Lee JY, Kauffman CA, de Repentigny L, Chapman SW, et al. The impact of culture isola-

tion of *Aspergillus* species: a hospital-based survey of aspergillosis. Clin Infect Dis. 2001;33(11):1824–33.
Phillips P, Weiner MH. Invasive aspergillosis diagnosed by immunohistochemistry with monoclonal and polyclonal reagents. Hum Pathol. 1987;18(10):1015–24.
Posch W, Steger M, Wilflingseder D, Lass-Flörl C. Promising immunotherapy against fungal diseases. Expert Opin Biol Ther. 2017;17(7):861–70.
Qureshi H, Hamid SS, Ali SS, Anwar J, Iqbal M, Khan NA. Is Aflatoxin B1 a biomarker for pathogenic potential of Aspergillus flavus? J Cell Sci Ther. 2014;5(6):188.
Raja NS, Singh NN. Disseminated invasive aspergillosis in an apparently immunocompetent host. J Microbiol Immunol Infect. 2006;39(1):73–7.
Raksha, Singh G, Urhekar AD. Virulence factors detection in Aspergillus isolates from clinical and environmental samples. J Clin Diagn Res. 2017;11(7):DC13–8.
Rambach G, Hagleitner M, Mohsenipour I, Lass-Flörl C, Maier H, Würzner R, et al. Antifungal activity of the local complement system in cerebral aspergillosis. Microbes Infect. 2005;7(13):1285–95.
Rambach G, Maier H, Vago G, Mohsenipour I, Lass-Flörl C, Defant A, et al. Complement induction and complement evasion in patients with cerebral aspergillosis. Microbes Infect. 2008;10(14–15):1567–76.
Rambach G, Dum D, Mohsenipour I, Hagleitner M, Würzner R, Lass-Flörl C, et al. Secretion of a fungal protease represents a complement evasion mechanism in cerebral aspergillosis. Mol Immunol. 2010;47(7–8):1438–49.
Ransohoff RM, Engelhardt B. The anatomical and cellular basis of immune surveillance in the central nervous system. Nat Rev Immunol. 2012;12(9):623–35.
Reed JA, Hemann BA, Alexander JL, Brigati DJ. Immunomycology: rapid and specific immunocytochemical identification of fungi in formalin-fixed, paraffin-embedded material. J Histochem Cytochem. 1993;41(8):1217–21.
Reinwald M, Buchheidt D, Hummel M, Duerken M, Bertz H, Schwerdtfeger R, et al. Diagnostic performance of an Aspergillus-specific nested PCR assay in cerebrospinal fluid samples of immunocompromised patients for detection of central nervous system aspergillosis. PLoS One. 2013a;8(2):e56706.
Reinwald M, Spiess B, Heinz WJ, et al. Aspergillus PCR-based investigation of fresh tissue and effusion samples in patients with suspected invasive aspergillosis enhances diagnostic capabilities. J Clin Microbiol. 2013b;51:4178–85.
Ricklin D, Hajishengallis G, Yang K, Lambris JD. Complement: a key system for immune surveillance and homeostasis. Nat Immunol. 2010;11(9):785–97.
Ruhnke M, Kofla G, Otto K, Schwartz S. CNS aspergillosis: recognition, diagnosis and management. CNS Drugs. 2007;21(8):659–76.
Sangoi AR, Rogers WM, Longacre TA, Montoya JG, Baron EJ, Banaei N. Challenges and pitfalls of morphologic identification of fungal infections in histologic and cytologic specimens. Am J Clin Pathol. 2009;131(3):364–75.
Schlam D, Canton J, Carreño M, Kopinski H, Freeman SA, Grinstein S, et al. Gliotoxin suppresses macrophage immune function by subverting phosphatidylinositol 3,4,5-trisphosphate homeostasis. MBio. 2016;7(2):e02242.
Schuetz AN, Cohen C. Aspergillus immunohistochemistry of culture-proven fungal tissue isolates shows high cross-reactivity. Appl Immunohistochem Mol Morphol. 2009;17(6):524–9.
Seres JL, Ono H, Benner EJ. Aspergillosis presenting as spinal cord compression. J Neurosurg. 1972;36(2):221–4.
Shamim MS, Siddiqui AA, Enam SA, Shah AA, Jooma R, Anwar S. Craniocerebral aspergillosis in immunocompetent hosts: surgical perspective. Neurol India. 2007;55(3):274–81.
Shankar SK, Mahadevan A, Sundaram C, Sarkar C, Chacko G, Lanjewar DN, et al. Pathobiology of fungal infections of the central nervous system with special reference to the Indian scenario. Neurol India. 2007;55(3):198–215.
Sharma BS, Khosla VK, Kak VK, Banerjee AK, Vasishtha RK, Prasad KS, et al. Intracranial fungal granuloma. Surg Neurol. 1997;47(5):489–97.
Sheth NK, Varkey B, Wagner DK. Spinal cord aspergillus invasion—complication of an aspergilloma. Am J Clin Pathol. 1985;84(6):763–9.
Singh NM, Husain S, Husain S, AST Infectious Diseases Community of Practice. Aspergillosis in solid organ transplantation. Am J Transplant. 2013;13(s4):228–41.
Spapen H, Spapen J, Taccone FS, Meersseman W, Rello J, Dimopoulos G, et al. Cerebral aspergillosis in adult critically ill patients: a descriptive report of 10 patients from the AspICU cohort. Int J Antimicrob Agents. 2014;43(2):165–9.
Speth C, Rambach G. Complement attack against Aspergillus and corresponding evasion mechanisms. Interdiscip Perspect Infect Dis. 2012;2012:463794.
Speth C, Rambach G, Würzner R, Lass-Flörl C. Complement and fungal pathogens: an update. Mycoses. 2008;51(6):477–96.
Streit WJ. Microglia as neuroprotective, immunocompetent cells of the CNS. Glia. 2002;40(2):133–9.
Sundaram C. Diagnostic utility of squash (smear) technique in the inflammatory lesions of central nervous system. Indian J Pathol Microbiol. 2003;46(4):569–72.
Sundaram C, Murthy JMK. Intracranial Aspergillus granuloma. Pathol Res Int. 2011;2011:157320.
Sundaram C, Ratnakar KS, Rao RR, Ranganadham P, Gayathri K, Dinakar I. Diffuse fulminant aspergillosis of the central nervous system. J Assoc Physicians India. 1989;37(2):186–7.
Sundaram C, Umabala P, Laxmi V, Purohit AK, Prasad VS, Panigrahi M, et al. Pathology of fungal infections of the central nervous system: 17 years' experience from Southern India. Histopathology. 2006;49(4):396–405.
Sundaram C, Goel D, Uppin SG, Seethajayalakshmi S, Borgohain R. Intracranial mycotic aneu-

rysm due to Aspergillus species. J Clin Neurosci. 2007;14(9):882–6.
Sundaram C, Shantveer G, Umabala P, Lakshmi V. Diagnostic utility of melanin production by fungi: study on tissue sections and culture smears with Masson-Fontana stain. Indian J Pathol Microbiol. 2014;57(2):217.
Sutton DA. Specimen collection, transport, and processing: mycology. In: Murray PR, Baron EJ, Jorgensen JH, Pfaller MA, Yolken RH, editors. Manual of clinical microbiology. 8th ed. Washington, DC: ASM Press; 2003. p. 1659–67.
Tarrand JJ, Lichterfeld M, Warraich I, Luna M, Han XY, May GS, Kontoyiannis DP. Diagnosis of invasive septate mold infections. A correlation of microbiological culture and histologic or cytologic examination. Am J Clin Pathol. 2003;119(6):854–8.
Tomee JF, Kauffman HF. Putative virulence factors of Aspergillus fumigatus. Clin Exp Allergy. 2000;30(4):476–84.
Tsai HF, Chang YC, Washburn RG, Wheeler MH, Kwon-Chung KJ. The developmentally regulated alb1 gene of Aspergillus fumigatus: its role in modulation of conidial morphology and virulence. J Bacteriol. 1998;180(12):3031–8.
Uppin MS, Anuradha SVN, Uppin SG, Paul TR, Prayaga AK, Sundaram C. Fungal infections as a contributing cause of death: an autopsy study. Indian J Pathol Microbiol. 2011;54(2):344–9.
Uppin MS, Challa S, Uppin SG, Alladi S, Yarlagadda JR. Cerebral Aspergillus arteritis with bland infarcts: a report of two patients with poor outcome. Neurol India. 2007;55(3):298–300.
Veerhuis R, Nielsen HM, Tenner AJ. Complement in the brain. Mol Immunol. 2011;48(14):1592–603.
Walsh TJ, Hier DB, Caplan LR. Aspergillosis of the central nervous system: clinicopathological analysis of 17 patients. Ann Neurol. 1985a;18(5):574–82.
Walsh TJ, Hier DB, Caplan LR. Fungal infections of the central nervous system: comparative analysis of risk factors and clinical signs in 57 patients. Neurology. 1985b;35(11):1654–7.
Walsh TJ, Petraitis V, Petraitiene R, Field-Ridley A, Sutton D, Ghannoum M, et al. Experimental pulmonary aspergillosis due to *Aspergillus terreus:* pathogenesis and treatment of an emerging fungal pathogen resistant to amphotericin B. J Infect Dis. 2003;188(2):305–19.
Zhou W, Li H, Zhang Y, Huang M, He Q, Li P, et al. Diagnostic value of galactomannan antigen test in serum and bronchoalveolar lavage fluid samples from patients with nonneutropenic invasive pulmonary aspergillosis. J Clin Microbiol. 2017;55(7):2153–61.

9 Candidiasis

M. Altay Atalay

Abbreviations

AIDS	Acquired immunodeficiency syndrome
CMC	Chronic mucocutaneous candidiasis
CNS	Central nervous system or Coagulase-negative staphylococci
CSF	Cerebrospinal fluid
CT	Computed tomography
CVC	Central venous catheter
DM	Diabetes mellitus
ESCMID	European Society of Clinical Microbiology and Infectious Diseases
GIT	Gastrointestinal tract
HIV	Human immunodeficiency virus
IC	Invasive candidiasis
ICU	Intensive care unit
IDSA	Infectious Diseases Society of America
IL	Interleukin
MRI	Magnetic resonance imaging
NAC	Non-albicans Candida
NPV	Negative predictive value
PPV	Positive predictive value
TPN	Total parenteral nutrition

M. A. Atalay (✉)
Department of Medical Microbiology, Erciyes University School of Medicine, Kayseri, Turkey

9.1 Introduction

Candidiasis can be seen at all ages worldwide and is manifested by the acute and/or chronic infections of the skin, mucosa, internal organs, and systems, which are caused by a genus of yeast called *Candida* species. *Candida* species are found in the mouth and the gastrointestinal tract (GIT) in approximately 30–50% of healthy individuals. They are also found in the genital system flora in 20–30% of the females. In addition, they live in the soil and on a wide variety of plants and foods. Their isolation from the soil is regarded as a sign of fecal contamination. Although there are more than 200 species of *Candida*, there are frequently isolated pathogens from human beings. Among them are *C. albicans* predominantly followed by *C. glabrata*, *C. tropicalis*, *C. parapsilosis*, *C. krusei*, *C. guilliermondii*, *C. lusitaniae*, *C. dubliniensis*, *C. pelliculosa*, *C. kefyr*, *C. lipolytica*, *C. famata*, *C. inconspicua*, *C. rugosa*, and *C. norvegensis*. Recently, another species of *Candida*, *Candida auris*, has been introduced, presenting with multidrug resistance and a high mortality rate as a dangerous health threat in some countries. Another recent development in the literature is renaming and the taxonomic rearrangement of *Candida* species. These rearrangements also include moving of a number of species to other genera. Some of these can be referred here as follows: *Candida krusei* → *Pichia kudriavzevii*, *Candida norvegensis* → *Pichia norvegensis*, *Candida guilliermondii* → *Meyerozyma guillier-*

M. Turgut et al. (eds.), *Fungal Infections of the Central Nervous System*,
https://doi.org/10.1007/978-3-030-06088-6_9

mondii, *Candida lusitaniae* → *Clavispora lusitaniae*, *Candida kefyr* → *Kluyveromyces marxianus*, and *Candida pelliculosa* → *Wickerhamomyces anomalus*. Furthermore, a group of following species of *Candida* including *C. glabrata*, *C. parapsilosis*, and *C. haemulonii* are today regarded as species complexes (Correia et al. 2006; Mersequel et al. 2015; Pfaller et al. 2005; Tavanti et al. 2005).

9.2 Epidemiology

Despite the fact that numerous species of *Candida* are isolated from animals at primitive levels and from the environment, the candidiasis infections in the human beings are usually of endogenous origin. In the human body, *Candida* species can be isolated from the GIT, oropharynx, vagina, and the skin. The leading species among these isolates is *C. albicans*. The variabilities in the rates of identified *C. albicans* isolates are influenced by personal characteristics of the individuals including their eating habits and ages. A study has reported that the rates of identified *C. albicans* isolates obtained from the oral cavity vary in a range from 1.9% to 41.4%. These rates have been found to be in a range of 0–55% and 2.2–68% for the GIT and vagina, respectively, in the same study (Odds 2010). While *C. tropicalis* species are isolated mostly from the oropharynx, *C. glabrata* species are isolated from the vagina and GIT. Moreover, it has been demonstrated that the colonization of the *Candida* species in the hospital inpatients is more common compared to healthy individuals. *Candida* species associated nosocomial infections may emerge with the involvement of the hospital personnel and via contaminated materials. The impact of these factors on the emergence of nosocomial infections has been determined by molecular diagnostic methods.

The prevalence of *Candida* infections has been reported to be on the rise in the last 20 years. The two major underlying causes of this fact are the pathological/iatrogenic immunosuppression and the increase in the use of broad-spectrum antibiotics. Another study reported that in 92% of all hematogenous infections, where *Candida* species were the causative microorganisms, the use of broad-spectrum antibiotics was identified, suppressing the normal bacterial flora and eliminating the effects of natural antagonists, which prevent the fungal colonization in the mucosa (Das et al. 2011). In addition, in a cohort study in which intraabdominal major surgical procedures were associated with *Candida* infections, it was reported that 50% of 107 patients with candidemia had recently undergone a surgical procedure (Block et al. 2009). Neutropenic patients suffering from acquired immunodeficiency syndrome (AIDS) and oncologic diseases are almost always reported to have oropharyngeal and esophageal candidiasis.

Recent epidemiologic studies have demonstrated that the frequency of candidiasis ranged from 1.2 to 25 in 100,000 patients (Arendrup 2010). *Candida* species are the fourth most common fungal agents associated with the hematogenous infections in the hospitals in the United States. More than 50% of the invasive *Candida* infections are due to non-albicans *Candida* (NAC) species (Pfalller et al. 2014). It has been observed that NAC species has received medical attention with increased rates of isolation approximately over the past 30 years. One of the underlying causes of this fact is explained by the evidence that the widespread use of azole derivatives, including fluconazole, leads to the excessive proliferation of the species such as *C. glabrata* and *C. krusei* in the perianal region and other areas of the body due to their relatively lower susceptibility to these antifungal agents. A prospective surveillance program including patients with invasive candidiasis determined a spurt in 2496 NAC infections between years 2004 and 2008. The species identified in these infection spurts are listed as follows according to their frequencies: *C. glabrata* complex (46.4%), *C. parapsilosis* complex (24.7%), *C. tropicalis* (13.9%), *C. krusei* (*Pichia kudriavzevii*; 5.5%), *C. lusitaniae* (*Clavispora lusitaniae*; 1.6%), *C. dubliniensis* (1.5%), and *Candida guilliermondii* (*Meyerozyma guilliermondii*; 0.4%). The same study has identified two or more *Candida* species in 4.4% of candidiasis cases. Although variations are observed in different studies, *C. albicans* is the most frequent agent isolated from candidiasis cases (Nieto et al. 2015).

9.3 Pathogenicity

An important feature of host defense against candidiasis is the intact skin barrier. Otherwise, an entry gate for these pathogenic microorganisms like *C. albicans* is created when the integrity of this barrier against the outer world is disrupted resulting from the insults due to medical devices or surgical procedures. The adherence capacities of the *Candida* species to epithelial cells (especially of *C. albicans*) or to the synthetic polymeric structures like intravascular or urethral catheters (*C. tropicalis*) have been associated with their virulence. Although these fungi present with their abilities to secrete proteases and lipases, facilitating their invasion, the clinical significance of these enzymes has not been clarified, yet (Matthews 1994).

The intensity of colonization by the associated agent plays an important role in the development of candidiasis. Candidiasis typically affects the inpatients who have stayed in the hospital for long-term periods. Fifty-one percent of the hematogenous *Candida* infections are associated with the patient acceptance to the intensive care unit (ICU) (Das et al. 2011). Another factor contributing to the pathogenesis is the presence of *Candida* species, which may cause biofilm formations in central venous catheters, contact lenses, intrauterine devices, and medical devices like pacemakers. The use of toremifene, a broad-spectrum antibiofilm compound, has been shown to reduce biofilm formation by *Candida* species. This is an important development for patients with recurrent infections associated with *Candida* and with other biofilm-forming bacteria, especially due to the presence of catheters (Donlan and Costerton 2002; Glockner 2011).

The clinical outcome of the infection is determined primarily by the state of host defense conditions. After the invasion of the dermis or the circulating blood by the pathogen, the primary defense systems are involved, consisting mainly of the neutrophils followed by the monocytes and eosinophils, which can terminate *Candida* species by oxidative and non-oxidative pathways. In particular, the risk proneness of the neutropenic patients for the development of candidiasis stresses the importance of neutrophils for the host defense systems against *Candida* species.

9.4 *Candida* Infections

Candida species cause numerous infections in the range from the mucosal colonization to multiple organ involvements.

9.4.1 Superficial *Candida* Infections

These infections usually originate from the own microbial flora of the individuals although they may be acquired contagiously on some occasions.

9.4.1.1 Oral Candidiasis

Oral candidiasis may present with various different clinical forms:

- *Acute pseudomembranous oral candidiasis*: It is most commonly encountered in breastfed infants and in the old-age individuals. Otherwise, these infections may occur in human immunodeficiency virus (HIV) (+) patients with a CD4 (+) cell count of <200/mm^3, in cancer patients, and in patients who use steroid inhalers. There are studies demonstrating the correlation between the frequencies of asymptomatic oral *Candida* carriage and HIV viremia in HIV-infected individuals. Furthermore, compared to CD4 cell counts, the high plasma levels of HIV-1 RNA identified during the early stages of HIV infections have been reported to be a better preliminary indicator for the development of oral candidiasis (Oberoi 2010). In patients infected with HIV, oral candidiasis has been associated with the long-term or intermittent use of fluconazole or other azole derivatives and with other patient factors including being over the age of 35, being addicted to intravenous substance use, and being black-raced. The most frequently isolated agent in oral candidiasis cases is *C. albicans*, followed by *C. glabrata* complex, *C. parapsilosis* complex, *C. tropicalis*, *C. krusei* (*Pichia kudriavzevii*), and *C. dubliniensis*. In the oropharyngeal candidiasis cases in the patients suffering from cancer, the most frequently isolated agents are particularly the fluconazole and itraconazole resistant clades of the *C. glabrata* complex. It has been reported that prophylaxis with fluconazole reduces the oropharyngeal *C. albicans* carriage rates from 46% to rates between 0% and 10% in leukemia patients who underwent bone marrow transplantation, whereas, it leads to the increased colonization rates of *C. glabrata* complex and *C. krusei* (*Pichia kudriavzevii*) mainly in the perianal region and in other parts of the body (Garcia-Cuesta et al. 2014).

- The clinical picture of the disease manifests with pseudomembranes appearing as white patches in the hard palate and gingiva and occasionally in the throat. The patches consist of desquamated epithelial cells, leukocytes, yeasts, and bacteria. Removal of these membranous structures results in bleeding from the underlying tissues. Oral candidiasis is usually self-limiting except in patients suffering from AIDS.
- *Chronic atrophic candidiasis*: This clinical form of oral candidiasis is also known as "denture stomatitis" in patients using dentures and having intraoral lesions. The most common manifestation is "angular cheilitis" identified by crusting in the corners of the lips.
- *Chronic hyperplastic candidiasis*: It is also known as candidal leukoplakia as well, and malignancies may develop from 15% to 20% of the lesions.

9.4.1.2 *Candida* Esophagitis

This disease, which can also be classified under deep candidiasis, may be associated with oropharyngeal candidiasis or may emerge as an independent entity. It is most common in patients suffering from AIDS. *C. albicans* is the most common underlying cause of fungal esophagitis followed by other *Candida* species including *C. tropicalis*, *C. krusei*, and *C. stellatoidea*, which have been reported as the other causative agents. A number of studies have identified risk factors for developing *C. albicans* esophagitis; however, the evidence for non- *C. albicans* species as the causative agents is limited (Kakati et al. 2015).

9.4.1.3 *Candida* Vulvovaginitis and Balanitis

Seventy-five percent of females suffer from at least one *candidal* vulvovaginitis episode in their life spans. Recurrences and persistent symptoms may occur in some cases due to treatment failures. *C. albicans* is the causative agent in 80% of the cases. It is followed by *C. glabrata* complex in 5% of the cases. In recent years, *C. africana* species have been reported as another causative agent of vaginitis in the literature. Diabetes mellitus (DM), pregnancy, and the use of broad-spectrum antibiotics are the most common significant risk factors. Itching, erythema, and burning sensation in the vagina and vulva and dysuria and dyspareunia are the common findings in patients suffering from this clinical condition. A thick and whey-like vaginal discharge may occur.

Penile candidiasis (balanitis) is most commonly associated with DM in men. Vulvovaginitis may occur in the sexual partners of females suffering from this type of infection. Patients with long-term catheter implementations may also develop chronic infections. Itching, erythema, and vesiculopustular lesions are evident in the glans penis (Achkar and Fries 2010).

9.4.1.4 Cutaneous *Candida* Infections

- Intertrigo is a common disease in obese females. Vesicles and pustules develop in occluded body areas prone to maceration such as the inguinal areas, areas under the breasts and axillae.
- The *candidal* infection of the skin between the toes presents with painful lesions due to the erythematous lesions and cracks in the skin. This clinical condition is often seen in individuals who are frequently in contact with water.

- Congenital cutaneous candidiasis is a rare clinical form seen in breastfed infants at birth or in the period just after the birth. This clinical form of the disease presents with vesiculopustular lesions on an erythematous base. Fifty percent of the cases are associated with the vaginal candidiasis of the mother.
- Diaper rash occurs in the perineal area of the infants. This condition is associated with the use of diapers and is rarely caused by *C. albicans* (Janniger et al. 2005).

9.4.1.5 Onychomycosis and Paronychia

Candida species are the causative agents in 5–10% of nail infections. The thumb and the middle finger are more commonly affected by this infection, which is more common in individuals who are more frequently in contact with water. *C. albicans* and *C. parapsilosis* are the major agents causing this infection. Candidal paronychia usually starts in the proximal parts of the nails, causing the nail bed to swell, and the condition eventually leads to the development of erythema and pain. The cuticle is separated from the nail bed. White, green, and black spots emerge in the proximal parts of the nail. Pitting is observed in the fingernails. Onycholysis and subungual hyperkeratosis may occur in distal *Candida* infections (Loo 2004).

9.4.1.6 Chronic Mucocutaneous Candidiasis (CMC)

CMC is an infection that occurs in association with congenital endocrinopathies or with the impairments of the cellular immune system, involving primarily the scalp, feet, and face. Nails and fingertips are sometimes involved, too. It may develop in the first 3 years of life and rarely turns into a deep infection. Interleukin-17 (IL-17) is produced by Th17 cells and is a significant factor affecting the mucosal immunity of the host against *Candida* species. It has been reported by the recent studies that any insults to the IL-17 immunity lead to the development of CMC (Okada et al. 2016).

9.4.2 Invasive *Candida* Infections

These infections are also referred as systemic candidiasis and may present with localized symptoms as well, including endophthalmitis, arthritis, or osteomyelitis.

9.4.2.1 Candidemia

This clinical condition is characterized by the cultivation of *Candida* species from the blood in the absence of any evident organ involvement. The most common symptom is the high fever. It must be remembered that the mortality rate is high (40–50%) in candidemia and candidemia may not be identified in approximately 50% of the individuals with organ involvement. One cannot argue that deep infections may develop in all patients with positive blood cultures; however, those patients should be treated to ameliorate the acute effects of the infection and to prevent any long-term sequelae. The major factors providing the grounds for candidemia in patients other than the newborns are the presence of central venous catheters, antibiotic use, antifungal treatment, relatively longer treatment periods in ICU, abdominal/pelvic operations, malignancy, total parenteral nutrition, immunosuppressive treatment, neutropenia, liver transplantation, DM, and *Candida* colonizations in multiple regions of the body including the patients without neutropenia. The most frequently isolated species in hematogenous infections is *C. albicans*; however, an increase in NAC species has been reported in the last decade. The most commonly identified NAC species are *C. glabrata* complex, *C. parapsilosis* complex, and *C. tropicalis*. Those species are followed by *C. krusei* (*Pichia kudriavzevii*), *C. lusitaniae* (*Clavispora lusitaniae*), *C. dubliniensis*, *C. guilliermondii* (*Meyerozyma guilliermondii*), *C. kefyr* (*Kluyveromyces marxianus*), *C. inconspicua*, and *C. lipolytica*. The major predisposing factor in cases with isolated NAC infections is reported as the previous use of antifungal agents (Pfaller and Diekema 2007; Bassetti et al. 2011).

9.4.2.2 Acute Disseminated Candidiasis

It is a fulminant infection usually with an antibacterial resistant fever. It can be seen in patients with and without neutropenia. The most common complications are meningitis, brain abscesses, renal abscesses, myocarditis, endocarditis, endophthalmitis, and cutaneous abscesses.

9.4.2.3 Chronic Disseminated Candidiasis

It develops during the neutropenic period in patients with leukemia. There may not be any evidence of organ involvement in the presence of persistent fever. The neutrophil count may return to normal levels; however, fever and weight loss persist. Hepatomegaly and splenomegaly can be seen. Alkaline phosphatase levels are usually very high. Multiple lesions are identified in computed tomography. Cultivation positivity of the biopsy samples is approximately 30%. Blood cultures are negative.

9.4.2.4 Gastrointestinal Candidiasis

It is a rare clinical condition with ulcer formation in the mucosa. It is most commonly seen in cancer patients at advanced stages and in patients suffering from AIDS. It is reported that, in newborns, diarrhea cases may be encountered associated with *C. albicans,* which can be treated with oral nystatin treatment (Parra-Herran et al. 2010).

9.4.2.5 Endocarditis

Two percent of all endocarditis cases develop due to *Candida* species. Those infections are on the rise in patients with prosthetic heart valves and in patients with intravenous substance dependency. Specific diagnostic findings include large pieces of vegetation and embolization of the greater vessels. Blood cultures and cultivations from the cloth samples obtained from the embolism cases are the pathognomonic evidence. However, filtering out of the yeast in the capillary bed following their entry to the circulation prevents them to enter the venous circulation. Eventually, their isolation rates from the blood are relatively lower (Rivoisy et al. 2018).

9.4.2.6 Myocarditis

Myocarditis occurs usually as a symptom of a hematogenously disseminated infection or as a complication of endocarditis. Approximately 50% of the patients with *Candida* myocarditis die of disseminated infection. Making the diagnosis can be a challenging process. Cardiac abscesses identified in patients with widespread candidiasis or candidemia are treated as the complications secondary to the existing infection. The isolation of the fungus from the lesions allows making the precise diagnosis (Einarsdóttir et al. 2002).

9.4.2.7 Thrombophlebitis

Thrombophlebitis is associated with the presence of intravascular devices. Partial or complete blockages are formed in greater vessels. Besides the clinical examination, venography and magnetic resonance imaging (MRI) are other useful tests. Fungi can be cultivated from the venous blood (Block et al. 2009).

9.4.2.8 Osteomyelitis

Osteomyelitis develops usually as a result of the hematogenous dissemination. Sometimes it may develop in association with aspiration or cortisone injections, and more rarely it may develop after a trauma (Fig. 9.1a, b). It is more common in cancer patients and in low birth weight infants. Blood cultures are usually negative. The confirmation of diagnosis requires examination of the biopsy samples and cultivation (Fig. 9.1c) (Kohli and Hadley 2005).

9.4.2.9 Arthritis

Arthritis develops as a result of direct inoculation of the microorganism following hematogenous spread, dissemination from an infected bone, or trauma. Usually larger joints are involved such as the shoulder and knee with the development of many nonspecific symptoms. Cultivation of the *Candida* species from the synovial fluid is important in making the diagnosis (Kohli and Hadley 2005).

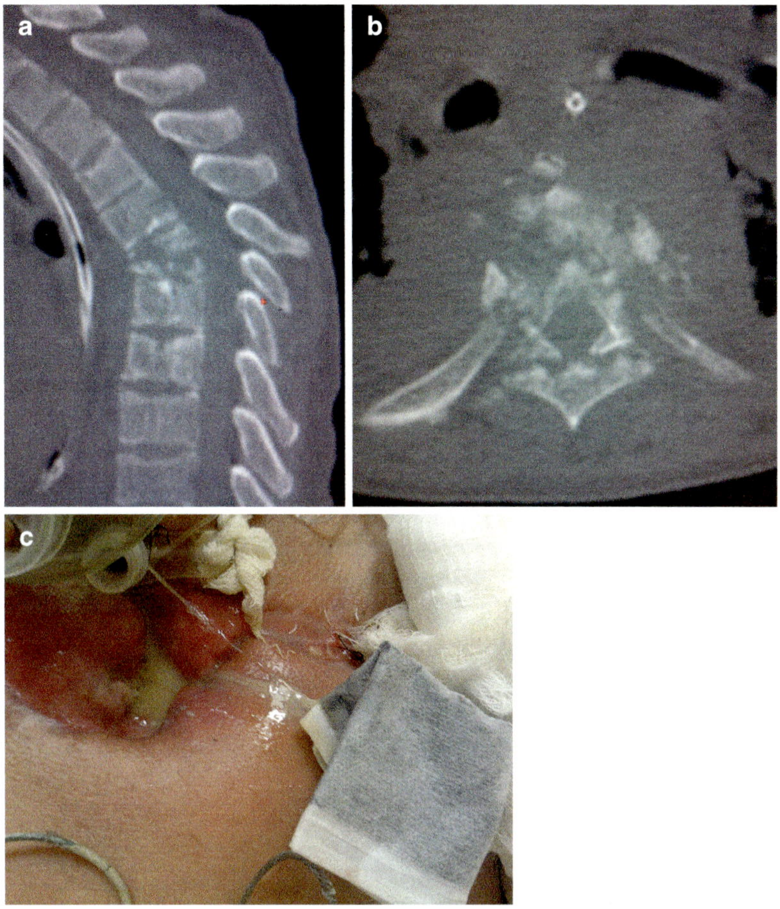

Fig. 9.1 The patient was a 39-year-old, homeless, chronic alcoholic, male individual. He fell 2 m to the ground, and he was treated in a Brazilian trauma hospital, where he showed signs of septic shock, hyperemia, and crackles in the sternal region, with 10 cm in diameter. Computed tomography (CT) of the spine revealed compression fracture of the thoracic vertebral body (**a**, **b**). The sternal bone fragment culture which was taken from the infected region was positive for *C. albicans* (**c**). (Courtesy of Á. Larocca, M.D.)

9.4.2.10 Endophthalmitis and Chorioretinitis

Their occurrences follow a hematogenous spread or ocular trauma. The most common ocular complications of candidemia are endogenous *Candida* chorioretinitis and endophthalmitis. Prospective studies report that those infections occur in 3.7–28% of patients with candidemia (Gauthier et al. 2005). The infection may start as chorioretinitis. Eventually, macula can be involved. Blindness may develop. Yellow-white lesions are seen in the retina at the examination of the fundus. The yeasts may be evident at the microscopic examination of the vitreous, and they may be cultivated from the vitreous biopsy specimens. Cultivation of *Candida* from blood confirms the diagnosis.

9.4.2.11 Central Nervous System Infections

Central nervous system (CNS) candidiasis is an uncommon clinical condition. It is usually seen in premature newborns and immunosuppressed patients. In recent years, especially autopsy studies have reported that there is a rise in the *Candida* infections of the CNS. The risk factors for this clinical condition are parenteral nutrition, aggressive chemotherapies, corticosteroid and immunosuppressant use, inappropriate use of broad-spectrum antibiotics, intravenous catheters, severe burns, being a newborn, abdominal surgery, and intravenous medication use. The most important causative agent of SSS infections is *C. albicans*. *Candida* meningitis may be a symptom of disseminated candidiasis, or it may develop as an independent clinical identity. The infection develops in low birth weight infants and in patients with ventriculoperitoneal shunts. It may occur associated with a hematogenous spread or with direct inoculation of the yeast in the subdural region due to trauma. There is usually a persistent fever unresponsive to antibiotics. However, fever may not be present if the patient receives steroid treatment. In patients with *Candida* meningitis, the examination of cerebrospinal fluid (CSF) reveals a white cell count of 50–200/mm^3 (neutrophilic or lymphocytic pleocytosis). In the CSF, the protein levels are increased (around 100 mg/dL), whereas the glucose levels are normal or low (they may be under 40 mg/dL in 60% of the patients). Gram staining and microscopic examination of CSF reveal yeasts in 40% of cases. The rate of positive cultivation is 80% with *C. albicans* in 90% of those cases. The most important indicator of the treatment success is achieving normal cell count and normal biochemical parameters in CSF, rather than its becoming sterile again. It will take 1–3 months for the cell count and biochemical parameters of CSF to return normal levels. *Candida* species are inclined to cause focal necrotic areas in the microcirculation and to cause microabscesses densely localized especially in the cerebellum, basal ganglia, and in the gray and white matter. Microabscesses are usually not visible in the CT examinations, whereas, MRI allows a better option for radiological examination. CT scans of patients with *Candida* meningitis are usually normal. However, hydrocephalus may be identified in approximately 20% of patients. In the differential diagnosis, herpes simplex encephalitis, tuberculous meningitis, and other fungal infections of the CNS associated with *Cryptococcus neoformans*/*Cryptococcus gattii* must be considered along with a noninfectious underlying cause, which is the subdural hematoma. *Candida* species may lead to non-specific lesions in CNS by affecting the vascular structures and causing bleeding, vasculitis, mycotic aneurysms, and thromboses in the smaller vessels. *Staphylococcus aureus* and tuberculosis infections and multiple sclerosis should be considered in the differential diagnosis of these lesions (Aldress et al. 2000; Portocarrero et al. 2000).

9.4.2.12 Urinary Tract Infections

It is well-known that DM, long-term antibiotic use, the use of Foley catheters, and the presence of other foreign bodies in the urinary tract are the risk factors. Fungus balls and infections may develop in the renal collecting system and in the lower urinary tract, respectively.

Renal candidiasis usually develops as the result of a hematogenous spread of the organism in 80% of the patients. Abscess formation is common. Masses of hyphae sometimes block the pelvis and ureters, leading to hydronephrosis or anuria.

Lower urinary tract infection usually develops due to a urethral catheter or by disseminating from the genital area or GIT. The patients are at risk if they have diabetes or injuries/anomalies in the urinary tract. Most cases of candiduria are asymptomatic.

Although the most common causative agent of the urinary tract infection is *C. albicans*, *C. glabrata* complex is isolated in 30% of the patients with urethral catheters and diabetes. The isolation of *C. tropicalis* from urine is accepted as the sign of disseminated candidiasis. The presence of leukocytes with accompanying yeasts in the urine of symptomatic patients shows an active infection of the upper urinary tract. Values of 10^3, 10^4, and 10^5 cfu/ml allow differentiating between neither upper and lower urinary tract infections nor colonization and active infection. However, the presence of only a few yeasts can be a significant finding when considered along with the general clinical condition of the patients without catheters. It is difficult to determine whether the infection is due to the bladder or kidney involvement. Besides the medical treatment with antifungal medications, all foreign bodies like catheters must be removed from the body, if possible, in the management of urinary tract infections (Sobel et al. 2011).

9.4.2.13 Pulmonary Candidiasis

Pulmonary candidiasis is a rare clinical manifestation. The infection develops as the result of a hematogenous spread and aspiration of the secretions in the mouth in neutropenic patients and low birth weight infants, respectively. No specific clinical and radiological evidence is identified. The identification of the presence of yeasts in the sputum or in the sample fluids obtained from bronchoscopic procedures is not pathognomonic as *Candida* species can be isolated in 3–85% of the sputum cultures due to oropharyngeal contaminations. The material obtained from the open pulmonary biopsies or from the percutaneous aspirations of the pulmonary lesions are the appropriate samples for examination (Kontoyiannis et al. 2002).

9.5 The Risk Factors for Candidemia and Invasive Candidiasis in the ICU Patients

Candidemias account for 50–70% of the invasive candida infections. *Candida* species rank the fourth after coagulase-negative staphylococci (CNS), *Staphylococcus aureus*, and enterococci in leading to 8–10% of nosocomial infections in the United States (25–50% of the cases are ICU patients), and they are the major causes of morbidity and mortality (Pappas 2006). Mortality due to candidemia is reported as 30%; however, it may reach rates of 50–70% in ICU patients. The most important risk factors for invasive candidiasis (IC) include prolonged periods of stay in the ICU, antibiotic use, hemodialysis, central venous catheters (CVCs), underlying major diseases, total parenteral nutrition (TPN), GIT perforations or operations, acute pancreatitis (invasive candidiasis occurs as a complication in 25% of cases), steroid or immunosuppressant use, mechanical ventilation, multiple blood transfusions, *Candida* species colonization in different areas of the body, and diabetes. The issue is bigger in the pediatric ICU patients, ranking the second in the septicemia cases in the United States. It has been reported that the most commonly associated risk factors with candidemia in this patient group include prolonged TPN, CVC, and topical antifungal use. In newborns, low birth weight (<1250 g), premature birth, low APGAR scores, *Candida* species colonization in different body regions or in catheters, H2 receptor blockers, GIT diseases, and congenital malformations are other risk factors. The microbiological diagnosis of invasive candidiasis in ICU patients can be established only during the late phases of infection despite the advanced technology. Retrospective studies associated the late diagnosis and timing of antifungal treatment with the increased mortality rates. Therefore, prediction models have been developed to identify the high-risk patients prone to invasive candidiasis. In order to assess the process after the colonization in patients undergoing surgical interventions, Pittet et al. (1994) proposed the term "*Candida* colonization index" in 1994. This index is the ratio of the number of different body regions colonized with the same strain of *Candida* species (culture positive) to the sum of the number of the body regions where samples for cultivation are collected. The threshold value is 0.5 meaning that the index will be increased if the ratio is above. Empirical treatments given to the patients with higher ratios above the threshold value achieved significant reductions in the incidence of invasive candidiasis. However, the model has some disadvantages including the very low levels of positive predictive value (PPV) and the increases in the laboratory workload. Nevertheless, the colonization index is important for the assessment of the early colonization dynamics in the ICU patients prone to invasive candidiasis. In addition, the higher negative predictive values (NPVs) indicate that the model will be useful in the prediction of the low-risk patients. Another concept in diagnosis is the "*Candida* score." For the first time in 2006, Leon et al. (2006) scored the risk assessments and suggested that colonization, major surgical procedures before being accepted in the ICU, evidence of severe sepsis, and TPN were the independent risk factors. The authors reported that they obtained a score by multiplying several factors with either 1 or 0 when these factors were present or absent respectively. They calculated the specificity and the sensitivity of estimating the possibility of the present disseminated infection when the score was >2.5. There are a number of studies on the colonization index and the *Candida* scores. The most important outcome is the higher NPV values in the assessment of those parameters, meaning that they do not allow making a diagnosis; however, they allow the exclusion of possible clinical entities in the differential diagnosis.

9.6 Treatment

Fungal Infection Study Groups of both the Infectious Diseases Society of America (IDSA) and European Society of Clinical Microbiology and Infectious Diseases (ESCMID) have published practice guidelines for the treatment of invasive candidiasis in various patient groups (Cornely et al. 2012; Cuenca-Estrella et al. 2012; Hope et al. 2012; Lortholary et al. 2012). The recent European guidelines recommend a 7–10-day treatment with fluconazole 100 mg/day as the first-line treatment for the treatment of oropharyngeal candidiasis of both adult and pediatric HIV-infected patients. Potential alternatives to fluconazole are listed in the guideline as follows: miconazole 10 or 50 mg/day for 7–14 days, itraconazole oral solution 100 or 200 mg/day for 14 days, and/or posaconazole 200 mg to be administered on the first day of the treatment continued with 100 mg/day (Lortholary et al. 2012). However, topical use of antifungal medications (e.g., amphotericin B lozenges or nystatin) has not been recommended due to their poor tolerability (bitter taste, side effects associated with GIS, the requirement for the administration of frequent doses) and lower efficacy. Echinocandins should not be preferred in the treatment of triazole-susceptible *Candida* species as they are more costly compared to fluconazole and only the parenteral forms of this medication are available. The ESCMID guideline recommends echinocandins (caspofungin, anidulafungin, and micafungin) as the first-line medications for the treatment of non-neutropenic adult candidemia patients (Hope et al. 2012). Compared to echinocandins, the effect sizes of liposomal amphotericin B and voriconazole are similar; however, they are recommended less frequently. On the other hand, fluconazole is recommended with marginal strength (Lortholary et al. 2012; Ullmann et al. 2012).

Alternatively, the first-line treatment with echinocandins in the hematogenous infections caused by *C. parapsilosis* has been shown to have no negative effects on the treatment outcomes. The ESCMID recommendations for fluconazole differ from the IDSA recommendations, and the 2009 IDSA guideline is being updated currently. In addition, both ESCMID and IDSA recommend the use of echinocandins in neutropenic patients (Fernández-Ruiz et al. 2014).

It is recommended as a standard modality that the treatment is continued for 14 days after termination of candidemia. If the patient is in a stable clinical condition and able to receive orally administered medications, the treatment is switched to fluconazole following a 10-day intravenous therapy in the lower line of treatment (Ullmann et al. 2012). Removal of any permanent intravenous catheters is recommended definitely. If removal of the catheter is not possible, treatment with liposomal amphotericin B or echinocandins may be started (Hope et al. 2012; Lortholary et al. 2012; Pappas et al. 2009).

For the treatment of CNS candidiasis, the recommended dose of lipid formulations of amphotericin B with or without flucytosine is 3–5 mg/kg. Flucytosine dose should be maintained at a level of 40–60 μg/ml. As a former line of treatment, a high-dose fluconazole treatment of 400–800 mg/day can be administered. The use of echinocandins in central nervous infections is limited due to their poor permeability through the blood-brain barrier although improvement with caspofungin has been reported in a patient with *Candida* meningitis resistant to amphotericin B deoxycholate and fluconazole (Cornely et al. 2012; Sugar and Liu 2000).

The appropriate treatment options to prevent the development of invasive candidiasis in high-risk neonates include fluconazole, nystatin, or alternatively lactoferrin ± *Lactobacillus*. The complication of invasive candidiasis in the newborn period is the development of the disseminated disease most likely including central nervous system infections. Amphotericin B deoxycholate, liposomal amphotericin B, amphotericin B lipid complex, fluconazole, miconazole, and caspofungin can be used in the treatment (Hope et al. 2012).

Although the efficacy of fluconazole has been established, primary antifungal prophylaxis is not recommended in Europe to prevent the development of oropharyngeal and esophageal candidiasis in HIV patients. The disadvantages of the primary prophylaxis include the possible drug interactions between the highly effective antiretroviral medications and azoles, development of resistance to fluconazole and/or other azoles, the presence of effective treatments for oropharyngeal candidiasis, cost, and potential toxic effects of triazoles. Thus, the best prophylaxis of oropharyngeal and esophageal candidiasis is the use of appropriate antiretroviral therapies (Lortholary et al. 2012).

Laser treatment has been used in the treatment of several diseases in dermatology in recent years. It has been reported that Nd-YAG laser therapy can be used as an alternative for patients disqualified to be treated with antifungal treatments (Naouri and Mazer 2013). Due to the capacity of *Candida* species to develop resistance to various treatment agents and due to some of the established toxic effects of the antifungal agents, attempts have been made in recent years to develop alternative medications. It is established that formic acid, as well as acetic acid, leads to apoptosis in *Candida* species. It has been reported that formic acid, a low-cost substance, can be used for treatment at low doses, although it is toxic at higher doses (Lastauskienė et al. 2014).

9.6.1 Antifungal Resistance

The mechanism of antifungal resistance is either primary or secondary. The development of resistance may be associated with single individual factors although it may be acquired as well due to the ability of the causative fungi to inhibit the antifungal mechanism of action of a specific drug and/or a class of drugs or due to the low concentrations of the drug (Cowen et al. 2014). *Candida* species are able to develop resistance against antifungal agents by (1) decreasing the intracellular concentrations of medications, (2) decreasing the concentrations and structures of targeted antifungal proteins, or (3) changing the sterol composition in the cell membrane (Perlin et al. 2015; Sanglard and Odds 2002). Recently, it has been suggested that CARD9 is a central regulator of neutrophil-dependent antifungal immunity in the CNS (Fig. 9.2) (Drummond and Lionakis 2018). 5-Flucytosine resistance occurs either by reducing the uptake of the drug into the cell or via

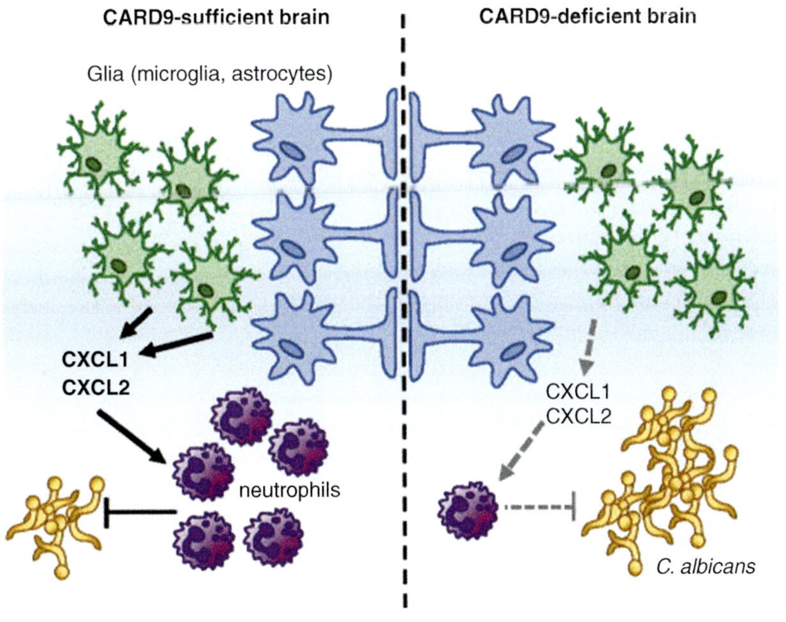

Fig. 9.2 Resident glial cells and recruited neutrophils may produce CXC chemokines upon *C. albicans*-infected brain in the CARD9-sufficient brain (left) and amplify neutrophil recruitment, resulting in control of fungal growth in the CNS, while there are important defects in the production of neutrophil recruitment and neutrophil-targeted chemokines in the CARD9-deficient glial cells (right), resulting in breakdown of control of fungal growth. (From Drummond and Lionakis (2018), with permission)

enzymatic changes involving the conversion of 5-flucytosine to 5-fluorouracil or of 5-fluorouracil to the 5-fluorouridine monophosphate. The examination of the azole resistance has revealed that various mechanisms may lead to the development of resistance by *Candida* species the against azole derivative drugs. The most common mechanisms are the excessive expression of the *MDR* or *CDR* encoded drug efflux pumps and the development of a point mutation in the gene encoding the target enzyme (ERG11). Echinocandin resistance is always acquired during treatment in susceptible *Candida* species. The mechanism of developing resistance is alterations in the amino acids in the HS1 and HS2 regions of the FKS subunit of glucan synthase, leading to a reduced drug sensitivity to this enzyme. Fungal adaptation to the effects of drugs develops due to the increased numbers of resistant FKS types in response to increased cellular stress. Primary resistance against the azole derivatives and/or echinocandins is most frequent with *C. glabrata complex* among *Candida* species (Alexander et al. 2013).

9.7 Conclusion

Candidiasis of CNS is uncommon and is one of the most serious consequences of invasive candidiasis. The risk factors include prematurity, immunosuppression, breach in mucocutaneous barrier as in patients on parenteral nutrition, patients with indwelling catheters or those receiving broad spectrum antibiotics or with prolonged ICU stay. Diagnosis of CNS candidiasis by imageology is difficult and differential diagnosis includes bacterial and tuberculous infections. High index of clinical suspicion is required for prompt diagnosis and treatment.

References

Achkar JM, Fries BC. *Candida* infections of the genitourinary tract. Clin Microbiol Rev. 2010;23:253–73.

Aldress K, Al Shaalan M, Memish Z, Alola S, Bannatyne R. *Candida* meningitis in children. Report of two cases. J Chemother. 2000;12:339–44.

Alexander BD, Johnson MD, Pfeiffer CD, Jiménez-Ortigosa C, Catania J, Booker R, Castanheira M, Messer SA, Perlin DS, Pfaller MA. Increasing echinocandin resistance in *Candida glabrata*: clinical failure correlates with presence of FKS mutations and elevated minimum inhibitory concentrations. Clin Infect Dis. 2013;56:1724–32.

Arendrup MC. Epidemiology of invasive candidiasis. Curr Opin Crit Care. 2010;16:445–52.

Bassetti M, Taramasso L, Nicco E, Molinari MP, Mussap M, Viscoli C. Epidemiology, species distribution, antifungal susceptibility and outcome of nosocomial candidemia in a tertiary care hospital in Italy. PLoS One. 2011;6:e24198.

Block AA, Thursky KA, Worth LJ, Slavin MA. Thrombolytic therapy for management of complicated catheter-related *Candida albicans* thrombophlebitis. Intern Med J. 2009;39:61–3.

Cornely OA, Bassetti M, Calandra T, Garbino J, Kullberg BJ, Lortholary O, Meersseman W, Akova M, Arendrup MC, Arikan-Akdagli S, Bille J, Castagnola E, Cuenca-Estrella M, Donnelly JP, Groll AH, Herbrecht R, Hope WW, Jensen HE, Lass-Flörl C, Petrikkos G, Richardson MD, Roilides E, Verweij PE, Viscoli C, Ullmann AJ, ESCMID Fungal Infection Study Group. ESCMID* guideline for the diagnosis and management of *Candida* diseases 2012: non-neutropenic adult patients. Clin Microbiol Infect. 2012;18:S19–37.

Correia A, Sampaio P, James S, Pais C. Candida bracarensis, sp. nov., a novel anamorphic yeast species phenotypically similar to *Candida glabrata*. Int J Syst Evol Microbiol. 2006;56:313–7.

Cowen LE, Sanglard D, Howard SJ, Rogers PD, Perlin DS. Mechanisms of antifungal drug resistance. Cold Spring Harb Perspect Med. 2014;5:a019752.

Cuenca-Estrella M, Verweij PE, Arendrup MC, Arikan-Akdagli S, Bille J, Donnelly JP, Jensen HE, Lass-Flörl C, Richardson MD, Akova M, Bassetti M, Calandra T, Castagnola E, Cornely OA, Garbino J, Groll AH, Herbrecht R, Hope WW, Kullberg BJ, Lortholary O, Meersseman W, Petrikkos G, Roilides E, Viscoli C, Ullmann AJ, ESCMID Fungal Infection Study Group. ESCMID* guideline for the diagnosis and management of *Candida* diseases 2012: diagnostic procedures. Clin Microbiol Infect. 2012;18:S9–18.

Das I, Nightingale P, Patel M, Jumaa P. Epidemiology, clinical characteristics, and outcome of candidemia: experience in a tertiary referral center in the UK. Int J Infect Dis. 2011;15:e759–63.

Donlan RM, Costerton JW. Biofilms: survival mechanisms of clinically relevant microorganisms. Clin Microbiol Rev. 2002;15:167–93.

Drummond RA, Lionakis MS. Candidiasis of the central nervous system in neonates and children with primary immunodeficiencies. Curr Fungal Infect Rep. 2018;12:92–7.

Einarsdóttir HM, Danielsen R, Gottfredsson M. Successful treatment of *Candida glabrata* myocarditis with voriconazole. Scand J Infect Dis. 2002;34:778–80.

Fernández-Ruiz M, Aguado JM, Almirante B, Lora-Pablos D, Padilla B, Puig-Asensio M, Montejo M, García-Rodríguez J, Pemán J, Ruiz Pérez de Pipaón M, Cuenca-Estrella M, CANDIPOP Project; GEIH-GEMICOMED (SEIMC); REIPI. Initial use of echinocandins does not negatively influence outcome in *Candida parapsilosis* bloodstream infection: a propensity score analysis. Clin Infect Dis. 2014;58:1413–21.

Garcia-Cuesta C, Sarrion-Pérez MG, Bagán JV. Current treatment of oral candidiasis: a literature review. J Clin Exp Dent. 2014;6:e576–82.

Gauthier GM, Nork TM, Prince R, Andes D. Subtherapeutic ocular penetration of caspofungin and associated treatment failure in *Candida albicans* endophthalmitis. Clin Infect Dis. 2005;41:e27–8.

Glockner A. Recurrent candidaemia and pacemaker wire infection with *Candida albicans*. Mycoses. 2011;54:S20–3.

Hope WW, Castagnola E, Groll AH, Roilides E, Akova M, Arendrup MC, Arikan-Akdagli S, Bassetti M, Bille J, Cornely OA, Cuenca-Estrella M, Donnelly JP, Garbino J, Herbrecht R, Jensen HE, Kullberg BJ, Lass-Flörl C, Lortholary O, Meersseman W, Petrikkos G, Richardson MD, Verweij PE, Viscoli C, Ullmann AJ, ESCMID Fungal Infection Study Group. ESCMID* guideline for the diagnosis and management of *Candida* diseases 2012: prevention and management of invasive infections in neonates and children caused by *Candida* spp. Clin Microbiol Infect. 2012;18:S38–52.

Janniger CK, Schwartz RA, Szepietowski JC, Reich A. Intertrigo and common secondary skin infections. Am Fam Physician. 2005;72:833–8.

Kakati B, Kotwal A, Biswas D, Sahu S. Fluconazole resistant Candida oesophagitis in immunocompetent patients: is empirical therapy justifiable? J Clin Diagn Res. 2015;9:16–8.

Kohli R, Hadley S. Fungal arthritis and osteomyelitis. Infect Dis Clin North Am. 2005;19:831–51.

Kontoyiannis DP, Reddy BT, Torres HA, Luna M, Lewis RE, Tarrand J, Bodey GP, II R. Pulmonary candidiasis in patients with cancer: an autopsy study. Clin Infect Dis. 2002;34:400–3.

Lastauskienė E, Zinkevičienė A, Girkontaitė I, Kaunietis A, Kvedarienė V. Formic acid and acetic acid induced a programmed cell death in pathogenic *Candida* species. Curr Microbiol. 2014;69:303–10.

León C, Ruiz-Santana S, Saavedra P, Almirante B, Nolla-Salas J, Alvarez-Lerma F, Garnacho-Montero J, León MA, EPCAN Study Group. A bedside scoring system ("*Candida* score") for early antifungal treatment in nonneutropenic critically ill patients with *Candida* colonization. Crit Care Med. 2006;34:730–7.

Loo DS. Cutaneous fungal infections in the elderly. Dermatol Clin. 2004;22:33–50.

Lortholary O, Petrikkos G, Akova M, Arendrup MC, Arikan-Akdagli S, Bassetti M, Bille J, Calandra T, Castagnola E, Cornely OA, Cuenca-Estrella M, Donnelly JP, Garbino J, Groll AH, Herbrecht R, Hope WW, Jensen HE, Kullberg BJ, Lass-Flörl C, Meersseman W, Richardson MD, Roilides E, Verweij PE, Viscoli C, Ullmann AJ, ESCMID Fungal Infection Study Group. ESCMID* guideline for the diagnosis and management of *Candida* diseases 2012: patients with HIV infection or AIDS. Clin Microbiol Infect. 2012;18:S68–77.

Matthews RC. Pathogenicity determinants of *Candida albicans*: potential targets for immunotherapy? Microbiology. 1994;140:1505–11.

Mersequel KB, Nishikaku A, Rodrigues AM, Padovan AC, e Ferreira RC, de Azevedo Melo AS, Briones MR, Colombo AL. Genetic diversity of medically important and emerging Candida species causing invasive infection. BMC Infect Dis. 2015;15:57.

Naouri M, Mazer JM. Finger onychomycosis due to *Candida tropicalis:* short-pulsed Nd:YAG laser therapy. Ann Dermatol Venereol. 2013;140:610–3.

Nieto MC, Telleria O, Cisterna R. Sentinel surveillance of invasive candidiasis in Spain: epidemiology and antifungal susceptibility. Diagn Microbiol Infect Dis. 2015;81:34–40.

Oberoi JK. Invasive candidiasis. JIMSA. 2010;23:25–8.

Odds FC. Molecular phylogenetics and epidemiology of *Candida albicans*. Future Microbiol. 2010;5:67–79.

Okada S, Puel A, Casanova JL, Kobayashi M. Chronic mucocutaneous candidiasis disease associated with inborn errors of IL-17 immunity. Clin Transl Immunology. 2016;5:e114.

Pappas PG. Invasive candidiasis. Infect Dis Clin North Am. 2006;20:485–506.

Pappas PG, Kauffman CA, Andes D, Benjamin DK Jr, Calandra TF, Edwards JE Jr, Filler SG, Fisher JF, Kullberg BJ, Ostrosky-Zeichner L, Reboli AC, Rex JH, Walsh TJ, Sobel JD, Infectious Diseases Society of America. Clinical practice guidelines for the management of candidiasis: 2009 update by the Infectious Diseases Society of America. Clin Infect Dis. 2009;48:503–35.

Parra-Herran CE, Pelaez L, Sola JE, Urbiztondo AK, Rodriguez MM. Intestinal candidiasis: an uncommon cause of necrotizing enterocolitis (NEC) in neonates. Fetal Pediatr Pathol. 2010;29:172–80.

Perlin DS, Shor E, Zhao Y. Update on antifungal drug resistance. Curr Clin Microbiol Rep. 2015;2:84–95.

Pfaller MA, Diekema DJ. Epidemiology of invasive candidiasis: a persistent public health problem. Clin Microbiol Rev. 2007;20:133–63.

Pfaller MA, Boyken L, Hollis RJ, Messer SA, Tendolkar S, Diekema DJ. In vitro activities of anidulafungin against more than 2500 clinical isolates of candida spp, including 315 isolates resistant to fluconazole. J Clin Microbiol. 2005;43:5425–7.

Pfalller MA, Andes DR, Diekema DJ, Horn DL, Reboli AC, Rotstein C, Franks B, Azie NE. Epidemiology and outcomes of invasive candidiasis due ton on-albicans species of Candida in 2,496 patients: data from the Prospective Antifungal Therapy (PATH) registry 2004–2008. PLoS One. 2014;9:e101510.

Pittet D, Monod M, Suter PM, Frenk E, Auckenthaler R. Candida colonization and subsequent infections in critically ill surgical patients. Ann Surg. 1994;220:751–8.
Portocarrero JS, Cecilia EP, Corral O, Romero-Vivas J, Picazo JJ. The central nervous system and infection by *Candida* species. Diagn Microbiol Infect Dis. 2000;37:169–79.
Rivoisy C, Vena A, Schaeffer L, Charlier C, Fontanet A, Delahaye F, Bouza E, Lortholary O, Munoz P, Lefort A, French Mycoses Study Group and Grupo de Apoyo al Manejo de las Endocarditis en España (GAMES). Prosthetic valve *Candida* spp. endocarditis: new insights into long-term prognosis—the ESCAPE study. Clin Infect Dis. 2018;66:825–32.
Sanglard D, Odds FC. Resistance of *Candida* species to antifungal agents: molecular mechanisms and clinical consequences. Lancet Infect Dis. 2002;2:73–85.
Sobel JD, Fisher JF, Kauffman CA, Newman CA. Candida urinary tract infections—epidemiology. Clin Infect Dis. 2011;52:433–6.
Sugar AM, Liu XP. Combination antifungal therapy in treatment of murine pulmonary mucormycosis: roles of quinolones and azoles. Antimicrob Agents Chemother. 2000;44:2004–6.
Tavanti A, Davidson AD, Gow NA, Maiden MC, Odds FC. *Candida orthopsilosis* and *Candida metapsilosis* spp. nov. to replace *Candida parapsilosis* groups II and III. J Clin Microbiol. 2005;43:284–92.
Ullmann AJ, Akova M, Herbrecht R, Viscoli C, Arendrup MC, Arikan-Akdagli S, Bassetti M, Bille J, Calandra T, Castagnola E, Cornely OA, Donnelly JP, Garbino J, Groll AH, Hope WW, Jensen HE, Kullberg BJ, Lass-Flörl C, Lortholary O, Meersseman W, Petrikkos G, Richardson MD, Roilides E, Verweij PE, Cuenca-Estrella M, ESCMID Fungal Infection Study Group. ESCMID* guideline for the diagnosis and management of Candida diseases 2012: adults with haematological malignancies and after haematopoietic stem cell transplantation (HCT). Clin Microbiol Infect. 2012;18:53–67.

Mucormycosis

10

A. Serda Kantarcioglu

Abbreviations

ABLC	AmB lipid complex
AIDS	Acquired immunodeficiency syndrome
Als	Agglutinin-like sequence
AmB	Amphotericin B
BHB	β-hydroxy butyrate
BHI	Brain heart infusion
CAS	Caspofungin
CNS	Central nervous system
CotH	Coating
CSF	Cerebrospinal fluid
CT	Computed tomography
DC	Dendritic cell
ECMM	European Confederation of Medical Mycology
EUCAST	European Committee on Antimicrobial Susceptibility Testing
G-CSF	Granulocyte colony-stimulating factor
GM-CSF	Granulocyte-macrophage colony-stimulating factor
GMS	Grocott methenamine silver
GRP	Glucose-regulated protein
HBO	Hyperbaric oxygen
H&E	Haematoxylin and eosin
HIV	Human immunodeficiency virus
IFN	Interferon
IL	Interleukin
ILC	Innate lymphocyte
ISA	Isavuconazole
ISHAM	International Society for Human and Animal Mycology
ITS	Internal transcribed spacer
iv	Intravenous
KOH	Potassium hydroxide
LAmB	Liposomal AmB
MALDI-TOF	Matrix-assisted laser desorption/ionization time-of-flight
MHC	Major histocompatibility complex
MIC	Minimal inhibitory concentration
MNC	Mononuclear cell
MRI	Magnetic resonance imaging
NK	Natural killer
NO	Nitric oxide
PAS	Periodic acid-Schiff
PCR	Polymerase chain reaction
PDGF	Platelet-derived growth factor
PL	Pectin lyase
PMN	Polymorphonuclear neutrophil
PRR	Pathogen recognition receptor/Pattern recognition receptor
PSZ	Posaconazole
RANTES	Regulated on activation, normal T cell expressed and secreted
RCM	Rhinocerebral mucormycosis
ROCM	Rhino-orbito-cerebral mucormycosis
SIG	Special Interest Group
TLR	Toll-like receptor
TNF	Tumour necrosis factor
Th 1	T-helper type 1
VRZ	Voriconazole

A. S. Kantarcioglu (✉)
Division of Mycology, Department of Medical Microbiology, Cerrahpasa Medical Faculty, Istanbul University-Cerrahpasa, Istanbul, Turkey

M. Turgut et al. (eds.), *Fungal Infections of the Central Nervous System*,
https://doi.org/10.1007/978-3-030-06088-6_10

10.1 Introduction

Development of cerebral mucormycosis as a complication of sino-orbital infection or direct involvement is a rarely encountered entity and can rapidly result in death. Rhinocerebral mucormycosis (RCM) is a necrotizing, angioinvasive, life-threatening infection of the nasal passages and sinus that can easily spread to the brain, oral cavity and eyes, caused by a wide range of fungi that belong to the *Mucorales* order of *Zygomycota* phylum of the Kingdom Fungi. More than 25 *Mucorales* species belonging to no fewer than 10 genera have been reported to infect humans (Dannaoui 2017).

A computerized search of the MEDLINE database (National Library of Medicine, Bethesda, Maryland, USA) was performed for cases reported in the literature between 1885 and 2018, with (by cross-referencing) the terms "zygomycetes", "*Mucorales*", "mucormycosis", "cerebral", "brain abscess", "meningitis", "central nervous system infection", "rhinocerebral infection", "rhino-orbito-cerebral infection", "disseminated" and "immunocompetent", "otherwise healthy" and "i.v. drug abusers". These keywords were used alone and/or in combination with an "and" statement. Additional cases were obtained by scanning the references cited in the original articles. Original full texts of all the relevant articles were obtained via MEDLINE, TUBITAK-ULAKBIM (Turkish Academic Network and Information Center) and other international libraries and were used for the analysis.

10.2 Taxonomy

Taxonomy of *Mucorales* has traditionally been based on the macroscopic and microscopic morphology of thallus and morphologic similarities of sexual reproductive structures. A large number of names were synonymysed.

The fungal order *Mucorales*, belonging to a section of lower fungi that until recently was referred to as zygomycetes, constitutes a phylogenetically ancient group of organisms. In the fungal tree of life, the group encompasses a number of widely spaced, ancestral lineages. Over time, mutations are hypothesized to have accumulated, which is reflected, e.g., in an immense degree of sequence diversity of evolutionary markers such as the ribosomal operon. By assessment of identical genes, mucoralean species are separated from each other at branches much longer than those of species of more recent fungi, such as *Aspergillus* or the dermatophytes (Hibbett et al. 2007).

Molecular studies revealed the diversity within and between species and the phylogeny, and taxonomy of the *Mucorales* have been substantially revised in recent years based on molecular data, and certain species have been reassigned to a different genus (Walther et al. 2013). Several new cryptic species have been identified within various genera, including *Lichtheimia* (formerly *Absidia*), *Mucor*, *Apophysomyces* and *Saksenaea*, and different morphological varieties have been shown in some biological species. Sequencing of internal transcribed spacer (ITS) region is the recommended method for accurate molecular identification and one of the most useful target for DNA barcoding of *Mucorales* species (Walther et al. 2013; Kwon-Chung 2012; Cornely et al. 2014).

10.3 Morphology, Biology and Genome

The *Mucorales* are characterized by aseptate (coenocytic), hyaline, irregularly branching hyphae, sexual reproduction with the formation of zygospores, and asexual reproduction with nonmotile sporangiospores. The asexual sporangiospores are formed in a globe-like structure called the sporangium on the apex of sporangiophore (Fig. 10.1a, b).

The sporangiospores then dispersed and, on appropriate conditions, germinate to produce a mycelial complex (Mendoza et al. 2015; Morace and Borghi 2012). These sporangiospores range from 3 to 11 µm in diameter and are easily aerosolized and cause infections in susceptible hosts when inhaled or introduced through the cutaneous percutaneous route. Most of the members of *Mucorales* are mesophilic (growing at 10–40 °C, with an optimum 20–35 °C). Some are thermo-

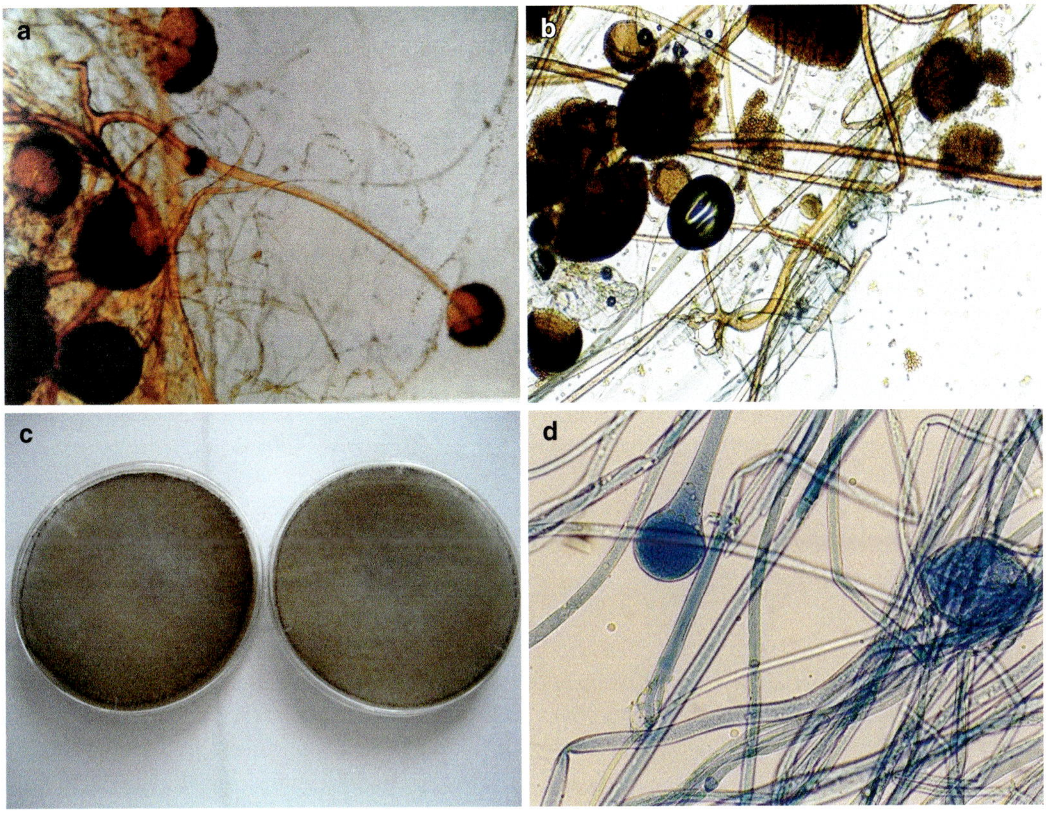

Fig. 10.1 Microscopical morphology of (**a**) Mucor sp., (**b**) Rhyzopus sp. (Lactophenol cotton blue stained, ×100), (**c**) Rhizopus arrhyzus on cooked sheep's blood agar as primary culture media, (**d**) Coenocytic hyphae and sporangium (Lactophenol cotton blue stained, ×100)

philic with a minimum growth temperature about 20 °C and maximum extending up to 60 °C. Others can grow at temperatures below 0 °C. Most of the pathogenic *Mucorales* are heterothallic, and in their sexual development, hyphae of the two different but compatible mating types, [(−) and (+)], sense each other and undergo fusion to form zygospores, which later germinate to form a sporangium at the apex culminating in sexual meiospores. However, in most species zygospore production is rarer due to the conditions necessary for their formation. The asexual sporangiospores are produced in massive quantities, and they are thought to be able to serve as the major source of dissemination and infection, whereas sexual zygospores are considered to be dormant (Mendoza et al. 2015; Muszewska et al. 2014). *Mucorales* produce wet and dry sporangiospores, the former disperse by air and the later are less prone to aerosolization. Spore size and hydrophilic/hydrophobic character impacts the dispersal of fungi.

Several members of *Mucorales* including *Rhizopus oryzae* (*R. arrhizus*), the most common environmental member of the *Mucoraceae* family and the most prevalent agent of mucormycosis, may, under particular in vitro or in vivo conditions, form a variety of cellular forms, branching mycelium, budding yeasts and spherule-like chlamydoconidia (Kantarcioğlu et al. 2006). Some species of order *Mucorales* are able to grow under anaerobic conditions, while most of them require aerobic conditions. During the transition of hyphae to yeast and vice versa of dimorphic *Mucorales*, there occurs a series of alterations in metabolism. Some of these alterations seem to be related only to a change in habitat, aerobic to anaerobic or the reverse (José

1985). Furthermore, while the majority of the *Mucorales* only grow at high water activities, some of them are able to grow in salt concentrations of at least 15%.

Several *Mucorales* genomes have been sequenced. Based on the sole gene count and genome size comparisons, *Rhizopus oryzae* (*R. arrhizus*) is an exception regarding the number of genes in the whole collection of currently sequenced *Mucorales*, with the average gene number of 11.000 genes. *R. oryzae* possess extraordinary genome plasticity owing to a whole genome duplication, which resulted in an elevated number of genes, including those involved in host-pathogen interactions (Muszewska et al. 2014).

10.4 Cell Wall and Biofilm Formation

Mucorales exhibit a special structure of cell wall. They differ in cell wall composition having less glucan and more chitin and without galactomannan compared with Ascomycota. *Mucorales* cell wall mainly composed of chitin and chitosan, the deacetylated homopolymer of chitin, as structural polysaccharides. Chitin is built of β-1,4 bonded N-acetyl glucosamine. The cell wall of *R. oryzae* and other *Mucorales* contains a high percentage of chitin and chitosan, which are synthesized by chitin synthases (23 genes) and chitin deacetylases (34 genes), respectively. Fungal hyphae grow at the tip. Therefore, specialized vesicles, the chitosomes, bring precursors of chitin and its synthesizing enzyme, chitin synthetase, to the outside of the membrane by exocytosis. The enzyme on the membrane catalyses glycosidic bond formations from the nucleotide sugar substrate, uridine diphospho-N-acetyl-D-glucosamine. The nascent polysaccharide chain is then cleaved by the enzyme chitin deacetylase. The enzyme catalyses the hydrolytic cleavage of the N-acetamido group in chitin. After this the chitosan polymer chain forms microfibrils. These fibres are embedded in an amorphous matrix consisting of proteins, glucans (which putatively cross-link the chitosan fibres), mannoproteins, lipids and other compounds (Muszewska et al. 2014; Li et al. 2011).

In vitro studies revealed the potential for biofilm formation for *R. oryzae*, *L. corymbifera* and *R. pusillus*, but not for *A. elegans* (Singh et al. 2011). The biofilm matrix is formed with glucosamine as the dominant dry component. *Rhizopus oryzae* is claimed to possess extraordinary genome plasticity owing to a whole genome duplication, which resulted in an elevated number of genes, including those involved in host-pathogen interactions (Muszewska et al. 2014; Lewis et al. 2012; Ma et al. 2009).

10.5 Ecology and Seasonality

The knowledge of pathogenic *Mucorales* ecology is often anecdotal and conflicting. The major mode of transmission might generally be inhalation of aerosolized sporangiospores. However, *Mucorales* very rarely found on nasal mucus, suggesting that spores in the mucus of airway mucosa are cleared by mucociliary transport or that there is a low level of airborne contamination (Richardson 2009). However, in susceptible hosts, infection may occur.

Mucorales are thermotolerant, fast-growing moulds and ubiquitous in nature and widely found on organic substrates including spoiled food and bread, over mature or decaying fruits and vegetable matter, crop debris and soil. The fungus grows and acquires nutrients from dead and decaying matter. Some species are parasites of plants causing soft rot, of insects, and small animals, while others form symbiotic relationships with plants. The fungus is also found on air, dust, compost piles and animal particularly herbivores' faeces and manure; however, human pathogenic Ascomycota are broadly encountered in air samples, whereas *Mucorales* are less abundant in both indoor and outdoor air samples in different geographic areas, in Poland (Ejdys 2001; Gniadek and Macura 2007), Lebanon (El-Herte et al. 2012), Turkey (Çolakoğlu 2003; Sen and Asan 2009; Asan et al. 2010) and even India (Sharma et al. 2001; Thirumala and Nathu 2013; Pavan and Manjunath 2014) where the disease incidence is relatively higher (Chakrabarti and Singh 2014). *Mucorales* are soilborne fungi and survive in the soil as spores. Unusual genera including *Apophysomyces* and *Saksenaea* are also soil saprophytes occurring mainly in tropical and subtropical climates (Gomes et al. 2011). The isolation of *Mucorales* from soil is probably influenced by soil characteristics. *Mucorales* are found soil rich in composite vegetation, decaying vegetables and fruits (Richardson 2009). Spore populations increase in the soil and severely decline during winter. Fruits that have fallen on the soil surface are infected through contact with infested soil. Throughout the fall and winter, spores are dislodged from the decaying fruit into the soil. Spores are also dispersed by mowing, which scatters pieces of infected fruit. The fungus survives best in cool, dry soils.

Fruit become most successful to infection 1 month before harvest. Fruits that are overmature are more susceptible to infection. *Rhizopus oryzae*, *Mucor racemosus*, *M. circinelloides*, *M. piriformis* and several other species of *Mucorales* are plant pathogens that causes a soft rot on sweet potatoes, tomatoes, apples, pears and other fruits and roots. All these fungi are saprophytic so they initially produce pectic enzymes that break down vegetable tissues. Once a spore lands on a wounded tissue, it germinates and starts growing on the surface, producing a thick mycelium which at the same time produces cell-degrading enzymes (pectinases, amylases) that denature the tissues in advance, thus leading to infection. The disease infection usually occurs in wounded areas after cracking of fruits during sale after harvest, transports, market shelf and storage when moisture conditions are favourable. Infected fruit may completely decay after about 2 months in cold storage. Decaying fruit become very juicy and within this juice are abundant spores of the fungus. *Rhizopus stolonifer* is more commonly known as black bread mould. *Mucorales* uses the soil and decaying fruits, and plant materials as a reservoir, and fungal spores can be inhaled from disturbed soil, decaying plants, raw vegetables or overmature fruits to form human mucormycosis.

Although mucormycosis is being reported globally, cases are relatively common in tropical and subtropical countries, where the climatic conditions favour the survival and growth of *Mucorales* in nature. Moisture is critical and there should be enough moisture (75–85%) for spores to germinate and mycelia to grow; therefore, seasonal variation in atmospheric conditions may affect the abundance of spores present in nature. Rainy seasons might permit high spore concentration in soil due to the washing of *Mucorales* spores from decaying plant material and precipitation, and winds might disperse them around in dust. Spores usually do not germinate at a higher relative humidity. The optimum temperature for sporulation, mycelial growth and spore germination is between 23 and 28 °C, while rotting and tuber decay develop between 15 and 23 °C; however, there are numerous reports of *Mucor* spp. causing decay of vegetables in cold storage. The high spore density of *Mucorales* depending on climatic conditions in soil and the outdoor or indoor environment close to human habitat may probably make easy to exposure and invasion of susceptible individuals.

Apophysomyces species complex, a recently emerged pathogen causing ROCM predominantly in healthy individuals, was found significantly associated with low nitrogen content of the soil in India (Prakash et al. 2016).

Mucorales are found occasionally in water-damaged buildings, as demonstrated by air sampling, and analysis of settled dust by quantitative polymerase chain reaction (PCR). Moreover, inhalation of sporangiospores in dust has been linked to outbreaks of RCM or pulmonary mucormycosis due to excavation, construction or contaminated air-conditioning filters. Whereas most *Mucorales* infections are community-acquired, nosocomial acquisition due to percutaneous routes of exposure is very important (Richardson 2009).

10.6 Etiologic Agents

Most cases of human infection are caused by members of Mucoraceae family, predominantly by *Rhizopus* species. *Rhizopus*, *Mucor* and *Lichtheimia* species (formerly *Absidia*) cause 70–80% of all mucormycosis cases, with *Lichtheimia* species as the second and third most abundant agent in Europe and the USA, respectively (Gomes et al. 2011; Roden et al. 2005; Skiada et al. 2011; Schwartze and Jacobsen 2014; Lanternier et al. 2012). Other common causative agents include species of *Apophysomyces*, *Rhizomucor*, *Cunninghamella* and *Saksenaea*. *Rhizopus oryzae* (*Rhizopus arrhizus*) is the most common environmental member of the genus. Approximately 60% of all the culture-proven cases of human mucormycosis and nearly 90% of the rhinocerebral cases are caused by *R. oryzae* (Richardson 2009; Murthy and Sundaram 2014). The fungus has been recovered as a saprobe from the nasal cavities and paranasal sinuses of healthy individuals (Kantarcioğlu et al. 2006) it becomes pathogenic under some particular conditions. *Mucorales* colonize a high number of patients but do not necessarily cause invasion (Bouza et al. 2006). *Apophysomyces elegans*, a saprophytic soil fungus, has recently emerged as a pathogen species that, unlike the other members of *Mucorales*, has been reported to cause rhino-orbitocerebral infections in immunocompetent individuals (Chakrabarti and Singh 2014; Liang et al. 2006; Singh et al. 2017). In English literature, the majority of patients with *A. elegans* ROCM had no predisposing conditions, except a few cases occurred following facial or head trauma (Liang et al. 2006; Singh et al. 2017; Wolkow et al. 2017). Although few in number, in English literature, four of the five reported cases of ROCM due to *Saksenaea* were in previously healthy individuals (Baradkar et al. 2008; Shatriah et al. 2012; Kaufman et al. 1988; Taj-Aldeen et al. 2012).

10.7 Epidemiology

Case series on mucormycosis have been reported from medical centres in India; reported cases were also reviewed in retrospective studies (Chakrabarti and Singh 2014; Roden et al. 2005; Petrikkos et al. 2014; Kennedy et al. 2016; Kontoyiannis et al. 2016; Rueping et al. 2009); central nervous system (CNS) or rhinocerebral was the most common site of *Mucorales* infection (14.6–69%): *Rhizopus* species, particularly *R. oryzae* (*R. arrhizus*), was the most frequent fungus isolated (Sundaram et al. 2005; Song et al. 2017), and case fatality rates were high.

CNS infection by the *Mucoraceae* was first described in 1885, in a man with multiple brain abscesses who died with widely disseminated infection (Paltauf 1885). In 1943, the description of three cases established the classic triad that characterizes most cases of mucormycosis: diabetes mellitus with ketoacidosis, naso-orbital necrotizing infection and meningoencephalitis (Gregory et al. 1943; Sepkowitz and Armstrong 1997). Shortly, thereafter, this was recognized as the most prevalent form of mucormycosis.

The emergence of mucormycosis is being reported globally, with a rise in the number of cases in patients with uncontrolled or poorly controlled diabetes. In recent years, mucormycosis appears to be increasing worldwide, but its exact prevalence and incidence remain unclear because of the difficulty to diagnose and neglect to report mainly in developing countries. A Working Group on zygomycosis was formed by the European Confederation of Medical Mycology (ECMM) in 2004 and collected cases of proven and probable zygomycosis in 13 European countries to analyse the clinical characteristics, microbiology, treatment practices and outcome of zygomycosis through a voluntary case registry, because no large prospective studies had been undertaken until then (Skiada et al. 2011; Petrikkos et al. 2014). Recent population-based studies and/or a few multicentre retrospective studies of proven and probable cases of mucormycosis (Chakrabarti and Singh 2014; Roden et al. 2005; Kennedy et al. 2016; Kontoyiannis et al. 2016; KÖMÜR et al. 2016; Bitar et al. 2009) suggested that mucormycosis has emerged as a prevalent infection after candidiasis and aspergillosis primarily in patients with underlying risk factors. In most studies, haematologic malignancy was reported as the most common underlying disease as well as uncontrolled diabetes mellitus in some other studies. While the majority of patients had at least one underlying condition, the others had no predisposing factors.

The fungus may affect one of several organ systems, most commonly the paranasal sinuses and the brain. Sinus involvement consisting of rhinocerebral, sinus and sino-orbital infections constituted the majority of infections followed by orbital and cerebral involvement. Rhinocerebral disease is the most common form of mucormycosis and occurs in the setting of diabetic ketoacidosis. ROCM is uncommon in patients with acquired immunodeficiency syndrome (AIDS). In patients with haematologic diseases, the infection most frequently occurs in neutropenic phase (Bouza et al. 2006). One of the most common underlying conditions in paediatric population was profound dehydration (Talmi et al. 2002; Sheikh and Amr 2011).

In the literature, seasonal variations in the incidence of mucormycosis with respect to temperature, rainfall and humidity have also been noted (Nithyanandam et al. 2003). Environmental factors, such as tropical and subtropical humid climate and high temperature typical for India, provide an optimum set-up for survival of these fungi (Chakrabarti and Singh 2014). Davies et al. (2017) reported an increased incidence of rhino-orbital-cerebral mucormycosis after Colorado flooding in the USA. The authors hypothesized that the combination of immunocompromised status and environmental exposure resulted in increased incidence (Davies et al. 2017). There are several reports suggesting that the incidence of mucormycosis increases in summer and early autumn (El-Herte et al. 2012; Talmi et al. 2002; Shpitzer et al. 2005; Al-Ajam et al. 2006). The authors reported their experience of 19 cases in Israel, that all except two cases presented between August and December, and hypothesized that ROCM may have seasonal incidence peaking in the fall and early winter (Talmi et al. 2002; Sheikh and Amr 2011). Then, the authors retrospectively analysed their own data during a 25-year period, trying to define the seasonal occurrence of RCM and a peak observed in the month of September; however, no association was noted between meteorologic conditions and the incidence of RCM (Shpitzer et al. 2005). El-Herte et al.'s (2012) review on the seasonal variation of the air concentration of spores of *Mucorales* and other fungi and the variation of clinical mucormycosis suggested ROCM may be closely related to high environmental exposure.

Zygomycete research in the scientific community is presently stimulated and coordinated on an international basis by the ECMM-ISHAM (International Society for Human and Animal Mycology) Working Group Zygomycoses, coordinated by George Petrikkos. The Working Group was founded in 2004 under ECMM. After organizing the first International Forum on Zygomycosis in 2008 at Cape Sounion, Greece, a supplement of Clinical Microbiology and Infection was published. A second Forum was held in 2010 at Porto Heli, Greece. A website was made in the same year (www.zygomyco.net) with a database where cases of mucormycosis can be submitted online. An overview of zygomycosis in Europe was published with 230 cases accrued by the registry of the Working Group (Skiada et al. 2011). The Working Group joined ISHAM in 2009. Several members of the group took part in a meeting in Chicago, organized by Thomas Walsh with the support of the Hank Schueler foundation, and a special issue of Clinical Infectious Diseases was published (Walsh et al. 2012). Subsequently a Special Interest Group (SIG) meeting was organized by Kerstin Voigt and Sybren de Hoog in conjunction with the International Mycological Congress on the Biology of Fungi (IMC9) held in Edinburgh, Scotland, August 2010. A follow-up meeting concentrating on zygomycete biodiversity took place in Utrecht, the Netherlands, March 2011. This meeting enabled fruitful discussions, inspiring an exchange of ideas and providing an updated view on this group of fungi. The outcome of this meeting formed the basis of the present special issue of *Persoonia*.

10.8 Pathogenesis

The pathogenesis of the infection is still poorly understood as well as the role of specific virulence determinants and the interaction with the host immune system. *Mucorales* are able to produce various proteins and metabolic products toxic to humans, but the pathogenic role of these potential virulence factors is still unknown.

10.8.1 Host Factors in Mucormycosis

10.8.1.1 Predisposing Factors, Underlying Conditions

Mucorales may cause CNS infections both in previously healthy individuals and having one or more underlying diseases and/or predisposing factors. Uncontrolled diabetes mellitus was the frequent underlying disease reported in cases caused by the more common genera of *Mucoraceae* (*Rhizopus*, *Mucor* and *Lichtheimia*). The other main risk factors are ketoacidosis (diabetic or other), renal failure, iatrogenic immunosuppression, use of corticosteroids or deferoxamine, defects in innate immunity, particularly of phagocytic effector cell functions, neutropenia due to cancer treatment, haematopoietic and solid organ transplantation, injectable drug use, disruption of mucocutaneous barriers by catheters and other devices and direct implant during neurosurgical procedures (Mendoza et al. 2015; Skiada et al. 2011; Liang et al. 2006; Kennedy et al. 2016; Rueping et al. 2009; Petrikkos et al. 2003).

Diabetic ketoacidosis and deferoxamine-treated patients are uniquely predisposed to mucormycosis. Haemodyalisis patients receiving the bacterial siderophore deferoxamine for treating iron overload are uniquely predisposed to highly lethal and frequently disseminated mucormycosis (Arizono et al. 1989). Deferoxamine prevents iron overload toxicity via efficiently chelating iron from the host; however, it is known that *Rhizopus* possess cell surface receptors to ferric-rich form of deferoxamine and ferrioxamine (Baldin and Ibrahim 2017).

Another predisposing factor of mucormycosis is considered the use of voriconazole (VRZ) in high-risk patients, either for prophylaxis or treatment of other fungal infections. Voriconazole has been shown to be inactive against *Mucorales* in vitro. During recent years *Mucorales* have emerged as agents of disease in hospitalized patients. Presumably this is partly due to prophylaxis against *Aspergillus fumigatus*, which reduces the frequency of *Aspergillus* infections (Voigt et al. 2013; Binder et al. 2014). However, in the literature, there were very few patients with ethmoidal sinus infection with orbital extension or brain involvement among VRZ-receiving patients, and all of them were also neutropenic (Marty et al. 2004; Vigouroux et al. 2005).

10.8.1.2 Previously Healthy Patients

Patients with no identifiable risk factors were also reported. Unlike RCM caused by the more common genera of *Mucoraceae* (*Rhizopus*, *Mucor and Lichtheimia*), RCM due to *A. elegans* appears to occur in immunocompetent patients. In addition, several cases occurred following facial or head trauma (Liang et al. 2006). The majority of the reported patients with RCM due to *Saksenaeceae* (though few) had no predisposing conditions (Wolkow et al. 2017; Sundaram et al. 2005).

From the first report of CNS infection by *Mucorales* up to April 2018, in the literature, 65 cases have been described in previously healthy patients (Sharma et al. 2001; Liang et al. 2006; Wolkow et al. 2017; Baradkar et al. 2008; Shatriah et al. 2012; Adelman and Aronson 1969; Bichile et al. 1985; Blodi et al. 1969; Chmel and Grieco 1973; Hameroff et al. 1970; Masucci et al. 1982; Pierce et al. 1982; Wetli et al. 1984; Woods and Hanna 1986; Kasantikul et al. 1987; Mackenzie et al. 1988; Miller et al. 1988; Oliveri et al. 1988; Stave et al. 1989; Fong et al. 1990; Riefler III et al. 1991; Bhattacharyya et al. 1992; Gollard et al. 1994; Hopkins et al. 1994; Siddiqi and Freedman 1994; Hussain et al. 1995; Radner et al. 1995; Rangel-Guerra et al. 1996; Fairley et al. 2000; Garcia-Covarrubias et al. 2001; Chakrabarti et al. 2003; Khor et al. 2003; Rao et al. 2006; Schütz et al. 2006; Verma et al. 2006; Elinav et al. 2009; Air et al. 2010; Tsung et al. 2010; El et al. 2011; Parsi et al. 2013; Sarrami et al. 2013; Angali et al. 2014; Reddy and Raju 2015; Ginsberg et al. 1987; Gaing et al. 1992; Terk et al. 1992; Bhadani et al. 2007; Watson et al. 1985; Pillai et al. 2016). Only three of the previously healthy patients were posttraumatic cases, one of them had a penetrating head injury

(Mackenzie et al. 1988), one had a history of closed-head trauma (Garcia-Covarrubias et al. 2001) and another one fell from a tractor and then fell into a water-filled ditch (Radner et al. 1995). Twenty-nine of the 65 previously healthy patients were i.v. drug abusers. Further three intravenous (i.v) drug abusers were human immunodeficiency virus (HIV)-positive patients (Cuadrado et al. 1988; Escobar and Del Brutto 1990), and one more i.v. drug abuser had cervix cancer (Scully et al. 2012). One of the previously healthy patients had a history of surgery for arteriovenous malformation (Rangel-Guerra et al. 1996), and one had cataract surgery and dental abscess (Wolkow et al. 2017). An unusual case was described in an immunocompetent host who had a previous history of primary cutaneous mucormycosis, but no cutaneous portal of entry had been identified (El et al. 2011). In an immunocompetent child with *Absidia* brain abscess, physicians had postulated that the previous aggressive use of antibiotics coupled with the breakdown of the gastrointestinal mucosa during severe diarrhoea might have led to mucormycosis (Tsung et al. 2010).

10.8.2 Virulence and Pathogenic Potential of *Mucorales*

In addition to host factors that predispose patients to mucormycosis, *Mucorales* possess virulence factors that enable the organism to cause disease. Although increasing frequency of causative agents of disease, little is known about the pathogenic potential of most mucoralean fungi. In general, adaptation, survival and replication with the host environment are likely to contribute to the virulence potential of fungi.

10.8.2.1 Spore Sizes

The small conidial size of fungi (e.g. *Aspergillus fumigatus*) is often regarded as a putative virulence factor because the size allows conidia to enter the host via respiration. Spore size of the *Mucorales* is variable, depending on the species 3–11 µm, but in general bigger than those of *A. fumigatus*, for example (Binder et al. 2014). However, the spores can be inhaled and cause disease in the human lungs and sinuses.

10.8.2.2 Stress and Temperature Tolerance

The clinically relevant species of *Mucorales* are thermotolerant and have the ability to grow at 37 °C, some even at higher temperatures (Table 10.1). However, no clinical correlation between growth speed at host temperature and differences in virulence potential was detected in a recent study (Schwartze et al. 2012).

The fungi require robust stress response to survive in human host. Wide variation in stress responses was noted in mucoralean fungi to both osmotic and oxidative stresses and acidic pH.

Table 10.1 Maximum growth temperature of the common etiologic agents of invasive mucormycosis belonging to *Mucorales* (De Hoog et al. 2000)

Family	Genus	Species	Maximum growth temperature (°C)
Mucoraceae	*Rhizopus*	*Oryzae*	>37
		Microsporus	>37
		Azygosporus	>37
		Schipperae	>37
	Mucor	*Circinelloides*	>37
		Indicus	>37
	Rhizomucor	*Pusillus*	>37
	Lichtheimia (Absidia)	*Corymbifera*	>37
	Apophysomyces	*Elegans*	>37
Cuninghamellaceae	*Cunninghamella*	*Bertholletiae*	>37
Saksenaeceae	*Saksenaea*	*Vasiformus*	>37
Syncephalastraseae	*Syncephalastrum*	*Racemosum*	>37

Rhizopus arrhizus (*R. oryzae*), the commonest cause of human infection, showed high stress tolerance in comparison with other species of *Mucorales* (Singh et al. 2016). The utilization of macronutrients, e.g. carbon sources, in the host affects growth in vivo and might thus contribute to virulence. Nutrients within the host are most likely available as complex molecules, e.g. proteins, rather than free amino acids.

10.8.2.3 Surface Proteins

Tissue invasion and destruction are important for mucormycosis. Primarily, interaction with blood vessels seems to play a crucial role in the pathogenesis of mucormycosis. *R. arrhizus* was shown to be able to invade endothelial cells with their subsequent damage as surveyed by in vitro assays (Schwartze et al. 2012; Ibrahim et al. 2005). It was also shown that invasion depends on specific recognition of the endothelial receptor glucose-regulated protein 78 (GRP78) which is a heat-shock protein involved in stress-related responses (Wang et al. 2009). This recognition causes host cellular death by induction of the endothelial cell-mediated fungus endocytosis (Baldin and Ibrahim 2017), and blocking of the interaction by anti-GRP78 antibodies protects diabetic ketoacidosis mice from mucormycosis (Liu et al. 2010) and results in strongly decreased mortality in mice (Schwartze et al. 2012; Liu et al. 2010). It was shown that when GRP78 is blocked other factors involved in *Rhizopus* interacting with endothelial cells such as the platelet-derived growth factor (PDGF) pathway are activated (Chibucos et al. 2016).

The fungal ligand that binds to GRP78 during invasion of the endothelium belongs to the spore-coating (CotH) protein family. CotH proteins are universally present in *Mucorales* and absent from any other organisms which the genome has been sequenced. In other pathogenic fungi, invasion of host cells is mediated by other cell surface proteins, such as agglutinin-like sequence (Als) proteins that have been reported to act as invasins for *C. albicans* and bind to different host receptors (cadherins), while *Aspergillus fumigatus* invasins thaumatin-like proteins (CalA) binds to integrins (Wächtler et al. 2012; Liu et al. 2016; Phan et al. 2007). Blocking the function of CotH proteins either biochemically by using anti-CotH antibodies or genetically by attenuating CotH expression reduces the ability of *Rhizopus delemar* to invade and injure endothelial cells in vitro and reduces disease severity in mice (Gebremariam et al. 2014). The most commonly isolated *Mucorales* from patients (*Rhizopus*, *Mucor* and *Lichtheimia*) contain three to seven copies of CotH, while those that are only occasionally the cause of the disease such as *Apophysomyces*, *Cunninghamella*, *Saksenaea* and *Syncephalastrum*) only contain one to two copies (Chibucos et al. 2016).

10.8.2.4 Factors Modulating GRP78-CotH Interactions

The unique predisposition of diabetic ketoacidosis patients and deferoxamine-treated patients to mucormycosis points to the importance of hyperglycaemia, iron and acidifying ketone bodies in the virulence of *Mucorales*. Diabetic patients suffer from an elevated concentration of glucose. Hyperglycaemia can induce excessive glycosylation of proteins such as transferrin and ferritin, diminishing their iron affinity (Ribes et al. 2000). On the other hand, in the presence of an acidotic condition due to accumulation of ketone bodies (e.g. β-hydroxy butyrate [BHB]), the low pH in the blood vessels strongly impairs the ability of transferring into chelate iron (Artis et al. 1982). Glucose, iron and BHB enhance the growth of fungus (Fu et al. 2004; Gebremariam et al. 2016) and also induce the expression of GRP78 and CotH, resulting in augmented fungal invasion and subsequent injury of the endothelium in vitro (Liu et al. 2010; Gebremariam et al. 2016). The role of GRP78-CotH interactions is currently unknown in the neutropenic host and the other patient populations susceptible to mucormycosis.

10.8.2.5 Toxin-Like Substances

It was shown that nonviable *Rhizopus*, killed by heat or chemicals, was able to cause a comparable amount of damage to endothelial cells as viable cells (Ibrahim et al. 2005). These results suggest the contribution of toxin-like substances in mucormycosis pathogenesis. Thus, it was speculated that the presence of toxin-like secondary metabolites produced from *Mucorales*, which mediate the interaction between the pathogen and the host (Baldin and Ibrahim 2017; Ibrahim et al. 2005).

10.8.2.6 Iron Uptake (Acquisition)

Iron is an essential element for cell growth and development, contributing to many vial processes of the cell. Pathogenic fungi can use multiple processes for obtaining iron from the host, and the level of available, unbound iron in serum plays a critical factor in predisposing patients with diabetic ketoacidosis to mucormycosis (Artis et al. 1982; Howard 1999; Boelaert et al. 1993). In mammalian hosts, iron is bound to host carrier proteins, such as transferrin, ferritin and lactoferrin, and this sequestration avoids toxic effect of free iron (Artis et al. 1982; Howard 1999). This strategy of limiting iron availability is also a major universal host defense mechanism against microbes and against *Mucorales* in particular, because *R. oryzae* grows poorly in normal serum unless exogenous iron is added (Artis et al. 1982; Boelaert et al. 1993). Patients with diabetic ketoacidosis have elevated levels of free iron in their serum. Patients receiving dialysis who are treated with the iron chelator deferoxamine are also susceptible to mucormycosis (Ibrahim et al. 2012). Fungi can obtain iron from the host by using high-affinity iron permeases or low-molecular-weight iron chelators (siderophores). *Rhizopus* is known to secrete rhizoferrin, a siderophore that supplies *Rhizopus* iron. Another mechanism by which fungi can obtain iron from the host is through use of heme. The *Rhizopus* genome project revealed two homologs of the heme oxygenase that may obtain iron from host haemoglobin and might explain the angioinvasive nature of *R. oryzae* (Ibrahim et al. 2012).

10.8.3 Host-Pathogen Interactions, Host Defense Against *Mucorales*

Human-infecting *Mucorales* are usually thermotolerant, which makes them able to invade internal body parts and form a chronic infection. The interplay between pathogens and hosts varies among fungal agents and the host condition. The innate immune system and its complex interplay with the adaptive immune system are important in the pathogenesis of chronic inflammatory diseases such as chronic rhinosinusitis due to *Mucorales* (Muszewska et al. 2014; Ooi et al. 2008). However, most of the mechanisms are known from in vitro studies or animal data and should be considered with caution as the inflammatory reaction may be different in humans.

10.8.3.1 Innate and Adaptive Immunity to *Mucorales*

The First Line of Defense

Aerosolized *Mucorales* sporangiospores may be inhaled and enter to the nose, deposited in the nasal turbinates and paranasal sinuses in immune-competent hosts. Among diabetic and other patients having predisposing conditions, the inhaled sporangiospores germinate to form hyphae that invade tissues causing locally destructive sinus, orbital and rhinocerebral infections (Spellberg et al. 2005). The first line of defense is the physical and chemical barriers of nasal mucosa. Nasal mucociliary clearance serves as the primary mechanism by which the airway epithelium removes pathogens from the airway lumen. Antimicrobial-rich mucus gel is composed by mucin proteins. Mucin produced by the mucus cells serves as sticky binding sites that trap inhaled pathogens. Physical obstruction of sinus ostia or mucostasis can cause hypoxic conditions within the cellular environment. However, some species of the order *Mucorales*, such as *Mucor* spp. and *Rhizopus* spp., are able to grow under anaerobic conditions. These near-anaerobic conditions may permit the survival of fermentative *Mucorales* species and significantly contribute to the pathogenesis of sinonasal mucormycosis (Hariri and Cohen 2016).

Sinonasal epithelial cells also generate and secrete antimicrobial compounds to directly counteract pathogens. These compounds have various antibacterial, antifungal and antiviral effects and include proteins such as defensins, cathelicidins and reactive oxygen and nitrogen species, e.g. nitric oxide (Abbas et al. 2014a, b). It is important for the immune system to be able to recognize the presence of these organisms. Host sinonasal epithelium plays an important role in initially recognizing the presence of microbes and responding by increasing production of antimicrobial peptides and cytokines, with recruitment of phagocytes and lymphocytes of the adaptive immune system, to eliminate the infection (Ooi et al. 2008).

To mount an appropriate immune response, there must be mechanisms by which the cells of the sinonasal epithelium can detect and react in a measured manner to potentially harmful threats in the airway. Pathogen recognition receptors (PRRs) recognize pathogen-associated molecular patterns (Ooi et al. 2008). Proper detection of these pathogens is significant for sinonasal epithelial cells to be able to prepare a defensive response. PRRs have been implicated as sensors able to detect the presence of the pathogens and certain compounds that they secrete. Activation of these receptors also triggers innate immune responses to prevent or counteract infection, including mucociliary clearance and the production and secretion of antimicrobial compounds (e.g. defensins) (Hariri and Cohen 2016).

Defensins are an antimicrobial peptide family distributed in epithelial cells and phagocytes. Members of both defensin subfamilies, α- and β-defensins, are expressed in sinonasal epithelial cells. They are capable of affecting membrane permeabilization in both bacteria and fungi. Cathelicidins are another major class of antimicrobial peptides. Cathelicidin LL-37 is produced in the human nasal mucosa. However, the effects of these two antimicrobial peptides on *Mucorales* should be investigated. Reactive oxygen and nitrogen species generated by the sinonasal epithelium can play an important role in upper airway innate immunity. Nitric oxide (NO) in the upper airway originates predominantly from the paranasal sinuses, particularly the maxillary sinuses, and provides protection against pathogens.

Sinonasal mucosal epithelial cells adhere to one another to form a physical barrier that protects the underlying sinonasal tissue from inhaled pathogens. Cell junctions are the intracellular connections responsible for cellular adhesion, which make such a physical barrier possible. *Mucorales* may harm the integrity of the sinonasal epithelial cell barrier by producing proteases (Ma et al. 2009) that can cleave tight junction proteins. The first line of defense against *Mucorales* is the upper sinonasal epithelial cells that are encountered at the initial site of infection. Intrinsically faulty or having dysfunction or damage in epithelial cells that extends to the basement membrane exposes extracellular matrix proteins. *R. oryzae* resting spores have been shown to adhere to the basement membrane proteins laminin and type IV collagen (Bouchara et al. 1996). Following adhesion to the basement membrane proteins, *Mucorales* spores germinate and invade host cells (Ghuman and Voelz 2017).

Innate Immune Response

Sporangiospores may colonize the mucus. Immune dysfunction, whether overt or subtle, is the key factor predisposing to fungal invasion of sinonasal tissues. Presumably, fungi are unable to penetrate the epithelial layer when the immune system is functioning normally (Hontelez et al. 2012). Following the successful crossing of physical barriers, *Mucorales* encounter cells of innate immune system, including macrophages, neutrophils, microglial and dendritic cells (DC), and lead to variable host responses. The main line of innate host response to filamentous fungi consists of circulating polymorphonuclear neutrophils (PMNs), mononuclear cells (MNCs) and macrophages. The function of these cells is both to damage the invading organisms and to regulate innate immune response through secretion of cytokines and chemokines.

Phagocytes are capable of damaging fungal spores and hyphae through oxygen-dependent and oxygen-independent mechanisms. The oxygen-dependent mechanisms consist of a series of reactions starting with the production of superoxide anion (Ooi et al. 2008; Delves and Roitt 2000), which is dismutated into hydrogen peroxide. Myeloperoxidase then catalyses the conversion of hydrogen peroxide and halides to generate hypohalides, such as hypochlorite and chloramines, which exert potent antifungal activities (Babior 2000; Hampton et al. 1998). Cationic peptides (defensins and cathelicidins) are part of the oxygen-independent pathway of phagocytic cells (De Lucca and Walsh 1999; Ramanathan et al. 2002; Yang et al. 2002). A variety of cytokines, chemokines, and growth factors play an important role in the host response against filamentous fungi (Romani 2004). Most of these in vitro studies have been performed with immune cells obtained from healthy volunteers, because their primary objective was to elucidate the basic properties of normal host response against fungal pathogens (Roilides et al. 2012).

Macrophages

Innate immune system acts to prevent pathogenic spread, resists the establishment of infection and triggers the adaptive immune response. Tissue macrophages and neutrophils will serve as functional effector cells. Macrophages ingest and then kill sporangiospores by non-oxydative mechanisms, thereby preventing their germination to hyphae (Roilides et al. 2012; Levitz et al. 1986). Mucoralean hyphae have often a bigger diameter than those of Ascomycota. Hyphae diameter and size determine the efficacy of phagocytosis by macrophages. Mainly the literature on *Mucorales*-macrophage interactions is limited and associated with murine or human pulmonary macrophages. However, based on their anatomical location, functional specialization and expression of surface markers, macrophages are characterized by a high degree of heterogenicity (Gordon and Taylor 2005; Gordon et al. 2014; Gordon and Plűddemann 2013). None of the available experiments were associated with sinus-resident macrophages and/or parenchymal macrophages (Ghuman and Voelz 2017).

Although macrophages are unable to kill fungal spores, macrophages, monocytes, and human neutrophils can damage and kill fungal hyphae without prior phagocytic uptake by means of oxidative stress and cationic peptides (Mendoza et al. 2015; Levitz et al. 1986; Chinn and Diamond 1982; Diamond and Clark 1982; Diamond et al. 1982; Waldorf 1989). *M. circinelloides* belongs to the order *Mucorales* and is a dimorphic fungus that grows as a budding yeast anaerobically and as a filamentous fungus aerobically. The larger sporangiospores germinate inside and lyse macrophages, whereas the smaller sporangiospores do not (Orlowski 1991; Lübbehüsen et al. 2003).

Polymorphonuclear Leucocytes

If germination of sporangiospores evades or escapes this first line of defense, functional neutrophils are required to damage hyphae and prevent their invasion of surrounding tissue (Diamond and Clark 1982). Neutrophils are the most abundant type of leucocytes found in the blood and are rapidly recruited to the site of pathogenic infection. These innate immune cells are able to phagocyte and destroy pathogens via cationic peptides and oxidative burst, in a nonspecific manner in healthy immune conditions (Abbas et al. 2014a, b). Neutrophils exhibit fungicidal activity mediated by the production of cationic peptide activity. It was found that *R. oryzae* spore developmental stage influences the efficacy of neutrophil-killing activity (Ibrahim et al. 2012).

Gil-Lamaignere et al. (2005) compared the antifungal function of human pectin lyase (PNL) against hyphae of *R. oryzae*, *R. microspores* and *Absidia corymbifera* and found that both PNL-oxidative burst in response to hyphae and PNL-induced hyphal damage were significantly lower in response to *Rhizopus* species than in response to *A. corymbifera*. Interferon-ϒ (IFN ϒ) and granulocyte-macrophage colony-stimulating factor (GM-CSF) augmented this activity in a time-dependent manner. IFN-ϒ significantly reduced interleukin-8 (IL-8) release in response to all species tested. Treatment of PNLs with the combination of cytokines enhanced the release of tumour necrosis factor-α (TNF-α) in response to *R. microspores* and *A. corymbifera* but not in response to *R. oryzae* hyphae. The authors suggested intergenus differences in host response to *Mucorales*. *Rhizopus* hyphae had been shown to induce the expression of *tlr*2 mRNA in human PNLs, which indicates that Toll-like receptor 2 (TLR2) contributes as a pattern recognition receptor (PRR) towards *Mucorales* recognition by these leucocytes. Following exposure to *Rhizopus* hyphae, neutrophil expression of pro-inflammatory genes such as TNF-α and il-1b was noted, which implies neutrophil activation in response to *Mucorales* (Gil-Lamaignere et al. 2005).

A number of pathogen-associated molecular patterns on the surface of fungal spores or hyphae bind to pattern recognition receptors of phagocytes and generate the molecular signal for the pro-inflammatory and antifungal activities of phagocytes. Toll-like receptors (TLRs) together with other receptors play a critical role in the recognition of the fungal patterns and the intracytoplasmic transduction of the signals (Diamond and Clark 1982).

Whereas *A. fumigatus* is recognized by both TLR2 and TLR4 (Roilides et al. 1993), hyphae of *R. oryzae* are recognized only by TLR2 (Roilides et al. 2012). Among secreted cytokines, *R. oryzae* has been shown to induce significantly more TNF-α and IL-6 release by healthy human MNCs than do *Aspergillus* spp. in vitro. This could be attributed to the specific composition of the cell wall of *R. oryzae*, which contains more chitin than *Aspergillus*.

Rhizopus oryzae is recognized by TLR2 and upregulates release of a number of cytokines and chemokines from phagocytes, among which are TNF-α and IL-6.11,12 (Skiada et al. 2011; Chamilos et al. 2008; Warris et al. 2005). Toll receptors in *Drosophila* play a significant role in innate immune response to *R. oryzae* (Roilides et al. 2014).

Chamilos et al. (2008) observed that human PMNs were less effective at damaging *R. oryzae* hyphae than *Aspergillus fumigatus* hyphae associated with impaired O2 release following exposure to both fungi. Exposure of human PMNs to hyphae of *R. oryzae* and *A. fumigatus* resulted in selective upregulation of TLR2 mRNA. They also found that human PMNs had a reduced capacity to induce oxidative damage against unopsonized hyphae of clinical *Mucorales* isolates in comparison with unopsonized hyphae of *A. fumigatus*.

Qualitative and quantitative abnormalities of neutrophils, monocytes and macrophages make patients predisposed to development of mucormycosis. For example, in patients with diabetes mellitus, monocytes and macrophages fail to suppress germination of sporangiospores. Diabetic ketoacidosis is associated with impairments in neutrophil function including chemotaxis, adherence and oxidative burst. Hyperglycaemia and ketoacidosis both impair phagocytic effector functions (Roilides et al. 2012; Simitsopoulou et al. 2010). Cortisone treatment, rendering murine models immunocompromised, revealed not only the inability of macrophages to kill *R. oryzae* spores but also the failure to inhibit spore germination (Waldorf et al. 1984a; Mowat and Baum 1971; Bagdade 1976; Bybee and Rogers 1964). Neutropenia may allow fungi to invade surrounding sinonasal tissues (Soler and Schlosser 2012).

DC-Mucorales Interaction

Dendritic cells (DCs) are found in tissue that has contact with the outside environment such as in the linings of the nose. Immature forms are also found in the blood. Once activated, DCs move to the lymph tissue to interact with T cells and B cells and help shape the adaptive immune response. Dendritic cells in the linings of the nose act as a major antigen-presenting cell for adaptive immune effectors and triggering the adaptive immune system. In a healthy immune setting and upon pathogen recognition, DC phagocytose pathogens, secrete pro-inflammatory cytokines and present pathogenic antigens to T and B lymphocytes (Abbas et al. 2014a, b; Ghuman and Voelz 2017). Chamilos et al. (2010) showed that in vitro DC activation does not occur in response to *Rhizopus* spores; however, hyphae were shown to induce a strong DC release of IL-23, which is known to drive T_h-17 responses, and TNF-α, which is known to upregulate T_h-1 responses (Ghuman and Voelz 2017). The authors demonstrated that *Mucorales* surface β-glucan was essential for DC activation by dectin-1 receptor and IL-23 production and T_h-17 responses by DCs in vitro (Ghuman and Voelz 2017; Chamilos et al. 2010).

Natural Killer Cells

Natural killer (NK) cells are lymphocytes in the same family as T and B cells, coming from a common progenitor. However, as cells of the innate immune system, NK cells are classified as group I innate lymphocytes (ILCs) and respond quickly to a wide variety of pathological challenges. NK cells secrete cytokines such as IFN-γ and TNF-α, which act on other immune cells like macrophage and DCs to enhance the immune response. While on patrol NK cells constantly contact other cells. Whether or not the NK cell kills these cells depends on a balance of signals from activating receptors and inhibitory receptors on the NK cell surface. Activating receptors recognize molecules that are expressed on the surface of infected cells and "switch on" the NK cell. Inhibitory receptors act as a check on NK cell killing. Most normal healthy cells express MHC I receptors which mark these cells as "self". Inhibitory receptors on the surface of the NK cell recognize cognate MHC I, and this "switches off" the NK cell, preventing it from killing. Infected cells often lose their MHC I, leaving them vulnerable to NK cell killing. Once the decision is made to kill, the NK cell releases cytotoxic granules containing perforin and granzymes, which leads to lysis of the target cell. Schmidt et al. (2016) demonstrated that both unstimulated and IL-2-prestimulated human NK cells damage *Rhizopus oryzae* hyphae but do not affect resting conidia. *Rhizopus* spores do not activate NK cells and were resistant to their fungicidal activity. In contrast, *Rhizopus* hyphae activate NK cells and were damaged by human NK cells through the release of perforin. They concluded that the damage of the fungus is mediated, at least in part, by perforin. *R. oryzae* hyphae decrease the secretion of immunoregulatory molecules by NK cells, such as IFN-γ and RANTES (regulated on activation, normal T cell expressed and secreted), indicating an immunosuppressive effect of the *Mucorales* hyphae.

The Effect of Immune Suppression

Finally, suppression of the immune system, such as from poorly controlled diabetes mellitus, chemotherapy, corticosteroids or prolonged neutropenia, may allow fungi to invade surrounding sinonasal tissues (Soler and Schlosser 2012). The patients with RCM often present with defects in innate immunity, particularly of phagocytic effector cell functions. For example, impaired macrophage and neutrophil function because of corticosteroid therapy might significantly increase susceptibility to *Mucorales* infection. Patients with diabetes mellitus, particularly those in ketoacidosis, are more likely to have *Mucorales* species. During ketoacidosis, the concentration of ketones in the patient's blood increases, leading to acidification. The decrease in pH increases the availability of free iron, an essential of growth factor for *Mucorales* (Mendoza et al. 2015).

Endothelial Interaction with Mucorales

Angioinvasion is a hallmark of mucormycosis. Penetration of the endothelial lining of vasculature results in vessel thrombosis and tissue necrosis and permits *Mucorales* to disseminate haematogenously (Ibrahim et al. 2005, 2012; Ben-Ami et al. 2009). Necrotic tissue can restrict the access of phagocytic effector cells or antifungals to infected areas, likely prohibiting fungal clearing and contributing to the organism's haematogenous dissemination via penetration of endothelial cells and the extracellular matrix of blood vessels (Ibrahim et al. 2012). Therefore, interactions between invading fungi and endothelial cells lining blood vessels represents a major step in the pathogenesis of mucormycosis (Baldin and Ibrahim 2017).

R. oryzae spores, germ tubes and hyphae adhere specifically to human umbilical vein cells *in vitro*, whereas only spores adhere to subendothelial matrix proteins. *R. oryzae* had also the ability to damage human umbilical vein cells irrespective of the organism's morphology and invade these cells by induced endocytosis. It was demonstrated that *R. oryzae* viable or nonviable spores and hyphae damage to human umbilical vein cells was possibly due to the presence of a toxin in *R. oryzae* and this damage required direct contact to and subsequent phagocytosis of the organism by human umbilical vein cells (Ibrahim et al. 2005). Liu et al. (2010) had identified glucose-regulated protein 78 (GRP78), a member of the Hsp70 chaperone family, and proposed that it was a required host receptor that mediates and damage of human endothelial cells by *R. oryzae* and invasion and damage of endothelial cells was in a receptor-dependent manner. It was shown that *Mucorales* internalization was host iron dependent (Liu et al. 2010). *R. oryzae* ungerminated spores, but not germinated spores or hyphae, attach to the matrix proteins laminin and type IV collagen in vitro (Bouchara et al. 1996).

T-Cell Response to Mucorales

In general, Th1-type cell-mediated immunity is required for clearance of a fungal infection, while Th2 immunity usually results in susceptibility to systemic infection or allergic responses. Th1 cells produce predominantly cytokines such as IFN-ϒ and IL-10 and promote protective cell-mediated immunity to fungi and phagocyte activation. In contrast, TH2 cells produce predominantly cytokines such as interleukins 3 and 4 (IL-3 and IL-4) and tend to promote antibody production (Ghuman and Voelz 2017; Blanco and Garcia 2008).

Mucorales-specific T cells can be found both in patients and in healthy individuals. Potenza et al. (2011) investigated *Mucorales*-specific T cells in patients with invasive mucormycosis and found that *Mucorales*-specific T cells belonging to both $CD4^+$ and $CD8^+$ subsets were present during infection. The authors also investigated *Mucorales*-specific cytokine profiles and found that IL-4, IFN-ϒ, IL-10 and IL-17 to be most abundantly produced. Additionally, IFN-ϒ-producing T cells were demonstrated to induce *Mucorales* hyphal damage.

Th17 cells produce IL-17 and implicate in mucosal immunity against fungi. In vitro stimulation of T cells by *R. oryzae* showed the generation of Th17 cells. Th17 cell production of IL-17 has an impact on neutrophil activity by acting as a chemoattractant and inducing the production of antifungal defensins by neutrophils (Chamilos et al. 2010).

Cytokines studied so far include the haematopoietic growth factors, granulocyte colony-stimulating factor (G-CSF) and granulocyte-macrophage colony-stimulating factor (GM-CSF), as well as IFN-γ. These cytokines have been shown to stimulate proliferation and differentiation of myeloid progenitor cells to neutrophils (G-CSF, GM-CSF) or monocytes and eosinophils (GM-CSF), to upregulate chemotaxis, phagocytosis and respiratory burst of phagocytic cells (neutrophils, monocytes, macrophages) (G-CSF, GM-CSF, IFN-γ) and to regulate/enhance protective T-helper type 1 (Th1) responses (IFN-γ) (Lohmeyer 1997; Roilides et al. 1998). Most of the data on the role of these cytokines in modifying host response against the *Mucorales* originate from in vitro and in vivo studies (Gil-Lamaignere et al. 2005; Liles et al. 1997; Pursell et al. 2003; Saoulidis et al. 2011), clinical evidence on their efficacy as adjunctive treatment in patients with mucormycosis remains limited (Roilides et al. 2014).

Interestingly, fungal morphology also affects the chemotactic potential of *R. oryzae* on neutrophils. Although inactive spores do not induce neutrophil migration, active spores and hyphae present a potent chemotactic signal (Waldorf and Diamond 1985). After encountering *R. oryzae* hyphae, human polymorphonuclear neutrophils activate the expression of Toll-like receptor 2 and NF-kB pathway-related genes (Chamilos et al. 2008). Additionally, dectin-1-dependent activation of interleukin 23 production by human dendritic cells induces pro-inflammatory Th17 responses (Chamilos et al. 2010). In contrast, macrophages from diabetic or corticosteroid-treated mice fail to inhibit spore germination (Waldorf et al. 1984a, b). Neutrophils from diabetic patients with hyperglycaemia and diabetic ketoacidosis retain the ability to damage fungal hyphae but show reduced responses to *R. oryzae* chemotactic factors (Chinn and Diamond 1982). This might interrupt downstream signalling and the activation of appropriate downstream cytokine responses.

10.9 Portal of Entry and Routes of Infection

The major mode of transmission might generally be inhalation of aerosolized sporangiospores. Based on radiologic and/or histologic observations, several routes of CNS invasion have been documented. Mainly, CNS involvement may occur from haematogenous spread or direct invasion, or direct inoculation.

Mucorales species fungus has a propensity for growing along the walls of blood vessels. *Mucorales* are vasotropic and vasoinvasion and neurotropism were considered the common pathologic features of invasive mucormycosis. Inhaled sporangiospores can be spread to the brain by the haematogenous route invading the intracranial vasculature. Cells of *Mucorales* may possess appropriate virulence factors or specific surface receptors to adhere the endothelial cell surface proteins, to cross the blood-brain-CSF barriers and escape the action of host mechanisms (Spellberg et al. 2005) and may extend to CNS via lumens and walls of vessels.

Apart from angioinvasion in RCM, direct spread through cribriform plate of the ethmoid bone into the anterior cranial fossa can occur (Melsom and Khangure 2000; Hosseini and Borghei 2005), and it was suggested that this represents perineural spread. *Mucorales* can spread up the nerve roots into the CNS (Parsi et al. 2013; McLean et al. 1996; Orguc et al. 2005; Margo et al. 2007). Histologically proven perineural extension of disease from cavernous sinus to pons along the trigeminal nerve with no apparent meningeal or intraparenchymal brain involvement was reported (McLean et al. 1996). Perineural invasion had been considered unusual but contrast-enhanced MRI studies have documented perineural invasion via the trigeminal nerve (Hosseini and Borghei 2005; Mohindra et al. 2007; Ghuman et al. 2015). High percentage of perineural invasion in patients with invasive mucormycosis was reported and hypothesized that perineural invasion was another possible mechanism involving extension of the fungi into CNS reported perineural invasion in 90% of biopsies that contained peripheral nerves (Cornely et al. 2014; Frater et al. 2001; Sravani et al. 2014).

Direct inoculation through penetrating head injury or during therapeutic or narcotic parenteral administration was also described. Brain involvement in the absence of sinus involvement had also been documented mainly in intravenous drug abusers (Sundaram et al. 2005; Spellberg et al. 2005). With instance of recycling of used syringes and catheters for i.v. administration, haematogenous inoculation of *Mucorales* spores can lead to primary CNS lesions, without overt predisposing factors.

Infection with *Apophysomyces* in previously healthy humans typically develops after traumatic implantation of the spores or inhalation into the sinuses (Wolkow et al. 2017).

10.10 Signs and Symptoms

Initial symptoms of RCM are nonspecific, involving sinus pain, headaches, nasal congestion, altered mental status, fever, soft tissue swelling and eye syndrome, lacrimation, irritation or periorbital anaesthesia. Unilateral vision disturbance and further changes involving ptosis, proptosis or loss of extraocular muscle function are signs of the progressing infection towards the retro-orbital region or the CNS. Necrotic black lesions on the hard palate, necrotic turbinates and septum perforation should be carefully inspected. Extension to the eyes is possible, leading to blurred vision or even complete loss of vision. From the eyes the disease can progress towards the central nervous system resulting in altered consciousness, cranial neuropathies or cerebral abscesses (Muszewska et al. 2014; Sheikh and Amr 2011; Binder et al. 2014; Spellberg et al. 2005; Teixeira et al. 2013). The most common presenting signs and symptoms of ROCM caused by *A. elegans* are similar to the classic features of those caused by other *Mucorales* species (Liang et al. 2006).

RCM progresses rapidly if not treated and extends to neighbouring tissues, causing thrombosis of the sphenopalatine vessels in the pterygopalatine fossa and/or anterior ethmoid vessels in the orbit, nasal ulceration and further necrosis associated with painful black-coloured eschar on the palate or mucosa of the nasal cavity, septum or osseous walls of the maxillary sinus, uni- or bilaterally (Hosseini and Borghei 2005).

10.11 Clinical Presentations

Rhino-orbito-cerebral disease defines an infection that originates in the paranasal sinuses with gradual and fast extension to the bony structures, eyes, facial soft tissues and the brain in a few days, following inhalation of spores. The angioinvasive nature of these fungi causes cerebral infections and brain abscesses; occasionally it may break out into the subarachnoid space (Gottfredsson and Perfect 2000). Chronic presentation of rhinocerebral mucormycosis was also described with indolent and slowly progressive course, often occurring over weeks to months (Sheikh and Amr 2011) (Fig. 10.2).

Brain involvement in RCM without sinus invasion had been reported in 37 i.v. drug abusers of 64 previously healthy patients. Meningitis due to *Mucorales* spp. in two (Sohail et al. 2001; Kasliwal et al. 2009) and *Absidia corymbifera* in one patient (Mackenzie et al. 1988) have been reported.

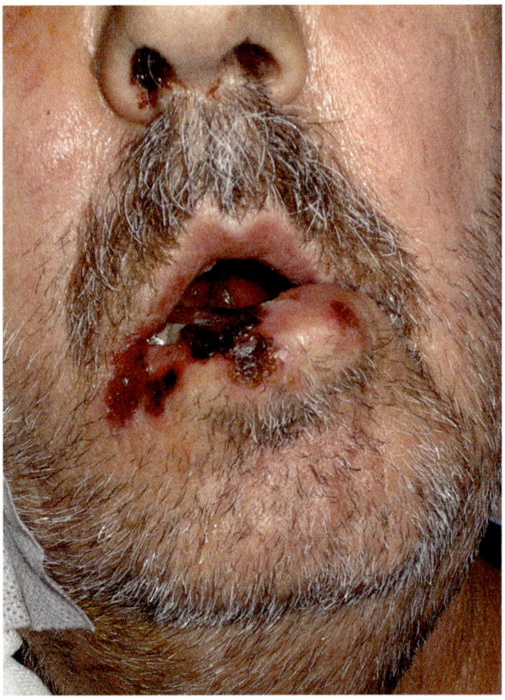

Fig. 10.2 Nasal and oral manifestations of a patient with ROCM

Most of the patients with RCM also developed acute ocular symptoms (Hosseini and Borghei 2005; Sponsler et al. 1992; Onerci et al. 1991; Weprin et al. 1998; Fisher et al. 1991; Langford et al. 1997; Aköz et al. 1999; Luna et al. 1996) as a result of invasion of the pterygopalatine fossa and inferior orbital fissure. Invasion of the optic nerve and/or central thrombosis of the retinal artery results in visual loss. Fundoscopic examination reveals retinal atrophy secondary to ischaemia. Paralysis of the ocular muscles may occur due to infiltration of the retrobulbar and extraocular muscles. This paralysis is usually complete, though at times it may be selective (Brown and Lau 2001). Both the involvement and lack of involvement of the lamina papyracea (orbital lamina) which is a smooth bone plate forming the lateral surface of the labyrinth of the ethmoid bone have been reported (Raj et al. 1998; Soto-Aguilar et al. 1997; deShazo et al. 1997). In such patients with ocular signs and no black necrosis of the nasal mucosa, CT scan of the brain may be normal, causing a delay in diagnosis. In these cases, biopsy and frozen sections from the nasal mucosa and/or sinuses can help achieve the diagnosis (Baldin and Ibrahim 2017; Langford et al. 1997; Ibrahim and Kontoyiannis 2013).

10.12 Radiology

The radiographic image of the ROCM could be mimicked by bacterial and fungal infections as well as tumours (Figs. 10.3 and 10.4). Scheckenbach et al. (2010) reported that initial CT scanning was not informative and most manifestations were not specific; according to Muszevska et al. (2014), only histopathology provides sufficient data to establish a reliable diagnosis. Contrast-enhanced magnetic resonance imaging (MRI) studies have documented perineural invasion via the trigeminal nerve (Parsi et al. 2013; McLean et al. 1996; Orguc et al. 2005; Margo et al. 2007; Sravani et al. 2014). The involvement of lymph nodes of the neck and the presence of lesions on MRI of the brain were documented particularly in immunocompetent i.v. drug users who have CNS infection (Hopkins et al. 1994).

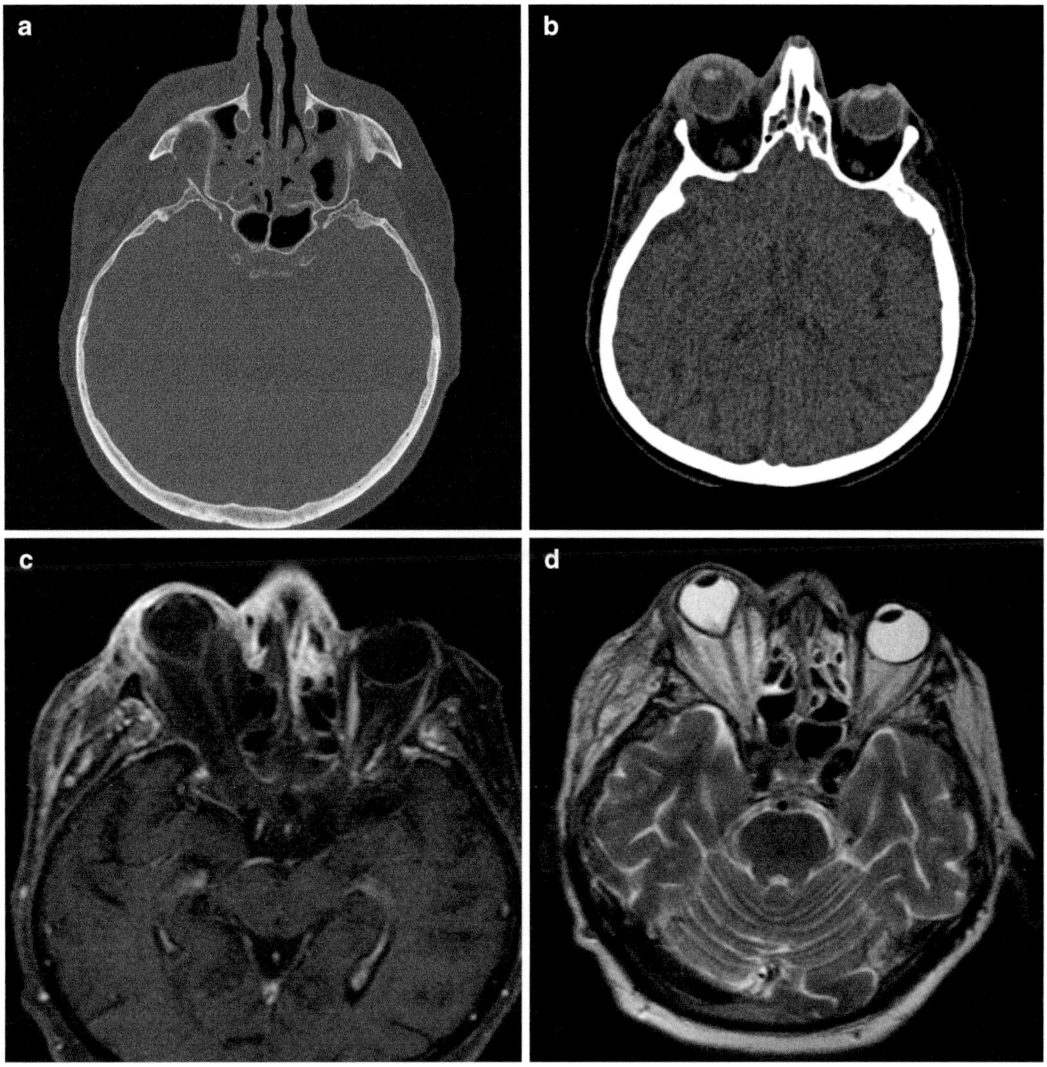

Fig. 10.3 (**a**) CT 1: Axial computer tomography scan of the sinuses showing mucosal thickening and opacification in the maxillary sinuses and ethmoid air cells with bony erosions of the medial wall of the maxillary sinuse suggesting invasive fungal sinusitis; (**b**) CT 2: Axial computer tomography scan showing proptosis and deformation of the right globe and soft tissue thickening of the right preseptal region. Also opacification of the ethmoid air cells; (**c**): MR T2: Axial T2 weighted MR scan showing mucosal thickening of the ethmoid air cells, inflammation of the intraconal and extraconal fat and extraoculer muscles extending to zygomatic region and invading ipsilateral cavernous sinüse; (**d**) MR T1C: Axial contrast enhanced fat suppressed T1 weighted MR scan showing soft tissue thickening and enhancement in the preseptal region of the right globe extending the zygomatic region, proptosis and deformation of the right globe. (Courtesy of Civan Islak, Prof, MD, University of Istanbul-Cerrahpasa, Cerrahpasa Medical Faculty Dept of Radiology)

There were several reported radiologic clues to diagnosis. Plain sinus radiographs seldom reveal an air-fluid level as seen in acute bacterial sinusitis; however, bony erosion might be found. Both CT scan and MRI of the brain may show characteristic changes, including sinus opacification, inflammatory changes in the paranasal sinuses, erosion of bone and obliteration of deep facial planes. Frontal lobe involvement may show little or no ring enhancement (Meyers et al. 1979).

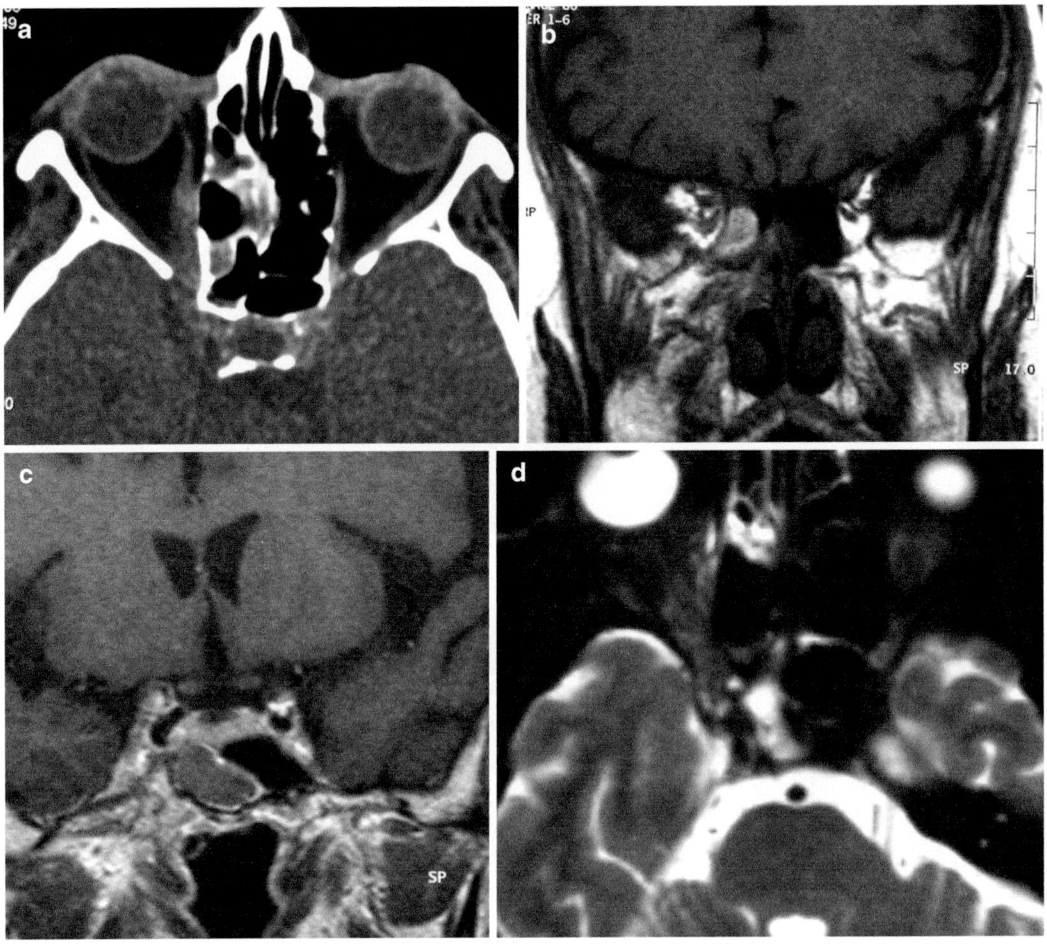

Fig. 10.4 (**a**) Axial computer tomography scan showing opacification and mucosal thickening of the ethmoid cellular airs extending to right sided extraconal fat and right cavernous sinuse; (**b**) Coronal nonenhanced T1 weighted MR scan showing fluid collection, mucosal thickening in right sfenoid sinuse suggesting sinusitis extending to ipsilateral cavernous sinus; (**c**) Coronal contrast enhanced T1 weighted MR scan showing collection of fluid in the right sfenoid sinüse; (**d**) Axial T2 weighted MR scan showing fluid collection, mucosal thickening in right sfenoid sinuse and ethmoid cellular airs suggesting sinusitis extending to extraconal fat and ipsilateral cavernous sinus. (Courtesy of Civan Islak, Prof, MD, University of Istanbul-Cerrahpasa, Cerrahpasa Medical Faculty Dept of Radiology)

Extension of the infection into the cavernous sinus, with cavernous sinus thrombosis and internal carotid artery narrowing, was well demonstrated on pre- and postgadolinium MRI scans. Infarctions in the anterior choroidal artery distribution suggested intracranial invasion of the infection, and watershed distribution of infarctions attested to the tenuousness of flow through a narrowed cavernous portion of carotid artery (Yousem et al. 1989). MRI demonstrated ischaemic optic nerve involvement due to ROCM in four case reports (Ghuman et al. 2015; Al-Shafai and Mikulis 2006; Mathur et al. 2007; Alsuhaibani et al. 2012).

Linear enhancement on MRI beginning at the orbital apex might be correlated with fungal tracking of the trigeminal and lacrimal nerves. Mucormycosis can spread considerable distances from its primary focus of infection along peripheral nerves, a phenomenon that can be identified clinically with contrast-enhanced MRI (Margo et al. 2007).

10.13 Histopathology

The diagnosis of mucormycosis is made on tissue section. Histopathological examination of tissue specimens that may allow differentiation between hyphae of *Aspergillus* or morphologically related fungi and hyphae of *Mucorales* seen by histopathological examination of tissue specimens is important for treatment decisions.

Hyphae usually vary from 6 to 30 μm in diameter, having often a bigger diameter than in Ascomycota, and are sparsely septate and irregularly branched. The organism characteristically invades the walls of adjacent blood vessels, causing thrombosis and infarction. Stains of fixed tissues with haematoxylin and eosin (H&E) or specialized fungal stains, such as Grocott methenamine silver (GMS) or periodic acid-Schiff (PAS) stains, show broad-based, ribbon-like, nonseptate hyphae with wide-angle branching (approximately 90°). The hyphae are often not well preserved and may become crinkled or gnarled in the tissue sections. This appearance of the hyphal elements is often described as resembling "crinkled cellophane" or "ribbon-like" (Cornely et al. 2014; Ribes et al. 2000; Lass-Flörl 2009). Cross-sections of hyphal elements often give tissues a vacuolated appearance. These cross-sections vary in diameter and may be confused with yeast cells. The H&E stain should always be confirmed with a more fungus-specific tissue stain such as GMS or PAS (Lass-Flörl 2009).

Acute suppurative inflammation predominates, with focal areas of granulomatous inflammation. Mucormycosis is characterized by prominent infarcts, angioinvasion and perineural invasion (Cornely et al. 2014; Frater et al. 2001). Perineural invasion was histologically identified in several patients diagnosed with RCM on tissue sections (Cornely et al. 2014; Sravani et al. 2014).

Immunohistochemistry is only marginally supported for the diagnosis of mucormycosis due to the lack of commercially available monoclonal antibodies and clinical validation.

10.14 Microbiology

10.14.1 Direct Microscopic Examination

Aspirated material from sinuses and biopsy material should be submitted for examination by clinical microbiology laboratory. Hyphae of the *Mucorales* may be difficult to observe on an unenhanced KOH wet mount and may not stain well with conventional Gram stain. The use of chitin-binding stains, such as calcofluor, fungifluor or blancofluor, may be used with a fluorescent microscope to identify hyphal elements on KOH wet mounts (Cornely et al. 2014; Lass-Flörl 2009). Direct microscopical examination may be undertaken using Giemsa-stained slide preparations of the imprinted tissue specimens (Fig. 10.5). By Giemsa technique, coenocytic hyphae may be stained eosinophilic (Kantarcioğlu et al. 2006). Hyphae of the *Mucorales* are typically broad, having a variable width (6–25 μm in diameter), ribbon-like and irregularly shaped, nonseptate (coenocytic) or sparsely septate, with branches often arising non-dichotomously in "right angles". The angle of branching is variable and includes wide-angle (90°) bifurcations.

A positive direct microscopy, especially from a sterile site, must be considered significant, even if the laboratory is unable to culture the fungus. The combined application of KOH and brighteners is possible (Lass-Flörl 2009). McDermott et al. (2010) recently reported the use of calcofluor-stained tissue as a rapid technique for intraoperative diagnosis and assessment of clean resected margins in lieu of frozen sections by pathology. The *Mucorales* are usually distinguishable histologically from other filamentous fungi, such as *Aspergillus* spp., *Fusarium* spp. and *Pseudallescheria boydii/ Scedosporium apiospermum* species complexes, which typically appear as slender dichotomously branching septate hyphae. Distinction by direct examination may allow AmB and other potentially life-saving therapeutic interventions to be initiated (Gamaletsou et al. 2012).

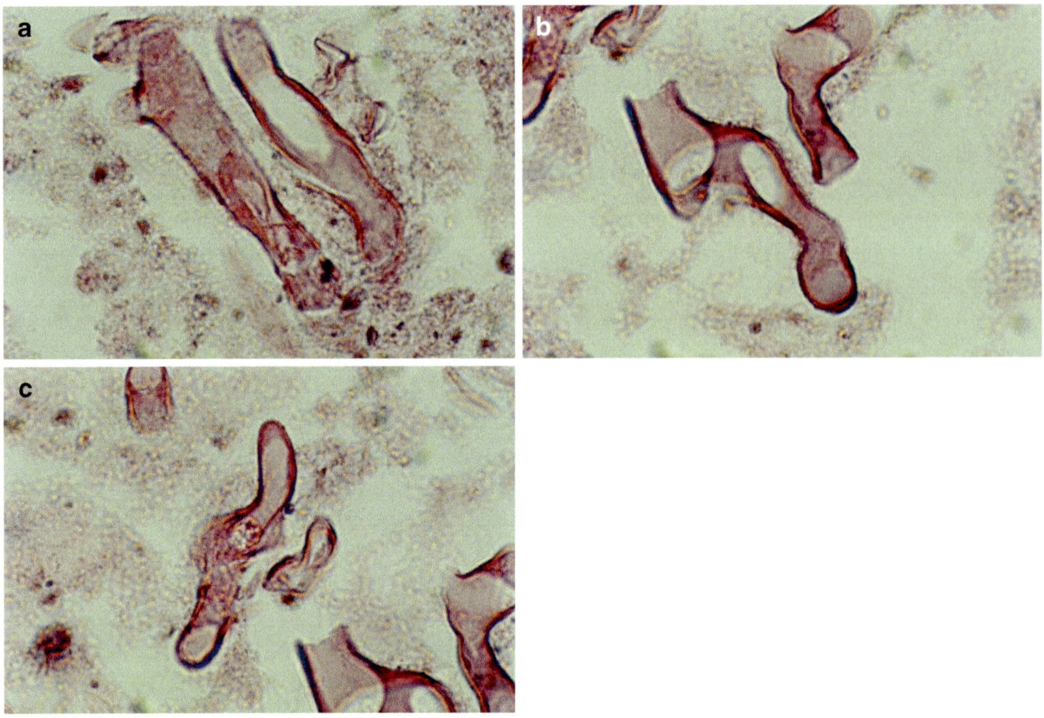

Fig. 10.5 (a-c) Fungal morphology in imprinted tissue preparations: broad coenocytic hyphae (Giemsa stained, ×100)

10.14.2 Molecular Diagnostics

Molecular assays for rapid and early detection of mucormycosis are being developed but remain investigational at this time. Currently, in the absence of a standardized test, the use of molecular methods on both fresh clinical material and paraffin slides for the diagnosis of mucormycosis is moderately supported. Fresh material is preferred over paraffin-embedded tissue because formalin damages DNA (Cornely et al. 2014).

10.14.3 Culture

Culture of specimens is considered an essential investigation. Although the sensitivity of culture is not optimal, it allows identification and susceptibility testing of the isolate in case of growth. These fungi can be difficult to recover. Blood cultures are of no benefit. *Mucorales* do not survive for more than a few hours at refrigerator temperatures; therefore, if culture is delayed, storage at room temperature is recommended *Mucorales* have primitive hyphae, which become easily damaged during biopsy procedures or tissue grinding in the laboratory. Thus they are not suitable for growing in culture despite their presence in microscopic or histopathological examinations (Lass-Flörl 2009). In any case, negative cultures do not rule out the infection.

It is recommended that the clinical material is inoculated onto Sabouraud dextrose agar and incubated at 30 °C and 37 °C for a minimum of 3–5 days. The growth of the *Mucorales* tends to be rapid, with mycelial elements expanding to cover the entire plate in only a few (1–7) days. The sporulating surface of the colonies may demonstrate variable degrees of colouration. Depending upon the order, species or individual isolate, *Mucorales* will demonstrate surface colouration varying from pure white to tan, brown, grey or even black. Brain heart infusion (BHI) broth with penicillin may be added to the normal battery when *Mucorales* are suspected. The use of broth provides optimal medium-specimen contact. Malt extract agar is an effective alternative to broth media for the isolation of

Mucorales. BHI broth may be used routinely by some ophthalmologists for corneal scrapings. *Mucorales* will grow rapidly, often filling the entire Petri dish within a few days (Fig. 10.1c, d). In any case, negative cultures do not rule out the infection. A culture result from a non-sterile body site is not in itself diagnostic of infection because these fungi are common in the environment (Lass-Flörl 2009; Torres-Narbona et al. 2007a, 2008).

10.14.4 Serology

There are no standardized assays available for the detection of *Mucorales*-specific antigens, and serological tests for mucormycosis cannot be recommended without further clinical evaluation and are not available for routine use at this time.

1,3-β-D-Glucan is a common component of the cell wall of a wide variety of fungi but not of the *Mucorales*. They are galactomannan negative. Therefore, serum tests based on these features are not recommended for the diagnosis of CNS mucormycosis.

10.14.5 Preoperative Cytology

Nonspecific signs of meningitis might be found in cerebrospinal fluid, although the culture yield was extremely low (Jones et al. 1981). Preoperative cytology is an effective technique to establish a diagnosis of mucormycosis and obviates the need for a preoperative biopsy. Frozen section is a specific and sensitive method to make a quick initial diagnosis of RCM (Sheikh and Amr 2011; Lackner et al. 2014; Hofman et al. 2003).

10.14.6 Genus and Species Identification

There is no strong evidence that identification to the genus/species level may be important to guide treatment. Identification to the species level is of interest for a better epidemiological knowledge of mucormycosis and may be of value for outbreak investigation. Identification to the genus and species level is strongly supported for a better epidemiological knowledge of the disease.

Recovery of *Mucorales* from cultures of clinical specimens allows not only for diagnosis but also for the identification of the causative organism to species level. Direct microscopy is not useful for species identification. Classical identification is based primarily on sporangial morphology. This includes the arrangement and number of sporangiospores, the shape, colour, presence or absence of columellae and apophyses as well as the arrangement of the sporangiophores and the presence or absence of rhizoids. Species can be differentiated by elements such as rhizoids, stolons and columella which are usually seen on lactophenol cotton blue-stained slides under microscope. Lactophenol cotton blue can be used to achieve better visualization (Fig. 10.1d) (Ribes et al. 2000). Growth temperature studies (25, 37, 45 °C) can be helpful in identifying culture characteristics. Sporulation may be stimulated by the use of nutrient-deficient media, such as cornmeal-glucose-sucrose-yeast extract agar or Czapek Dox agar.

Carbon assimilation is moderately supported, and molecular identification is strongly supported in comparison with morphology. The best technique for molecular identification is ITS sequencing. There are currently limited data for MALDI-TOF as an identification method. Molecular techniques are more reliable than phenotypic identification of *Mucorales* in culture to the species level. Sequencing of ITS is currently the best molecular technique for species identification. Carbon assimilation profiles using the commercialized kits ID32C and API 50 CH (bioMerieux, Marcy l'Etoile, France) allowed precise and accurate identification of *Mucorales* to the species level (Schwarz et al. 2007). Alternative techniques such as matrix-assisted laser desorption/ ionization time-of-flight (MALDI-TOF) mass spectrometry are promising but not yet validated for all species (Cornely et al. 2014). Although MALDI-TOF identification of *Mucorales* seems promising, more data are needed to validate this technique and commercially available databases should be validated (Dolatabadi et al. 2015).

10.15 Antifungal Susceptibility

10.15.1 In Vitro Susceptibility Testing

European Committee on Antimicrobial Susceptibility Testing (EUCAST) and CLSI (M38-A2) (CLSI 2008; EUCAST 2017) reference microdilution methods are used as standard assays for antifungal susceptibility testing of *Mucorales*. Using methods other than the reference assays such as Etest (Caramalho et al. 2015; Torres-Narbona et al. 2007b; Khan et al. 2009) or XTT assay (Antachopoulos et al. 2006; Spreghini et al. 2010) remains investigational. With these fungi it is often difficult to achieve accurate and consistent endpoints. As the interpretive minimal inhibitory concentrations (MIC) breakpoints have not yet been defined for zygomycetes/*Mucorales* and the correlations between clinical response and MIC values for a given strain are uncertain, the use of antifungal susceptibility testing in mucormycosis for routine clinical decisions is not recommended at this time (Cornely et al. 2014). Except for posaconazole, moderate (<80%) correlation of Etest and Sensititre YeastOne with the CLSI M38-A2 method was noted in antifungal susceptibility testing of *Mucorales* (Cornely et al. 2014; CLSI 2008). Rapid (within 6–8 h) susceptibility testing can be achieved with the XTT assay (Antachopoulos et al. 2006). Currently, there are no validated MIC breakpoints for any of the drugs against fungal genera in *Mucorales*, and so determination of susceptibility categories (S, I and R) is not possible. A correlation between the generated MIC and clinical outcome was addressed in only a few studies.

AmB, which is the antifungal of choice for this mycosis, was the most active agent against all isolates, with the exception of those belonging to the genera *Cunninghamella* and *Apophysomyces*. High drug MICs for *Cunninghamella* species have been reported before (Gomez-Lopez et al. 2001; Ortín et al. 2004; Honda 1998; Zeilender et al. 1990). Terbinafine was active against all species tested, except for *R. oryzae*, *M. circinelloides* and *R. variabilis*. Azole drugs showed various levels of activity. Itraconazole showed activity against only *R. pusillus* and *Lichtheimia corymbifera*. Similar results have been found in other studies (Dannaoui et al. 2003; Rogers 2008). Itraconazole has also shown good activity in animal models of infection with *L. corymbifera* (Dannaoui et al. 2002; Mosquera et al. 2001). Therefore, itraconazole could be useful for some cases of mucormycosis when susceptible strains are involved. Voriconazole has no in vitro activity against these fungi. In addition, it has been shown that patients with leukaemia and bone marrow transplant recipients on VRZ prophylaxis can develop breakthrough infections caused by *Mucorales* species (Kontoyiannis et al. 2005). Ravuconazole showed some activity against *M. corymbifer*, *R. pusillus*, *R. oryzae*, *R. microsporus* and *Actinomucor elegans*, although isolates resistant to this drug were found in most of the species. Posaconazole was the azole drug which showed the best in vitro activity (Alastruey-Izquierdo et al. 2009).

In a retrospective analysis of 16 patients infected with *A. elegans*, an AmB MIC of <1 lg/mL correlated with recovery. Of those infected with strains with an AmB MIC of ≥1 lg/mL, 43% failed to respond (Chakrabarti et al. 2010). Animal studies for determination of in vitro-in vivo correlation are also limited. In murine models of infections due to *Rhizopus microsporus* (Rodríguez et al. 2009) and *R. oryzae* (Rodríguez et al. 2008, 2009), posaconazole was shown to be more effective in infections due to strains with an MIC of 0.25 lg/mL compared with those with an MIC of 2 lg/mL. On the other hand, a low minimum fungicidal concentration, i.e. 0.5 lg/mL of posaconazole, was associated with response in mice infected with *R. oryzae*. High posaconazole minimum fungicidal concentration values, i.e. >16 lg/mL, correlated with clinical failure in a similar murine model (Spreghini et al. 2010).

Antifungal susceptibility testing of the strains in the order *Mucorales* has been performed mostly for epidemiological purposes. The data presented in these studies provide significant clues for the expected susceptibility profiles and are useful to evaluate genus-, species- and strain-based variations in susceptibility. Fluconazole, voriconazole, echinocandins and flucytosine lack meaningful in vitro activity against *Mucorales*. In general, AmB and posaconazole are the most active drugs in vitro. The comparative activities of AmB and posaconazole may vary depending on the genus and species of the infecting strain. AmB, posaconazole and isavuconazole are currently the most active agents against *Mucorales*; however, their activity remains suboptimal, and new therapeutic strategies are needed. Combination therapy could be a promising approach (Dannaoui 2017; Alastruey-Izquierdo et al. 2009; Rodríguez et al. 2009; Sun et al. 2002; Almyroudis et al. 2007; Arikan et al. 2008; Vitale et al. 2011).

Species-specific differences in azole and terbinafine susceptibilities are noted particularly for *Rhizopus* and *Mucor* (Dannaoui et al. 2003; Rodríguez et al. 2009; Vitale et al. 2011). Strain-based variations have also been described, as for posaconazole susceptibility of *R. oryzae* strains (Rodríguez et al. 2009).

Despite the lack of preference for its use in treatment of mucormycosis, itraconazole MICs are relatively low for a number of strains, including those of *Rhizomucor* (Alastruey-Izquierdo et al. 2009; Vitale et al. 2011) and *Lichtheimia* (Dannaoui et al. 2003; Alastruey-Izquierdo et al. 2009; Sun et al. 2002; Vitale et al. 2011). Efficacy of combination therapy was addressed in murine models of mucormycosis. Improved survival was observed with the combination of AmB lipid complex and caspofungin (CAS) compared with monotherapy and untreated controls in diabetic ketoacidotic mice infected with a more virulent brain isolate of *R. oryzae*. However, improved organ clearance was not achieved with combination therapy (Spellberg et al. 2005). In a murine model of disseminated mucormycosis caused by *R. oryzae*, posaconazole was combined with AmB at low dose (0.3 mg/kg/day) prolonged survival, and reduced tissue burden was observed compared with monotherapy and controls. However, it was not superior to AmB (0.8 mg/kg/day) alone (Rodríguez et al. 2008). In vitro combination studies have also been performed to explore the interaction of antifungal agents against members of the order *Mucorales*.

10.16 Treatment and Outcome

CNS mucormycosis is perhaps one of the most aggressive fungal infections of humans, and the early cases were uniformly fatal. The first survivor, reported by Harris in 1955, was a 14-year-old girl with diabetes who was treated successfully by rigid control of her diabetes and administration of systemic iodides (Harris 1955).

AmB was the drug of choice for primary treatment of mucormycosis. Antifungal therapy was considered as essential part of a combined therapeutic approach also involving surgical debridement of all devitalized tissue and reversal of underlying predisposing conditions. AmB deoxycholate had been used as standard treatment when no alternative was available (Walsh et al. 2012; Jacobs et al. 2002). The efficacy of AmB has been reproducibly demonstrated in both laboratory (in vitro and in vivo) investigations and in clinical studies (Antachopoulos et al. 2006; Spreghini et al. 2010; Dannaoui et al. 2003; Chakrabarti et al. 2010; Rodríguez et al. 2009; Sun et al. 2002; Arikan et al. 2008; Rodriguez-Tudela et al. 2003). Although interpretive breakpoints for determination of in vitro susceptibility to AmB have not been determined, apparent in vitro resistance, with elevated MICs, may be observed in clinical isolates, especially among *Cunninghamella* species (Alastruey-Izquierdo et al. 2009; Vitale et al. 2011; Pastor et al. 2010). These in vitro properties are consistent with the poor prognosis of mucormycosis caused by *Cunninghamella bertholletiae*, where among 34 reported cases, overall mortality was 76% (Orguc et al. 2005).

Liposomal AmB (LAmB) may be superior to AmB lipid complex (ABLC) for CNS infection as evidenced by higher CNS concentrations and more rapid clearance of fungus in animal models (Groll et al. 2000). The optimal dosage of lipid formulations is unknown. Based on in vivo and in vitro data, the initial dosage may be 5.0 mg/kg/day. Higher dosages of LAmB (e.g. 7.5–10 mg/kg/day) may allow for greater CNS penetration and may be safely achieved in immunocompromised patients (Walsh et al. 2001) and may be appropriate for CNS mucormycosis (Walsh et al. 2012; Jacobs et al. 2002). Despite this aggressive medical approach, surgical resection of infected CNS tissue is usually necessary. Reversal of immunosuppression, recovery from neutropenia and control of diabetes mellitus are also important cornerstones of therapy of cerebral mucormycosis. Local irrigation and intracavitary/interstitial and intrathecal administration of AmB have been attempted in cases unresponsive to conventional therapy. Intrathecal AmB is not indicated in treatment of cerebral mucormycosis due to complications that outweigh any putative benefits (Jacobs et al. 2002).

Although combination treatment with an AmB formulation and CAS has been described as successful in a limited number of predominantly diabetic patients with ROCM (Reed et al. 2008), low penetration of CAS into CSF following intravenous administration of standard doses was reported in humans (Strenger et al. 2017) confirming published data from animal studies. In models of neutropenic and ketoacidotic mice, the combination of LAmB and posaconazole (PSZ) also did not improve survival rates or reduce fungal tissue burden (Ibrahim et al. 2009).

PSZ was the first drug in the azole class to show a broad spectrum of activity against the *Mucorales* species (Alastruey-Izquierdo et al. 2009) and had proven to be useful in combination with AmB to treat RCM or patients for whom treatment with AmB alone has failed (Rueping et al. 2009; Mullane et al. 2007; Perkhofer et al. 2008) hypothesized that inflammatory disturbance of the blood-brain barrier may facilitate the penetration of PSZ into the CSF and the cerebral abscess fluid. Based on their clinical data, the authors proposed that PSZ may be an option in the treatment of cerebral fungal infections, as has been formerly suggested by the promising results from a clinical trial by Pitisuttithum et al. (2005).

Isavuconazole (ISA) was reported having a significant effect in the CNS as demonstrated in animal models (Falci and Pasqualotto 2013). Peixoto et al. (2014) reported that after failing PSZ and being intolerant to AmB, a patient with disseminated mucormycosis including CNS infection was treated successfully with ISA for over 6 months. The authors proposed that ISA may become an option to treat patients with mucormycosis, especially those who cannot tolerate AmB therapy.

Hyperbaric oxygen (HBO) is sometimes used as adjunctive therapy in management of mucormycosis (Kantarcioğlu et al. 2006). In vitro studies had previously demonstrated that high pressures (10 atm absolute, ATA) of 100% oxygen were reported as fungicidal for some *Mucorales*, including *Rhizopus* spp. in vitro (Gamaletsou et al. 2012). However, HBO mode of therapy was not recommended for routine primary treatment of mucormycosis (Jacobs et al. 2002).

ESCMID and ECMM Joint Clinical Guidelines focus on the diagnosis and management of mucormycosis. Imaging is strongly recommended to determine the extent of disease. For adults and children, surgical debridement was recommended whenever possible in addition to immediate first-line antifungal treatment with liposomal or ABLC with a minimum dose of 5 mg/kg/day. AmB deoxycholate was recommended better avoided because of its toxicity and severe adverse effects. For salvage treatment posaconazole prophylaxis 200 mg four times daily was strongly recommended in this guide. Reversal of predisposing conditions was underlined in patients with ongoing neutropenia, controlling hyperglycaemia and ketoacidosis in diabetic patients and limiting glucocorticosteroids to the minimum dose required. The authors recommended against using deferasirox in haematological patients outside clinical trials and marginally support a recommendation for deferasirox in diabetic patients. HBO is supported with marginal strength only. Furthermore, continuing treatment until complete response demonstrated on imaging and permanent reversal of predisposing factors was strongly recommended (Cornely et al. 2014).

10.17 Conclusion

Mucormycosis involving CNS often leads to a rapid fatal outcome. ROCM has a mortality rate of 40–50%; and 70% of survivors are left with residual defects. The factors related to a lower survival rate were reported as delayed diagnosis and treatment, hemiparesis or hemiplegia, bilateral sinus involvement, leukaemia, renal disease and treatment with deferoxamine (Sheikh and Amr 2011). The prognosis of cerebral mucormycosis is poor with 5-year survival rates of just 20–45%.3 (Orguc et al. 2005). Severely immunosuppressed patients (e.g. because of transplantation, malignancies, steroids or neutropenia) with mucormycosis were often prone to fatal outcome, and prolonged neutropenia was one of the most important disadvantages among these groups of patients. Corticosteroid therapy was another important disadvantage that increases fatality rate by causing either defects in macrophages and neutrophils.

References

Abbas AK, Lichtman AH, Pillai S. Cellular and molecular immunology E-book. Philadelphia, PA: Elsevier Health Sciences; 2014a.

Abbas AK, Lichtman AH, Pillai S. Basic immunology: functions and disorders of the immune system. Philadelphia, PA: Elsevier Health Sciences; 2014b.

Adelman LS, Aronson SM. The neuropathologic complications of narcotics addiction. Bull N Y Acad Med. 1969;45(2):225.

Air EL, et al. Isolated cerebellar mucormycosis, slowly progressive over 1 year in an immunocompetent patient. Surg Neurol Int. 2010;1:81.

Aköz T, Civelek B, Akan M. Rhinocerebral mucormycosis: report of two cases. Ann Plast Surg. 1999;43(3):309–12.

Al-Ajam M, et al. Mucormycosis in the eastern Mediterranean: a seasonal disease. Epidemiol Infect. 2006;134(2):341–6.

Alastruey-Izquierdo A, et al. In vitro activity of antifungals against Zygomycetes. Clin Microbiol Infect. 2009;15(s5):71–6.

Almyroudis NG, et al. In vitro susceptibilities of 217 clinical isolates of zygomycetes to conventional and new antifungal agents. Antimicrob Agents Chemother. 2007;51(7):2587–90.

Al-Shafai L, Mikulis D. Diffusion MR imaging in a case of acute ischemic optic neuropathy. Am J Neuroradiol. 2006;27(2):255–7.

Alsuhaibani AH, Al-Thubaiti G, Al Badr FB. Optic nerve thickening and infarction as the first evidence of orbital involvement with mucormycosis. Middle East Afr J Ophthalmol. 2012;19(3):340.

Angali RK, et al. Fatal rhino-orbito-cerebral mucormycosis in a healthy individual. J Oral Maxillofac Pathol. 2014;18(3):460.

Antachopoulos C, et al. Rapid susceptibility testing of medically important zygomycetes by XTT assay. J Clin Microbiol. 2006;44(2):553–60.

Arikan S, et al. Comparative in vitro activities of posaconazole, voriconazole, itraconazole, and amphotericin B against Aspergillus and Rhizopus, and synergy testing for Rhizopus. Sabouraudia. 2008;46(6):567–73.

Arizono K, et al. A case report of rhinocerebral mucormycosis in hemodialysis patient receiving deferoxamine. Nihon Jinzo Gakkai Shi. 1989;31(1):99–103.

Artis WM, et al. A mechanism of susceptibility to mucormycosis in diabetic ketoacidosis transferrin and iron availability. Diabetes. 1982;31(12):1109–14.

Asan A, Okten SS, Sen B. Airborne and soilborne microfungi in the vicinity Hamitabat Thermic Power Plant in Kirklareli City (Turkey), their seasonal distributions and relations with climatological factors. Environ Monit Assess. 2010;164(1–4):221–31.

Babior BM. Phagocytes and oxidative stress. Am J Med. 2000;109(1):33–44.

Bagdade J. Phagocytic and microbicidal function in diabetes mellitus. Acta Endocrinol Suppl (Copenh). 1976;205:27.

Baldin C, Ibrahim AS. Molecular mechanisms of mucormycosis—the bitter and the sweet. PLoS Pathog. 2017;13(8):e1006408.

Baradkar V, et al. Fatal rhino-orbito-cerebral infection caused by Saksenaea vasiformis in an immunocompetent individual: first case report from India. Indian J Med Microbiol. 2008;26(4):385.

Ben-Ami R, et al. A clinicopathological study of pulmonary mucormycosis in cancer patients: extensive angioinvasion but limited inflammatory response. J Infect. 2009;59(2):134–8.

Bhadani PP, et al. A rare presentation of invasive rhino-orbital mucormycosis in an immunocompetent young girl: a case report. Indian J Pathol Microbiol. 2007;50(4):785–6.

Bhattacharyya AK, et al. Rhinocerebral mucormycosis: an unusual case presentation. J Laryngol Otol. 1992;106(1):48–9.

Bichile LS, Abhyankar SC, Hase N. Chronic mucormycosis manifesting as hydrocephalus. J Neurol Neurosurg Psychiatry. 1985;48(11):1188.

Binder U, Maurer E, Lass-Flörl C. Mucormycosis—from the pathogens to the disease. Clin Microbiol Infect. 2014;20(s6):60–6.

Bitar D, et al. Increasing incidence of zygomycosis (mucormycosis), France, 1997–2006. Emerg Infect Dis. 2009;15(9):1395.

Blanco JL, Garcia ME. Immune response to fungal infections. Vet Immunol Immunopathol. 2008;125(1–2):47–70.

Blodi FC, Hannah FT, Wadsworth JA. Lethal orbitocerebral phycomycosis in otherwise healthy children. Am J Ophthalmol. 1969;67(5):698–705.
Boelaert JR, et al. Mucormycosis during deferoxamine therapy is a siderophore-mediated infection. In vitro and in vivo animal studies. J Clin Invest. 1993;91(5):1979–86.
Bouchara J, et al. Attachment of spores of the human pathogenic fungus Rhizopus oryzae to extracellular matrix components. Eur J Cell Biol. 1996;70(1):76–83.
Bouza E, Munoz P, Guinea J. Mucormycosis: an emerging disease? Clin Microbiol Infect. 2006;12(s7):7–23.
Brown RB, Lau SK. Case 3-2001: a 59-year-old diabetic man with unilateral visual loss and oculomotor-nerve palsy. N Engl J Med. 2001;344(4):286–93.
Bybee JD, Rogers DE. The phagocytic activity of polymorphonuclear leukocytes obtained from patients with diabetes mellitus. Transl Res. 1964;64(1):1–13.
Caramalho R, et al. Etest cannot be recommended for in vitro susceptibility testing of Mucorales. Antimicrob Agents Chemother. 2015;59(6):3663–5.
Chakrabarti A, Singh R. Mucormycosis in India: unique features. Mycoses. 2014;57(s3):85–90.
Chakrabarti A, et al. Apophysomyces elegans: an emerging zygomycete in India. J Clin Microbiol. 2003;41(2):783–8.
Chakrabarti A, et al. Apophysomyces elegans: epidemiology, amplified fragment length polymorphism typing, and in vitro antifungal susceptibility pattern. J Clin Microbiol. 2010;48(12):4580–5.
Chamilos G, et al. Zygomycetes hyphae trigger an early, robust proinflammatory response in human polymorphonuclear neutrophils through toll-like receptor 2 induction but display relative resistance to oxidative damage. Antimicrob Agents Chemother. 2008;52(2):722–4.
Chamilos G, et al. Generation of IL-23 producing Dendritic Cells (DCs) by airborne fungi regulates fungal pathogenicity via the induction of TH-17 responses. PLoS One. 2010;5(9):e12955.
Chibucos MC, et al. An integrated genomic and transcriptomic survey of mucormycosis-causing fungi. Nat Commun. 2016;7:12218.
Chinn R, Diamond RD. Generation of chemotactic factors by Rhizopus oryzae in the presence and absence of serum: relationship to hyphal damage mediated by human neutrophils and effects of hyperglycemia and ketoacidosis. Infect Immun. 1982;38(3):1123–9.
Chmel H, Grieco MH. Cerebral mucormycosis and renal aspergillosis in heroin addicts without endocarditis. Am J Med Sci. 1973;266(3):225–31.
CLSI C. Reference method for broth dilution antifungal susceptibility testing of filamentous fungi; approved standard—second edition—document M38-A2. Wayne, PA: CLSI; 2008.
Çolakoğlu G. Airborne fungal spores at the Belgrad forest near the city of Istanbul (Turkey) in the year 2001 and their relation to allergic diseases. J Basic Microbiol. 2003;43(5):376–84.
Cornely O, et al. ESCMID and ECMM joint clinical guidelines for the diagnosis and management of mucormycosis 2013. Clin Microbiol Infect. 2014;20:5–26.
Cuadrado LM, et al. Cerebral mucormycosis in two cases of acquired immunodeficiency syndrome. Arch Neurol. 1988;45(1):109–11.
Dannaoui E. Antifungal resistance in Mucorales. Int J Antimicrob Agents. 2017;50(5):617–21.
Dannaoui E, et al. Efficacy of antifungal therapy in a nonneutropenic murine model of zygomycosis. Antimicrob Agents Chemother. 2002;46(6):1953–9.
Dannaoui E, et al. In vitro susceptibilities of zygomycetes to conventional and new antifungals. J Antimicrob Chemother. 2003;51(1):45–52.
Davies BW, et al. Increased incidence of rhino-orbital-cerebral mucormycosis after Colorado flooding. Ophthalmic Plast Reconstr Surg. 2017;33(3S):S148–51.
De Hoog G, et al. Atlas of clinical fungi. 2nd ed. Utrecht: Centraalbureau voor Schimmelcultures; 2000.
De Lucca AJ, Walsh TJ. Antifungal peptides: novel therapeutic compounds against emerging pathogens. Antimicrob Agents Chemother. 1999;43(1):1–11.
Delves PJ, Roitt IM. The immune system. N Engl J Med. 2000;343(1):37–49.
Diamond RD, Clark RA. Damage to Aspergillus fumigatus and Rhizopus oryzae hyphae by oxidative and nonoxidative microbicidal products of human neutrophils in vitro. Infect Immun. 1982;38(2):487–95.
Diamond RD, Haudenschild CC, Erickson NF 3rd. Monocyte-mediated damage to Rhizopus oryzae hyphae in vitro. Infect Immun. 1982;38(1):292–7.
Dolatabadi S, et al. Differentiation of clinically relevant Mucorales Rhizopus microsporus and R. arrhizus by matrix-assisted laser desorption ionization time-of-flight mass spectrometry (MALDI-TOF MS). J Med Microbiol. 2015;64(7):694–701.
Ejdys E. Environment of school as potential place of interindividual transmissions. Wiad Parazytol. 2001;47(3):353–8.
El JB, et al. Erysipelas of the face revealing a mucormycosis. J Mycol Med. 2011;21(3):202–5.
El-Herte RI, Baban TA, Kanj SS. Mucormycosis: a review on environmental fungal spores and seasonal variation of human disease. Adv Infect Dis. 2012;2(03):76.
Elinav H, et al. Rhinocerebral mucormycosis in patients without predisposing medical conditions: a review of the literature. Clin Microbiol Infect. 2009;15(7):693–7.
Escobar A, Del Brutto OH. Multiple brain abscesses from isolated cerebral mucormycosis. J Neurol Neurosurg Psychiatry. 1990;53(5):431–3.
EUCAST, T.S.o.A.S.T.A.o.t.E.E.C.f.A.S.T., EUCAST Definitive Document E.Def 9.2 in Method for the determination of broth dilution minimum inhibitory concentrations of antifungal agents for conidia forming mould. Basel, Switzerland, 2014: EUCAST; 2017.
Fairley C, et al. Survival after rhino-orbital-cerebral mucormycosis in an immunocompetent patient. Ophthalmology. 2000;107(3):555–8.

Falci DR, Pasqualotto AC. Profile of isavuconazole and its potential in the treatment of severe invasive fungal infections. Infect Drug Resist. 2013;6:163.
Fisher EW, et al. Rhinocerebral mucormycosis: use of liposomal amphotericin B. J Laryngol Otol. 1991;105(7):575–7.
Fong K, Seneviratne E, McCormack J. Mucor cerebral abscess associated with intravenous drug abuse. Intern Med J. 1990;20(1):74–7.
Frater JL, Hall GS, Procop GW. Histologic features of zygomycosis: emphasis on perineural invasion and fungal morphology. Arch Pathol Lab Med. 2001;125(3):375–8.
Fu Y, et al. Cloning and functional characterization of the Rhizopus oryzae high affinity iron permease (rFTR1) gene. FEMS Microbiol Lett. 2004;235(1):169–76.
Gaing A, Corbalan F, Weinberger J. Phycomycosis (mucormycosis) in differential diagnosis of cerebral mass lesions in intravenous drug users. Mt Sinai J Med. 1992;59(1):69.
Gamaletsou MN, et al. Rhino-orbital-cerebral mucormycosis. Curr Infect Dis Rep. 2012;14(4):423–34.
Garcia-Covarrubias L, et al. Rhino-orbitocerebral mucormycosis attributable to Apophysomyces elegans in an immunocompetent individual: case report and review of the literature. J Trauma. 2001;50(2):353–7.
Gebremariam T, et al. CotH3 mediates fungal invasion of host cells during mucormycosis. J Clin Invest. 2014;124(1):237–50.
Gebremariam T, et al. Bicarbonate correction of ketoacidosis alters host-pathogen interactions and alleviates mucormycosis. J Clin Invest. 2016;126(6):2280–94.
Ghuman H, Voelz K. Innate and adaptive immunity to Mucorales. J Fungi. 2017;3(3):48.
Ghuman MS, et al. Bilateral optic nerve infarction in rhino-cerebral mucormycosis: a rare magnetic resonance imaging finding. J Neurosci Rural Pract. 2015;6(3):403.
Gil-Lamaignere C, et al. Interferon-γ and granulocyte-macrophage colony-stimulating factor augment the activity of polymorphonuclear leukocytes against medically important zygomycetes. J Infect Dis. 2005;191(7):1180–7.
Ginsberg F, et al. Isolated cerebral mucormycosis: case report with CT and pathologic correlation. Am J Neuroradiol. 1987;8(3):558–60.
Gniadek A, Macura A. Intensive care unit environment contamination with fungi. Adv Med Sci. 2007;52:283–7.
Gollard R, et al. Isolated cerebral mucormycosis: case report and therapeutic considerations. Neurosurgery. 1994;34(1):174–7.
Gomes MZ, Lewis RE, Kontoyiannis DP. Mucormycosis caused by unusual mucormycetes, non-Rhizopus, -Mucor, and -Lichtheimia species. Clin Microbiol Rev. 2011;24(2):411–45.
Gomez-Lopez A, et al. In vitro susceptibility of clinical isolates of Zygomycota to amphotericin B, flucytosine, itraconazole and voriconazole. J Antimicrob Chemother. 2001;48(6):919–21.
Gordon S, Plüddemann A. Tissue macrophage heterogeneity: issues and prospects. In: Seminars in immunopathology. New York: Springer; 2013.
Gordon S, Taylor PR. Monocyte and macrophage heterogeneity. Nat Rev Immunol. 2005;5(12):953.
Gordon S, Plüddemann A, Martinez Estrada F. Macrophage heterogeneity in tissues: phenotypic diversity and functions. Immunol Rev. 2014;262(1):36–55.
Gottfredsson M, Perfect JR. Fungal meningitis. In: Seminars in neurology. New York: Thieme Medical Publishers, Inc.; 2000.
Gregory J, Golden A, Haymaker W. Muconnycosis of the central nervous system. A report of three cases. Bull Johns Hopkins Hosp. 1943;6:405–15.
Groll AH, et al. Comparative efficacy and distribution of lipid formulations of amphotericin B in experimental *Candida albicans* infection of the central nervous system. J Infect Dis. 2000;182(1):274–82.
Hameroff SB, Eckholdt JW, Lindenberg R. Cerebral phycomycosis in a heroin addict. Neurology. 1970;20(3):261–5.
Hampton MB, Kettle AJ, Winterbourn CC. Inside the neutrophil phagosome: oxidants, myeloperoxidase, and bacterial killing. Blood. 1998;92(9):3007–17.
Hariri BM, Cohen NA. New insights into upper airway innate immunity. Am J Rhinol Allergy. 2016;30(5):319.
Harris JS. Mucormycosis: report of a case. Pediatrics. 1955;16(6):857–67.
Hibbett DS, et al. A higher-level phylogenetic classification of the fungi. Mycol Res. 2007;111(5):509–47.
Hofman V, et al. Usefulness of frozen section in rhinocerebral mucormycosis diagnosis and management. Pathology. 2003;35(3):212–6.
Honda A. A murine model of zygomycosis by Cunninghamella bertholletiae. Mycopathologia. 1998;144(3):141–6.
Hontelez S, et al. Molecular view on PRR cross-talk in antifungal immunity. Cell Microbiol. 2012;14(4):467–74.
Hopkins RJ, et al. Cerebral mucormycosis associated with intravenous drug use: three case reports and review. Clin Infect Dis. 1994;19(6):1133–7.
Hosseini SMS, Borghei P. Rhinocerebral mucormycosis: pathways of spread. Eur Arch Otorhinolaryngol. 2005;262(11):932–8.
Howard DH. Acquisition, transport, and storage of iron by pathogenic fungi. Clin Microbiol Rev. 1999;12(3):394–404.
Hussain S, et al. Rhinocerebral invasive mycosis: occurrence in immunocompetent individuals. Eur J Radiol. 1995;20(2):151–5.
Ibrahim AS, Kontoyiannis DP. Update on mucormycosis pathogenesis. Curr Opin Infect Dis. 2013;26(6):508.
Ibrahim AS, et al. Rhizopus oryzae adheres to, is phagocytosed by, and damages endothelial cells in vitro. Infect Immun. 2005;73(2):778–83.
Ibrahim AS, et al. Posaconazole mono-or combination therapy for treatment of murine zygomycosis. Antimicrob Agents Chemother. 2009;53(2):772–5.
Ibrahim AS, et al. Pathogenesis of mucormycosis. Clin Infect Dis. 2012;54(Suppl 1):S16–22.

Jacobs S, Gonzalez CE, Walsh TJ. Mucormycosis and entomophthoramycosis. 2002. http://www.antimicrobe.org/new/f13.asp.

Jones PG, et al. Focal intracranial mucormycosis presenting as chronic meningitis. JAMA. 1981;246(18):2063–4.

José R-H. Dimorphism on Mucor species with emphasis on M. rouxii and M. bacilliformis. In: Szaniszlo PJ, editor. Fungal dimorphism with emphasis on fungi pathogenic for humans. New York: Springer US, Plenum Press; 1985. p. 361–86.

Kantarcioğlu AS, et al. A Rhizopus oryzae strain isolated from resected bone and soft tissue specimens from a sinonasal and palatal mucormycosis case. Report of a case and in vitro experiments of yeastlike cell development. Med Mycol. 2006;44(6):515–21.

Kasantikul V, Shuangshoti S, Taecholarn C. Primary phycomycosis of the brain in heroin addicts. Surg Neurol. 1987;28(6):468–72.

Kasliwal MK, et al. Bilateral anterior cerebral artery aneurysm due to mucormycosis. J Clin Neurosci. 2009;16(1):156–9.

Kaufman L, Padhye A, Parker S. Rhinocerebral zygomycosis caused by Saksenaea vasiformis. J Med Vet Mycol. 1988;26(4):237–41.

Kennedy K, et al. Mucormycosis in Australia: contemporary epidemiology and outcomes. Clin Microbiol Infect. 2016;22(9):775–81.

Khan ZU, et al. Mucor circinelloides as a cause of invasive maxillofacial zygomycosis: an emerging dimorphic pathogen with reduced susceptibility to posaconazole. J Clin Microbiol. 2009;47(4):1244–8.

Khor B, et al. Rhinocerebral mucormycosis in Taiwan. J Microbiol Immunol Infect. 2003;36(4):266–9.

KÖMÜR S, et al. Mucormycosis: a 10-year experience at a tertiary care center in Turkey. Turk J Med Sci. 2016;46(1):58–62.

Kontoyiannis DP, et al. Zygomycosis in a tertiary-care cancer center in the era of Aspergillus-active antifungal therapy: a case-control observational study of 27 recent cases. J Infect Dis. 2005;191(8):1350–60.

Kontoyiannis DP, et al. Prevalence, clinical and economic burden of mucormycosis-related hospitalizations in the United States: a retrospective study. BMC Infect Dis. 2016;16(1):730.

Kwon-Chung KJ. Taxonomy of fungi causing mucormycosis and entomophthoramycosis (zygomycosis) and nomenclature of the disease: molecular mycologic perspectives. Clin Infect Dis. 2012;54(Suppl 1):S8–S15.

Lackner M, Caramalho R, Lass-Flörl C. Laboratory diagnosis of mucormycosis: current status and future perspectives. Future Microbiol. 2014;9(5):683–95.

Langford JD, McCartney DL, Wang RC. Frozen section-guided surgical debridement for management of rhino-orbital mucormycosis. Am J Ophthalmol. 1997;124(2):265–7.

Lanternier F, et al. A global analysis of mucormycosis in France: the RetroZygo Study (2005–2007). Clin Infect Dis. 2012;54(Suppl 1):S35–43.

Lass-Flörl C. Zygomycosis: conventional laboratory diagnosis. Clin Microbiol Infect. 2009;15(s5):60–5.

Levitz SM, et al. In vitro killing of spores and hyphae of Aspergillus fumigatus and Rhizopus oryzae by rabbit neutrophil cationic peptides and bronchoalveolar macrophages. J Infect Dis. 1986;154(3):483–9.

Lewis RE, et al. How does antifungal pharmacology differ for mucormycosis versus aspergillosis? Clin Infect Dis. 2012;54(Suppl 1):S67–72.

Li CH, et al. Sporangiospore size dimorphism is linked to virulence of Mucor circinelloides. PLoS Pathog. 2011;7(6):e1002086.

Liang KP, et al. Rhino-orbitocerebral mucormycosis caused by Apophysomyces elegans. J Clin Microbiol. 2006;44(3):892–8.

Liles WC, et al. Granulocyte colony-stimulating factor administered in vivo augments neutrophil-mediated activity against opportunistic fungal pathogens. J Infect Dis. 1997;175(4):1012–5.

Liu M, et al. The endothelial cell receptor GRP78 is required for mucormycosis pathogenesis in diabetic mice. J Clin Invest. 2010;120(6):1914–24.

Liu H, et al. Aspergillus fumigatus CalA binds to integrin alpha5beta1 and mediates host cell invasion. Nat Microbiol. 2016;2:16211.

Lohmeyer J. Role of hemopoietic growth factors and cytokines in host defense against fungal infections. Mycoses. 1997;40(s2):37–9.

Lübbehüsen TL, Nielsen J, McIntyre M. Morphology and physiology of the dimorphic fungus Mucor circinelloides (syn. M. racemosus) during anaerobic growth. Mycol Res. 2003;107(2):223–30.

Luna JD, et al. Intraconal amphotericin B for the treatment of rhino-orbital mucormycosis. Ophthalmic Surg Lasers. 1996;27(8):706–8.

Ma L-J, et al. Genomic analysis of the basal lineage fungus Rhizopus oryzae reveals a whole-genome duplication. PLoS Genet. 2009;5(7):e1000549.

Mackenzie D, Soothill J, Millar J. Meningitis caused by Absidia corymbifera. J Infect. 1988;17(3):245–8.

Margo CE, et al. Rhinocerebral mucormycosis with perineural spread. Ophthalmic Plast Reconstr Surg. 2007;23(4):326–7.

Marty FM, Cosimi LA, Baden LR. Breakthrough zygomycosis after voriconazole treatment in recipients of hematopoietic stem-cell transplants. N Engl J Med. 2004;350(9):950–2.

Masucci EF, et al. Cerebral mucormycosis (phycomycosis) in a heroin addict. Arch Neurol. 1982;39(5):304–6.

Mathur S, Karimi A, Mafee M. Acute optic nerve infarction demonstrated by diffusion-weighted imaging in a case of rhinocerebral mucormycosis. Am J Neuroradiol. 2007;28(3):489–90.

McDermott NE, et al. Successful treatment of periodontal mucormycosis: report of a case and literature review. Oral Surg Oral Med Oral Pathol Oral Radiol Endod. 2010;109(3):e64–9.

McLean FM, Ginsberg LE, Stanton CA. Perineural spread of rhinocerebral mucormycosis. Am J Neuroradiol. 1996;17(1):114–6.
Melsom S, Khangure M. Craniofacial mucormycosis following assault: an unusual presentation of an unusual disease. J Med Imaging Radiat Oncol. 2000;44(1):104–6.
Mendoza L, et al. Human fungal pathogens of Mucorales and Entomophthorales. Cold Spring Harb Perspect Med. 2015;5(4):a019562.
Meyers BR, et al. Rhinocerebral mucormycosis: premortem diagnosis and therapy. Arch Intern Med. 1979;139(5):557–60.
Miller NS, et al. Fungal infection associated with intravenous drug abuse: a case of localized cerebral phycomycosis. J Clin Psychiatry. 1988;49:320–2.
Mohindra S, et al. Rhinocerebral mucormycosis: the disease spectrum in 27 patients. Mycoses. 2007;50(4):290–6.
Morace G, Borghi E. Invasive mold infections: virulence and pathogenesis of Mucorales. Int J Microbiol. 2012;2011 https://doi.org/10.1155/2012/349278.
Mosquera J, et al. Treatment of Absidia corymbifera infection in mice with amphotericin B and itraconazole. J Antimicrob Chemother. 2001;48(4):583–6.
Mowat AG, Baum J. Chemotaxis of polymorphonuclear leukocytes from patients with diabetes mellitus. N Engl J Med. 1971;284(12):621–7.
Mullane K, et al. Posaconazole salvage therapy allows successful allogeneic hematopoietic stem cell transplantation in patients with refractory invasive mold infections. Transpl Infect Dis. 2007;9(2):89–96.
Murthy JMK, Sundaram C. Chapter 95—Fungal infections of the central nervous system. In: Biller J, Ferro JM, editors. Handbook of clinical neurology. Amsterdam: Elsevier; 2014. p. 1383–401.
Muszewska A, Pawłowska J, Krzyściak P. Biology, systematics, and clinical manifestations of Zygomycota infections. Eur J Clin Microbiol Infect Dis. 2014;33(8):1273–87.
Nithyanandam S, et al. Rhino-orbito-cerebral mucormycosis. A retrospective analysis of clinical features and treatment outcomes. Indian J Ophthalmol. 2003;51(3):231–6.
Oliveri S, et al. Rhizopus arrhizus in Italy as the causative agent of primary cerebral zygomycosis in a drug addict. Eur J Epidemiol. 1988;4(3):284–8.
Onerci M, et al. Rhinocerebral mucormycosis with extension to the cavernous sinus. A case report. Rhinology. 1991;29(4):321–4.
Ooi EH, Wormald P-J, Tan LW. Innate immunity in the paranasal sinuses: a review of nasal host defenses. Am J Rhinol. 2008;22(1):13–9.
Orguc S, et al. Rhinocerebral mucormycosis: perineural spread via the trigeminal nerve. J Clin Neurosci. 2005;12(4):484–6.
Orlowski M. Mucor dimorphism. Microbiol Rev. 1991;55(2):234–58.
Ortín X, et al. Cunninghamella bertholletiae infection (mucormycosis) in a patient with acute T-cell lymphoblastic leukemia. Leuk Lymphoma. 2004;45(3):617–20.
Paltauf A. Mycosis mucorina. Arch Pathol Anat Physiol. 1885;102(3):543–64.
Parsi K, et al. Perineural spread of rhino-orbitocerebral mucormycosis caused by Apophysomyces elegans. Ann Indian Acad Neurol. 2013;16(3):414.
Pastor FJ, et al. In vitro and in vivo antifungal susceptibilities of the Mucoralean fungus Cunninghamella. Antimicrob Agents Chemother. 2010;54(11):4550–5.
Pavan R, Manjunath K. Qualitative analysis of indoor and outdoor airborne fungi in cowshed. J Mycol. 2014;2014 https://doi.org/10.1155/2014/985921.
Peixoto D, et al. Isavuconazole treatment of a patient with disseminated mucormycosis. J Clin Microbiol. 2014;52(3):1016–9.
Perkhofer S, et al. Posaconazole enhances the activity of amphotericin B against hyphae of zygomycetes in vitro. Antimicrob Agents Chemother. 2008;52(7):2636–8.
Petrikkos G, et al. Mucormycosis: ten-year experience at a tertiary-care center in Greece. Eur J Clin Microbiol Infect Dis. 2003;22(12):753–6.
Petrikkos G, Skiada A, Drogari-Apiranthitou M. Epidemiology of mucormycosis in Europe. Clin Microbiol Infect. 2014;20:67–73.
Phan QT, et al. Als3 is a *Candida albicans* invasin that binds to cadherins and induces endocytosis by host cells. PLoS Biol. 2007;5(3):e64.
Pierce PF, et al. Zygomycetes brain abscesses in narcotic addicts with serological diagnosis. JAMA. 1982;248(21):2881–2.
Pillai P, Cyriac R, Rajeevan PS. Cerebral mucormycosis and endophthalmitis following dengue in a immunocompetent female. J Assoc Physicians India. 2016;64(1):54.
Pitisuttithum P, et al. Activity of posaconazole in the treatment of central nervous system fungal infections. J Antimicrob Chemother. 2005;56(4):745–55.
Potenza L, et al. Mucorales-specific T cells emerge in the course of invasive mucormycosis and may be used as a surrogate diagnostic marker in high-risk patients. Blood. 2011;118(20):5416–9.
Prakash H, et al. The environmental source of emerging apophysomyces variabilis infection in India. Sabouraudia. 2016;54(6):567–75.
Pursell K, et al. Impaired phagocyte respiratory burst responses to opportunistic fungal pathogens in transplant recipients: in vitro effect of r-metHuG-CSF (Filgrastim). Transpl Infect Dis. 2003;5(1):29–37.
Radner AB, Witt MD, Edwards JE Jr. Acute invasive rhinocerebral zygomycosis in an otherwise healthy patient: case report and review. Clin Infect Dis. 1995;20(1):163–6.
Raj P, Vella E, Bickerton R. Successful treatment of rhinocerebral mucormycosis by a combination of aggressive surgical debridement and the use of systemic liposomal amphotericin B and local therapy with nebulized amphotericin—a case report. J Laryngol Otol. 1998;112(4):367–70.
Ramanathan B, et al. Cathelicidins: microbicidal activity, mechanisms of action, and roles in innate immunity. Microbes Infect. 2002;4(3):361–72.

Rangel-Guerra RA, et al. Rhinocerebral and systemic mucormycosis. Clinical experience with 36 cases. J Neurol Sci. 1996;143(1):19–30.

Rao SS, et al. Sinoorbital mucormycosis due to Apophysomyces elegans in immunocompetent individuals—an increasing trend. Am J Otolaryngol. 2006;27(5):366–9.

Reddy RHK, Raju S. Isolated cerebral mucormycosis in an immunocompetent patient—a case report. Indian J Neurosurg. 2015;4(01):038–41.

Reed C, et al. Combination polyene-caspofungin treatment of rhino-orbital-cerebral mucormycosis. Clin Infect Dis. 2008;47(3):364–71.

Ribes JA, Vanover-Sams CL, Baker DJ. Zygomycetes in human disease. Clin Microbiol Rev. 2000;13(2):236–301.

Richardson M. The ecology of the Zygomycetes and its impact on environmental exposure. Clin Microbiol Infect. 2009;15(Suppl 5):2–9.

Riefler J III, Batbouta J, Uphoff DF. Rhizopus brain abscess: report of a case and review of the literature. Mil Med. 1991;156(9):497–9.

Roden MM, et al. Epidemiology and outcome of zygomycosis: a review of 929 reported cases. Clin Infect Dis. 2005;41(5):634–53.

Rodríguez MM, et al. Posaconazole combined with amphotericin B, an effective therapy for a murine disseminated infection caused by Rhizopus oryzae. Antimicrob Agents Chemother. 2008;52(10):3786–8.

Rodríguez MM, et al. Correlation of in vitro activity, serum levels, and in vivo efficacy of posaconazole against Rhizopus microsporus in a murine disseminated infection. Antimicrob Agents Chemother. 2009;53(12):5022–5.

Rodriguez-Tudela J, et al. Interlaboratory evaluation of hematocytometer method of inoculum preparation for testing antifungal susceptibilities of filamentous fungi. J Clin Microbiol. 2003;41(11):5236–7.

Rogers TR. Treatment of zygomycosis: current and new options. J Antimicrob Chemother. 2008;61(Suppl 1):i35–40.

Roilides E, et al. Enhancement of oxidative response and damage caused by human neutrophils to Aspergillus fumigatus hyphae by granulocyte colony-stimulating factor and gamma interferon. Infect Immun. 1993;61(4):1185–93.

Roilides E, et al. The role of immunoreconstitution in the management of refractory opportunistic fungal infections. Med Mycol. 1998;36:12–25.

Roilides E, Kontoyiannis DP, Walsh TJ. Host defenses against zygomycetes. Clin Infect Dis. 2012;54(Suppl 1):S61–6.

Roilides E, Antachopoulos C, Simitsopoulou M. Pathogenesis and host defence against Mucorales: the role of cytokines and interaction with antifungal drugs. Mycoses. 2014;57(s3):40–7.

Romani L. Immunity to fungal infections. Nat Rev Immunol. 2004;4(1):11.

Rueping MJ, et al. Forty-one recent cases of invasive zygomycosis from a global clinical registry. J Antimicrob Chemother. 2009;65(2):296–302.

Saoulidis S, et al. Antifungal activity of posaconazole and granulocyte colony-stimulating factor in the treatment of disseminated zygomycosis (mucormycosis) in a neutropaenic murine model. Mycoses. 2011;54(5):e486–92.

Sarrami AH, et al. Fatal disseminated mucormycosis in an immunocompetent patient: a case report and literature review. Int J Prev Med. 2013;4(12):1468.

Scheckenbach K, et al. Emerging therapeutic options in fulminant invasive rhinocerebral mucormycosis. Auris Nasus Larynx. 2010;37(3):322–8.

Schmidt S, et al. Natural killer cell-mediated damage of clinical isolates of mucormycetes. Mycoses. 2016;59(1):34–8.

Schütz P, et al. Fatal rhino-orbito-cerebral zygomycosis caused by Apophysomyces elegans in a healthy patient. J Oral Maxillofac Surg. 2006;64(12):1795–802.

Schwartze VU, Jacobsen ID. Mucormycoses caused by Lichtheimia species. Mycoses. 2014;57(s3):73–8.

Schwartze VU, et al. Lichtheimia species exhibit differences in virulence potential. PLoS One. 2012;7(7):e40908.

Schwarz P, et al. Carbon assimilation profiles as a tool for identification of zygomycetes. J Clin Microbiol. 2007;45(5):1433–9.

Scully MA, et al. SWAN MRI revealing multiple microhemorrhages secondary to septic emboli from mucormycosis. Neurology. 2012;79(18):1932–3.

Sen B, Asan A. Fungal flora in indoor and outdoor air of different residential houses in Tekirdag City (Turkey): seasonal distribution and relationship with climatic factors. Environ Monit Assess. 2009;151(1–4):209–19.

Sepkowitz K, Armstrong D. Space-occupying fungal lesions. In: Scheld WM, Whitley RJ, Durack DT, editors. Infections of the central nervous system, vol. 2. Philadelphia, PA: Lippincott-Raven Press; 1997. p. 741–62.

Sharma RR, et al. Fatal rhino-orbito-cerebral mucormycosis in an apparently normal host: case report and literature review. J Clin Neurosci. 2001;8(6):583–6.

Shatriah I, et al. Rhino-orbito-cerebral mucormycosis in an immunocompetent patient: case report and review of literature. Middle East Afr J Ophthalmol. 2012;19(2):258.

deShazo RD, et al. A new classification and diagnostic criteria for invasive fungal sinusitis. Arch Otolaryngol Head Neck Surg. 1997;123(11):1181–8.

Sheikh SS, Amr SS. Fungal infections of the central nervous system. In: Rai M, editor. Progress in mycology. New York: Springer Science & Business Media; 2011.

Shpitzer T, et al. Seasonal variations in rhino-cerebral Mucor infection. Ann Otol Rhinol Laryngol. 2005;114(9):695–8.

Siddiqi SU, Freedman JD. Isolated central nervous system mucormycosis. South Med J. 1994;87(10):997–1000.

Simitsopoulou M, et al. Cunninghamella bertholletiae exhibits increased resistance to human neutrophils with or without antifungal agents as compared to Rhizopus spp. Med Mycol. 2010;48(5):720–4.

Singh R, Shivaprakash M, Chakrabarti A. Biofilm formation by zygomycetes: quantification, structure and matrix composition. Microbiology. 2011;157(9):2611–8.

Singh P, et al. Stress response in medically important Mucorales. Mycoses. 2016;59(10):628–35.

Singh ND, et al. Apophysomyces elegans caused rhino-orbito mucormycosis: an emerging infection in immunocompetent individuals: case series with review of the literature. J Microbiol Infect Dis. 2017;7(04):207–12.

Skiada A, et al. Zygomycosis in Europe: analysis of 230 cases accrued by the registry of the European Confederation of Medical Mycology (ECMM) Working Group on Zygomycosis between 2005 and 2007. Clin Microbiol Infect. 2011;17(12):1859–67.

Sohail M, et al. Acute fulminant fungal sinusitis: clinical presentation, radiological findings and treatment. Acta Trop. 2001;80(2):177–85.

Soler ZM, Schlosser RJ. The role of fungi in diseases of the nose and sinuses. Am J Rhinol Allergy. 2012;26(5):351.

Song Y, et al. Mucormycosis in renal transplant recipients: review of 174 reported cases. BMC Infect Dis. 2017;17(1):283.

Soto-Aguilar M, et al. Classification of and criteria for the diagnosis of invasive fungal sinusitis. J Investig Med. 1997;45:3A.

Spellberg B, Edwards J, Ibrahim A. Novel perspectives on mucormycosis: pathophysiology, presentation, and management. Clin Microbiol Rev. 2005;18(3):556–69.

Sponsler TA, et al. Ocular invasion in mucormycosis. Surv Ophthalmol. 1992;36(5):345–50.

Spreghini E, et al. In vitro and in vivo activities of posaconazole against zygomycetes with various degrees of susceptibility. J Antimicrob Chemother. 2010;65(10):2158–63.

Sravani T, et al. Rhinocerebral mucormycosis: pathology revisited with emphasis on perineural spread. Neurol India. 2014;62(4):383–6.

Stave GM, Heimberger T, Kerkering TM. Zygomycosis of the basal ganglia in intravenous drug users. Am J Med. 1989;86(1):115–7.

Strenger V, et al. Low penetration of caspofungin into cerebrospinal fluid following intravenous administration of standard doses. Int J Antimicrob Agents. 2017;50(2):272–5.

Sun QN, et al. In vitro activities of posaconazole, itraconazole, voriconazole, amphotericin B, and fluconazole against 37 clinical isolates of zygomycetes. Antimicrob Agents Chemother. 2002;46(5):1581–2.

Sundaram C, et al. Cerebral zygomycosis. Mycoses. 2005;48(6):396–407.

Taj-Aldeen S, et al. Rare pediatric rhino-orbital infection caused by Saksenaea vasiformis. Infection. 2012;40(6):703–7.

Talmi YP, et al. Rhino-orbital and rhino-orbito-cerebral mucormycosis. Otolaryngol Head Neck Surg. 2002;127(1):22–31.

Teixeira CA, et al. Rhinocerebral mucormycosis: literature review apropos of a rare entity. BMJ Case Rep. 2013;2013:bcr2012008552.

Terk MR, et al. MR imaging in rhinocerebral and intracranial mucormycosis with CT and pathologic correlation. Magn Reson Imaging. 1992;10(1):81–7.

Thirumala S, Nathu MP. Original research article study of fungal spores diversity, in Malebenur region of Karnataka, India. Int J Curr Microbiol App Sci. 2013;2(3):44–8.

Torres-Narbona M, et al. Impact of zygomycosis on microbiology workload: a survey study in Spain. J Clin Microbiol. 2007a;45(6):2051–3.

Torres-Narbona M, et al. In vitro activities of amphotericin B, caspofungin, itraconazole, posaconazole, and voriconazole against 45 clinical isolates of zygomycetes: comparison of CLSI M38-A, Sensititre YeastOne, and the Etest. Antimicrob Agents Chemother. 2007b;51(3):1126–9.

Torres-Narbona M, et al. Workload and clinical significance of the isolation of zygomycetes in a tertiary general hospital. Med Mycol. 2008;46(3):225–30.

Tsung L, et al. Intraventricular amphotericin for absidiomycosis in an immunocompetent child. Hong Kong Med J. 2010;16(2):137–40.

Verma A, Brozman B, Petito CK. Isolated cerebral mucormycosis: report of a case and review of the literature. J Neurol Sci. 2006;240(1):65–9.

Vigouroux S, et al. Zygomycosis after prolonged use of voriconazole in immunocompromised patients with hematologic disease: attention required. Clin Infect Dis. 2005;40(4):e35–7.

Vitale RG, et al. Antifungal susceptibility and phylogeny of opportunistic members of Mucorales. J Clin Microbiol. 2011; https://doi.org/10.1128/JCM.06133-11.

Voigt K, et al. The zygomycetes in a phylogenetic perspective. Persoonia. 2013;30:i.

Wächtler B, et al. *Candida albicans*-epithelial interactions: dissecting the roles of active penetration, induced endocytosis and host factors on the infection process. PLoS One. 2012;7(5):e36952.

Waldorf AR. Pulmonary defense mechanisms against opportunistic fungal pathogens. Immunol Ser. 1989;47:243–71.

Waldorf AR, Diamond RD. Neutrophil chemotactic responses induced by fresh and swollen Rhizopus oryzae spores and Aspergillus fumigatus conidia. Infect Immun. 1985;48(2):458–63.

Waldorf AR, Levitz SM, Diamond RD. In vivo bronchoalveolar macrophage defense against Rhizopus oryzae and Aspergillus fumigatus. J Infect Dis. 1984a;150(5):752–60.

Waldorf A, Ruderman N, Diamond R. Specific susceptibility to mucormycosis in murine diabetes and bronchoalveolar macrophage defense against Rhizopus. J Clin Invest. 1984b;74(1):150–60.

Walsh TJ, et al. Safety, tolerance, and pharmacokinetics of high-dose liposomal amphotericin B (AmBisome) in patients infected with Aspergillus species and other filamentous fungi: maximum tolerated dose study. Antimicrob Agents Chemother. 2001;45(12):3487–96.

Walsh TJ, et al. Early clinical and laboratory diagnosis of invasive pulmonary, extrapulmonary, and disseminated mucormycosis (zygomycosis). Clin Infect Dis. 2012;54(Suppl 1):S55–60.

Walther G, et al. DNA barcoding in Mucorales: an inventory of biodiversity. Persoonia. 2013;30:11.

Wang M, et al. Role of the unfolded protein response regulator GRP78/BiP in development, cancer, and neurological disorders. Antioxid Redox Signal. 2009;11(9):2307–16.

Warris A, et al. Cytokine responses and regulation of interferon-gamma release by human mononuclear cells to Aspergillus fumigatus and other filamentous fungi. Sabouraudia. 2005;43(7):613–21.

Watson DF, et al. Isolated cerebral phycomycosis presenting as focal encephalitis. Arch Neurol. 1985;42(9):922–3.

Weprin BE, et al. Long-term survival in rhinocerebral mucormycosis: case report. J Neurosurg. 1998;88(3):570–5.

Wetli CV, et al. Fungal cerebritis from intravenous drug abuse. J Forensic Sci. 1984;29(1):260–8.

Wolkow N, et al. Chronic orbital and calvarial fungal infection with Apophysomyces variabilis in an immunocompetent patient. Surv Ophthalmol. 2017;62(1):70–82.

Woods KF, Hanna BJ. Brain stem mucormycosis in a narcotic addict with eventual recovery. Am J Med. 1986;80(1):126–8.

Yang D, et al. Mammalian defensins in immunity: more than just microbicidal. Trends Immunol. 2002;23(6):291–6.

Yousem DM, et al. MR findings in rhinocerebral mucormycosis. J Comput Assist Tomogr. 1989;13(5):878–82.

Zeilender S, et al. Fatal Cunninghamella bertholletiae infection in an immunocompetent patient. Chest. 1990;97(6):1482–3.

Histoplasmosis and Coccidioidomycosis

11

María del Rocío Reyes-Montes, Maria Lucia Taylor, Esperanza Duarte-Escalante, and María Guadalupe Frías-De-León

Abbreviations

AIDS	Acquired immune deficiency syndrome
CF	Complement fixation
CNS	Central nervous system
CSF	Cerebrospinal fluid
ECM	Extracellular matrix
EIA	Enzyme immunoassay
ELISA	Enzyme-linked immunosorbent assay
EORTC/MSG	European Organization for Research and Treatment of Cancer/Invasive Fungal Infections Cooperative Group and the National Institute of Allergy and Infectious Diseases Mycoses Study Group
FDA	Food and Drug Administration
GMS	Gomori methenamine silver
HE	Hematoxylin-eosin
HIV	Human immunodeficiency virus
ID	Double immunodiffusion
IFN	Interferon
IL	Interleukin
ITS	Internal transcribed spacer
PAS	Periodic acid-Schiff
PCR	Polymerase chain reaction
PMN	Polymorphonuclear
PRRs	Recognition receptors
qPCR	Real-time quantitative
RAPD	Random amplified polymorphic DNA
ROS	Reactive oxygen species
Sag	Serum antigens
STAT3	Signal transducer and activator of transcription 3
TLRs	Toll-like receptors
TNF	Tumor necrosis factor
UAg	Urinary antigen
USA	United States of America

11.1 Histoplasmosis

11.1.1 Introduction

Histoplasmosis is caused by a dimorphic fungus that corresponds to the species *Histoplasma capsulatum*, although nowadays the studies aimed to identify new phylogenetic species must be taken into account (Kasuga et al. 2003; Taylor et al. 2000a; Teixeira et al. 2016). Sepulveda et al. (Sepúlveda et al. 2017) suggested that the genus *Histoplasma* includes at least four species,

M. del Rocío Reyes-Montes · M. L. Taylor
E. Duarte-Escalante
Microbiology and Parasitology Department, School of Medicine, Universidad Nacional Autónoma de México, Mexico City, Mexico

M. G. Frías-De-León (✉)
Research Unit, Hospital Regional de Alta Especialidad de Ixtapaluca, Ixtapaluca, Estado de México, Mexico

M. Turgut et al. (eds.), *Fungal Infections of the Central Nervous System*, https://doi.org/10.1007/978-3-030-06088-6_11

H. capsulatum sensu stricto Darling 1906, *H. mississippiensis* sp. nov., *H. ohiense* sp. nov., and *H. suramericanum* sp. nov., through a study of population genetics and a phylogenetic analysis of the whole genome of *Histoplasma* isolates from geographic areas where histoplasmosis is endemic.

Fungal infections of the central nervous system (CNS), among which the histoplasmosis stands out, are potentially deadly and have occurred with greater frequency since the 1970s due to the increase in the use of corticosteroids, cytotoxic drugs, and antibiotics, as well as the acquired immune deficiency syndrome (AIDS) epidemic (Chakrabarti 2007). The infections may appear as meningitis, mass lesions, or abscesses.

11.1.2 Epidemiology

Histoplasmosis is a fungal infection of broad geographic distribution (Kauffman 2007), which affects more than 60 countries (Bracca et al. 2003), with predominance in the Americas, East Asia, Oceania, and sub-Saharan Africa (Farina et al. 2005). The endemic areas are of a mild, subtropical, or humid tropical climate, proximate to courses of freshwater. The soils that facilitate the massive growth of *H. capsulatum* mycelia and give origin to the so-called epidemic foci often contain excrement of blackbirds such as starlings, poultry, or bats. In most American countries, the high prevalence of this mycosis is associated with the increase of patients with immunosuppression caused by different conditions such as AIDS, neoplasms, diabetes, and people undergoing organ transplantation among others and to the great ubiquity of the fungus in nature, since it has been detected both in enclosed places (caves, mines, etc.) and open spaces (parks, avenues, etc.) which define areas of high and low risk of acquisition of the infection. The activities that are associated with the infection of the fungus include agriculture, exposure to poultry houses or caves, remodeling or demolition of old buildings, and felling and cleaning of sites where birds or bats are found (Taylor et al. 2000b).

The real incidence of histoplasmosis is unknown because its notification is not mandatory; most data derives from publications, personal experience of experts, or through surveys of histoplasmin intradermal tests. In the United States of America (USA), histoplasmosis has been described as the most common endemic mycosis. Benedict and Mody (Benedict and Mody 2016) assessed the epidemiological characteristics of histoplasmosis outbreaks between 1938 and 2013. From 105 outbreaks, 2850 cases of histoplasmosis were reported in various locations of 26 US and Puerto Rico states. The locations of the outbreaks were generally consistent with the known distribution of histoplasmosis; there were only a few outbreaks in states where it is believed to be a low level of endemicity such as Florida, Minnesota, New York, North Dakota, and South Carolina. Outside of the USA, the incidence of histoplasmosis is highest in Mexico, Honduras, Guatemala, Nicaragua, Panama, several islands of the Caribbean, Jamaica, Puerto Rico, Martinique, Cuba, Argentina, Brazil, Uruguay, Peru, Colombia, Venezuela (Ferreira and Borges 2009), and Spain (Rodriguez-Tudela et al. 2015). In European countries, histoplasmosis is considered to be an emerging mycosis, as a consequence of increased immigration and of European tourism to American and African countries (Antinori et al. 2006; Buitrago and Cuenca-Estrella 2012; Gascon et al. 2000). In Asia, there are recognized cases in India, Malaysia, Singapore, Indonesia, Thailand, Vietnam, and Japan (Randhawa 1970).

Data on the prevalence of histoplasmosis in Israel, Syria, Saudi Arabia, Lebanon, Qatar, Iran, Iraq, Pakistan, and India are uncertain. The cutaneous histoplasmin hypersensitivity tests have shown a negative or very low sensitivity so it has been suggested that the low reactivity is caused by cross-reactions with fungi antigenically related to *H. capsulatum* (Randhawa 1970).

In Africa there is very few information regarding this topic; however, in Zimbabwe, South Africa, Uganda, and Tanzania, some cases have been reported in patients with AIDS (Cottle et al. 2013; Gumbo et al. 2001; Lofgren et al. 2012).

Recent data indicate approximately 100,000 cases of disseminated histoplasmosis per year around the world, which illustrates the importance of this mycosis (Bongomin et al. 2017).

11.1.3 Pathogenesis and Pathology

The infection caused by *H. capsulatum* occurs when microconidia are inhaled, penetrating the body mainly through the airways. Subsequently, the macroconidia are transformed into the yeast phase and replicated within the macrophages, causing the beginning of a lung infection. The infection is usually asymptomatic in healthy individuals unless a large inoculum has been inhaled (Loulergue et al. 2007). In most immunocompetent patients, the infection is acute, self-limited, and is resolved with the development of cell-mediated immunity (Knox and Hage 2010), leaving only residual calcifications in the lung and sometimes the spleen (a benign form of histoplasmosis). In these patients, the induction of adaptive immunity, particularly the Th1 response, is required for activation of macrophages to increase their fungicide capabilities and stimulate the formation of granulomas (Kauffman 2007, 2008), thus carrying out an efficient elimination of the fungus through the oxygen-dependent mechanisms (reactive oxygen intermediates), which cause the so-called respiratory burst, and reactive nitrogen intermediates that generate nitric oxide, which is toxic for some microorganisms and tumor cells (Lane et al. 1994; Newman 1999). Besides, the independent mechanisms of oxygen that relate to the production of certain proteins already formed and accumulated in the granules, such as lysozymes, lactoferrin, and cationic proteins called defensins, cathepsin G, and azurocidin (Newman et al. 2000), also come into action, providing protection against reinfection. In patients with alterations of the cellular immune response, the infection caused by *H. capsulatum* is usually not controlled, and there is a tendency to progressive dissemination (Horwath et al. 2015). The infection spreads to various organs, which mainly include the bone marrow, liver, spleen, and adrenal glands (Kauffman 2007), and finally hematogenous dissemination.

11.1.4 Clinical Features

The clinical manifestations of histoplasmosis vary depending on the immune status of the host and the size of the inoculum. The disease is usually asymptomatic or manifests as an acute respiratory disease that is self-limited in immunocompetent persons, but it can cause a serious disease with progressive lung disease or disseminated infection, especially in immunocompromised individuals with impaired T-cell immunity, like patients with human immunodeficiency virus (HIV) infection who are treated with inhibitors of the tumor necrosis factor (TNF)-α and patients with interferon (IFN)-γ receptor deficiency (Hage et al. 2010; Zerbe and Holland 2005). The dissemination can be hematogenous toward the skin, adrenal glands, and endocardium, and in some cases, the progressive disseminated histoplasmosis secondarily affects the CNS (Dines et al. 1979). Between 25% and 50% of patients with histoplasmosis can present CNS symptoms (Goodwin et al. 1981; Wheat et al. 1990, 2005; Wheat and Kauffman 2003; Zerbe and Holland 2005). The clinical syndrome includes subacute or chronic meningitis, focal brain or spinal cord injuries, stroke syndromes, and encephalitis (Machado et al. 1993; Saccente 2008; Wheat et al. 1990). Patients with CNS histoplasmosis present fever, confusion, headache, lethargy, weakness, hydrocephalus, and focal neurologic deficits that resembles a stroke (Enarson et al. 1978; Wheat et al. 2005).

11.1.5 Diagnosis

The tests for laboratory diagnosis include culture, microscopic exam ination, detection of antibodies, antigen detection through the enzyme-linked immunosorbent assay (ELISA), and methods of molecular diagnostics, based on the polymerase chain reaction (PCR).

The direct microscopic examination and culture on Sabouraud medium are the gold standard for histoplasmosis diagnosis. *H. capsulatum* can be identified in cultures after the sample has been inoculated in a suitable medium and incubated long enough to allow the fungus growth or in body fluids and tissue samples using different stains and direct microscopy. The adequate stain to identify *H. capsulatum* in clinical samples is calcofluor white. The culture sensitivity for the detection of the fungus depends on the clinical manifestation (pulmonary versus disseminated), host immunity, and the burden of disease. Patients with disseminated histoplasmosis have a higher rate of positive cultures (74%) than patients with acute pulmonary histoplasmosis (42%) (Hage et al. 2015). In patients with HIV/AIDS, the cultures of samples from airways can be positive in up to 90%, while blood cultures may be positive in up to 50% (Kauffman 2007). In the histopathological examination of *H. capsulatum*, consideration must be given to microorganisms with similar morphology, such as *Cryptococcus* spp., *Blastomyces dermatitidis*, *Candida glabrata*, *Pneumocystis jirovecii*, *Coccidioides* spp., *Talaromyces* (formerly *Penicillium marneffei*), *Leishmania* spp., *Toxoplasma gondii*, and *Trypanosoma cruzi*. For the correct identification, specific histochemical stains such as Gomori methenamine silver (GMS) and periodic acid-Schiff (PAS) should be used, which are the most useful to visualize *H. capsulatum* in tissue preparations (Fig. 11.1) (Knox and Hage 2010). The microscopic examinations, as well as the histopathology, require a good level of experience, in order to identify correctly *H. capsulatum* and discard similarities with other microorganisms.

The serological test used in the diagnosis of histoplasmosis is the double immunodiffusion (ID) which detects the presence of serum antibodies that precipitate in the agar gel after

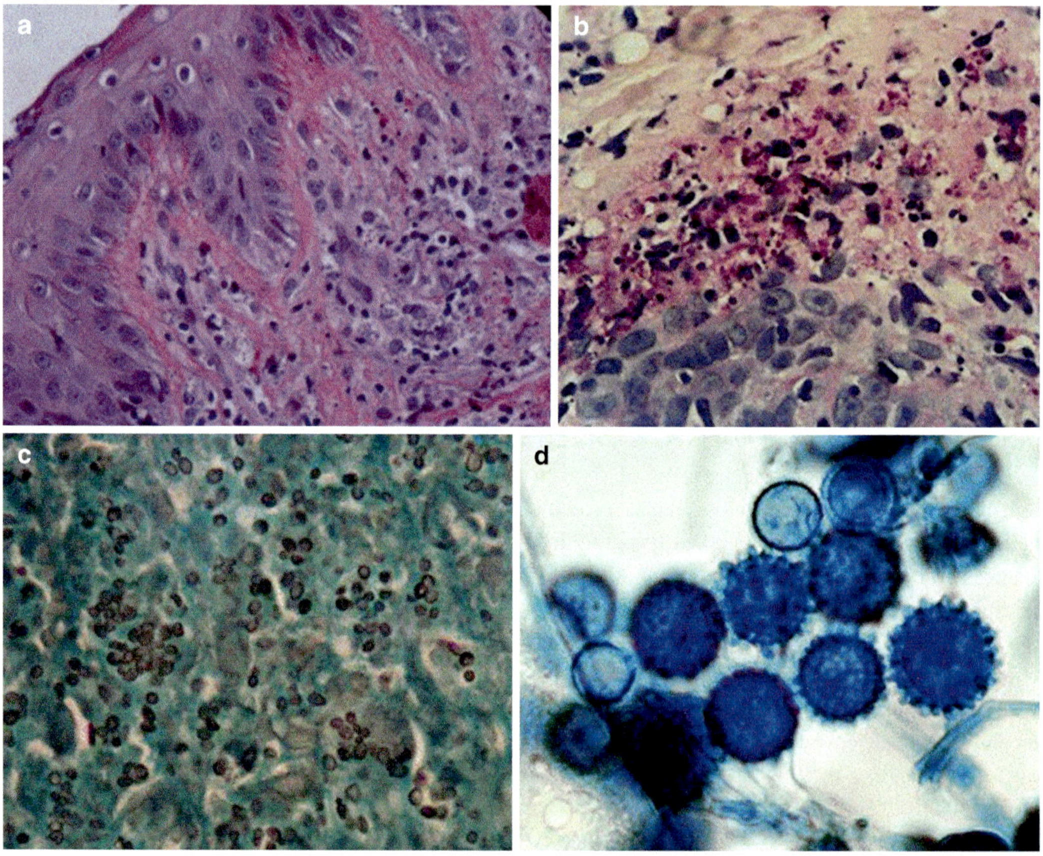

Fig. 11.1 (**a**) Numerous yeast cells. Hematoxylin and eosin stain; (**b**) numerous yeast cells PAS stain positive; (**c**) numerous yeast cell of *Histoplasma* GMS; and (**d**) characteristic macroconidia (echinulate conidia) of *Histoplasma capsulatum*. (From Chang and Meaux (2015), with permission)

bonding with antigens H and M of *H. capsulatum*. The band M is detected in the majority of patients with acute histoplasmosis (80%) but persists for long periods of time; the band H is rarely seen (20%), but when present, it confirms the acute infection. The ID is an inexpensive technique but has variable sensitivity and specificity, with predictive values of 86–100% according to the antigen used, and has low sensitivity in immunocompromised patients who produce low levels of immunoglobulins. The complement fixation (CF) test is more sensitive than the ID technique (90% versus 80%, respectively). Through CF, a titre 1:8 results positive, indicating prior exposure to *H. capsulatum*, while a titre ≥1:32 is suggestive of active infection (Wheat et al. 1990). The ELISA technique is widely used in patients with acute pulmonary histoplasmosis or disseminated histoplasmosis (Kasuga et al. 2003). This test is used in the detection of antigens in urine samples and/or serum. The sensitivity and specificity of the urinary antigen detection (UAg) and testing of serum antigens (SAg) vary depending on the type and extent of the infection. The detection of the UAg is more sensitive than the SAg in patients with disseminated histoplasmosis (Wheat and Kauffman 2003), so Libert et al. (2018) support the detection of UAg to discard suspected histoplasmosis.

Nowadays, molecular techniques have had greater acceptance because of their sensitivity, specificity, and speed. In the last two decades, several molecular assays using different molecular markers for the detection of *H. capsulatum* in clinical samples through PCR have been developed (Babady et al. 2011; Bialek et al. 2002; Bracca et al. 2003; Dantas et al. 2013; Frías De León et al. 2012; Gago et al. 2014; Guedes et al. 2003; Haynes et al. 1995; Martagon-Villamil et al. 2003; Tang et al. 2006; Ueda et al. 2003). Due to its high sensitivity and specificity, the Hcp100 marker is used in the diagnosis of histoplasmosis (Bialek et al. 2002). This molecular marker was validated on clinical samples by Muñoz et al. (2010), showing sensitivity and specificity of 100% and 95.2%, respectively. Another marker described for the detection of *H. capsulatum* is named 1281–1283(220), which was designed from random amplified polymorphic DNA (RAPD) patterns of fungal isolates from different countries in the Americas. This marker has been tested through PCR simplex in clinical and environmental samples with good specificity (Frías De León et al. 2012). Buitrago et al. (2013) conducted a multicenter study to validate the Hcp100, and 1281–1283(220) markers, in comparison with the amplification by real-time quantitative PCR (qPCR) of the rDNA ITS1. The authors showed that the marker detected by qPCR was the most sensitive, followed by Hcp100 and 1281–1283(220). Therefore, molecular methods are useful for the histoplasmosis diagnosis, although these methods have not been approved yet for routine clinical use by the Food and Drug Administration (FDA).

11.1.6 Treatment Options

The treatment of CNS histoplasmosis should be aggressive and prolonged. Daily treatment with liposomal amphotericin B 5.0 mg/kg, until adding up to a total of 175 mg/kg administered for 4–6 weeks, is recommended. Subsequently, treatment should be switched to high doses of itraconazole (200 mg two or three times a day) or fluconazole (600–800 mg per day) for at least 1 year, until the detection of antigens becomes negative in cerebrospinal fluid (CSF). In patients with severe immunodeficiencies, such as AIDS, maintenance therapy is needed for life (Wheat et al. 2007).

11.2 Coccidioidomycosis

11.2.1 Introduction

Coccidioidomycosis is caused by the fungi *Coccidioides immitis* and *C. posadasii* (Fisher et al. 2002). The infection is acquired by susceptible hosts through the inhalation of its arthroconidium present in the soil of endemic areas, which include arid and semiarid regions of the Southwestern USA, Northern Mexico, Central

America, and some regions of South America (Hector and Laniado-Laborín 2005).

Although 60% of the infections are subclinical and self-limited, approximately 1% of these result in infections with extrapulmonary dissemination, especially in immunocompromised patients, in which the dissemination to the CNS is associated with high morbidity and mortality (Adam et al. 2009). In addition, neurological manifestations caused by *Coccidioides* spp. in the CNS are variables, from meningitis to meningoencephalitis and meningomyelitis (Adam et al. 2009). CNS coccidioidomycosis should be considered in the differential diagnosis of patients with neurological symptoms, especially if they are immunosuppressed and live in regions where the disease is endemic.

11.2.2 Epidemiology

The geographical distribution of *Coccidioides* is restricted to the American continent in endemic regions that include the USA (Arizona, California, New Mexico, Nevada, Utah, Washington, and Texas), Mexico, and some areas in Guatemala, Honduras, Venezuela, Brazil, Argentina, and Paraguay (Hector and Laniado-Laborín 2005). In the USA, the annual incidence of coccidioidomycosis is variable; however, it has increased in recent years with a rate that goes from 5.3 per 100.000 inhabitants in 1998 to a rate of 42.6 in 2011 (Centers for Disease Control and Prevention (CDC) 2013). The rate of positive skin prick tests for *Coccidioides* is found in ranges of 50–70% in Kern County, including the City of Bakersfield and neighboring counties of Tulare and Kings. On the other hand, unlike *C. immitis*, *C. posadasii* has a wider region of endemicity which includes the central and southern Arizona in west Texas and southern New Mexico. The region with a higher concentration of *C. posadasii* is Arizona, where most of the skin prick tests and positive cases of coccidioidomycosis occur in the Maricopa County (including the city of Phoenix), Pima (including the City of Tucson), and Pinal Counties. It is also present, sporadically, in sites in the southern part of Utah and Nevada (Brown et al. 2013). However, recent studies suggest that the geographic range of *Coccidioides* spp. extends toward the north, particularly in the state of Washington, where several cases were reported in 2010 and 2011, without the patients reporting recent travels to endemic areas (Marsden-Haug et al. 2013, 2014).

In the rest of the American continent, the species associated with coccidioidomycosis is *C. posadasii*. However, the actual incidence is unknown because it is not mandatory to report this disease; furthermore, it has been poorly studied. In Mexico, the coccidioidomycosis data is restricted to the publication of clinical cases and retrospective studies in different hospital centers (Baptista Rosas and Riquelme 2007; Laniado-Laborin 2007; Mondragón-González et al. 2005; Muñoz-Hernández et al. 2004, 2008); however, it is suggested that the current situation of the disease may have followed a development like that of the USA (Nguyen et al. 2013). Therefore, Hector et al. (2011) propose that the coccidioidomycosis is an emerging disease in Mexico due to the increase in the rate of infection recorded in recent years.

In Central and South America, the epidemiological situation is no different, as there are few studies on this disease. In Brazil, Cordeiro et al. (2009), through a serological survey with 229 volunteers in the northeastern part of the country, found a 7.42% of positive samples and showed a direct relationship with endemic areas. In Argentina, Canteros et al. (2010) performed a retrospective study of the coccidioidomycosis cases from 1892 to 2009, finding an increase in the number of cases in this period, so they proposed that the disease is emerging in the country.

In endemic regions of the USA, the most affected people are the construction and farm workers, military personnel, archaeologists, excavators, inmates, and officers in correctional facilities. Also, it is known that in these endemic regions, the epidemics have occurred after dust storms, earthquakes, and excavations where the dispersion of arthroconidia is facilitated (Stockamp and Thompson III 2016).

In Mexico, the majority of coccidioidomycosis cases are acquired in the place of residence (endemic areas), although some cases are related to migration to the USA, where the disease is acquired (Baptista Rosas and Riquelme 2007). While in Brazil, an association between the infection caused by *Coccidioides* spp. and armadillo (*Dasypus novemcinctus*) hunters in endemic areas has been demonstrated (Brillhante et al. 2012).

The main risk factor for acquiring the infection and developing the disease is exposure to dust by occupational or recreational causes in endemic areas. It has also been described that the disease is more common in men, as well as in African Americans and Filipinos, and in patients with immunocompromised caused by different reasons such as HIV, transplant recipients, and renal failure, among others (Laniado-Laborin 2007).

A recent work concludes that the major risk factors for the development of disseminated coccidioidomycosis are exogenous immunosuppression (caused by steroids biological products), pregnancy, race/ethnicity, and discrete genetic defects, such as defects in the interleukin-12/IFN-γ pathway and the signal transducer and activator of transcription 3 (STAT3) (Odio et al. 2017).

11.2.3 Pathogenesis and Pathology

The initial encounter between *Coccidioides* spp. and the host begins when the arthroconidium of the fungus is inhaled by a susceptible host, who visits or lives in endemic areas, and they reach the lungs and alveoli. Epithelial cells of the lung are equipped with pattern recognition receptors (PRRs), such as Toll-like receptors (TLRs) and dectin-1, which are capable of inducing immediate effector responses besides influencing the regulation of alveolar macrophages. In the lungs, the innate immune cells recognize components of the fungus through multiple receivers, inducing phagocytosis and the production of reactive oxygen species (ROS). In a matter of hours, *Coccidioides* induces an influx of activated polymorphonuclear (PMN) cells, which, at the same time, can increase the formation of spherules. The PMN responds in a similar manner to macrophages, that is, surrounding the arthroconidia without eliminating them. There is evidence that the phagosome-lysosome fusion does not occur, thus preventing the arthroconidia to come into contact with the lytic enzymes of the PMN (Frey and Drutz 1986). Hence, the arthroconidia grow and transform into immature spherules, which induce phagocytosis and the production of ROS, TLR-2, and Dectin-1, as well as the signals mediated by MyD88 and intracellular adapters, which lead to the activation of the transcription factor NF-kB that produces proinflammatory cytokines such as TNF and macrophage inflammatory protein 2 (MIP-2) and interleukin 6 (IL-6), which are essential effectors of the cellular response of the Th1 and Th17. The dectin-1 also mediates the production of cytokines Th1 and Th17, IL-23, IL-17A, IL-22, IL-12, and IFN. In addition, the spherules increase the expression of the RNAm and other factors for evasion in the host. In the following days (two or three), the spherules undergo a nuclear division and mature into large septate cells (30–80 μm) that contain endospores. These spherules are too large to be phagocyted; besides, they produce an alkaline extracellular matrix (ECM) that prevents contact with PMN. In the fourth or fifth day, the spherules break to release mature endospores. Host response is to attract PMNs and macrophages, which phagocyte the endospores easily. However, phagocytosis can present some drawbacks, as the endospores can remain in large bunches joined by fibrillary structures coming from the outside wall of the spherule and protected by the ECM. From this moment on continues the parasitic cycle of the fungus in the host (Smith et al. 2013). Furthermore, dissemination of the fungus can occur through the bloodstream or lymphatic stream toward any anatomical site of the host, including the CNS (Johnson and Einstein 2006), frequently causing meningitis, a clinical picture of great relevance due to the high rates of morbidity and mortality.

11.2.4 Clinical Features

Meningitis caused by *Coccidioides* spp. is the most important disseminated form, due to the high risk that represents for the host. Meningitis occurs in almost one-third of the immunocompromised patients, in most cases, in weeks or months after the primary infection. The most common symptom is headache. The patient can have altered mental states, with or without fever, personality changes, nausea, and vomiting. In addition, walking abnormalities and neurologic deficits may occur in some cases (Johnson and Einstein 2006; Sharma 2010). On the other hand, there may be some complications of meningitis, which include hydrocephalus, myocardial infarction, vasculitis, and abscesses. The vasculitis is of great importance since it is characterized by cerebral infarction due to inflammatory changes in the walls of small- and medium-sized brain arteries and veins that lead to vascular insufficiency and neurologic deficits that threaten the patient's life (Tager et al. 2017). In addition to meningitis and vasculitis, brain inflammation can occur as a result of the fungus dissemination along the walls of vessels or perivascular spaces (Shih and Koeller 2015). It has also been described that it is common for coccidioidomycosis to extend into the spinal cord as microscopic foci of the disease, although it is rare that discrete lesions develop in the CNS (Bañuelos et al. 1996).

On the other hand, the pattern of neuroimaging of coccidioidomycosis is similar to that of meningitis caused by tuberculosis, which shows a thick exude and an abnormal increase in basal cisterns and the subarachnoid space which can further evolve into hydrocephalus or vasculitis (Shih and Koeller 2015). It has also been described the presence of subarachnoid hemorrhage as a result of granulomatous inflammation of large vessels (Shih and Koeller 2015).

11.2.5 Diagnosis

According to the criteria of the European Organization for Research and Treatment of Cancer/Invasive Fungal Infections Cooperative Group and the National Institute of Allergy and Infectious Diseases Mycoses Study Group (EORTC/MSG), the diagnosis of invasive fungal infections is made based on a combined interpretation of risk factors, clinical symptoms, and results of images. In particular, the symptoms of CNS invasion by *Coccidioides* spp. are nonspecific, so the diagnosis is complicated. On the other hand, biopsies of the CNS are considered too risky in severely ill patients, especially in populations of patients with hematological low platelet counts or neutropenia. However, the biopsy material stained with hematoxylin-eosin (HE), GMS, or PAS is useful for the diagnosis (Góralska et al. 2018).

Coccidioidal meningitis is usually diagnosed by the detection of anti-*Coccidioides* antibodies in the CSF, in an 80% of cases, through serological tests as ID, CF, or enzyme immunoassay (EIA) (Kassis et al. 2015; Stockamp and Thompson III 2016). In addition, the analysis of CSF usually shows an elevated white blood cell count with a mixed or lymphocytic pleocytosis and a high level of protein (occasionally quantifiable in grams per deciliter instead of milligrams per deciliter) and a low blood glucose level.

A recent study showed that the quantitative test of *Coccidioides* antigen detection in CSF, performed in microtiter plates coated with anti-*Coccidioides* antibodies, is effective in the diagnosis of coccidioidal meningitis, as it showed a 93% sensitivity and a 100% specificity (Kassis et al. 2015).

Although the imaging studies are useful to evaluate the complications associated with meningitis, the initial characteristics of the disease can be difficult to distinguish from other causes, especially with tuberculosis and even autoimmune diseases, without detailed evidence (Stockamp and Thompson III 2016).

11.2.6 Treatment Options

In the case of CNS coccidioidomycosis, fluconazole has become the most commonly used primary therapy at a dose of 400 mg/day, although higher doses have been suggested which can range from initial doses of 400 mg/day or 800–1200 mg every 24 h, as they can decrease the rate of therapeutic failure. Also, the itraconazole has been used as primary therapy, usually in doses of

200 mg every 12 h, with fatty foods and an acidic drink to increase absorption. However, the intrathecal amphotericin B deoxycholate is the original gold standard. It can be administered via direct lumbar or cisternal injection, and it is currently used as rescue therapy upon failure of the azoles. The therapy often begins with low doses that increase gradually unless the patient experience symptoms or signs of toxicity (Galgiani et al. 2016).

11.3 Conclusion

Meningitis caused by *Histoplasma* spp. and *Coccidioides* spp. has increased in the last decades. These mycoses have a high morbidity and mortality mainly due to a delay in the diagnosis and treatment failure. The success of the treatment for CNS mycosis is based on maintaining a high index of clinical suspicion as well as the identification of the fungus.

References

Adam RD, Elliott SP, Taljanovic MS. The spectrum and presentation of disseminated coccidioidomycosis. Am J Med. 2009;122:770–7.

Antinori S, Magni C, Nebuloni M, Parravicini C, Corbellino M, Sollima S, Galimberti L, Ridolfo AL, Wheat LJ. Histoplasmosis among human immunodeficiency virus-infected people in Europe: report of 4 cases and review of the literature. Medicine (Baltimore). 2006;85(1):22–36.

Babady NE, Buckwalter SP, Hall L, Le Febre KM, Binnicker MJ, Wengenack NL. Detection of *Blastomyces dermatitidis* and *Histoplasma capsulatum* from culture isolates and clinical specimens by use of real-time PCR. J Clin Microbiol. 2011;49:3204–8.

Bañuelos AF, Williams PL, Johnson RH, Bibi S, Fredricks DN, Gilroy SA, Bhatti SU, Aguet J, Stevens DA. Central nervous system abscesses due to *Coccidioides* species. Clin Infect Dis. 1996;22:240–50.

Baptista Rosas RC, Riquelme M. Epidemiología de la coccidioidomicosis en México. Rev Iberoam Micol. 2007;24:100–5.

Benedict K, Mody RK. Epidemiology of histoplasmosis outbreaks, United States, 1938–2013. Emerg Infect Dis. 2016;22(3):370–8.

Bialek R, Feucht A, Aepinus C, Just-Nubling G, Robertson VJ, Knobloch J, Hohle R. Evaluation of two nested PCR assays for detection of *Histoplasma capsulatum* DNA in human tissue. J Clin Microbiol. 2002;40:1644–7.

Bongomin F, Gago S, Oladel RO, Denning DW. Global and multi-national prevalence of fungal diseases-estimate precision. J Fungi (Basel). 2017;3(4):57.

Bracca A, Tosello ME, Girardini JE, Amigot SL, Gomez C, Serra E. Molecular detection of *Histoplasma capsulatum* var. *capsulatum* in human clinical samples. J Clin Microbiol. 2003;41:1753–5.

Brillhante RS, Moreira Filho RE, Rocha MF, Castelo-Branco Dde S, Fechine MA, Lima RA, Picanço YV, Cordeiro Rde A, Camargo ZP, Queiroz JA, Araujo RW, Mesquita JR, Sidrim JJ. Coccidioidomycosis in armadillo hunters from the state of Ceará, Brazil. Mem Inst Oswaldo Cruz. 2012;107(6):813–5.

Brown J, Benedict K, Park BJ, Thompson GR III. Coccidioidomycosis: epidemiology. Clin Epidemiol. 2013;5:185–97.

Buitrago MJ, Cuenca-Estrella M. Current epidemiology and laboratory diagnosis of endemic mycoses in Spain. Enferm Infecc Microbiol Clin. 2012;30(7):407–13.

Buitrago MJ, Canteros CE, Frías De León G, González Á, Marques-Evangelista De Oliveira M, Muñoz CO, Ramirez JA, Toranzo AI, Zancope-Oliveira R, Cuenca-Estrella M. Comparison of PCR protocols for detecting *Histoplasma capsulatum* DNA through a multicenter study. Rev Iberoam Micol. 2013;30:256–60.

Canteros CE, Toranzo A, Ibarra-Camou B, David V, Carrizo SG, Santillán-Iturres A, Serrano J, Fernández N, Capece P, Gorostiaga J, Chacón YA, Tonelli R, Boscaro G, Abiega C, Mendieta S, Fernández C, Fernández A, Vitale R, Santos P, Pizarro MR, López-Joffre MC, Lee W, Mazza M, Posse G, Tiraboschi IN, Negroni R, Davel G. Coccidioidomycosis in Argentina, 1892–2009. Rev Argent Microbiol. 2010;42:261–8.

Centers for Disease Control & Prevention (CDC). Increase in reported coccidioidomycosis—United States, 1998–2011. MMWR Morb Mortal Wkly Rep. 2013;62(12):217–21.

Chakrabarti A. Epidemiology of central nervous system mycoses. Neurol India. 2007;55:191–7.

Chang P, Meaux T. Progressive disseminated histoplasmosis and HIV/AIDS: a dermatological perspective. Curr Fungal Infect Rep. 2015;9:213–9.

Cordeiro RA, Fechine MA, Brilhante RS, Rocha MF, da Costa AK, Nagao MA, de Camargo ZP, Sidrim JJ. Serologic detection of coccidioidomycosis antibodies in northeast Brazil. Mycopathologia. 2009;167(4):187–90.

Cottle LE, Gkrania-Klotsas E, Williams HJ, Brindle HE, Carmichael AJ, Fry G, Beeching NJ. A multinational outbreak of histoplasmosis following a biology field trip in the Ugandan rainforest. J Travel Med. 2013;20(2):83–7.

Dantas KC, Freitas RS, Moreira AP, Silva MV, Benard G, Vasconcellos C, Criado PR. The use of nested polymerase chain reaction (nested PCR) for the early diagnosis of *Histoplasma capsulatum* infection in serum and whole blood of HIV-positive patients. An Bras Dermatol. 2013;88:141–3.

Dines DE, Payne WS, Bernatz PE, Pairolero PC. Mediastinal granuloma and fibrosing mediastinitis. Chest. 1979;75(3):320–4.

Enarson DA, Keys TF, Onofrio BM. Central nervous system histoplasmosis with obstructive hydrocephalus. Am J Med. 1978;64:895–6.

Farina C, Rizzi M, Ricci L, Gabbi E, Caligaris S, Goglio A. Imported and autochthonous. Histoplasmosis in Italy: new cases and old problems. Rev Iberoam Micol. 2005;22:169–71.

Ferreira MS, Borges AS. Histoplasmose. Rev Soc Brasil Med Trop. 2009;42:192–8.

Fisher MG, Koening GI, White TJ, Taylor JW. Molecular and phenotypic description of *Coccidioides posadasii* sp. Nov., previously recognized as the non-California population of *Coccidioides immitis*. Mycologia. 2002;94:73–84.

Frey CL, Drutz DJ. Influence of fungal surface components on the interaction of *Coccidioides immitis* with polymorphonuclear neutrophils. J Infect Dis. 1986;153(5):933–43.

Frías De León MG, Arenas López G, Taylor ML, Acosta Altamirano G, Reyes-Montes MR. Development of specific sequence characterized amplified region markers for detecting *Histoplasma capsulatum* in clinical and environmental samples. J Clin Microbiol. 2012;50:673–9.

Gago S, Esteban C, Valero C, Zaragoza O, Puig de la Bellacasa J, Buitrago MJ. A multiplex real-time PCR assay for identification of *Pneumocystis jirovecii*, *Histoplasma capsulatum*, and *Cryptococcus neoformans*/*Cryptococcus gattii* in samples from AIDS patients with opportunistic pneumonia. J Clin Microbiol. 2014;52:1168–76.

Galgiani JN, Ampel NM, Blair JE, Catanzaro A, Geertsma F, Hoover SE, Johnson RH, Kusne S, Lisse J, MacDonald JD, Meyerson SL, Raksin PB, Siever J, Stevens DA, Sunenshine R, Theodore N. Executive summary: 2016 Infectious Diseases Society of America (IDSA) Clinical Practice Guideline for the treatment of coccidioidomycosis. Clin Infect Dis. 2016;63(6):e112–46.

Gascon J, Torres JM, Luburich P, Ayuso JR, Xaubet A, Corachan M. Imported histoplasmosis in Spain. J Travel Med. 2000;7:89–91.

Goodwin RA, Loyd JE, Des Prez RM. Histoplasmosis in normal host. Medicine (Baltimore). 1981;60:231–66.

Góralska K, Blaszkowska J, Dzikowiec M. Neuroinfections caused by fungi. Infection. 2018; https://doi.org/10.1007/s15010-018-1152-2.

Guedes HL, Guimarães AJ, De Medeiros-Muniz M, Pizzini CV, Hamilton AJ, Peralta JM, Deepe GS Jr, Zancopé-Oliveira RM. PCR assay for identification of *Histoplasma capsulatum* based on the nucleotide sequence of the M antigen. J Clin Microbiol. 2003;41:535–9.

Gumbo T, Just-Nubling G, Robertson V, Latif AS, Borok MZ, Hohle R. Clinicopathological features of cutaneous histoplasmosis in human immunodeficiency virus-infected patients in Zimbabwe. Trans R Soc Trop Med Hyg. 2001;95(6):635–6.

Hage CA, Bowyer S, Tarvin SE, Helper D, Kleiman MB, Wheat LJ. Recognition, diagnosis, and treatment of histoplasmosis complicating tumor necrosis factor blocker therapy. Clin Infect Dis. 2010;50:85–92.

Hage CA, Azar MM, Bahr N, Loyd J, Wheat LJ. Histoplasmosis: up-to-date evidence-based approach to diagnosis and management. Semin Respir Crit Care Med. 2015;36:729–45.

Haynes K, Westerneng T, Fell J, Moens W. Rapid detection and identification of pathogenic fungi by polymerase chain reaction amplification of large subunit ribosomal DNA. J Med Vet Mycol. 1995;3:319–25.

Hector RF, Laniado-Laborín R. Coccidioidomycosis a fungal disease of the Americas. PLoS Med. 2005;2(1):e2.

Hector RF, Rutherford GW, Tsang CA, Erhart LM, McCotter O, Anderson SM, Komatsu K, Tabnak F, Vugia DJ, Yang Y, Galgiani JN. The public health impact of coccidioidomycosis in Arizona and California. Int J Environ Res Public Health. 2011;8:1150–73.

Horwath MC, Fecher RA, Deepe GS Jr. *Histoplasma capsulatum*, lung infection and immunity. Future Microbiol. 2015;10:967–75.

Johnson RH, Einstein HE. Coccidioidal meningitis. Clin Infect Dis. 2006;42:103–7.

Kassis C, Zaidi S, Kuberski T, Moran A, Gonzalez O, Hussain S, Hartmann-Manrique C, Al-Jashaami L, Chebbo A, Myers RA, Wheat LJ. Role of *Coccidioides* antigen testing in the cerebrospinal fluid for the diagnosis of coccidioidal meningitis. Clin Infect Dis. 2015;61(10):1521–6.

Kasuga T, White TJ, Koenig G, McEwen J, Restrepo A, Castañeda E, Da Silva Lacaz C, Heins-Vaccari EM, De Freitas RS, Zancopé-Oliveira RM, Qin Z, Negroni R, Carter DA, Mikami Y, Tamura M, Taylor ML, Miller GF, Poonwan N, Taylor JW. Phylogeography of the fungal pathogen *Histoplasma capsulatum*. Mol Ecol. 2003;12:3383–401.

Kauffman CA. Histoplasmosis: a clinical and laboratory update. Clin Microbiol Rev. 2007;20:115–32.

Kauffman CA. Diagnosis of histoplasmosis in immunosuppressed patients. Curr Opin Infect Dis. 2008;21(4):421–5.

Knox KS, Hage CA. Histoplasmosis. Proc Am Thorac Soc. 2010;7(3):169–72.

Lane T, Wu-Hsieh B, Howard D. Antihistoplasma effect to activate mouse splenius macrophages involves production of reactive nitrogen intermediates. Infect Immun. 1994;62:1940–5.

Laniado-Laborin R. Expanding understanding of epidemiology of coccidioidomycosis in the Western hemisphere. Ann N Y Acad Sci. 2007;1111:19–34.

Libert D, Procop GW, Ansari MQ. *Histoplasma* urinary antigen testing obviates the need for coincident serum antigen testing. Am J Clin Pathol. 2018;149:362–8.

Lofgren SM, Kirsch EJ, Maro VP, Morrisey AB, Msuya LJ, Kinabo GD, Saganda W, Diefenthal HC, Ramadhani HO, Wheat LJ, Crump JA. Histoplasmosis among hospitalized febrile patients in northern Tanzania. Trans R Soc Trop Med Hyg. 2012;106(8):504–7.

Loulergue P, Bastides F, Baudouin V, Chandenier J, Mariani-Kurkdjian P, Dupont B, Viard JP, Dromer F, Lortholary O. Literature review and case histories of *Histoplasma capsulatum* var. *duboisii* infections in HIV-infected patients. Emerg Infect Dis. 2007;13(11):1647–52.

Machado LR, Nóbrega JPS, Livramento JA, Vianna LS II, Spina-França A. Histoplasmosis of the central nervous system: clinical features in eight patients. Arq Neuropsiquiatr. 1993;51:209–12.

Marsden-Haug N, Goldoft M, Ralston C, Limaye AP, Chua J, Hill H, Jecha L, Thompson GR 3rd, Chiller T. Coccidioidomycosis acquired in Washington State. Clin Infect Dis. 2013;56:847–50.

Marsden-Haug N, Hill H, Litvintseva AP, Engelthaler DM, Driebe EM, Roe CC, Ralston C, Hurst S, Goldoft M, Gade L, Wohrle R, Thompson GR, Brandt ME, Chiller T, Centers for Disease Control and Prevention (CDC). *Coccidioides immitis* identified in soil outside of its known range—Washington, 2014. MMWR Morb Mortal Wkly Rep. 2014;63:450.

Martagon-Villamil J, Shrestha N, Sholtis M, Isada CM, Hall GS, Bryne T, Lodge BA, Reller LB, Procop GW. Identification of *Histoplasma capsulatum* from culture extracts by real-time PCR. J Clin Microbiol. 2003;41:1295–8.

Mondragón-González R, Méndez-Tovar LJ, Bernal-Vázquez E, Hernández-Hernández F, López-Martínez R, Manzano-Gayosso P, Ríos-Rosas C, Contreras-Pérez C, Anides-Fonseca AE. Detección de infección por *Coccidioides immitis* en Coahuila, México. Rev Argent Microbiol. 2005;37:135–8.

Muñoz C, Gómez BL, Tobón A, Arango K, Restrepo A, Correa MM, Muskus C, Cano LE, González A. Validation and clinical application of a molecular method for identification of *Histoplasma capsulatum* in human specimens in Colombia, South America. Clin Vaccine Immunol. 2010;17:62–7.

Muñoz-Hernández B, Castañón LR, Calderón I, Vázquez ME, Manjarrez ME. Parasitic mycelial forms of *Coccidioides* species in Mexican patients. J Clin Microbiol. 2004;42:1247–9.

Muñoz-Hernández B, Martínez-Rivera MA, Palma Cortés G, Tapia-Díaz A, Manjarrez Zavala ME. Mycelial forms of *Coccidioides* spp. in the parasitic phase associated to pulmonary coccidioidomycosis with type 2 diabetes mellitus. Eur J Clin Microbiol. 2008;27:813–20.

Newman S. Macrophages in host defense against *Histoplasma capsulatum*. Trends Microbiol. 1999;7(2):67–71.

Newman S, Gootee L, Gabay J, Selsted M. Identification of constituents of human neutrophil azurophil granules that mediate fungistasis against *Histoplasma capsulatum*. Infect Immun. 2000;68(19):5668–72.

Nguyen C, Barker BM, Hoover S, Nix DE, Ampel NM, Frelinger JA, Orbach MJ, Galgiani JN. Recent advances in our understanding of the environmental, epidemiological, immunological, and clinical dimensions of coccidioidomycosis. Clin Microbiol Rev. 2013;26(3):505–25.

Odio CD, Marciano BE, Galgiani JN, Holland SM. Risk factors for disseminated coccidioidomycosis, United States. Emerg Infect Dis. 2017;23(2):308–11.

Randhawa HS. Occurrence of histoplasmosis in Asia. Mycopathol Mycol Appl. 1970;41(1):75–89.

Rodriguez-Tudela JL, Alastruey-Izquierdo A, Gago S, Cuenca-Estrella M, León C, Miro JM, Nuñez Boluda A, Ruiz Camps I, Sole A, Denning DW, University of Manchester in association with the LIFE program. Burden of serious fungal infections in Spain. Clin Microbiol Infect. 2015;21(2):183–9.

Saccente M. Central nervous system histoplasmosis. Curr Treat Options Neurol. 2008;10:161–7.

Sepúlveda VE, Márquez R, Turissini DA, Goldman WE, Matute DR. Genome sequences reveal cryptic speciation in the human pathogen *Histoplasma capsulatum*. MBio. 2017;8(6):e01339–7.

Sharma RR. Fungal infections of the nervous system: current perspective and controversies in management. Int J Surg. 2010;8:591e601.

Shih RY, Koeller KK. Bacterial, fungal, and parasitic infections of the central nervous system: radiologic-pathologic correlation and historical perspectives. Radiographics. 2015;35(4):1141–69.

Smith JA, Riddell J, Kauffman CA. Cutaneous manifestations of endemic mycoses. Curr Infect Dis Rep. 2013;15:440–9.

Stockamp NW, Thompson GR III. Coccidioidomycosis. Infect Dis Clin North Am. 2016;30:229–46.

Tager D, Hatch A, Segar J, Roller B, Al Mohajer M, Zangeneh TT. Coccidioidal meningitis complicated by central nervous system vasculitis in a patient with leukemia. Med Mycol Case Rep. 2017;16:8–11.

Tang YW, Li H, Durkin MM, Sefers SE, Meng S, Connolly PA, Stratton CW, Wheat LJ. Urine polymerase chain reaction is not as sensitive as urine antigen for the diagnosis of disseminated histoplasmosis. Diagn Microbiol Infect Dis. 2006;53:46–51.

Taylor JW, Jacobson DJ, Kroken S, Kasuga T, Geiser DM, Hibbett DS, Fischer MC. Phylogenetic species recognition and species concepts in fungi. Fungal Genet Biol. 2000a;31(1):21–32.

Taylor ML, Reyes-Montes MR, Chávez-Tapia CB, Curiel-Quesada E, Duarte-Escalante E, Rodríguez-Arellanes G. Ecology and molecular epidemiology findings of *Histoplasma capsulatum*, in Mexico. In: Benedik M, editor. Research advances in microbiology. Global Research Network: Kerala; 2000b. p. 29–35.

Teixeira MM, Patané JS, Taylor ML, Gómez BL, Theodoro RC, de Hoog S, Engelthaler DM, Zancopé-Oliveira RM, Felipe MS, Barker BM. Worldwide phylogenetic distributions and population dynamics of the genus *Histoplasma*. PLoS Negl Trop Dis. 2016;10(6):e0004732.

Ueda Y, Sano A, Tamura M, Inomata T, Kamei K, Yokoyama K, Kishi F, Ito J, Mikami Y, Miyaji M, Nishimura K. Diagnosis of histoplasmosis by detection of the internal transcribed spacer region of fungal rRNA gene from a paraffin-embedded skin sample from a dog in Japan. Vet Microbiol. 2003;94:219–24.

Wheat LJ, Kauffman CA. Histoplasmosis. Infect Dis Clin North Am. 2003;17:1–19.

Wheat LJ, Batteiger BJ, Sathapatayavongs B. *Histoplasma capsulatum* infections of the central nervous system: a clinical review. Medicine (Baltimore). 1990;69:244–60.

Wheat LJ, Musial CE, Jenny-Avital E. Diagnosis and management of central nervous system histoplasmosis. Clin Infect Dis. 2005;40:844–52.

Wheat LJ, Freifeld AG, Kleiman MB, Baddley JW, McKinsey DS, Loyd JE, Kauffman CA, Infectious Diseases Society of America. Clinical practice guidelines for the management of patients with histoplasmosis: 2007 update by the Infectious Diseases Society of America. Clin Infect Dis. 2007;45(7):807–25.

Zerbe CS, Holland SM. Disseminated histoplasmosis in persons with interferon-gamma receptor 1 deficiency. Clin Infect Dis. 2005;41:e38–41.

Cryptococcosis

12

Anita Mahadevan and Shankar Krishna Susarla

Abbreviations

AIDS	Acquired immunodeficiency syndrome
ART	Antiretroviral therapy
BBB	Blood-brain barrier
CM	Cryptococcal meningitis
CNS	Central nervous system
CSF	Cerebrospinal fluid
DC	Dendritic cell
EFA	Early fungicidal activity
HAART	Highly active antiretroviral therapy
GalXM	Galactoxylomannan
GXM	Glucuronoxylomannan
HIV	Human immunodeficiency virus
IL	Interleukin
INOS	Inducible nitric oxide synthase
IRD	Immune restoration disease
IRIS	Immune reconstitution inflammatory syndrome
MP	Mannoprotein
MRI	Magnetic resonance imaging
TNF	Tumor necrosis factor

A. Mahadevan (✉) · S. K. Susarla
Department of Neuropathology, National Institute of Mental Health and Neurosciences (NIMHANS), Bangalore, India

12.1 Introduction

A large number of fungi can cause meningitis in humans, which include yeasts (such as *Cryptococcus* and *Candida*), filamentous fungi (such as *Aspergillus* and *Zygomycetes*), dematiaceous molds (*Phaeohyphomycetes*), and dimorphic fungi (such as *Histoplasma* spp., *Coccidioides*, *Paracoccidioides*, and *Blastomyces*). They are uniformly fatal unless detected early, with institution of prompt and effective treatment. *Cryptococcus* is considered an opportunistic pathogen as it causes disease in the immunocompromised host. This so-called "sugar-coated" yeast is a unique model of eukaryotic virulence which has helped in understanding fungal pathogenesis, developing robust diagnostic tests, and standardizing treatment modalities.

12.2 Epidemiology

There have been three waves of epidemics in this infection. The first peak in incidence was in the mid-1980s with the advent of acquired immunodeficiency syndrome (AIDS). Cryptococcal meningitis (CM) was reported in 8% of patients with human immunodeficiency virus (HIV)/AIDS in the USA and as much as 40% of these patients in other parts of the world (Powderly 2000). A recent epidemiologic analysis projected that there are around one million cases of cryptococcal

M. Turgut et al. (eds.), *Fungal Infections of the Central Nervous System*,
https://doi.org/10.1007/978-3-030-06088-6_12

meningitis in AIDS patients each year that are responsible for over 600,000 annual deaths (Park et al. 2009).

In India, CM is reported as the most common opportunistic infection of the CNS in patients with HIV/AIDS (Wadia et al. 2001; Satishchandra et al. 2000). At our institute in south India, cryptococcal meningitis at autopsy was seen in 31.3% of cases (Shankar et al. 2005). Its overall incidence declined with the availability of highly active antiretroviral therapy (HAART), though cryptococcosis is responsible for 15–44% of deaths in HIV/AIDS patients in sub-Saharan Africa and remains one of the most common AIDS-defining illnesses in India, Brazil, and Thailand.

A second outbreak started with the increase in successful solid organ transplantation and the expanding armamentarium of immunosuppressive drugs for treatment of cancers and connective tissue diseases such as anti-tumor necrosis factor (TNF), anti-CD54 monoclonal, antibodies, etc. (Pyrgos et al. 2013). *C. neoformans* accounted for 10% of fungal infections in transplant recipients (Singh and Forrest 2009; Hosseini-Moghaddam and Husain 2010).

A third outbreak of infection with *C. gattii* occurred in Vancouver and Pacific Northwest islands (1999–2003) that has been attributed to the emergence of hypervirulent *C. gattii* strains due to climatic changes (Billmyre et al. 2014).

12.3 Mycology

The genus name of *Cryptococcus* was derived from the Greek words "kryptos" meaning hidden and "kokkos" meaning berry. It exists ubiquitously in the environment with worldwide distribution. It was first isolated from peach juice samples in 1894 (Sanfelice 1894). More than 50 species of the genus *Cryptococcus* exist, but only two are associated with human disease: *C. neoformans* and *C. gattii*. The polysaccharide capsule has antigenic determinants, based on which five serotypes are described: serotypes A, D, and AD (*C. neoformans*) and serotypes B and C (*C. gattii*) that are responsible for human infections.

Genomic analyses established that serotypes A and D are distinct strains, called *C. neoformans* var. *grubii* and *C. neoformans* var. *neoformans*, respectively. *C. neoformans* var. *grubii* (serotype A) is the most common causative agent of the central nervous system (CNS) disease in HIV/AIDS with high mortality and morbidity. The different strains have varying epidemiological features. In low-income countries, most cases of cryptococcosis are caused by serotype A (*C. neoformans* var. *grubii*), whereas, in the West, it is restricted to infections in HIV-positive patients only. In contrast, serotype D (*C. neoformans* var. *neoformans*) is a predominant strain found in Western Europe and is uncommon in the rest of the world. In our institute in south India, *Cryptococcus neoformans* was the common isolate in HIV-associated cryptococcosis. The majority of isolates from HIV-positive patients from India are serotype A var. *grubii* consistent with the serotype prevalent worldwide (Banerjee et al. 2004; Kwon-Chung and Bennett 1984) and a few reports of var. *gattii* (Chakrabarti et al. 1997; Banerjee et al. 2001).

C. gattii (serotypes B and C) causes 70–80% of cryptococcal infections among immunocompetent hosts restricted to tropical and subtropical areas. However, a recent outbreak (1999–2003), involving patients with apparently normal immune system, was reported in some areas of Canada and Northwest USA. The incidence of cryptococcal infection does not significantly differ in relation to age, race, or occupation (Kidd et al. 2004).

12.4 Ecologic Niches

There are environmental niches where *Cryptococcus* is most frequently isolated. The *C. neoformans* var. *neoformans* has a global distribution. It is mainly isolated from debris around pigeon roosts and soil contaminated with decaying pigeon or chicken droppings. The pigeons by themselves are not infected. *C. gattii* is isolated from several trees especially the *Eucalyptus* spp. and therefore more common in the tropics and subtropical regions (Kwon-Chung and Bennett 1984; Litvintseva et al. 2011).

In our institute, a study conducted by the department of Neuromicrobiology revealed that the predominant source of cryptococci in the environment in our geographical location was pigeon excreta (33%) followed by soil contaminated with pigeon/bird droppings (13%), while soil surrounding eucalyptus trees, the tree bark and leaves of eucalyptus tree was less common (Nagarathna et al., personal communication).

Predilection for these ecological niches is attributed to the requirement for certain compounds in the environment for its replication. The human fungal pathogen *Cryptococcus* can complete its sexual cycle during a pathogenic association with plants, as the inositol found in plants stimulates sexual reproduction in *Cryptococcus* species accounting for the predilection for growth in eucalyptus trees (Xue et al. 2007). Similarly sexual reproduction of *C. neoformans* occurs in media enriched with pigeon guano, accounting for its ecological niche in pigeon droppings (Nielsen et al. 2007).

The recent outbreak of *C. gattii* infection in immunocompetent individuals in Vancouver Island, Canada, and the Pacific Northwest suggests evolution of host range, geographic location, and virulence of this pathogen and its emergence as a travel-associated pathogen (Byrnes et al. 2009).

12.5 Pathogenesis

C. neoformans is an opportunistic pathogen as immunosuppressed individuals are more susceptible to infection. The fungal structure is responsible for establishing an infection and survival in the human host, while its virulence factors contribute to pathogenicity. However, the outcome of the infection is determined by the immune status of the host. The most devastating infections develop in patients with defective cell-mediated immunity, such as AIDS, solid organ transplantation, reticuloendothelial malignancy, corticosteroid treatment, long-term immunosuppressive therapy, advanced renal and liver diseases, rheumatological diseases, and sarcoidosis, but not in subjects with neutropenia or immunoglobulin deficiency (Buchanan and Murphy 1998). Paradoxically, treatment efforts to reverse the immunodeficiency, e.g., through antiretroviral therapy, worsen symptoms through an exuberant inflammatory response: the immune reconstitution inflammatory syndrome (IRIS).

There are three basic steps for fungi to successfully infect the brain—establish local infection, disseminate into the bloodstream, and cross the blood-brain barrier to reach the CNS.

12.5.1 Step 1: Local Infection

12.5.1.1 Host Factors

Basidiospores of cryptococci that are the result of sexual reproduction are the infectious forms of the yeast that reach the pulmonary alveoli following inhalation. Containment of the fungus within the lung requires cell-mediated, innate immunity, and antibody responses (Eisenman et al. 2007). The first line of defense is phagocytosis mediated by macrophages and complement (Feldmesser et al. 2001). Other factors include CD4+ and CD8+ T cells and cytokines including TNF-α, interferon (IFN)-γ, and interleukin (IL)-18 (Huffnagle and Lipscomb 1998). The first critical step for successful control of *C. neoformans* infection in the lung is polarization of CD4+ T cells toward T-helper 1 (Th1) phenotype by IFN-γ production and monocyte-derived dendritic cell (DC) recruitment (Drummond 2017). Th1 cells stimulate "classic activation" of macrophages (M1) and production of inducible nitric oxide synthase (iNOS) for fungal killing (Hole and Wormley 2016). Phagocytosis by alveolar macrophages is initiated by antibody and complement mediated (opsonin/non-opsonin dependent) interaction between epitopes on the cryptococcal polysaccharide capsule with the cell surface receptors—such as mannose, dectin-1, CD14, and Toll-like receptor 4 (Garcia-Rodas and Zaragoza 2012). Once phagocytosed, the phagosomes containing cryptococci fuse with lysosomes, and CD4+ T cells stimulate killing via IFN-γ and iNOS. CD4+ T-cell depletion as occurs in AIDS prevents killing of the cryptococci within macrophages, allowing it to survive and replicate.

12.5.1.2 Pathogen Factors

The protective host mechanisms are counteracted by *C. neoformans*' complex survival mechanisms (Coelho et al. 2014). The most well studied is its ability to block phagocytosis. This is achieved by various mechanisms: through blocking maturation of phagosomes, neutralizing acidification of the phagosome (Smith et al. 2015), or lysosome damage. The *C. neoformans* has evolved a non-lytic extrusion mechanism (termed vomocytosis) following phagocytosis which allows both the host and the parasite to survive. This is prevented by actin polymerization and extracellular signal regulated kinase (ERK)5 signaling in macrophages (Gilbert et al. 2017; Johnston and May 2010). Intracellular macrophage parasitism facilitates replication and dissemination to the CNS.

12.5.2 Step 2: Dissemination

12.5.2.1 Host Factors

If the macrophages fail to kill the yeasts by phagocytosis, they will serve as niche for fungal replication within phagosomes. The cryptococci are then released from the macrophage, either by host macrophages bursting or by extrusion without lysis (Ma et al. 2006; Alvarez and Casadevall 2006, 2007). Once in the bloodstream, host defense can rapidly clear the pathogen. An experimental inoculation into the bloodstream via tail vein of a mouse found that only 1–2% of yeasts survived after 30 min (Chang et al. 2004). The yeast can bypass the host defenses if immediately phagocytosed by another macrophage, thereby avoiding clearance. The macrophages can cross the blood brain barrier (BBB) to deliver the yeasts into the brain where replication causes meningoencephalitis.

12.5.2.2 Pathogen Factors: Virulence

Cryptococcus neoformans has several virulence factors, which include the polysaccharide capsule, soluble extracellular constituents (cryptococcal products), melanin and laccase production, mannitol production, and factors such as superoxide dismutase, proteases, phospholipase B, and lysophospholipase.

Ability to tolerate body temperature of 37 °C is the most essential feature of the fungus. Thermotolerance is linked to cell integrity and controlled by several signaling pathways—calcineurin pathway (Kraus et al. 2005) and the protein kinase C1-activated mitogen-activated protein (MAP) kinase pathway (Gerik et al. 2005). Importance of the calcineurin pathway for CNS invasion is exemplified by lack of CNS involvement in renal transplant recipients on tacrolimus therapy (Singh et al. 2007). Tacrolimus is a natural macrolide antifungal agent which is toxic to *C. neoformans* in vitro by inhibiting calcineurin at 37 °C, but not at 24 °C. Thus, temperature-dependent inhibition of tacrolimus prevents crossing the blood-brain barrier which may prevent CNS infection but allow the growth of fungus at cooler body sites like the skin, soft tissues, and bone. These patients are therefore more likely to have cutaneous, soft tissue, and osteoarticular rather than CNS infection.

12.5.3 Capsule

Unlike other pathogenic fungi, *Cryptococcus neoformans* is a yeast that does not exhibit filamentous growth or dimorphism, except during the mating process (Kozubowski and Heitman 2012). Although some pseudohyphal forms have occasionally been described during infection, this is a rare phenomenon (Gazzoni et al. 2010). The capsule of *C. neoformans* is its key virulence factor. Mutants lacking the capsule are typically avirulent (Chang and Kwon-Chung 1994). Capsule formation is induced in the presence of CO_2, phospholipids, and low-iron conditions (Granger et al. 1985; Chrisman et al. 2011; Jung et al. 2006).

The capsule is a complex polysaccharide that surrounds the cell body of the fungus. It has multiple functions. It protects the yeast in stress conditions, such as dehydration, free radicals, and antimicrobial compounds, and protects the fungus from phagocytosis (Zaragoza et al. 2008). It also exerts deleterious effects on the host immune response (Zaragoza et al. 2009). Capsular formation inhibits antibody (Ab) production, depletes complement, inhibits leukocyte migration, and induces apoptosis in macrophages and T cells (Lipovsky et al. 2000; Monari et al. 2006; Ellerbroek et al. 2002). The striking variations in capsule structure and size result in multiple phenotypic forms that differ in their recognition by the host immune system (Zaragoza 2011).

The three morphological and phenotypic variations include changes in capsule structure, size, and the total size of the cell, by the formation of cryptococcal giant/titan cells or microforms. These changes facilitate fungal survival, adaptation, escape from immune destruction and phagocytosis, dissemination, and long-term survival.

12.5.4 Capsule Size: Phenotypic Switching

Variation in capsule size can occur in different stages of the disease. Following first contact with the host, there is capsule enlargement ("early" response) to escape phagocytosis and ensure intracellular survival. The capsular rearrangements prevent recognition by immune cells. It also assists in systemic dissemination and crossing of the BBB. Production of micro-cells facilitates both dissemination and brain invasion. In later stages, there is formation of fungal giant/titan cells (a "late" response), a key factor that ensures long-term survival. In immunocompetent hosts, the infection is controlled, but the fungal cells are not completely cleared and go into a dormant/latent state (Dromer et al. 2007). The variation of *Cryptococcus* cell morphology as smooth, mucoid, or wrinkled form has been described (Guerrero and Fries 2008). The smooth *C. gattii* cells produced smaller capsules that were more efficient in crossing the BBB to cause CNS infection (Jain et al. 2006). The large number of different yeast forms also plays a role in the immune reconstitution inflammatory syndrome (IRIS) or immune restoration disease (IRD). This occurs in HIV patients who rapidly recover their immune system following the initiation of the HAART. An exaggerated inflammatory response is elicited, producing sudden worsening of symptoms and deterioration. IRIS is common following infection with *Mycobacterium tuberculosis* and *C. neoformans* (French 2009).

12.5.5 Capsule Structure

The major component of the cryptococcal polysaccharide capsule is the high molecular weight complex polysaccharide, glucuronoxylomannan (GXM), constituting 90–95% of the total mass (Cherniak et al. 1980). The remaining 5–10% is formed by galactoxylomannan (GalXM) (Cherniak et al. 1982). GXM has a chain of mannose residues, with substitutions of xylose and glucuronic acid, while GalXM has a chain of galactose with substitutions of xylose and mannose along with a small proportion of mannoproteins (MPs) (Levitz and Specht 2006). The GXM is distributed throughout the whole capsule, whereas GXMGal and MPs localize close to the cell wall (De Jesus et al. 2010).

The *C. neoformans* capsule is a double-edged sword. While on the one hand, it can protect the fungus from host defenses, on the other hand, it promotes effective clearance of the fungus from tissues. The capsule protects *C. neoformans* from phagocytosis and killing by neutrophils, monocytes, or macrophages (Kozel and Mastroianni 1976; Kozel and Gotschlich 1982; Vecchiarelli et al. 1994a). The capsule being strong negatively charged causes electrostatic repulsion of the negatively charged host effector cells, reducing cell-cell interactions required for clearance of the cryptococci (Nosanchuk and Casadevall 1997).

12.5.5.1 Role of Capsule in Promoting Host Defense: Immunosuppressive Effect

The capsules of serotype A and D isolates are chemotactic for neutrophils, and complement is fixed by cryptococcal capsules by the alternative pathway (Kozel and Pfrommer 1986). C3b and

C3bi once deposited on the surface of the cryptococci trigger phagocytosis by binding to CR3 receptors on leukocytes (Griffin 1981). The cryptococcal capsule can mask the C3b and C3bi deposits, thereby preventing complement-mediated killing (Kozel et al. 1984). The capsule can also prevent opsonization by antibodies to GXM, by blocking the Fc portion of the antibody (Kozel et al. 1988). The thicker the capsule, the greater is its protective capacity.

Encapsulated isolates effectively impair T-cell response (Collins and Bancroft 1991), especially the proliferative responses in T cells due to reduced secretion of interleukin-1 (IL-1) (Vecchiarelli et al. 1994b) and proinflammatory cytokines such as TNF-α, IL-1ß, and IL-6 by monocytes and macrophages (Delfino et al. 1996, 1997). The reduction in TNF-α in infections in turn prevents the induction of protective immunity, with disease progression.

Minimal host tissue responses are observed in patients with disseminated cryptococcosis. This is due to inhibition of leukocyte migration, by the capsular products GXM, GalXM, and MP (Dong and Murphy 1995). GXM stimulates neutrophils to shed L-selectin, necessary for initiating neutrophil migration into tissues (Dong and Murphy 1996). The levels of cryptococcal antigen in serum and CSF correlate with the severity of disease, response to therapy, and prognosis (Diamond and Bennett 1974). Denning et al. suggested that high cryptococcal antigen concentrations could change the osmolality of the CSF, affecting outflow and adsorption of CSF via the arachnoid villi and increasing intracranial pressure. The increased pressure may be responsible for the severe headaches, visual loss, and early death (Denning et al. 1991). The release of mannitol by *C. neoformans* contributes to increased intracranial pressure and restricting its use in reducing CSF pressure (Staib 1962).

A characteristic that differentiates pathogenic isolates from nonpathogenic isolates of *Cryptococcus* species is the organism's ability to form a brown to black pigment on a medium (such as birdseed or caffeic acid agar) containing diphenolic compounds. This melanin-like compound is produced by *C. neoformans* isolates with phenoloxidase activity (Shaw and Kapica 1972). Conversion of dihydroxyphenols such as 3,4-dihydroxyphenylalanine (DOPA) to dopaquinone is catalyzed by a phenoloxidase and is a rate-limiting step. *C. neoformans* lacks the tyrosinase enzyme required for endogenous production of dihydroxyphenol. Hence, to produce melanin, a *C. neoformans* isolate has to find diphenolic compounds from its growth environment and catalyze conversion of these compounds into melanin intermediates. The brain is rich in catecholamines such as DOPA and is a favorite target for infection by *C. neoformans*. However, the brain is not a preferred niche for growth as the organism cannot use catecholamines as a sole carbon source (Polacheck et al. 1990) but may serve as a place for the organisms to survive. Production of melanin from brain catecholamines protects the fungus from oxidative damage by scavenging free radicals. But melanized yeast cells are less susceptible to amphotericin B contributing to the difficulty to effectively treat infections in immunocompromised hosts (Wang and Casadevall 1994). Melanin also "cloaks" *C. neoformans* from recognition by host effector cells to mount a protective T-cell response (Huffnagle et al. 1995). Fortunately though, phenoloxidase activity in *C. neoformans* is greatly diminished at 37 °C body temperature; thereby, there is no melanin production in vivo (Jacobson and Emery 1991) as demonstrated with Fontana-Masson stains (Kwon-Chung et al. 1981). Laccase, a key enzyme in melanin biosynthesis, plays a role in virulence (Zhu and Williamson 2004).

Production of D-mannitol, a potent scavenger of hydroxyl radicals, may contribute to the survival of *C. neoformans* in the host as it protects from heat, osmotic stress, and damage by reactive oxygen intermediates (Wong et al. 1990). High concentrations of D-mannitol in the CNS may also contribute to brain edema. It is not known whether different isolates of *C. neoformans* vary in mannitol production.

Similarly, production of superoxide dismutase (SOD) by cryptococci, which is scavenger of free radicals, is increased at 37 °C which compensates for the decrease in melanin production (Jacobson et al. 1994).

Extracellular phospholipase activity produced by *C. neoformans* assists in invasion of host tissue by disrupting host cell membranes and allowing cryptococcal yeast forms to penetrate into host tissues (Chen et al. 1997).

Urease production by cryptococci contributes to dissemination to the central nervous system (CNS) (Olszewski et al. 2004). Real-time imaging microscopy demonstrated that urease does not affect the trapping of the yeast in the capillary but is important for transmigration of yeast cells. Release of ammonia by the product of urease causes local damage to endothelium, increasing permeability and promoting transmigration.

Fungal inositol transporters play an important role as virulence factor. The human brain contains abundant free inositol, at concentrations of 200-fold higher than plasma concentrations (Fisher et al. 2002). During brain infection, *Cryptococcus* utilizes inositol as a source of carbon for metabolism and replication (Healy et al. 1977). *Cryptococcus* has been detected within microglia in the CNS which have inositol (Lee et al. 1996a, b). An unusually large inositol transporter gene family with over ten members has been identified in *Cryptococcus*, having an important role in fungal virulence (Xue et al. 2007, 2010). Fungal inositol is important for crossing the BBB. Inositol sphingolipid synthesis and breakdown are important for the fungus to survive within activated macrophages (Luberto et al. 2001; Shea et al. 2006).

In summary, virulent isolates of *C. neoformans* must be able to produce small particles capable of entry into the alveolar spaces, multiply at 37 °C at a pH of 7.3–7.4, in an atmosphere of approximately 5% CO_2, must have an intact calcineurin pathway, and must be a PICT-mating type. The ability to produce a large capsule and shed great amounts of capsular material into the body fluids makes the organism highly virulent. Other factors, such as melanin, mannitol, superoxide dismutase, protease, and phospholipase production, enhance the pathogenicity of *C. neoformans*. The effectiveness of many of these cryptococcal virulence factors depends on the status of the host's defense mechanisms.

12.5.6 Step 3: CNS Infection—Crossing the BBB

Penetration of blood-brain barrier (BBB) is the key step to cause CNS infection.

Three major pathways can be used to cross the BBB—transcellular, paracellular, or the Trojan horse pathway. Evidence suggests that *C. neoformans* primarily uses the transcellular route (Chang et al. 2004; Sabiiti and May 2012; Liu et al. 2012; Jong et al. 2012). Real-time imaging in mice has demonstrated internalization of the fungus by the vascular endothelium from the luminal surface of blood vessels, its transmigration across the cytoplasm of endothelial cell, and exit on the abluminal side of the BBB into the brain (Shi et al. 2010). Findings of transmission and scanning electron microscopy demonstrate that *C. neoformans* induces reorganization of host cell actin cytoskeletal structures and microvilli-like protrusions to gain entry into the brain microvascular endothelial cells (Sabiiti and May 2012). Invasion occurs through the lipid rafts-endocytic pathway using the ganglioside GM1, CD44 cell surface glycoprotein, and intracellular kinase-DYRK3 (dual-specificity tyrosine phosphorylation-regulated kinase 3) (Jong et al. 2008; Huang et al. 2011). The fungal ligand hyaluronic acid directly interacts with CD44 from lipid rafts for adhesion and invasion of endothelial cells. Real-time imaging elegantly demonstrated that both yeast cells stop moving suddenly once they reach mouse brain capillaries of smaller diameter, and only viable cells cross the capillary wall (Shi et al. 2010).

The presence of cryptococci within macrophage-like cells within and outside the capillaries in infected brain sections from human and experimental mice demonstrates that *C. neoformans* was transported within phagocytes across the BBB via the "Trojan horse" pathway (Chretien et al. 2002; Santangelo et al. 2004; Charlier et al. 2009). Paracellular crossing of the BBB by injury to the brain endothelium and opening up of tight junctions can facilitate entry of *C. neoformans* into the CNS. This is facilitated by changes in capsule structure and secretion of proteases by the fungus (Charlier et al. 2005;

Xu et al. 2014). Occludin, marker of tight junctions, rapidly degrades altering integrity of endothelial tight junction.

The reason for the remarkable neurotropism for the CNS is not clear. Experimental model of systemic cryptococcosis that closely mimics human infection has provided valuable insights into the pathogenesis. *Cryptococcus* is a facultative intracellular pathogen. It survives within macrophages and replicates and escapes the hostile host environment (Feldmesser et al. 2000). Yeast cells escape from phagocytic cells by active phagosomal extrusion and invasion of other macrophages.

The capsular polysaccharide, mannitol, the mating type, melanin, phenotypic switching, phospholipase, prostaglandins, and urease are important for neurotropism and CNS invasion (Perfect and Casadevall 2002). Fungal cell morphology and capsule morphology are important in crossing the BBB. The giant/titan forms cannot be phagocytosed, preventing systemic dissemination as well as BBB invasion. The *Cryptococcus* cell morphology can be smooth, mucoid, or wrinkled. The smooth *C. gattii* cells are more efficient in crossing BBB due to their smaller capsules (Guerrero and Fries 2008; Jain et al. 2006).

Other cell surface and secreted proteins important for CNS invasion include extracellular phospholipase B (Feldmesser et al. 2000; Cox et al. 2001; Maruvada et al. 2012), urease (Olszewski et al. 2004), and laccase (Qiu et al. 2012). Ligand-receptor interaction between capsular hyaluronic acid and CD44 receptor promotes adhesion of vascular endothelium in the brain (Jong et al. 2008; Long et al. 2012). A proteomic approach examining the cryptococcal cell surface proteins identified an assortment of proteases and free radical-inducing proteins modulating CNS invasion (Long et al. 2012; Eigenheer et al. 2007). One of the key candidate proteins is a fungalysin metalloprotease belonging to the M36 peptidase class of proteases mediating host-fungus interaction that are unique to some fungi. The fungalysin class of metalloprotease in *A. fumigatus* breaks down elastin in the connective tissue of the lung and arteries (Markaryan et al. 1994). Steen et al. identified a similar metalloprotease in a rabbit model of cryptococcal meningitis (Steen et al. 2003). (Mpr1) in the extracellular proteome of *C. neoformans* (CnMpr1) also belonging to the same M36 class of fungalysins (Vu et al. 2014). *C. neoformans* lacking *MPR1* (*mpr1Δ*) failed to cross the BBB due to its failure to adhere to the brain endothelium.

12.6 Pathology

Infection is initiated by inhalation of the sexual form of yeast cells (measuring <4 μm dia meter) from the environment of *dust containing excreta of pigeons*. There is no human-to-human transmission.

The organism is a basidiomycete (*Filobasidiella neoformans*) that exists in two forms: the vegetative form, as a yeast measuring 2.5–10 μm dia meter, and the sexual form (basidiospores), measuring 1.8–3 μm in diameter. The basidiospores, which are the infectious form of *C. neoformans*, which is a desiccated form of the yeast, being smaller than 4 μm, can enter the pulmonary alveoli to establish pulmonary infection (Velagapudi et al. 2009).

12.7 Pulmonary Infection

The inhaled spores lodge with the alveolar spaces of the lung. *Cryptococcus* can colonize the respiratory tract. Once in the lungs, the yeast cells become rehydrated and acquire the characteristic polysaccharide capsule and convert to encapsulated blastoconidia (Fig. 12.1f). The encapsulated yeasts, by the antiphagocytic and immunosuppressive properties of the capsule, avoid phagocyte recognition and prevent leukocyte migration allowing fungal replication. In the presence of intact T-cell immunity, the primary pulmonary infection may be in dormant form or mimic influenza-like respiratory infection that resolves spontaneously. An epidemiological survey found that almost all adults in

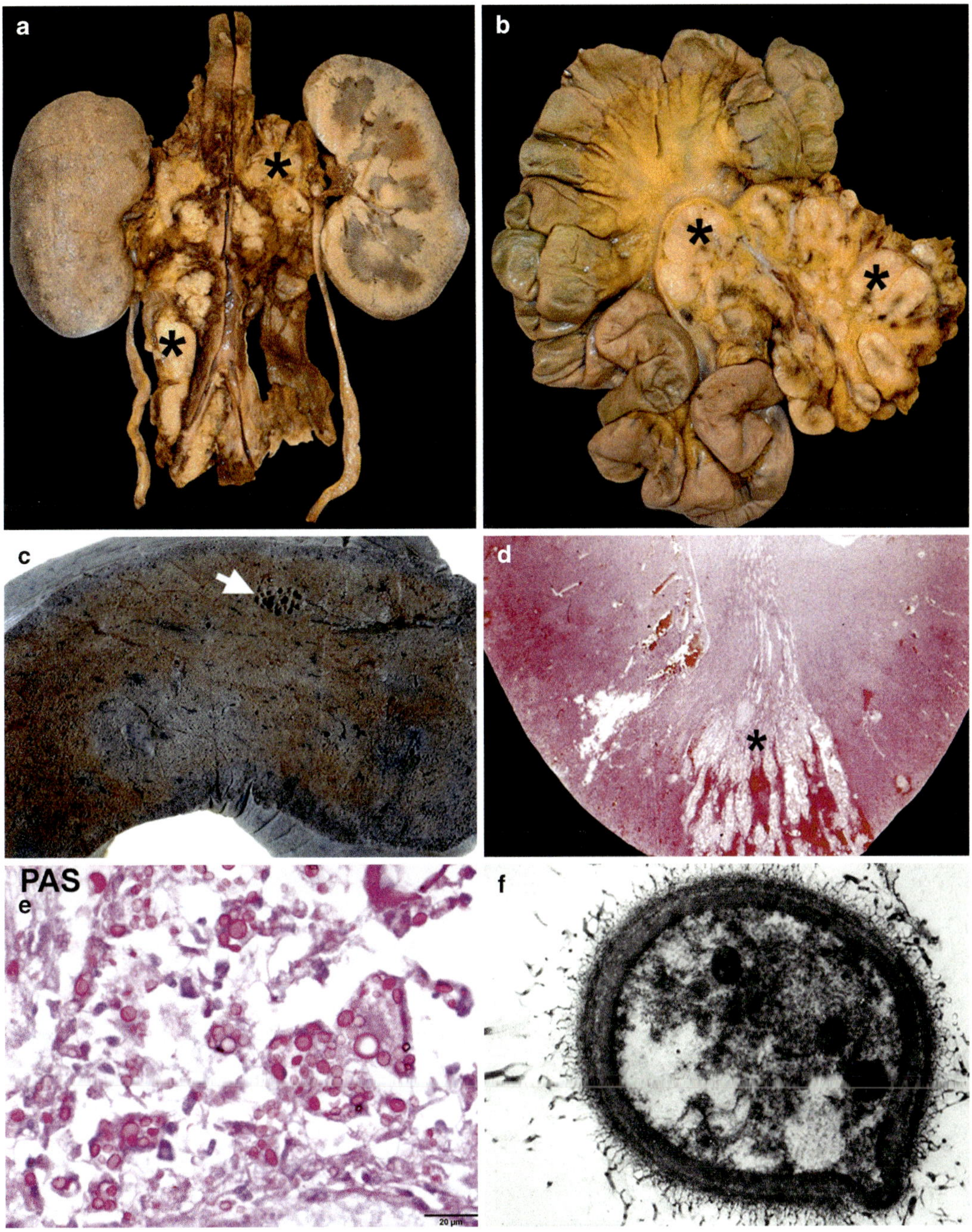

Fig. 12.1 Systemic involvement in disseminated cryptococcosis. (**a**) Para-aortic lymph nodes enlarged and infiltrated by cryptococci (*). Also note small cryptococcal nodules on subcapsular surface of the right kidneys resembling tubercles. (**b**) Cryptococcal lymphadenitis involving mesenteric nodes (*). (**c**) Pulmonary cryptococcal lesions seen as small honeycomb-like aggregates of cryptococci (*). (**d**) Photomicrograph from the kidney shows collections of cryptococci in the renal cortex, extending into the medulla along medullary rays (*). (**e**) Budding yeast forms of cryptococci highlighted on periodic acid-Schiff stain. (**f**) Electron micrograph demonstrating cryptococcal capsule and the intracellular organellar details (**d**: H&E stain ×Obj.10; **e**: PAS stain ×Obj.40; **f**: Uranyl acetate-lead citrate ×14,000)

New York have antibodies to *C. neoformans*, indicating exposure to this organism (Chen et al. 1999). When host T-cell-mediated IMMUNITY is impaired, the dormant form is reactivated and disseminates hematogenously to cause systemic infection, preferentially to the central nervous system, causing cryptococcal meningitis. Other common sites of dissemination include the kidneys, spleen, lymph nodes, skin, adrenals, bone, eye, and prostate gland (Fig. 12.1a–e). The inflammatory reaction is usually minimal or granulomatous.

Charlier et al. using a mouse model of disseminated meningoencephalitis delineated the sequential events following crossing of the blood-brain barrier (BBB). Mice sacrificed at 1, 6, 24, and 48 h post-intravenous inoculation revealed that crossing of the BBB occurred early following inoculation. This did not involve the choroid plexus but instead occurred at the level of the cortical capillaries, damaging the microvascular structures. Their findings in fact suggest that seeding of the leptomeninges is not the primary event. The cryptococci were trapped at the level of microvasculature within the brain, with rupture into the perivascular spaces and secondary extension into the subarachnoid space. There are alterations in cryptococcal capsule structure and cell size, induced by the structure of the local capillary network. The rapid changes in capsule structure help evade host immune response to control cryptococcal infection.

CNS cryptococcosis may present as encephalitis, meningitis, or cerebral space-occupying lesions. CNS involvement may occur several years after inhalation of infecting particles.

The brain on external examination has a characteristic glistening mucoid exudate with pooling of CSF in subarachnoid space (Fig. 12.2a). When subacute or chronic, accompanying hydrocephalus is seen due to chronic fibrosing leptomeningitis along the base.

Histologically, the subarachnoid space is widened by the cryptococci floating in pools of mucin, aggregating around the vessels. The inflammation is minimal with predominant foamy histiocytes, with ingested yeast forms (Fig. 12.2c). In less than 10% of cases, large mucoid intraparenchymal lesions in the basal ganglia can be seen produced by the expansion of Virchow-Robin spaces by gelatinous collections of cryptococci producing "pseudocystic lesions" or "soap bubble appearance" (Fig. 12.2d–f). These are most frequently seen in the thalamus and the gray white junction and less frequently in the brainstem, suggesting entrapment around the end arteries of the pial, lenticulostriate, and thalamostriate vessels corresponding to hypointense lesions on magnetic resonance imaging (MRI).

The CNS involvement differs between HIV-positive and HIV-negative patients. In AIDS patients, the brain shows numerous extracellular cryptococci without significant inflammatory cell response in subarachnoid (Fig. 12.2c, g–i] space with grossly visible pseudocystic parenchymal lesions in basal ganglia that are common (Fig. 12.2d–f). In HIV-positive patients, cryptococcal cell wall maybe pigmented due to melanin production. The immune depletion also allows the cryptococci to accumulate within the brain, predominantly extracellularly.

In immunocompetent hosts, a granulomatous inflammation containing yeast forms is usually seen. Lymphocytic infiltrates are of T cells (CD45RO+). The yeast forms are also fewer and predominantly intracellular phagocytosed within giant cells and macrophages confined to the subarachnoid space. Reactive astrocytosis is minimal. Cryptococomas with large granulomatous lesions having a honeycomb appearance due to aggregates of mucoid yeast forms of cryptococci may be seen. Granulomatous response is prominent with giant cells ingesting multiple cryptococci. Focal reactive astrocytosis has been documented (Tripathi et al. 2014). Vasculitis is uncommon unlike tuberculous pathology.

Special stains that highlight the cell wall of the fungus include periodic acid Schiff and Gomori methenamine silver stains, whereas the mucopolysaccharide-rich capsule is highlighted by mucicarmine stain (Fig. 12.2g–i). The polysaccharide capsular antigen is seen to spread into the interstitial space. In an experimental study in mice, Radhakrishnan et al. demonstrated that administration of hyaluronidase depolymerizes the capsular mucopolysaccharide eliciting a florid granulomatous response in the brain

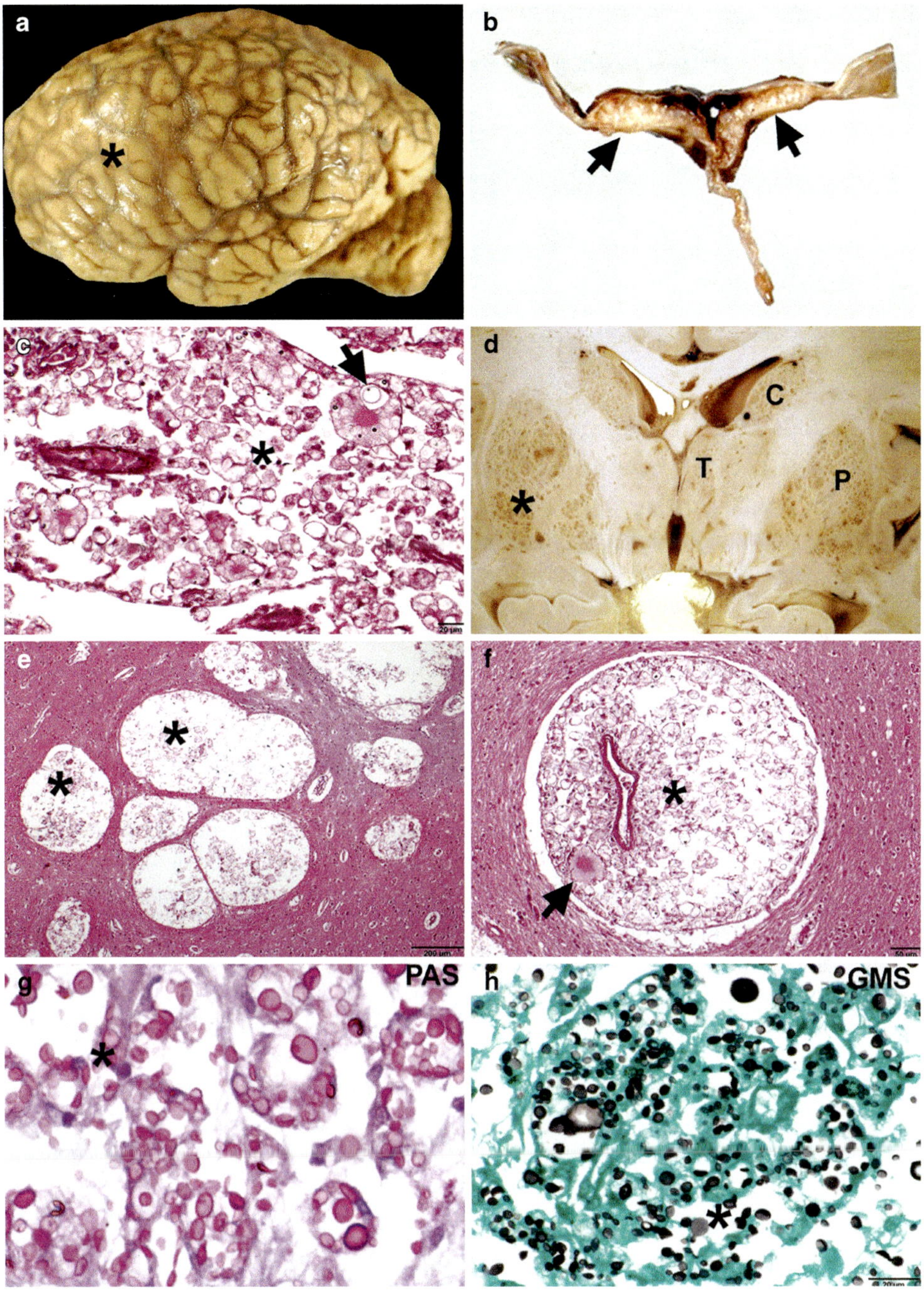

Fig. 12.2 Cryptococcal meningitis. Thick, glistening, gelatinous mucoid exudate seen along the superolateral convexity of the brain (**a**, *). The cryptococci are filling the arachnoidal granulations along the dural venous sinuses (**b**, arrows). On microscopy, numerous budding yeast forms are seen phagocytosed by macrophages and giant cells (arrows) in subarachnoid space (**c**). Multiple punched-out pseudocystic parenchymal lesions are seen in caudate (C), putamen (P), and thalamus producing a soap bubble appearance (**d**, *). These are seen on microscopy as expansion of Virchow-Robin spaces by collections of cryptococci (**e**, **f**, *). The cryptococcal cell wall and budding forms are highlighted by periodic acid-Schiff stain (**g**) and Gomori methenamine silver (**g**), while the mucopolysaccharide-rich capsule of *Cryptococcus* is highlighted on mucicarmine stains (**h**). Note the marked phenotypic variation in sizes and capsule thickness of the yeasts (**c**, **e**, **f**: H&E stain; **g**: PAS stain; **h**: Gomori methenamine silver stain; **i**: Mucicarmine stain. Magnification = scale bar)

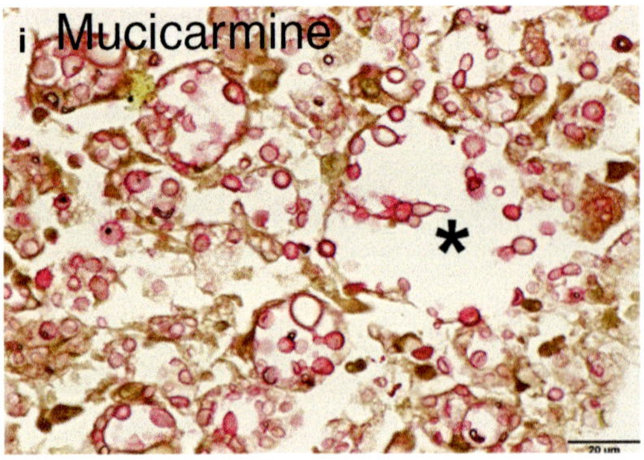

Fig. 12.2 (continued)

(Radhakrishnan et al. 1982). Severe headache and elevated intracranial pressure in the absence of cerebral edema are commonly reported in more than 50% cases of cryptococcal meningitis in association with HIV infection (Saag et al. 2000). Plugging of the dural venous sinuses and the arachnoid villi by the myxoid capsule-rich cryptococci was seen in our autopsy study (Saag et al. 2000) (Fig. 12.2b). The resultant obstruction to venous drainage causes impedance to CSF circulation and "dynamic hydrocephalic attacks" that remain undetectable on MRI. Lumbar drainage of large volumes of CSF produces dramatic relief of symptoms (Shankar et al. 2007). In HIV-associated cryptococcal meningitis, there is poor CSF inflammatory cell response, with pools of extracellular cryptococci yielding high positive culture of cryptococci from extraneural sites and systemic dissemination (Khanna et al. 1996). In this study that compared HIV-positive and HIV-negative cases, those with HIV had poorer CSF cell response, the mean CD4 count at presentation was 91 cells/μl, and the median survival after diagnosis was 22 months. Other poor prognostic factors identified were altered mental status, positive blood cultures, CSF antigen titer above 1:1024, positive CSF India ink, CSF white cell count below 20 cells/mm^3, and elevated CSF pressures.

Unlike tuberculous meningitis, the paucity of inflammation and vasculitis makes complications, such as cerebral infarction, rare. In HIV-negative cases, the incidence of cerebral infarction is approximately 4% (Tjia et al. 1985). Evidence of arteritis on angiography has been observed in a patient with cryptococcal meningitis. Immune-mediated vasospasm and hydrocephalus stretch the already compressed vessels in the parenchyma by the cryptococcal perivascular collections (Leite et al. 2004).

The damage-response framework (DRF) hypothesis of microbial pathogenesis which holds that host damage results from immune response to pathogen is also implicated in the pathological changes in cryptococcosis (Pirofski and Casadevall 2017). In fact, experimental inoculation in mice demonstrates that $CD4^+$ T-cell-mediated response initiated for fungal clearance is also a major contributor to tissue damage (Neal et al. 2017). The DRF classify most microbes into six pathogen classes. *C. neoformans* was first classified as a class 2 pathogen, which included "pathogens that cause damage either in hosts with weak immune responses or in the setting of normal immune responses" (Casadevall and Pirofski 1999). But the emergence of immune reconstitution inflammatory syndrome (IRIS)-associated cryptococcosis in patients with HIV/AIDS following initiation of antiretroviral therapy (ART) suggested that heightened immune response can contribute to the pathology of cryptococcosis. Thus, classification of *C. neoformans* as a class 2 pathogen needed to be revisited (Shankar et al. 2007).

12.8 Immune Reconstitution Inflammatory Syndrome (IRIS)

With the advent of HAART, the incidence of *C. neoformans* infection in HIV-infected patients has declined, and immunocompromised organ transplant recipients are at a higher risk. However, patients with immune reconstitution inflammatory syndrome (IRIS) can develop cryptococcal meningitis. These patients on commencing antiretroviral therapy either develop increased severity of an existing opportunistic infection ("paradoxical" IRIS) or present with a new opportunistic infection ("unmasking" IRIS). The pathology of IRIS is complex but revolves around ART-triggered recovery of the immune response in a previously immunosuppressed tissue environment with high microbial loads, and consequent potential immunopathology reflected by florid inflammatory response with predominant CD8+ T cells.

Cryptococcal IRIS occurs in 10–20% of HIV patients with median period of 4–9 weeks following ART initiation and presents with recurrence of signs and symptoms of meningitis (Jarvis et al. 2014). Risk factors for development of IRIS include low CSF cell counts (<5/μl), low levels of proinflammatory cytokines (IFN- γ, TNF- α, IL-6, and IL-8), and increase in chemokines in CSF (CCL2/MCP-1, CCL3/MIP-1α) (Boulware et al. 2010; Jarvis et al. 2015).

12.9 Prognostic Factors

High Th1 immune response reflected by high CSF levels of IFN-γ, TNF-α, and IL-6 are associated with low CSF fungal load, faster clearance on antifungal therapy, and good survival (Jarvis et al. 2014; Siddiqui et al. 2005). Flow cytometric studies have shown that the phenotype of CD4 T cells is more important in determining outcome, and not just the CD4 counts. Good survival was associated with higher counts of IFN-γ and TNF-α secreting CD4+ T cells.

Immune signature in non-survivors was low Th1 and higher Th2 cytokines—IL-10, IL-6, and CXCL10 in CSF, with neutrophilia. In addition, there was evidence of widespread systemic monocyte deactivation characterized by decreased HLA-DR expression (Siddiqui et al. 2005). This paralleled high plasma concentration of the capsular polysaccharide glucuronoxylomannan (GXM). GXM deactivates monocytes and T-cell responses (Retini et al. 1998).

High intracranial pressure (≥30 cm H_2O) was associated with fewer T cells, a higher fungal burden, and larger size of *Cryptococcus*. The absence of effective Th1 response produces a higher CSF fungal load at baseline due to monocyte deactivation, excessive CNS chemokine production, and slower fungal clearance on antifungal therapy, with increased CSF fungal load at the end of antifungal therapy. This high residual cryptococcal antigen load probably drives IRIS when CD4 counts rise due to antiretroviral therapy (ART).

Scriven et al. (Scriven et al. 2017) hypothesize that the shift in macrophage phenotype is driven directly by reduction in the HIV viral load and high CD206 expression. CD206 (mannose receptor) is a marker of "alternative activation" of macrophages, stimulated by T-helper 2 (Th2) CD4+ T cells producing IL-4 and IL-13. Dysregulation of Th2 responses leading to high levels of activated macrophages in the CSF may be the common pathogenetic pathway for paradoxical and unmasking cryptococcal IRIS.

Immunomodulation with steroid therapy increases the risk of a poor outcome as it is found to slow the clearance of *Cryptococcus* from CSF leading to higher mortality and morbidity (Beardsley et al. 2016). Augmentation with IFN-γ has demonstrated benefits in faster fungal clearance when coupled with effective antifungal therapy.

12.10 Diagnosis

Diagnostic tests employing detection of cryptococcal capsular polysaccharide in serum and CSF by latex agglutination or enzyme-linked immunosorbent assay (ELISA) have superseded the classic India ink test in CSF wherein the capsule is negatively stained by India ink (Fig. 12.3a). The antigen test has an overall sensitivity and specificity of 93–100% and 93–98%, respectively. The false-positive rate is less than 1% and is usually due to technical reasons (e.g., cross-reactivity with antigens from *Trichosporon* species). These tests can sometimes be positive prior to viable cryptococcal colonies in cultures. Culture remains the gold standard for confirmation of diagnosis producing characteristic creamy, smooth, mucoid colonies of *Cryptococcus* on Sabouraud dextrose agar medium. Caffeic acid agar medium will highlight black-colored colonies in case of pathogenic *Cryptococcus* strains (Fig. 12.3b, c).

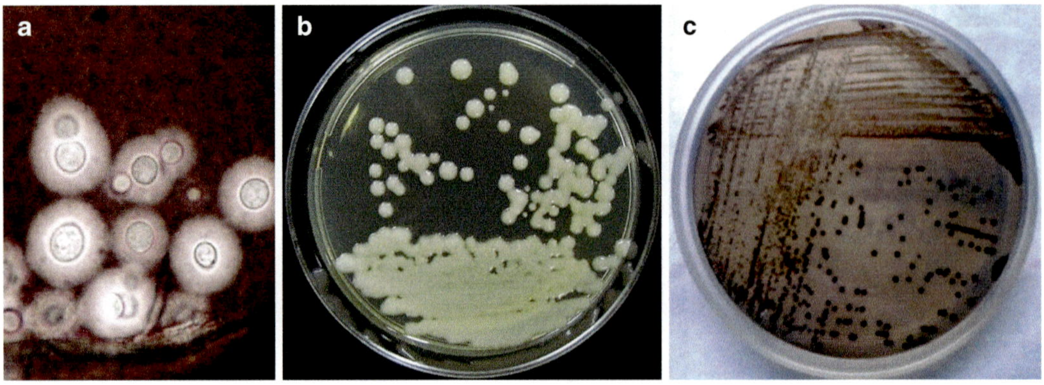

Fig. 12.3 Diagnostic tests. (**a**) India ink preparation in CSF highlights negatively stained cryptococci with thick capsules. (**b**) Characteristic creamy, smooth, mucoid colonies of *Cryptococcus* on Sabouraud dextrose agar medium. (**c**) Caffeic acid agar medium highlights black-colored colonies in case of pathogenic *Cryptococcus* strains. (Courtesy: Dr. Nagarathna Chandrashekar, Professor, Department of Neuromicrobiology, NIMHANS, Bangalore)

A lateral flow assay (LFA) has been recently introduced (Hansen et al. 2013). It is a semiquantitative test and has several advantages including rapid turnaround time, with potential bedside use or "point of care" and low cost, thereby making it useful in resource-restricted countries. It has excellent concordance with latex agglutination, ELISA, and cultures. It can even detect *C. gattii* infections not detected by the other serological tests. The tests also offer prognostic information. Baseline high titers of polysaccharide antigen in serum or CSF (>1:1024) reflect high fungal burden and poor prognosis (Khanna et al. 1996). High counts of viable yeasts in CSF are a predictor of death during systemic antifungal therapy (Jarvis et al. 2014). However, caution needs to be exercised in using polysaccharide antigen titers to make therapeutic decisions as elimination kinetics of the antigen in the host are not precise.

The viable quantitative CSF yeast count is useful for therapeutic monitoring as it is an index of the early fungicidal activity (EFA) with serial quantitative CSF yeast measurements during antifungal treatment (Day et al. 2013). This test however is still a research tool and is not yet available for routine clinical practice. Evaluation of EFA as a potential surrogate marker in cryptococcal meningitis is important in validation of novel anti-cryptococcal agents.

12.11 Treatment

The antifungal agents for treatment of cryptococcosis include amphotericin B (and its liposomal derivatives), 5-fluorocytosine (5FC), and fluconazole used singly or in combination. In cryptococcal meningitis, treatment is in three phases: an initial 2-week induction therapy with amphotericin B, followed by 8-week consolidation therapy and maintenance therapy with fluconazole, continued for 6–12 months and/or until restoration of host immunity (Perfect et al. 2010). Amphotericin B is fungicidal while fluconazole is fungistatic.

12.12 Conclusion

Human fungal diseases constitute a significant global health problem particularly in resource-poor countries. There is an urgent need for better diagnostic tools and a wider array of therapies to treat these dangerous infections. An enhanced understanding of the pathomechanisms of how fungi establish infections and the immune mechanisms operating for its elimination will enable us to develop the targeted therapy and improve outcome. Although immunopathogenic mechanisms of *Cryptococcus* species are the most studied, there remain many unanswered questions as to how these pathogens are controlled within the nervous system. Unravelling answers to these questions will provide new insights into organ-specific fungal pathogenesis and help develop effective treatment reducing morbidity and mortality.

References

Alvarez M, Casadevall A. Phagosome extrusion and host-cell survival after Cryptococcus neoformans phagocytosis by macrophages. Curr Biol. 2006;16:2161–5.

Alvarez M, Casadevall A. Cell-to-cell spread and massive vacuole formation after Cryptococcus neoformans infection of murine macrophages. BMC Immunol. 2007;8:16.

Banerjee U, Dutta K, Diwedi MSS. Cryptococcosis due to C. neoformans var. gattii: a short review and Indian clinical scenario. Nat J Infect Dis. 2001;2:32–6.

Banerjee U, Datta K, Casadevall A. Serotype distribution of Cryptococcus neoformans in patients in a tertiary care center in India. Med Mycol. 2004;42:181–6.

Beardsley J, Wolbers M, Kibengo FM, Ggayi A-BM, Kamali A, Cuc NTK, et al. Adjunctive dexamethasone in HIV-associated cryptococcal meningitis. N Engl J Med. 2016;374:542–54.

Billmyre RB, Croll D, Li W, Mieczkowski P, Carter DA, Cuomo CA, et al. Highly recombinant VGII Cryptococcus gattii population develops clonal outbreak clusters through both sexual macroevolution and asexual microevolution. MBio. 2014;5:e01494–14.

Boulware DR, Bonham SC, Meya DB, Wiesner DL, Park GS, Kambugu A, et al. Paucity of initial cerebrospinal fluid inflammation in cryptococcal meningitis is associated with subsequent immune reconstitution inflammatory syndrome. J Infect Dis. 2010;202:962–70.

Buchanan KL, Murphy JW. What makes Cryptococcus neoformans a pathogen? Emerg Infect Dis. 1998;4:71–83.

Byrnes EJ, et al. First reported case of Cryptococcus gattii in the Southeastern USA: implications for travel-associated acquisition of an emerging pathogen. PLoS One. 2009;4(6):e5851.

Casadevall A, Pirofski LA. Host-pathogen interactions: redefining the basic concepts of virulence and pathogenicity. Infect Immun. 1999;67:3703–13.

Chakrabarti A, Jatana M, Kumar P, Chatha L, Kaushal A, Padhye AA. Isolation of Cryptococcus neoformans var. gattii from Eucalyptus camaldulensis in India. J Clin Microbiol. 1997;35:3340–2.

Chang YC, Kwon-Chung KJ. Complementation of a capsule-deficient mutation of Cryptococcus neoformans restores its virulence. Mol Cell Biol. 1994;14:4912–9.

Chang YC, Stins MF, McCaffery MJ, Miller GF, Pare DR, Dam T, et al. Cryptococcal yeast cells invade the central nervous system via transcellular penetration of the blood-brain barrier. Infect Immun. 2004;72:4985–95.

Charlier C, Chretien F, Baudrimont M, Mordelet E, Lortholary O, Dromer F. Capsule structure changes associated with Cryptococcus neoformans crossing of the blood-brain barrier. Am J Pathol. 2005;166:421–32.

Charlier C, Nielsen K, Daou S, Brigitte M, Chretien F, Dromer F. Evidence of a role for monocytes in dissemination and brain invasion by Cryptococcus neoformans. Infect Immun. 2009;77:120–7.

Chen SC, Wright LC, Santangelo RT, Muller M, Moran VR, Kuchel PW, et al. Identification of extracellular phospholipase B, lysophospholipase, and acyltransferase produced by Cryptococcus neoformans. Infect Immun. 1997;65:405–11.

Chen LC, Goldman DL, Doering TL, Pirofski LA, Casadevall A. Antibody response to Cryptococcus neoformans proteins in rodents and humans. Infect Immun. 1999;67:2218–24.

Cherniak R, Reiss E, Slodki ME, Plattner RD, Blumer SO. Structure and antigenic activity of the capsular polysaccharide of Cryptococcus neoformans serotype A. Mol Immunol. 1980;17:1025–32.

Cherniak R, Reiss E, Turner SH. A galactoxylomannan antigen of Cryptococcus neoformans serotype A. Carbohydr Res. 1982;103:239–50. Available from: http://www.sciencedirect.com/science/article/pii/S0008621500806862

Chretien F, Lortholary O, Kansau I, Neuville S, Gray F, Dromer F. Pathogenesis of cerebral Cryptococcus neoformans infection after fungemia. J Infect Dis. 2002;186:522–30.

Chrisman CJ, Albuquerque P, Guimaraes AJ, Nieves E, Casadevall A. Phospholipids trigger Cryptococcus neoformans capsular enlargement during interactions with amoebae and macrophages. PLoS Pathog. 2011;7:e1002047.

Coelho C, Bocca AL, Casadevall A. The intracellular life of Cryptococcus neoformans. Annu Rev Pathol. 2014;9:219–38.

Collins HL, Bancroft GJ. Encapsulation of Cryptococcus neoformans impairs antigen-specific T-cell responses. Infect Immun. 1991;59:3883–8.

Cox GM, McDade HC, Chen SC, Tucker SC, Gottfredsson M, Wright LC, et al. Extracellular phospholipase activity is a virulence factor for Cryptococcus neoformans. Mol Microbiol. 2001;39:166–75.

Day JN, Chau TTH, Wolbers M, Mai PP, Dung NT, Mai NH, et al. Combination antifungal therapy for cryptococcal meningitis. N Engl J Med. 2013;368:1291–302.

De Jesus M, Nicola AM, Chow S-K, Lee IR, Nong S, Specht CA, et al. Glucuronoxylomannan, galactoxylomannan, and mannoprotein occupy spatially separate and discrete regions in the capsule of Cryptococcus neoformans. Virulence. 2010;1:500–8.

Delfino D, Cianci L, Migliardo M, Mancuso G, Cusumano V, Corradini C, et al. Tumor necrosis factor-inducing activities of Cryptococcus neoformans components. Infect Immun. 1996;64:5199–204.

Delfino D, Cianci L, Lupis E, Celeste A, Petrelli ML, Curro F, et al. Interleukin-6 production by human monocytes stimulated with Cryptococcus neoformans components. Infect Immun. 1997;65:2454–6.

Denning DW, Armstrong RW, Lewis BH, Stevens DA. Elevated cerebrospinal fluid pressures in patients with cryptococcal meningitis and acquired immunodeficiency syndrome. Am J Med. 1991;91:267–72.

Diamond RD, Bennett JE. Prognostic factors in cryptococcal meningitis. A study in 111 cases. Ann Intern Med. 1974;80:176–81.

Dong ZM, Murphy JW. Intravascular cryptococcal culture filtrate (CneF) and its major component, glucuronoxylomannan, are potent inhibitors of leukocyte accumulation. Infect Immun. 1995;63:770–8.

Dong ZM, Murphy JW. Cryptococcal polysaccharides induce L-selectin shedding and tumor necrosis factor receptor loss from the surface of human neutrophils. J Clin Invest. 1996;97:689–98.

Dromer F, Mathoulin-Pelissier S, Launay O, Lortholary O. Determinants of disease presentation and outcome during cryptococcosis: the CryptoA/D study. PLoS Med. 2007;4:e21.

Drummond RA. Neuro-immune mechanisms of anti-cryptococcal protection. J Fungi (Basel). 2017;4:4.

Eigenheer RA, Jin Lee Y, Blumwald E, Phinney BS, Gelli A. Extracellular glycosylphosphatidylinositol-anchored mannoproteins and proteases of Cryptococcus neoformans. FEMS Yeast Res. 2007;7:499–510.

Eisenman HC, Casadevall A, McClelland EE. New insights on the pathogenesis of invasive Cryptococcus neoformans infection. Curr Infect Dis Rep. 2007;9:457–64.

Ellerbroek PM, Hoepelman AIM, Wolbers F, Zwaginga JJ, Coenjaerts FEJ. Cryptococcal glucuronoxylomannan inhibits adhesion of neutrophils to stimulated endothelium in vitro by affecting both neutrophils and endothelial cells. Infect Immun. 2002;70:4762–71.

Feldmesser M, Kress Y, Novikoff P, Casadevall A. Cryptococcus neoformans is a facultative intracellular pathogen in murine pulmonary infection. Infect Immun. 2000;68:4225–37.

Feldmesser M, Kress Y, Casadevall A. Intracellular crystal formation as a mechanism of cytotoxicity in murine pulmonary Cryptococcus neoformans infection. Infect Immun. 2001;69:2723–7.

Fisher SK, Novak JE, Agranoff BW. Inositol and higher inositol phosphates in neural tissues: homeostasis, metabolism and functional significance. J Neurochem. 2002;82:736–54.

French MA. HIV/AIDS: immune reconstitution inflammatory syndrome: a reappraisal. Clin Infect Dis. 2009;48:101–7.

Garcia-Rodas R, Zaragoza O. Catch me if you can: phagocytosis and killing avoidance by Cryptococcus neoformans. FEMS Immunol Med Microbiol. 2012;64:147–61.

Gazzoni AF, Oliveira F d M, Salles EF, Mayayo E, Guarro J, Capilla J, et al. Unusual morphologies of Cryptococcus spp. in tissue specimens: report of 10 cases. Rev Inst Med Trop Sao Paulo. 2010;52:145–9.

Gerik KJ, Donlin MJ, Soto CE, Banks AM, Banks IR, Maligie MA, et al. Cell wall integrity is dependent on the PKC1 signal transduction pathway in Cryptococcus neoformans. Mol Microbiol. 2005;58:393–408.

Gilbert AS, Seoane PI, Sephton-Clark P, Bojarczuk A, Hotham R, Giurisato E, et al. Vomocytosis of live pathogens from macrophages is regulated by the atypical MAP kinase ERK5. Sci Adv. 2017;3:e1700898.

Granger DL, Perfect JR, Durack DT. Virulence of Cryptococcus neoformans. Regulation of capsule synthesis by carbon dioxide. J Clin Invest. 1985;76:508–16.

Griffin FMJ. Roles of macrophage Fc and C3b receptors in phagocytosis of immunologically coated Cryptococcus neoformans. Proc Natl Acad Sci U S A. 1981;78:3853–7.

Guerrero A, Fries BC. Phenotypic switching in Cryptococcus neoformans contributes to virulence by changing the immunological host response. Infect Immun. 2008;76:4322–31.

Hansen J, Slechta ES, Gates-Hollingsworth MA, Neary B, Barker AP, Bauman S, et al. Large-scale evaluation of the immuno-mycologics lateral flow and enzyme-linked immunoassays for detection of cryptococcal antigen in serum and cerebrospinal fluid. Clin Vaccine Immunol. 2013;20:52–5.

Healy ME, Dillavou CL, Taylor GE. Diagnostic medium containing inositol, urea, and caffeic acid for selective growth of Cryptococcus neoformans. J Clin Microbiol. 1977;6:387–91.

Hole C, Wormley FLJ. Innate host defenses against Cryptococcus neoformans. J Microbiol. 2016;54:202–11.

Hosseini-Moghaddam SM, Husain S. Fungi and molds following lung transplantation. Semin Respir Crit Care Med. 2010;31:222–33.

Huang S-H, Long M, Wu C-H, Kwon-Chung KJ, Chang YC, Chi F, et al. Invasion of Cryptococcus neoformans into human brain microvascular endothelial cells is mediated through the lipid rafts-endocytic pathway via the dual specificity tyrosine phosphorylation-regulated kinase 3 (DYRK3). J Biol Chem. 2011;286:34761–9.

Huffnagle GB, Lipscomb MF. Cells and cytokines in pulmonary cryptococcosis. Res Immunol. 1998;149:387–96. Available from: http://www.sciencedirect.com/science/article/pii/S0923249498807621

Huffnagle GB, Chen GH, Curtis JL, McDonald RA, Strieter RM, Toews GB. Down-regulation of the afferent phase of T cell-mediated pulmonary inflammation and immunity by a high melanin-producing strain of Cryptococcus neoformans. J Immunol. 1995;155:3507–16.

Jacobson ES, Emery HS. Temperature regulation of the cryptococcal phenoloxidase. J Med Vet Mycol. 1991;29:121–4.

Jacobson ES, Jenkins ND, Todd JM. Relationship between superoxide dismutase and melanin in a pathogenic fungus. Infect Immun. 1994;62:4085–6.

Jain N, Guerrero A, Fries BC. Phenotypic switching and its implications for the pathogenesis of Cryptococcus neoformans. FEMS Yeast Res. 2006;6:480–8.

Jarvis JN, Bicanic T, Loyse A, Namarika D, Jackson A, Nussbaum JC, et al. Determinants of mortality in a combined cohort of 501 patients with HIV-associated Cryptococcal meningitis: implications for improving outcomes. Clin Infect Dis. 2014;58:736–45.

Jarvis JN, Meintjes G, Bicanic T, Buffa V, Hogan L, Mo S, et al. Cerebrospinal fluid cytokine profiles predict risk of early mortality and immune reconstitution inflammatory syndrome in HIV-associated cryptococcal meningitis. PLoS Pathog. 2015;11:e1004754.

Johnston SA, May RC. The human fungal pathogen Cryptococcus neoformans escapes macrophages by a phagosome emptying mechanism that is inhibited by Arp2/3 complex-mediated actin polymerisation. PLoS Pathog. 2010;6:e1001041.

Jong A, Wu C-H, Shackleford GM, Kwon-Chung KJ, Chang YC, Chen H-M, et al. Involvement of human CD44 during Cryptococcus neoformans infection of brain microvascular endothelial cells. Cell Microbiol. 2008;10:1313–26.

Jong A, Wu C-H, Gonzales-Gomez I, Kwon-Chung KJ, Chang YC, Tseng H-K, et al. Hyaluronic acid receptor CD44 deficiency is associated with decreased Cryptococcus neoformans brain infection. J Biol Chem. 2012;287:15298–306.

Jung WH, Sham A, White R, Kronstad JW. Iron regulation of the major virulence factors in the AIDS-associated pathogen Cryptococcus neoformans. PLoS Biol. 2006;4:e410.

Khanna N, Chandramuki A, Desai A, Ravi V. Cryptococcal infections of the central nervous system: an analysis of predisposing factors, laboratory findings and outcome in patients from South India with special reference to HIV infection. J Med Microbiol. 1996;45:376–9.

Kidd SE, Hagen F, Tscharke RL, Huynh M, Bartlett KH, Fyfe M, et al. A rare genotype of Cryptococcus gattii caused the cryptococcosis outbreak on Vancouver Island (British Columbia, Canada). Proc Natl Acad Sci U S A. 2004;101:17258–63.

Kozel TR, Gotschlich EC. The capsule of Cryptococcus neoformans passively inhibits phagocytosis of the yeast by macrophages. J Immunol. 1982;129:1675–80.

Kozel TR, Mastroianni RP. Inhibition of phagocytosis by cryptococcal polysaccharide: dissociation of the attachment and ingestion phases of phagocytosis. Infect Immun. 1976;14:62–7.

Kozel TR, Pfrommer GS. Activation of the complement system by Cryptococcus neoformans leads to binding of iC3b to the yeast. Infect Immun. 1986;52:1–5.

Kozel TR, Highison B, Stratton CJ. Localization on encapsulated Cryptococcus neoformans of serum components opsonic for phagocytosis by macrophages and neutrophils. Infect Immun. 1984;43:574–9.

Kozel TR, Pfrommer GS, Guerlain AS, Highison BA, Highison GJ. Role of the capsule in phagocytosis of Cryptococcus neoformans. Rev Infect Dis. 1988;10(Suppl 2):S436–9.

Kozubowski L, Heitman J. Profiling a killer, the development of Cryptococcus neoformans. FEMS Microbiol Rev. 2012;36:78–94.

Kraus PR, Nichols CB, Heitman J. Calcium- and calcineurin-independent roles for calmodulin in Cryptococcus neoformans morphogenesis and high-temperature growth. Eukaryot Cell. 2005;4:1079–87.

Kwon-Chung KJ, Bennett JE. Epidemiologic differences between the two varieties of Cryptococcus neoformans. Am J Epidemiol. 1984;120:123–30.

Kwon-Chung KJ, Hill WB, Bennett JE. New, special stain for histopathological diagnosis of cryptococcosis. J Clin Microbiol. 1981;13:383–7.

Lee SC, Dickson DW, Casadevall A. Pathology of cryptococcal meningoencephalitis: analysis of 27 patients with pathogenetic implications. Hum Pathol. 1996a;27:839–47.

Lee SC, Casadevall A, Dickson DW. Immunohistochemical localization of capsular polysaccharide antigen in the central nervous system cells in cryptococcal meningoencephalitis. Am J Pathol. 1996b;148:1267–74.

Leite AGB, Vidal JE, Bonasser Filho F, Nogueira RS, de Oliveira ACP. Cerebral infarction related to cryptococcal meningitis in an HIV-infected patient: case report and literature review. Braz J Infect Dis. 2004;8:175–9.

Levitz SM, Specht CA. The molecular basis for the immunogenicity of Cryptococcus neoformans mannoproteins. FEMS Yeast Res. 2006;6:513–24.

Lipovsky MM, Tsenova L, Coenjaerts FE, Kaplan G, Cherniak R, Hoepelman AI. Cryptococcal glucuronoxylomannan delays translocation of leukocytes across the blood-brain barrier in an animal model of acute bacterial meningitis. J Neuroimmunol. 2000;111:10–4.

Litvintseva AP, Xu J, Mitchell TG. Population structure and ecology of Cryptococcus neoformans and Cryptococcus gattii. In: Cryptococcus. Washington, DC: American Society of Microbiology; 2011. p. 97–111. https://doi.org/10.1128/9781555816858.ch08.

Liu T-B, Perlin DS, Xue C. Molecular mechanisms of cryptococcal meningitis. Virulence. 2012;3:173–81.

Long M, Huang S-H, Wu C-H, Shackleford GM, Jong A. Lipid raft/caveolae signaling is required for Cryptococcus neoformans invasion into human brain microvascular endothelial cells. J Biomed Sci. 2012;19:19.

Luberto C, Toffaletti DL, Wills EA, Tucker SC, Casadevall A, Perfect JR, et al. Roles for inositol-phosphoryl ceramide synthase 1 (IPC1) in pathogenesis of C. neoformans. Genes Dev. 2001;15:201–12.

Ma H, Croudace JE, Lammas DA, May RC. Expulsion of live pathogenic yeast by macrophages. Curr Biol. 2006;16:2156–60.

Markaryan A, Morozova I, Yu H, Kolattukudy PE. Purification and characterization of an elastinolytic metalloprotease from Aspergillus fumigatus and immunoelectron microscopic evidence of secretion of this enzyme by the fungus invading the murine lung. Infect Immun. 1994;62:2149–57.

Maruvada R, Zhu L, Pearce D, Zheng Y, Perfect J, Kwon-Chung KJ, et al. Cryptococcus neoformans phospholipase B1 activates host cell Rac1 for traversal across the blood-brain barrier. Cell Microbiol. 2012;14:1544–53.

Monari C, Bistoni F, Vecchiarelli A. Glucuronoxylomannan exhibits potent immunosuppressive properties. FEMS Yeast Res. 2006;6:537–42.

Neal LM, Xing E, Xu J, Kolbe JL, Osterholzer JJ, Segal BM, et al. CD4(+) T cells orchestrate lethal immune pathology despite fungal clearance during Cryptococcus neoformans meningoencephalitis. MBio. 2017;8 https://doi.org/10.1128/mBio.01415-17.

Nielsen K, De Obaldia AL, Heitman J. Cryptococcus neoformans mates on pigeon guano: implications for the realized ecological niche and globalization. Eukaryot Cell. 2007;6:949–59.

Nosanchuk JD, Casadevall A. Cellular charge of Cryptococcus neoformans: contributions from the capsular polysaccharide, melanin, and monoclonal antibody binding. Infect Immun. 1997;65:1836–41.

Olszewski MA, Noverr MC, Chen G-H, Toews GB, Cox GM, Perfect JR, et al. Urease expression by Cryptococcus neoformans promotes microvascular sequestration, thereby enhancing central nervous system invasion. Am J Pathol. 2004;164:1761–71.

Park BJ, Wannemuehler KA, Marston BJ, Govender N, Pappas PG, Chiller TM. Estimation of the current global burden of cryptococcal meningitis among persons living with HIV/AIDS. AIDS. 2009;23: 525–30.

Perfect JR, Casadevall A. Cryptococcosis. Infect Dis Clin N Am. 2002;16:837–74. v–vi

Perfect JR, Dismukes WE, Dromer F, Goldman DL, Graybill JR, Hamill RJ, et al. Clinical practice guidelines for the management of cryptococcal disease: 2010 update by the Infectious Diseases Society of America. Clin Infect Dis. 2010;50:291–322.

Pirofski LA, Casadevall A. Immune-mediated damage completes the parabola: Cryptococcus neoformans pathogenesis can reflect the outcome of a weak or strong immune response. MBio. 2017;8:6–10.

Polacheck I, Platt Y, Aronovitch J. Catecholamines and virulence of Cryptococcus neoformans. Infect Immun. 1990;58:2919–22.

Powderly WG. Cryptococcal meningitis in HIV-infected patients. Curr Infect Dis Rep. 2000;2:352–7.

Pyrgos V, Seitz AE, Steiner CA, Prevots DR, Williamson PR. Epidemiology of cryptococcal meningitis in the US: 1997–2009. PLoS One. 2013;8:e56269.

Qiu Y, Davis MJ, Dayrit JK, Hadd Z, Meister DL, Osterholzer JJ, et al. Immune modulation mediated by cryptococcal laccase promotes pulmonary growth and brain dissemination of virulent Cryptococcus neoformans in mice. PLoS One. 2012;7:e47853.

Radhakrishnan VV, Mathai A, Shanmugham J, Mathews GJ. The role of hyaluronidase in experimental cryptococcal infections. Surg Neurol. 1982;17:239–44.

Retini C, Vecchiarelli A, Monari C, Bistoni F, Kozel TR. Encapsulation of Cryptococcus neoformans with glucuronoxylomannan inhibits the antigen-presenting capacity of monocytes. Infect Immun. 1998;66:664–9.

Saag MS, Graybill RJ, Larsen RA, Pappas PG, Perfect JR, Powderly WG, et al. Practice guidelines for the management of cryptococcal disease. Infectious Diseases Society of America. Clin Infect Dis. 2000;30:710–8.

Sabiiti W, May RC. Capsule independent uptake of the fungal pathogen Cryptococcus neoformans into brain microvascular endothelial cells. PLoS One. 2012;7:e35455.

Sanfelice F. Contributo alla morfologia e biologia dei blastomiceti che si sviluppano nei succhi di alcuni frutti. Ann Ig. 1894;4:463–95.

Santangelo R, Zoellner H, Sorrell T, Wilson C, Donald C, Djordjevic J, et al. Role of extracellular phospholipases and mononuclear phagocytes in dissemination of cryptococcosis in a murine model. Infect Immun. 2004;72:2229–39.

Satishchandra P, Nalini A, Gourie-Devi M, Khanna N, Santosh V, Ravi V, et al. Profile of neurologic disorders associated with HIV/AIDS from Bangalore, south India (1989–96). Indian J Med Res. 2000;111:14–23.

Scriven JE, Graham LM, Schutz C, Scriba TJ, Wilkinson KA, Wilkinson RJ, et al. The CSF immune response in HIV-1-associated cryptococcal meningitis: macrophage activation, correlates of disease severity, and effect of antiretroviral therapy. J Acquir Immune Defic Syndr. 2017;75:299–307.

Shankar SK, Mahadevan A, Satishchandra P, Kumar RU, Yasha TC, Santosh V, et al. Neuropathology of HIV/AIDS with an overview of the Indian scene. Indian J Med Res. 2005;121:468–88.

Shankar SK, Mahadevan A, Sundaram C, Sarkar C, Chacko G, Lanjewar DN, et al. Pathobiology of fungal infections of the central nervous system with special reference to the Indian scenario. Neurol India. 2007;55:198–215.

Shaw CE, Kapica L. Production of diagnostic pigment by phenoloxidase activity of Cryptococcus neoformans. Appl Microbiol. 1972;24:824–30.

Shea JM, Kechichian TB, Luberto C, Del Poeta M. The cryptococcal enzyme inositol phosphosphingolipid-phospholipase C confers resistance to the antifungal effects of macrophages and promotes fungal dissemination to the central nervous system. Infect Immun. 2006;74:5977–88.

Shi M, Li SS, Zheng C, Jones GJ, Kim KS, Zhou H, et al. Real-time imaging of trapping and urease-dependent transmigration of Cryptococcus neoformans in mouse brain. J Clin Invest. 2010;120:1683–93.

Siddiqui AA, Brouwer AE, Wuthiekanun V, Jaffar S, Shattock R, Irving D, et al. IFN-gamma at the site of infection determines rate of clearance of infection in cryptococcal meningitis. J Immunol. 2005;174:1746–50.

Singh N, Forrest G. Cryptococcosis in solid organ transplant recipients. Am J Transplant. 2009;9(Suppl 4):S192–8.

Singh N, Alexander BD, Lortholary O, Dromer F, Gupta KL, John GT, et al. Cryptococcus neoformans in organ

transplant recipients: impact of calcineurin-inhibitor agents on mortality. J Infect Dis. 2007;195:756–64.
Smith LM, Dixon EF, May RC. The fungal pathogen Cryptococcus neoformans manipulates macrophage phagosome maturation. Cell Microbiol. 2015;17:702–13.
Staib F. Cryptococcus neoformans and Guizotia abyssinica (syn. G. oleifera D.C.). (Colour reaction for Cr. neoformans.). Zeitschrift Hyg Infekt. 1962;148:466–75.
Steen BR, Zuyderduyn S, Toffaletti DL, Marra M, Jones SJM, Perfect JR, et al. Cryptococcus neoformans gene expression during experimental cryptococcal meningitis. Eukaryot Cell. 2003;2:1336–49.
Tjia TL, Yeow YK, Tan CB. Cryptococcal meningitis. J Neurol Neurosurg Psychiatry. 1985;48:853–8.
Tripathi S, Patro I, Mahadevan A, Patro N, Phillip M, Shankar SK. Glial alterations in tuberculous and cryptococcal meningitis and their relation to HIV co-infection—a study on human brains. J Infect Dev Ctries. 2014;8:1421–43.
Vecchiarelli A, Pietrella D, Dottorini M, Monari C, Retini C, Todisco T, et al. Encapsulation of Cryptococcus neoformans regulates fungicidal activity and the antigen presentation process in human alveolar macrophages. Clin Exp Immunol. 1994a;98:217–23.
Vecchiarelli A, Dottorini M, Pietrella D, Monari C, Retini C, Todisco T, et al. Role of human alveolar macrophages as antigen-presenting cells in Cryptococcus neoformans infection. Am J Respir Cell Mol Biol. 1994b;11:130–7.
Velagapudi R, Hsueh Y-P, Geunes-Boyer S, Wright JR, Heitman J. Spores as infectious propagules of Cryptococcus neoformans. Infect Immun. 2009;77:4345–55.
Vu K, Tham R, Uhrig JP, Thompson GR 3rd, Na Pombejra S, Jamklang M, et al. Invasion of the central nervous system by Cryptococcus neoformans requires a secreted fungal metalloprotease. MBio. 2014;5:e01101–14.
Wadia RS, Pujari SN, Kothari S, Udhar M, Kulkarni S, Bhagat S, et al. Neurological manifestations of HIV disease. J Assoc Physicians India. 2001;49:343–8.
Wang Y, Casadevall A. Growth of Cryptococcus neoformans in presence of L-dopa decreases its susceptibility to amphotericin B. Antimicrob Agents Chemother. 1994;38:2648–50.
Wong B, Perfect JR, Beggs S, Wright KA. Production of the hexitol D-mannitol by Cryptococcus neoformans in vitro and in rabbits with experimental meningitis. Infect Immun. 1990;58:1664–70.
Xu C-Y, Zhu H-M, Wu J-H, Wen H, Liu C-J. Increased permeability of blood-brain barrier is mediated by serine protease during Cryptococcus meningitis. J Int Med Res. 2014;42:85–92.
Xue C, Tada Y, Dong X, Heitman J. The human fungal pathogen Cryptococcus can complete its sexual cycle during a pathogenic association with plants. Cell Host Microbe. 2007;1:263–73.
Xue C, Liu T, Chen L, Li W, Liu I, Kronstad JW, et al. Role of an expanded inositol transporter repertoire in Cryptococcus neoformans sexual reproduction and virulence. MBio. 2010;1:e00084–10.
Zaragoza O. Multiple disguises for the same party: the concepts of morphogenesis and phenotypic variations in Cryptococcus neoformans. Front Microbiol. 2011;2:181.
Zaragoza O, Chrisman CJ, Castelli MV, Frases S, Cuenca-Estrella M, Rodriguez-Tudela JL, et al. Capsule enlargement in Cryptococcus neoformans confers resistance to oxidative stress suggesting a mechanism for intracellular survival. Cell Microbiol. 2008;10:2043–57.
Zaragoza O, Rodrigues ML, De Jesus M, Frases S, Dadachova E, Casadevall A. The capsule of the fungal pathogen Cryptococcus neoformans. Adv Appl Microbiol. 2009;68:133–216.
Zhu X, Williamson PR. Role of laccase in the biology and virulence of Cryptococcus neoformans. FEMS Yeast Res. 2004;5:1–10.

Blastomycosis and Phaeohyphomycosis

13

María Guadalupe Frías-De-León, Erick Martínez-Herrera, María del Rocío Reyes-Montes, and Gustavo Acosta-Altamirano

Abbreviations

AIDS	Acquired immune deficiency syndrome
CNS	Central nervous system
CSF	Cerebrospinal fluid
GMS	Gomori methenamine silver
HE	Hematoxylin-eosin
HIV	Human immunodeficiency virus
PAS	Periodic acid-Schiff
PCR	Polymerase chain reaction
PMN	Polymorphonuclear
USA	United States of America

13.1 Blastomycosis

13.1.1 Introduction

Blastomycosis is a systemic fungal infection, endemic from the center of the United States of America (USA) and south from Canada, which affects humans and animals, mainly dogs, and is caused by a fungus dimorphic with two species defined: *Blastomyces dermatitidis* and *B. gilchristii* (Bentley et al. 2013; Brown et al. 2013; Gilchrist 1894). The ecological niche of these fungi is the floor of the moist forested areas, where fungi grow in the mycelial form (septate hyphae and ovoid conidia) (21 °C), but is converted to the yeast phase at body temperature or in the laboratory to 32–35 °C (Bradsher et al. 2003; Brown et al. 2013). Blastomycosis is acquired by inhalation, mainly affecting lungs, but may also occur as an extrapulmonary disease. The most common extrapulmonary involvement is the skin, followed by bony, prostatic, and central nervous system (CNS) involvement (Chander et al. 2007; Saccente and Woods 2010). The involvement of the CNS is a serious but rare manifestation of blastomycosis, which may occur as meningitis, intracranial mass lesions, or abscesses in the spinal cord or the epidural space (Chander et al. 2007; Saccente and Woods 2010). Most cases of CNS blastomycosis occur in patients with immunocompromised and have been associated with concomitant infection at other sites; the reports of CNS blastomycosis insulated are scarce (Bariola et al. 2010). The high rate of mortality associated with this manifestation of the blastomycosis is due to the delay in diagnosis and, therefore, an inappropriate treatment (Bradsher et al. 2003). So it is important to consider the blastomycosis in the list of differential diagnoses for lung and skin infections and other organic systems in patients of endemic area (Bradsher 1997).

M. G. Frías-De-León (✉) · E. Martínez-Herrera
G. Acosta-Altamirano
Research Unit, Hospital Regional de Alta Especialidad de Ixtapaluca,
Ixtapaluca, Estado de México, Mexico

M. del Rocío Reyes-Montes
Microbiology and Parasitology Department, School of Medicine, Universidad Nacional Autónoma de México, Mexico City, Mexico

M. Turgut et al. (eds.), *Fungal Infections of the Central Nervous System*,
https://doi.org/10.1007/978-3-030-06088-6_13

13.1.2 Epidemiology

Blastomycosis is rare, most cases occur in the Ohio and Mississippi river valleys and in the southeast of the USA, as well as in the Midwestern states and provinces bordering the Great Lakes in Canada and areas adjacent to San Lorenzo river (Michigan, Wisconsin, Minnesota, Ontario) (De Groote et al. 2000). In states where blastomycosis is reportable, the annual incidence rates are approximately 1–2 cases per 100,000 inhabitants. Wisconsin may have the highest incidence of blastomycosis of any state, with annual rates that vary from 10 to 40 cases per 100,000 people in some northern counties (Centers for Disease Control and Prevention n.d.). For this reason, although the disease is not notifiable at the national level in the USA, since 1984, it was designated as a reportable condition in Wisconsin, as well as in Arkansas, Louisiana, Michigan, and Minnesota. In Canada, the annual incidence of blastomycosis in Ontario, Quebec, Manitoba, Saskatchewan, and Kenora is approximately 0.62 cases per 100,000 inhabitants, with areas that have rates of hospitalization of 0.3–0.6 cases per 100,000 inhabitants (Cottle et al. 2013). Only six states and two Canadian provinces have mandatory reporting of the disease, so epidemiological patterns of this disease have not been widely characterized (Castillo et al. 2016; Centers for Disease Control and Prevention n.d.). In Ontario, the disease is not notifiable since 1989, but recently there has been an average annual increase in the rate of blastomycosis which could be indicative of genuine increases in the incidence of the disease (Litvinjenko and Lunny 2017).

The cases of blastomycosis occur throughout the year without a significant seasonal peak and are reported more often in men than in women, between 35 and 55 years of age, which is probably related to the increased risk for outdoor exhibitions during work or recreation (forestry workers or hunters) (Chapman et al. 1997). It has been reported that the incidence is higher among African-American populations in the USA and aboriginal people in Canada (Cano et al. 2003; Crampton et al. 2002). Asian residents, especially immigrants from Hmong ethnic group, have reported an infection rate 12 times greater than in Wisconsin native. These facts increase speculation that there are genetic factors that predispose to the disease (Castillo et al. 2016).

Rarely have been reported cases outside the endemic area, as in Florida, Colorado, Hawaii, Israel, India, Africa, Central, and South America (Cano et al. 2003; Carlos et al. 2010; Chapman et al. 1997; Crampton et al. 2002; De Groote et al. 2000; Dworkin et al. 2005; Litvinjenko and Lunny 2017; Randhawa et al. 2013; Roy et al. 2013; Vasquez et al. 1998). In cases reported in Africa, the distributions of age and sex of the patients are similar to those in North America. However, in the African patient, bone involvement is more frequent than that of the CNS. It is important to mention that in Africa there is an apparent absence of disease in dogs. Also, it has been seen that the *B. dermatitidis* isolates from the two continents are closely related but differ in some aspects (Carman et al. 1989; Cooper et al. 1988). Within the endemic areas for blastomycosis, incidence rates of disease vary because of the type of soil (proximity to watercourses, pH, and organic content) in each region, since the humid atmosphere and acid pH are the characteristics most favorable to *B. dermatitidis* growth (Klein et al. 1987).

13.1.3 Pathogenesis and Pathology

Blastomycosis is caused by inhalation of aerosolized conidia of *Blastomyces* spp., although rarely the infection can occur through a puncture in the skin with contaminated material (Chapman et al. 1997; Litvinjenko and Lunny 2017; Saccente and Woods 2010; Smith et al. 2013). The conidia that reach the pulmonary alveoli are susceptible to be phagocyted by macrophages and neutrophils of the innate immune system. To escape innate defenses, the conidia are converted into yeast. This conversion provides resistance to phagocytosis and induces the expression of virulence factors critical to the pathogenicity, immune evasion, and proliferation; among these are the virulence factor of immune modulation (BAD1) on the cell surface and the reduction of beta(1.3)-D-glucan that prevents the recognition of the yeast by receiver's dectin-1 in innate immune cells (Koneti et al. 2008; Richer et al. 2014). The yeasts develop and multiply in the lower lobes of the lungs or pass toward the interstitial tissue, generating an inflammatory response with polymorphonuclear (PMN) leukocytes, with suppurative changes and granuloma formation. Bronchial lesions are common and destroy the mucosa with dissemination to the lung underlying. After conversion to the phase of yeast, the organisms can disseminate through hemathogenic way toward other body sites, especially the skin, bone/joints, genitourinary system, and CNS (Bradsher and Bariola 2011; Saccente and Woods 2010). T-cell activation is necessary for control of this disease (Wüthrich et al. 2011). It has been speculated that in some people, the fungal structures can remain viable and reactivate to cause disease extrapulmonary even after several years (Castillo et al. 2016).

13.1.4 Clinical Features

Blastomycosis can be presented as a subclinical disease, a progressive pulmonary or extrapulmonary disease, or both (Bradsher et al. 2003; Chapman et al. 1997). Disseminated extrapulmonary infection can affect nearly all organs, including the CNS, although infrequently. Infections have also been reported in the eye, endocrine glands, larynx, breast, uterus, and peritoneum (Bradsher and Bariola 2011; Litvinjenko and Lunny 2017).

CNS involvement occurs in 5–10% of patients with disseminated infection but has been observed in up to 33% of the autopsies of patients with blastomycosis (Bariola et al. 2010; Litvinjenko and Lunny 2017; Saccente and Woods 2010). Patients with acquired immune deficiency syndrome (AIDS) and blastomycosis are more likely to manifest affectation of the CNS (40%) (Castillo et al. 2016). CNS involvement also appears to be common in children; it has been informed of this complication in 15% of cases, which frequent manifestation are mass lesions or abscesses (Brick et al. 2013).

The manifestations of CNS blastomycosis include chronic meningitis, acute meningitis, and intracranial abscesses. The variety of symptoms include headache, fever, altered mental status, stiff neck, nausea, vomiting, vision changes, seizures, or focal neurologic deficits, such as dysphasia and paresthesia of the extremities, according to the affected area (Lyons and Andriole 1986).

In cases of chronic meningitis, the cerebrospinal fluid (CSF) reveals a predominantly neutrophilic pleocytosis lymphocytic or high protein and glucose normal to low (Bariola et al. 2010). Although meningitis is the most common manifestation of CNS blastomycosis, solitary mass lesions are not an uncommon presentation; some patients have presented focal neurologic deficits as a result of single lesions of intracranial mass (Chander et al. 2007; Roos et al. 1987). Meningitis usually presents with headache, meningismus, photophobia, papilledema, decreased consciousness, and, in advanced cases, seizures or complications with the increased intracranial pressure. Fungal meningitis may have a variable severity and can be clinically indistinguishable from bacterial causes of chronic meningitis. Fungal abscesses generally present with focal neurologic abnormality, headache, and/or seizures, which is the consequence of the local destruction or compression of the brain tissue. It should be noted that fungal and bacterial syndromes overlap, so a careful review of the risk factors of the guest should raise suspicion of a fungal cause which will lead the assessment and appropriate management of patients (Scully et al. 2008).

13.1.5 Diagnosis

Blastomycosis should be considered in the differential diagnosis of pneumonia lobar or segmental subacute, especially in residents or visitors from endemic areas. However, even in hyperendemic counties, diagnosis may be missed or delayed

(Baumgardner et al. 2011; Pfaff et al. 2014). This disease should be considered especially in patients with a history of outdoor recreational activities and with manifestations of pneumonitis refractory to initial antibiotic treatment.

The gold standard in the diagnosis of blastomycosis of the CNS is the cultivation of CSF or ventricular fluid, since the CSF culture obtained by lumbar puncture is slightly sensitive (Bariola et al. 2010). It is important that cultures are maintained for at least 4 weeks before you discard the presence of the fungus, and the colonies can be identified using DNA probes or DNA amplification by polymerase chain reaction (PCR) (Babady et al. 2011). Another diagnosis option is the histopathological examination which allows the observation of yeasts of double wall (Patel et al. 2010). It is also recommended to include a magnetic resonance imaging before the biopsy for culture and histopathology (Bush et al. 2013). The hematoxilin-eosin (HE) and Gomori methenamine silver (GMS) stains may increase the sensitivity of detection, while periodic acid-Schiff (PAS), in situ hybridization, and other histochemical stains can help differentiate *B. dermatitidis* from other fungi (Mukhopadhyay and Gal 2010). The diagnosis may also be based on the demonstration of budding yeast of broad base by direct microscopic examination of clinical samples not stained. The serological tests are not useful. The WI-1 antigen, a protein in the cell wall of yeast, has been used to diagnose blastomycosis by radioimmunoassay in endemic areas (Centers for Disease Control and Prevention n.d.).

The sampling of CSF is indicated in all patients with meningitis and may show a predominance of neutrophils in the case of blastomycosis. Care is required before taking samples of the CSF to ensure that increased intracranial pressure do not place the patient in an undue risk of lumbar puncture (Davis et al. 2007). The meningitis caused by *B. dermatitidis* is associated with a CSF pleocytosis. The protein level in CSF is generally high, while the glucose level is typically normal or reduced. The neurosurgical procedure, excluding the lumbar puncture, has been shown to be useful to carry out the diagnosis of CNS blastomycosis (Bariola et al. 2010; Ward et al. 1995).

13.1.6 Treatment Options

The guidelines of the Infectious Diseases Society of America for the treatment of blastomycosis emphasize that all patients with blastomycosis should receive antifungal therapy, regardless of the clinical presentation, due to the high probability of progression or recurrence of infection if not treated (Chapman et al. 2008). The recommended treatment for patients with CNS blastomycosis is the lipid formulation of amphotericin B, 5 mg/kg daily for 4–6 weeks or until the CNS symptoms have improved, followed by a reduction therapy with azole antifungals for at least a year (Bradsher et al. 2003). Of the azole antifungals, voriconazole is the ideal because it achieves good concentrations in CSF and has an excellent activity against the fungus, while the itraconazole, although it has good activity against *B. dermatitidis*, levels in CSF are low (Bush et al. 2013). The fluconazole has excellent penetration into the CSF and has proven to be effective at high doses (400–800 mg) in the treatment of blastomycosis of the CNS in some patients (Brick and Agger 2011; Pappas et al. 1997; Pearson et al. 1992). Posaconazole fails to reach appropriate levels in the CSF so it should not be used. Depending on the response to therapy and the immune status of patients with CNS blastomycosis, lifetime therapy with an azole antifungal may be needed to prevent relapse (Centers for Disease Control and Prevention n.d.; Chapman et al. 2008). For patients with CNS blastomycosis with lesions of intracranial mass, surgical removal may be curative (Roos et al. 1987).

13.2 Phaeohyphomycosis

13.2.1 Introduction

Phaeohyphomycosis is caused by filamentous, ubiquitous, opportunist fungi which can produce melanin, the reason they were previously known as black fungi or dematiaceous, currently called pheoid fungi (Gottfredsson and Perfect 2000; Matsumoto et al. 1994; Revankar et al. 2004; Rinaldi 1996). These fungi can produce superficial, subcutaneous, or systemic infections, in both immunocompetent and immunosuppressed patients (Rinaldi 1996). Infection of CNS is rare and shown as brain abscesses or meningitis (Gottfredsson and Perfect 2000).

13.2.2 Epidemiology

The largest number of phaeohyphomycosis cases has been reported in the USA, affecting people of any age and ethnicity, without occupational or gender predisposition, although some authors have reported that it predominates in adult men (Brandt and Warnock 2003; Emmens et al. 1996). Among the factors that predispose to this mycosis are solid organ and bone marrow transplants, neutropenia, therapies based on systemic steroids, traumas, intravenous drug abuse, leukemia, the use of catheters, chronic sinusitis, and human immunodeficiency virus (HIV) infection (Ben-Ami et al. 2009; Emmens et al. 1996; Gómez and Cardona-Castro 2016). It has been observed that the disease also is frequently found in immunocompetent persons without obvious risk factors, in whom the mortality rate is high (Ben-Ami et al. 2009).

The fungi more related to CNS phaeohyphomycosis are *Cladophialophora bantiana* and *Ramichloridium mackenziei*; however, there are many other fungi that can cause the disease, like *Ochroconis gallopavum*, *Bipolaris spicifera*, *Fonsecaea pedrosoi*, *Chaetomium strumarium*, *Bipolaris hawaiiensis*, *Chaetomium atrobrunneum*, *Exophiala castellanii*, *Wangiella dermatitidis*, *Acrophialophora fusispora*, *Cladosporium cladosporioides*, *Cladophialophora modesta*, *Curvularia pallescens*, *Exophiala jeanselmei*, *Microascus cinereus*, *Myceliophthora thermophila*, *Rhinocladiella atrovirens*, *Scedosporium prolificans*, *Scopulariopsis brumptii*, *Cladophialophora* species, *Exophiala* species, *Nodulisporium* species, and *Scopulariopsis* species (Chakrabarti et al. 2016; Revankar et al. 2004).

13.2.3 Pathogenesis and Pathology

Little is known about the mechanisms of pathogenicity that these pheoid fungi use to produce infection. It is known that the melanin, a component of its cell wall, is one of the main factors of virulence, and its function is to protect the fungus of free radicals and the sodium hypochlorite that phagocytic cells release to the environment with the oxidative stress. Another feature that helps to prevent any type of action on the plasma membrane is the union of the melanin to hydrolytic enzymes (Hamilton and Gomez 2002; Jacobson 2000; Revankar and Sutton 2010). The pheoid fungi also have enzymes (peptidases, hyaluronidases, proteases, and chitin synthase) that confer them ability to survive and cause infection. In the case of CNS infections, one of the hypotheses that have been proposed is that these fungi penetrate through the airways by inhalation of conidia, causing mainly a pulmonary asymptomatic clinical picture; subsequently the hematogenous dissemination occurs from the lungs and by neurotropism spreads to the brain. The CNS phaeohyphomycosis can also be acquired by traumatic inoculation of the fungus and later dissemination to the brain (Brandt and Warnock 2003; Dixon et al. 1987). Its incubation period is unknown.

13.2.4 Clinical Features

The frequent forms in which the CNS phaeohyphomycosis presents are single brain abscess, meningitis, encephalitis, myelitis, or arachnoiditis (Litchevski et al. 2014; Ochiai et al. 2012). The most common clinical findings in these patients are headaches, seizures, neurological deficits, fever, altered mental status, nausea, vomiting, and meningismus (Litchevski et al. 2014; Revankar et al. 2004).

13.2.5 Diagnosis

There are laboratory methods to identify the fungi responsible for phaeohyphomycosis; however, there may be inconveniences as to determine whether they are causal agents of the disease since they can be found as contaminants in the environment. Therefore, a high clinical suspicion of mycosis is needed in order to confirm the pheoid fungus (Revankar 2006; Revankar and Sutton 2010).

When a CNS phaeohyphomycosis is suspected, it is recommended to perform a brain tomography which may reveal frontal nodular lesions that occupy the space with edema, compatible with a brain abscess. In the case of performing radiology, an encapsulated mass that presents granulation tissue, fibrosis, lymphocytes, neutrophils, giant cells, and, the most important finding, fungal elements scattered or within multinuclear giant cells can be visualized (Gómez and Cardona-Castro 2016; Sundaram et al. 2006). One of the practices that are recommended when it comes to a nonmalignant brain abscess is to perform a craniotomy with a total resection. The histopathological examination using Gram, GMS, or HE stain reveals dematiaceous hyphae (Sundaram et al. 2006). Another option for the diagnosis of phaeohyphomycosis is the cultivation of samples of brain abscesses in an agar free of inhibitors (agar Sabouraud without antibiotics and actidione). Currently, the PCR is one of the most noted resources used for the identification of fungi to a species level (Gómez and Cardona-Castro 2016; Revankar 2006).

13.2.6 Treatment Options

There is no ideal treatment for CNS phaeohyphomycosis; however, it has been reported that the treatment that has given better results for survival, both in brain injuries and in disseminated infections, is the combination of azoles (itraconazole, voriconazole, or posaconazole) and amphotericin B, either with an echinocandin or flucytosine. It has been proved that total removal of brain abscesses give better results than partial removals, even though survival is still low, approximately of 30% (Gómez and Cardona-Castro 2016; Revankar 2006). Al Abdely et al. (2005) have reported that the use of azoles is not universal but depends on the etiologic agent, for example, posaconazole is effective in cases of brain abscess by *R. mackenziei*. In the case of infections caused by *C. bantiana*, voriconazole is more effective in immunocompetent patients that in immunocompromised individuals (Fica et al. 2003; Levin et al. 2004; Lyons et al. 2005).

13.3 Conclusion

The CNS mycoses by *Blastomyces* spp. and phaeoid fungi have a high morbidity and mortality due to a delay in diagnosis and the failed treatment. The successful treatment of the CNS mycosis is based on maintaining a high index of suspicion in immunocompromised patients that present an altered mental state or symptoms similar to meningitis and who live or have traveled to an endemic region. Furthermore it is important for the specific identification of the pathogen for the adequate pharmacological treatment of the patients.

References

Al Abdely HM, Alkhunaizi AM, Al Tawfiq JA, Hassounah M, Rinaldi MG, Sutton DA. Successful therapy of cerebral phaeohyphomycosis due to *Ramichloridium mackenziei* with the new triazole posaconazole. Med Mycol. 2005;43(1):91–5.

Babady NE, Buckwalter SP, Hall L, Le Febre KM, Binnicker MJ, Wengenack NL. Detection of *Blastomyces dermatitidis* and *Histoplasma capsulatum* from culture isolates and clinical specimens by use of real-time PCR. J Clin Microbiol. 2011;49:3204–8.

Bariola JR, Perry P, Pappas PG, Proia L, Shealey W, Wright PW, et al. Blastomycosis of the central nervous system: a multicenter review of diagnosis and treatment in the modern era. Clin Infect Dis. 2010;50:797–804.

Baumgardner DJ, Temte JL, Gutowski E, Agger WA, Bailey H, Burmester JK, et al. The differential diagnosis of pulmonary blastomycosis using case vignettes: a Wisconsin Network for Health Research (WiNHR) study. WMJ. 2011;110(2):68–73.

Ben-Ami R, Lewis RE, Raad II, Kontoyiannis DP. Phaeohyphomycosis in a tertiary care cancer center. CID. 2009;48:1033–41.

Bentley RT, Reese MJ, Heng HG, Long Lin T, Shimonohara N, Fauber A. Ependymal and periventricular magnetic resonance imaging changes in four dogs with central nervous system blastomycosis. Vet Radiol Ultrasound. 2013;54(5):489–96.

Bradsher RW. Clinical features of blastomycosis. Semin Respir Infect. 1997;12(3):229–34.

Bradsher RW, Bariola JR. Blastomycosis. In: Kauffman CA, Pappas PG, Sobel JD, et al., editors. Essentials of clinical mycology. 2nd ed. New York: Springer; 2011. p. 337–48.

Bradsher RW, Chapman SW, Pappas PG. Blastomycosis. Infect Dis Clin North Am. 2003;17(1):21–40.

Brandt ME, Warnock DW. Epidemiology, clinical manifestations, and therapy of infections caused by dematiaceous fungi. J Chemother. 2003;15(Suppl 2):36–47.

Brick KE, Agger WA. Successful treatment of brainstem blastomycosis with fluconazole. Clin Med Res. 2011;10(2):72–4.

Brick KE, Drolet BA, Lyon VB, Galbraith SS. Cutaneous and disseminated blastomycosis: a pediatric case series. Pediatr Dermatol. 2013;30:23–8.

Brown EM, McTaggart LR, Zhang SX, Low DE, Stevens DA, Richardson SE. Phylogenetic analysis reveals a cryptic species *Blastomyces gilchristii*, sp. nov. within the human pathogenic fungus *Blastomyces dermatitidis*. PLoS One. 2013;8(3):e59237.

Bush JW, Wuerz T, Embil JM, Del Bigio MR, McDonald PJ, Krawitz S. Outcomes of persons with blastomycosis involving the central nervous system. Diagn Microbiol Infect Dis. 2013;76:175–81.

Cano MV, Ponce-de-Leon GF, Tippen S, Lindsley MD, Warwick M, Hajjeh RA. Blastomycosis in Missouri: epidemiology and risk factors for endemic disease. Epidemiol Infect. 2003;131:907–14.

Carlos WG, Rose AS, Wheat LJ, Norris S, Sarosi GA, Knox KS, et al. Blastomycosis in Indiana: digging up more cases. Chest. 2010;138:1377–82.

Carman WF, Frean JA, Crewe-Brown HH, Culligan GA, Young CN. Blastomycosis in Africa. A review of known cases diagnosed between 1951 and 1987. Mycopathologia. 1989;107(1):25–32.

Castillo CG, Kauffman CA, Miceli MH. Blastomycosis. Infect Dis Clin North Am. 2016;30(1):247–64.

Centers for Disease Control & Prevention. Blastomycosis. Atlanta, GA: CDC. https://www.cdc.gov/fungal/diseases/blastomycosis/. Accessed 13 July 2018.

Chakrabarti A, Kaur H, Rudramurthy M, Appannanavar SB, Patel A, Mukherjee KK, et al. Brain abscess due to *Cladophialophora bantiana*: a review of 124 cases. Med Mycol. 2016;54:111–9.

Chander B, Deb P, Sarkar C, Garg A, Mehta VS, Sharma MC. Cerebral blastomycosis: a case report. Indian J Pathol Microbiol. 2007;50(4):821–4.

Chapman SW, Lin AC, Hendricks KA, Nolan RL, Currier MM, Morris KR, et al. Endemic blastomycosis in Mississippi: epidemiological and clinical studies. Semin Respir Infect. 1997;12:219–28.

Chapman SW, Dismukes WE, Proia LA, Bradsher RW, Pappas PG, Threlkeld MG, et al. Clinical practice guidelines for the management of blastomycosis: 2008 update by the Infectious Diseases Society of America. Clin Infect Dis. 2008;46:1801–12.

Cooper K, Lalloo UG, Naran HK. Cerebral blastomycosis. A report of 2 cases. S Afr Med J. 1988;74(10):521–4.

Cottle LE, Gkrania-Klotsas E, Williams HJ, Brindle HE, Carmichael AJ, Fry G, et al. A multinational outbreak of histoplasmosis following a biology field trip in the Ugandan rainforest. J Travel Med. 2013;20(2):83–7.

Crampton TL, Light RB, Berg GM, Meyers MP, Schroeder GC, Hershfield ES, et al. Epidemiology and clinical spectrum of blastomycosis diagnosed at Manitoba hospitals. Clin Infect Dis. 2002;34:1310–6.

Davis JA, Costello DJ, Venna N. Laboratory investigation of fungal infections of the central nervous system. Neurol India. 2007;55:233–40.

De Groote MA, Bjerke R, Smith H, Rhodes LV III. Expanding epidemiology of blastomycosis: clinical features and investigation of 2 cases in Colorado. Clin Infect Dis. 2000;30:582–4.

Dixon DM, Merz WG, Elliott HL, Macleay S. Experimental central nervous system phaeohyphomycosis following intranasal inoculation of *Xylohypha bantiana* in cortisone-treated mice. Mycopathologia. 1987;100:145–53.

Dworkin MS, Duckro AN, Proia L, Semel JD, Huhn G. The epidemiology of blastomycosis in Illinois and factors associated with death. Clin Infect Dis. 2005;41:e107–11.

Emmens RK, Richardson D, Thomas W, Hunter S, Hennigar RA, Wingard JR, et al. Necrotizing cerebritis in an allogeneic bone marrow transplant recipient due to *Cladophialophora bantiana*. J Clin Microbiol. 1996;30:1330–2.

Fica A, Diaz MC, Luppi M, Olivares R, Saez L, Baboor M, Vasquez P. Unsuccessful treatment with voriconazole of a brain abscess due to *Cladophialophora bantiana*. Scand J Infect Dis. 2003;35(11–12):892–3.

Gilchrist TC. Protozoan dermatitidis. J Cutan Gen Dis. 1894;12:496.

Gómez LV, Cardona-Castro N. Feohifomicosis, una infección fúngica oportunista emergente. Rev CES Med. 2016;30(1):66–77.

Gottfredsson M, Perfect JR. Fungal meningitis. Semin Neurol. 2000;20(3):307–22.

Hamilton AJ, Gomez BL. Melanins in fungal pathogens. J Med Microbiol. 2002;51:189–91.

Jacobson ES. Pathogenic roles for fungal melanins. Clin Microbiol Rev. 2000;13:708–17.

Klein BS, Vergeront JM, DiSalvo AF, Kaufman L, Davis JP. Two outbreaks of blastomycosis along rivers in Wisconsin: isolation of *Blastomyces dermatitidis* from riverbank soil and evidence of its transmission along waterways. Am Rev Respir Dis. 1987;136:1333–8.

Koneti A, Linke MJ, Brummer E, Stevens DA. Evasion of innate immune responses: evidence for mannose binding lectin inhibition of tumor necrosis factor alpha production by macrophages in response to *Blastomyces dermatitidis*. Infect Immun. 2008;76:994–1002.

Levin TP, Baty DE, Fekete T, Truant AL, Suh B. *Cladophialophora bantiana* brain abscess in a solid-organ transplant recipient: case report and review of the literature. J Clin Microbiol. 2004;42(9):4374–8.

Litchevski V, Goldschmidt A, Nass D, Rahav G, Cohen ZR. Cerebral phaeohyphomycosis in an immunocompetent patient: a case report and literature summary. Clin Neurol Neurosurg. 2014;124:179–81.

Litvinjenko S, Lunny D. Blastomycosis hospitalizations in northwestern Ontario: 2006–2015. Can Commun Dis Rep. 2017;43(10):200–5.

Lyons RW, Andriole VT. Fungal infections of the CNS. Neurol Clin. 1986;4(1):159–70.

Lyons MK, Blair JE, Leslie KO. Successful treatment with voriconazole of fungal cerebral abscess due to *Cladophialophora bantiana*. Clin Neurol Neurosurg. 2005;107(6):53–4.

Matsumoto T, Ajello L, Matsuda T, Szaniszlo PJ, Walsh TJ. Developments in hyalohyphomycosis and phaeohyphomycosis. J Med Vet Mycol. 1994;32(Suppl 1):329–49.

Mukhopadhyay S, Gal AA. Granulomatous lung disease: an approach to the differential diagnosis. Arch Pathol Lab Med. 2010;134:667–90.

Ochiai H, Kawano H, Minato S, Yoneyama T, Shimao Y. Cerebral phaeohyphomycosis: case report. Neuropathology. 2012;32(2):202–6.

Pappas PG, Bradsher RW, Kauffman CA, Cloud GA, Thomas CJ, Campbell GD Jr, et al. Treatment of blastomycosis with higher doses of fluconazole. The National Institute of Allergy and Infectious Diseases Mycoses Study Group. Clin Infect Dis. 1997;25:200–5.

Patel AJ, Gattuso P, Reddy VB. Diagnosis of blastomycosis in surgical pathology and cytopathology: correlation with microbiologic culture. Am J Surg Pathol. 2010;34:256–61.

Pearson GJ, Chin TW, Fong IW. Case report: treatment of blastomycosis with fluconazole. Am J Med Sci. 1992;303(5):313–5.

Pfaff BL, Agger WA, Volk TJ. Blastomycosis diagnosed in a nonhyperendemic area. WMJ. 2014;113(1):11–8.

Randhawa HS, Chowdhary A, Kathuria S, Roy P, Misra DS, Jain S, et al. Blastomycosis in India: report of an imported case and current status. Med Mycol. 2013;51:185–92.

Revankar SG. Phaeohyphomycosis. Infect Dis Clin North Am. 2006;20(3):609–20.

Revankar SG, Sutton DA. Melanized fungi in human disease. Clin Microbiol Rev. 2010;23(4):884–928.

Revankar SG, Sutton DA, Rinaldi MG. Primary central nervous system phaeohyphomycosis: a review of 101 cases. CID. 2004;38:206–16.

Richer SM, Smedema ML, Durkin MM, Brandhorst TT, Hage CA, Connolly PA, et al. Development of a highly sensitive and specific blastomycosis antibody enzyme immunoassay using *Blastomyces dermatitidis* surface protein BAD-1. Clin Vaccine Immunol. 2014;21:143–6.

Rinaldi MG. Phaeohyphomycosis. Dermatol Clin. 1996;14(1):147–53.

Roos KL, Bryan JP, Maggio WW, Jane JA, Scheld WM. Intracranial blastomycoma. Medicine (Baltimore). 1987;66(3):224–35.

Roy M, Benedict K, Deak E, Kirby MA, McNiel JT, Sickler CJ, et al. A large community outbreak of blastomycosis in Wisconsin with geographic and ethnic clustering. Clin Infect Dis. 2013;57:655–62.

Saccente M, Woods GL. Clinical and laboratory update on blastomycosis. Clin Microbiol Rev. 2010;23:267–81.

Scully EP, Baden LR, Katz JT. Fungal brain infections. Curr Opin Neurol. 2008;21:347–52.

Smith JA, Riddell J, Kauffman CA. Cutaneous manifestations of endemic mycoses. Curr Infect Dis Rep. 2013;15:440–9.

Sundaram C, Umabala P, Laxmi V, Purohit AK, Prasad VSSV, Panigrahi M, et al. Pathology of fungal infections of the central nervous system: 17 years' experience from Southern India. Histopathology. 2006;49(4):396–405.

Vasquez JE, Mehta JB, Agrawal R, Sarubbi FA. Blastomycosis in northeast Tennessee. Chest. 1998;114:436–43.

Ward BA, Parent AD, Raila F. Indications for the surgical management of central nervous system blastomycosis. Surg Neurol. 1995;43(4):379–88.

Wüthrich M, Gern B, Hung CY, Ersland K, Rocco N, Pick-Jacobs J, et al. Vaccine-induced protection against 3 systemic mycoses endemic to North America requires Th17 cells in mice. J Clin Invest. 2011;121:554–68.

Cladophialophora bantiana

14

Hurriyet Deniz Ozgun, Darren L. Jacobs, and Steven A. Toms

Abbreviations

AFLP	Amplified fragment length polymorphism
CNS	Central nervous system
CT	Computed tomography
CSF	Cerebrospinal fluid
DHN	Dihydroxynaphthalene
DOPA	Dihydroxyphenylalanine
ITS	Internal transcribed spacer
MRI	Magnetic resonance imaging
PCR	Polymerase chain reaction
UV	Ultraviolet

H. D. Ozgun
Acıbadem Mehmet Ali Aydınlar University, İstanbul, Turkey

Department of Neurosurgery, Lifespan Health System, Providence, RI, USA
e-mail: hurriyet.ozgun@live.acibadem.edu.tr

D. L. Jacobs
Department of Neurosurgery, Geisinger Health System, Danville, PA, USA
e-mail: dljacobs@geisinger.edu

S. A. Toms (✉)
Department of Neurosurgery, Lifespan Health System, Providence, RI, USA

Brown University Alpert Medical School, Providence, RI, USA
e-mail: steven.toms@lifespan.org

14.1 Introduction

Cladophialophora bantiana is a thermotolerant multinucleated saprophytic black mold that reproduces asexually via unicellular conidia. It is considered a hyphomycete, because its conidia are not surrounded (Ajantha et al. 2011). Some *C. bantiana* produce budding cells and dark hyphae; due to this it is sometimes called "black yeast-like fungi" (Seyedmousavi et al. 2014). It is an ubiquitous (Salama et al. 1997) fungus that grows in humid and warm environments (Chakrabarti 2007) such as soil and woody plant materials, which predisposes human interaction (Kuan et al. 2016). *C. bantiana* is the most common cause of non-traumatic fungal central nervous system (CNS) infection in immunocompetent humans (Ajantha et al. 2011) and most commonly manifests as clinical infection in the CNS. It is thought that the route of entry is primarily via inhalation and secondarily by hematogenous spread even though soil exposure was not commonly reported in reported cases (Levin et al. 2004). Direct inoculation of the CNS also is another possible but rare cause of infection (Salama et al. 1997).

According to the taxonomical ranking of *Cladophialophora bantiana*, it belongs to the phylum *Ascomycota* and the subphylum *Pezizomycotina*. It is in the class *Eurotiomycetes* and subclass *Chaetothyriomycetidae*. *C. bantiana* is included in the order *Chaetothyriales* and in the family *Herpotrichiellaceae* (http://

M. Turgut et al. (eds.), *Fungal Infections of the Central Nervous System*,
https://doi.org/10.1007/978-3-030-06088-6_14

www.mycobank.org/Biolomics.aspx?Table=Mycobank&Rec=48324&Fields=All). This family of fungi has evolved different features than other ascomycetes families, which may be due to rapid diversification of this family after becoming a human pathogen (De Hoog 2000). Lacking conidiophores, "shield cells," or prominent hila are differentiating properties of *Chaetothyriales* order which differentiates *Cladophialophora* species from morphologically similar *Cladosporium* species (Revankar and Sutton 2010).

Melanin present in *C. bantiana* is a potential virulence factor for pathogenesis of CNS infections. Melanin has already been shown to be a prominent feature in other neurotropic fungi, such as *Cryptococcus neoformans* and *Wangiella dermatitidis* (Revankar et al. 2004). Furthermore, murine models of the fungus without melanin reduce the virulence of *C. bantiana* considerably (Revankar et al. 2004). It has been hypothesized that the mechanism of CNS localization shares mechanistic properties with that of malignant melanoma in its predilection for CNS metastasis (Ajantha et al. 2011).

There are several hypotheses regarding the mechanisms behind the virulence of melanin. Some believe that melanin is protective to *C. bantiana* because it prevents the free radicals and hypochlorite that are produced by phagocytes. It binds to hydrolytic enzymes to inhibit phagocytes actions on its plasma membrane (Revankar et al. 2004). It is further hypothesized that melanin-recognizing receptors on blood brain barrier might lead to the easy passage of melanin to brain parenchyma (Revankar et al. 2004). Melanin also protects the fungi against ultra violet (UV) radiation and it may be the underlying cause of thermotolerant characteristics of dematiaceous fungi (Langfelder et al. 2003).

There are some structural and biochemical differences between human and fungal melanin. Human melanin is derived from tyrosine and fungal melanin is derived mostly from acetate derivatives (Revankar et al. 2004). Fungal melanin can be derived from L-3,4-dihydroxyphenylalanine (DOPA)-melanin or from 1,8-dihydroxynaphthalene (DHN)-melanin, which is synthesized through pentaketide metabolism (Langfelder et al. 2003), during fungal spore formation (Kuan et al. 2016) by oxidative polymerization of phenolic compounds (De Hoog 2000). In various fungi, melanin synthesis is linked to cAMP-dependent signaling pathway (Langfelder et al. 2003). Fungal melanin is located either as embedded in the cell wall or attached to the outer side, which is classified as cell wall-bound melanin. However, human melanin is localized within specialized cells (melanocytes) and intracellular vacuoles (melanosomes) (Langfelder et al. 2003).

Although melanin-containing fungi other than *C. bantiana* do not invade CNS as often, it remains unclear as to whether the melanin itself is necessary and sufficient for the neurotropism and pathogenicity of these fungi (Ajantha et al. 2011). For example, there are some nonpathogenic fungi that contain DHN-melanin. Thus, factors other than melanin may be important for its virulence, such as thermotolerance and the stage of melanin production or melanin localizations (Langfelder et al. 2003). To reach a conclusion about whether melanin mainly is behind the pathogenesis of CNS localization of *C. bantiana*, further experiments disrupting DHN-melanin biosynthesis pathway are warranted (De Hoog 2000).

Although not specific to dematiaceous fungi (Perfect et al. 2003), melanin is the reason behind the darkly pigmented appearance, which gives a specific name to its infection: phaeohyphomycosis (Kuan et al. 2016). Phaeohyphomycosis means "condition of dark hyphal fungus," which comes from the Greek word "phaios" meaning dark or dusky (Satton et al. 2009), and is a rare condition when compared to other infections (Jayakeerthi et al. 2004). Besides *C. bantiana*, the major cause of cerebral fungal abscess cases (Jayakeerthi et al. 2004) include many other neurotropic (plesiomorph characteristic) fungi including *Exophiala (Wangiella) dermatitidis*, *Ramichloridium mackenziei*, *Myceliophthora thermophila*, *Acrophialophora fusispora*, *Microascus cinereus*, and *Ochroconis gallopava* (De Hoog 2000; Langfelder et al. 2003). Overall, 48% of the cerebral phaeohyphomycosis cases reported were caused by *C. bantiana*, with a mortality of 71% (Lakshmi et al. 2008). Although there are no strong predilections described for *C. bantiana* infections, genetic susceptibilities such as mutations in the CARD9 gene, use of corticosteroids, and decreases in cytokine production may be found in some cases of cerebral phaeohyphomycosis (Seyedmousavi et al. 2014).

14.2 Discovery of *C. bantiana*

Cladophialophora bantiana was discovered by Guido Banti in 1911, who was an anatomy professor and a physician at the University of Florence at the time. Banti had a female patient with fatal cerebral phaeohyphomycosis. Later in her autopsy, Banti spotted numerous dark brown nodules similar to melanotic sarcoma, along with phaeoid mycelium and long chained 5–10 conidia. After Banti, Pier Andrea Saccardo named the samples that he received from Banti as *Torula bantiana*.

In 1960 Dante Borelli, a medical mycologist, named *Torula bantiana* as *Cladosporium trichoides*, which was a synonym for *Cladosporium bantianum*, and observed that it could grow at 42 °C. In 1961 Rafaele Stiglioni proved that this fungus belonged to *Cladosporium* genus by using the drawings of *Torula* of dematiaceous hyphae and photomicrographs of histological preparations of Banti. In 1963 another group of scientists denied *Torula bantiana* belonging to *Cladosporium* genus. Between 1981 and 1983 variations in size were noticed, which built up on to the question if they were two different types of fungi.

In 1984, it was discovered that the two fungi had same antigens, and in 1986 Borelli claimed that they were thermotolerant, which lead to the conclusion that they were cospecific. In 1992 again the same question was raised; however in 1995 Sybren G. De Hoog and colleagues ended the discussion by concluding that *Torula bantiana* und *Cladophialophora bantiana* were the same organism (De Hoog 1995).

The *C. bantiana* differ from related fungi in another important aspect important to their growth. Due to the carbohydrate active enzyme (CAZyme) content in *C. bantiana* genome, rather than cellulose, they decompose hemicellulose and pectin components, which are abundant in plant cell wall (Kuan et al. 2016). Finally, direct gene sequencing and polymerase chain reaction (PCR) have been useful in identifying species of similar fungi. Historically, the introns in the 18S rRNA gene subunit of species have been used for random target PCR in phylogenetic identification of species and have also been used to identify *C. bantiana* and predict neurotropic behavior (van den Ende and De Hoog 1999).

The youngest *C. bantiana* case noted in the literature was a 6-day-old neonate with a skin fungal infection (Jayakeerthi et al. 2004). The youngest *C. bantiana* abscess in the CNS was documented in a 6-month-old boy (Jayakeerthi et al. 2004). *C. bantiana* presents itself mostly in the immunocompetent young males, especially in second and third decades of life (Jayakeerthi et al. 2004). In cerebral phaeohyphomycosis male predominance is 76% and the mean age is 38. The majority of patients (52%) had no identifiable underlying medical conditions (Satton et al. 2009). A total of 77 (76%) of 101 cases were in men, and 24 cases (25%) were in women. Predilection for race or geographic location has not yet been identified (Jayakeerthi et al. 2004).

14.3 Clinical Presentation of Infection

Phaeohyphomycosis can cause four types of diseases, which are superficial, cutaneous and corneal, subcutaneous, and systemic. *C. bantiana* is observed in systemic phaeohyphomycosis (Satton et al. 2009), although it can rarely cause cutaneous or subcutaneous infections (Kuan et al. 2016). Systemic phaeohyphomycosis (disseminated infection) often leads to cerebral disease (Perfect et al. 2003), which is rare in animals, and the transmission to humans from animals has not been reported yet (Rantala et al. 2015).

C. bantiana presents non-specifically with chronic headaches in 59% of the cases (Satton et al. 2009). Fewer (54%) present with localizing signs due to mass effect causing focal neurological deficits (Satton et al. 2009), such as weakness in the limbs, altered mental status, increased tone, numbness, hemiplegia, hemiparesis, cranial nerve deficits, facial palsy, slurring of speech, decreased hearing, positive Babinski sign, papilledema, diplopia, motor aphasia, fever, seizures, and rarely chronic meningitis. These manifestations can precede diagnosis from weeks to years (Trinh et al. 2003) based on the disease burden, clinical severity, and impact on the patient's daily routine.

14.4 Radiological Findings

Contrast enhanced computed tomography (CT) scans reveal brain abscess in 87% and 71% are single lesion when radiographically identified. The second most common CT finding is chronic meningitis, occurring in 9% of cases (Satton et al. 2009). Clinical cases show focal and irregularly shaped (Emmens et al. 1996) ring-enhancing mass lesions on CT and magnetic resonance imaging (MRI) (Garzoni et al. 2008) (see Figs. 14.1, 14.2, and 14.3). Most

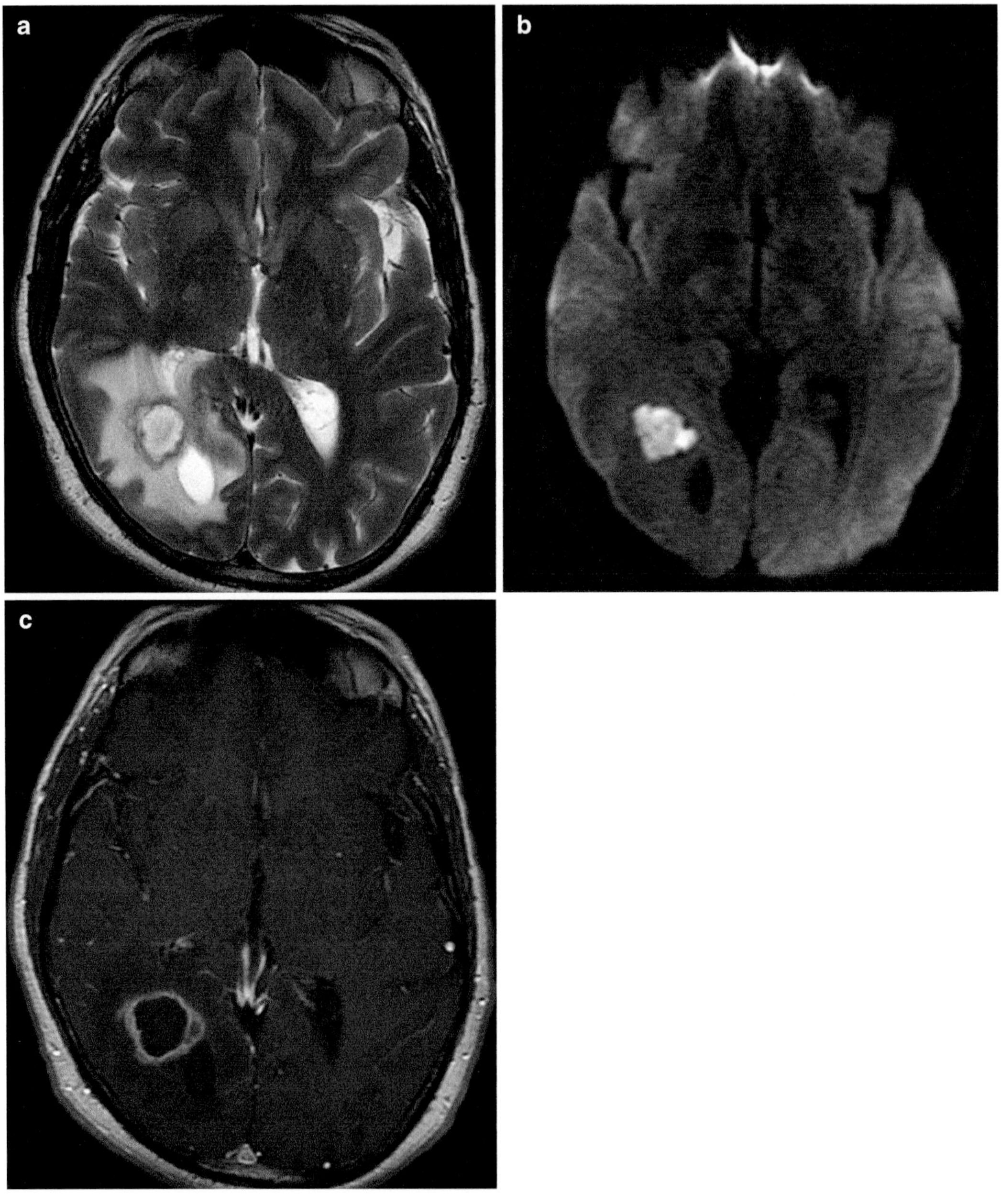

Fig. 14.1 MRI of brain in a *C. bantiana* patient showing a ring and a cystic lesion with a large amount of edema on T2-weighted (**a**) with restricted diffusion on diffusion-weighted imaging (**b**). The lesion demonstrated ring enhancement on T1-weigted imaging with gadolinium (**c**)

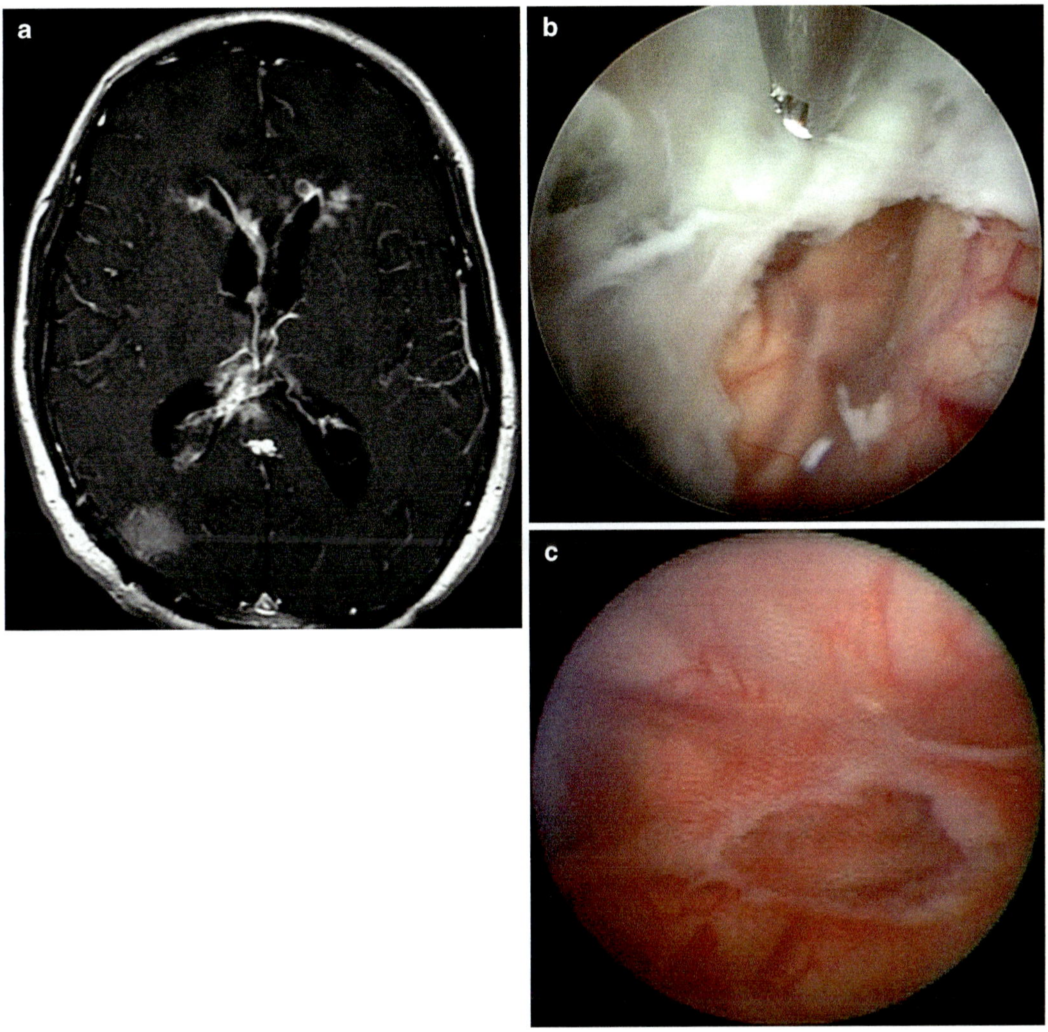

Fig. 14.2 A case of *C. bantiana* ventriculitis shows diffuse ependymal enhancement on T1-weighted imaging with gadolinium (**a**). Endoscopic exploration showed extensive arachnoidal adhesions (**b**) and fungal plaques on the ependymal wall (**c**)

scans demonstrate cerebral vasogenic (Trinh et al. 2003) edema, which might cause sulcal effacement. *C. bantiana* will often show contrast enhancement and necrotic lesions with ring enhancement on T1-weighted MRI images with gadolinium (Levin et al. 2004). Larger abscesses may show midline shift in the brain due to mass effect (Salama et al. 1997). The differential diagnosis based on CT and/or MRI includes metastases, high-grade gliomas (Emmens et al. 1996), and bacterial brain abscesses (Garzoni et al. 2008). In immunocompromised people, wider list of differential diagnosis should be considered, such as opportunistic infections and lymphomas (Garzoni et al. 2008).

The abscesses are typically confined to one hemisphere generally and they are more likely to occur in the frontal lobe of the brain (Ajantha et al. 2011). Given the likely hematological spread of the pathogen to the brain, this localization preference should not be surprising, although cases of *C. bantiana* have been observed in choroid plexus, thalamus, diencephalon, and cerebellum. In the rare case in which they localize in pons or brainstem, the consequences may be rapidly fatal

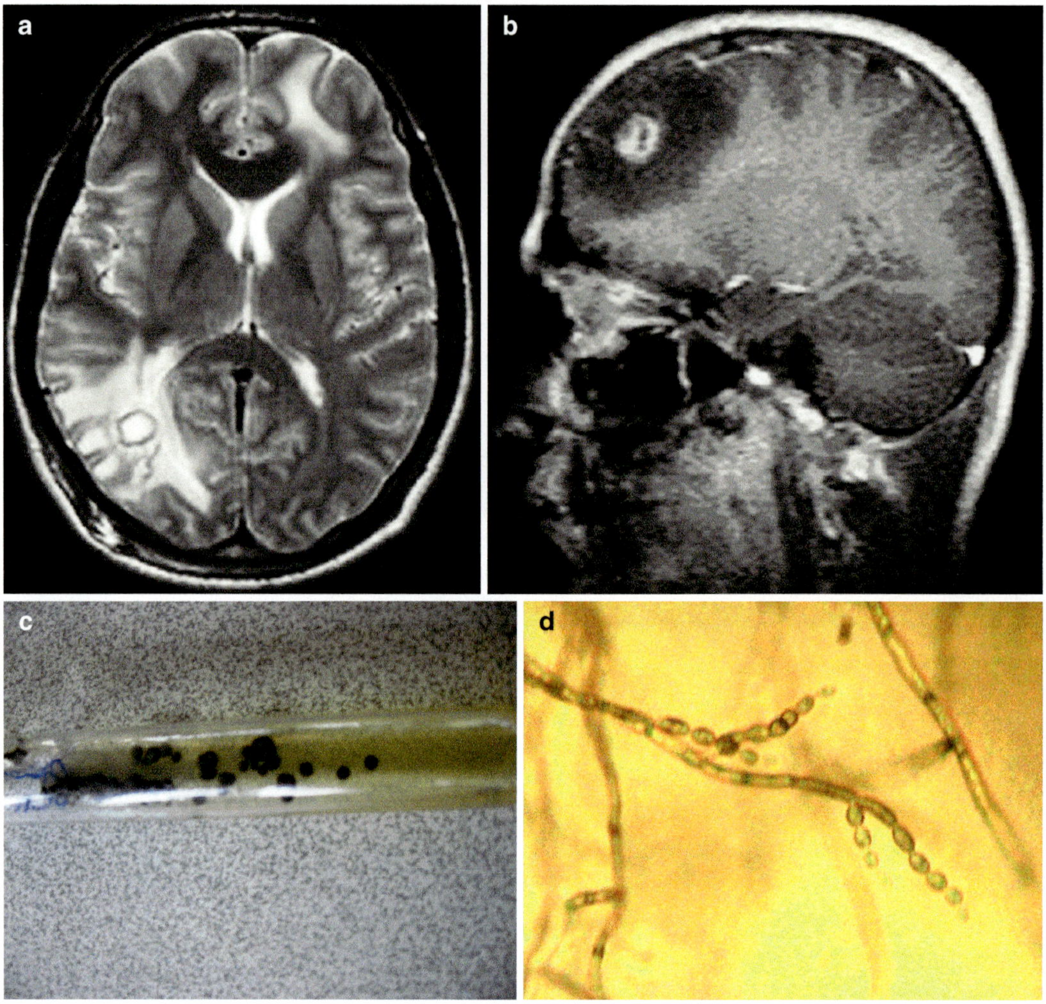

Fig. 14.3 MRI of brain in a *C. bantiana* patient showing a space-occupying lesion in the right parietal lobe and left frontal lobe (**a**, **b**). Surface colors of all media including Sabouraud dextrose agar medium with cycloheximide were olive-gray to black and contained velvety colonies (**c**). Lemon-like very long and integrated chains of conidium with poor branching in cornmeal Tween 80 agar as well as growth at 42 °C in passages, positive urease test result, and cycloheximide resistance suggested *C. bantiana* (**d**). The isolate was confirmed as *C. bantiana* based on its DNA sequence analysis (Courtesy of M. A. Atalay, M.D.)

secondary to respiratory failure (Emmens et al. 1996).

14.5 Diagnosis (Biopsy/Surgery/Culture)

C. bantiana is mostly commonly diagnosed with a surgical procedure, such as a stereotactic brain biopsy or cyst aspiration (Garzoni et al. 2008). Unfortunately, sometimes the disease is so extensive that it is not identified until a post mortem analysis often revealing extensive necrotizing cerebritis (Emmens et al. 1996). Since *C. bantiana* may be inhaled and since it can affect even immunocompetent people, it should be treated according to the rules of biosafety level 3, which requires a biosafety cabinet, negative airflow into the laboratory, and protective laboratory clothing such as respiratory protection (Rantala et al. 2015; Badali et al. 2010). The staff who handle the specimen must protect themselves accordingly (Ajantha et al. 2011).

During surgical resection or biopsy, the dark pigmentation of the tissue is apparent grossly. Microscopically, *C. bantiana* frozen sections should reveal pleomorphic cells, branching hyphae (Ahmad et al. 2017), and multinucleated giant cells (Salama et al. 1997; Emmens et al. 1996). Permanent sections of hematoxylin and eosin and Gomori silver methenamine should reveal multinucleated giant cells composed of fungi (Ahmad et al. 2017), giant cells, and inflammation (Lakshmi et al. 2008) but no focal demyelination (Trinh et al. 2003). Lactophenol cotton blue staining shows darkly pigmented and septate fungal hyphae, 2–3 mm in diameter (Jayakeerthi et al. 2004) and long, wavy, sparsely branching, dry, strongly coherent chains of oval (Ahmad et al. 2017) conidia (Kuan et al. 2016; Badali et al. 2008). The fungal and bacterial brain abscesses can be differentiated neuropathologically via the invasion of the capsule and beyond, which occurs in fungal abscesses but not in bacterial ones (Revankar and Sutton 2010). In the case of melanin not being visible with the usual stains, Fontana-Masson stain, which is specific to melanin (Ajantha et al. 2011), can be used to highlight the pigment (Satton et al. 2009).

The fungal media preferred, the temperature to grow, and the duration of growth should be considered, to prevent misdiagnosis or failure to diagnose. *C. bantiana* can be observed with microscopic wet mount examination or KOH wet mount (Kuan et al. 2016; Seyedmousavi et al. 2014) and can grow in conventional fungal media, such as potato dextrose, oatmeal, and malt agar. Sabouraud agar is not the first choice because it cannot develop the dark color of *C. bantiana* (see Fig. 14.3). However, it can grow on cycloheximide-rich media. It is urease positive and it is non-proteolytic on casein agar (Ajantha et al. 2011). The fungus grows with a moderate rate, which takes 7–8 days to see and 15 days to mature (Ajantha et al. 2011). The high growth temperature of 42 °C is a virulence factor (Ajantha et al. 2011) and a differentiating characteristic of saprophytic fungi (Lakshmi et al. 2008). The fungi's thermal stress-responsive proteins have contributed to its ability to survive in the human body (Kuan et al. 2016).

In addition to morphology and growth temperature, phylogenetic analysis (Kuan et al. 2016) and molecular identification methods are more reliable ways to differentiate *C. bantiana* from other fungi. Identification of *C. bantiana* based on DNA can be done via amplified fragment length polymorphism (AFLP). This method detects genomic restriction fragments by PCR amplification, by selectively amplifying primers without needing prior sequence information (Badali et al. 2010). When genetic analysis is needed for diagnosis, DNA extraction using malt agars cetyltrimethylammonium bromide method may be used (Moller et al. 1992). Species can be confirmed by internal transcribed spacer (ITS) sequencing, which is used for identification based on molecular systematics and DNA and has low variability in *C. bantiana* (Rantala et al. 2015; van den Ende and De Hoog 1999). 558 base pair intron at position 1768 in the small-subunit rDNA gene (Badali et al. 2010) is considered strictly specific to *C. bantiana* (Kantarcıoğlu and De Hoog 2004). For definite diagnosis, results also should be compared to deposits in GenBank and database of CBS (Fungal Biodiversity Center) on black fungi (Rantala et al. 2015).

14.6 Treatment (Surgery/Antifungals)

Although there is no consensus about a standard anti-fungal therapy yet, maximal surgical resection, wherever possible, seems to improve survival in *C. bantiana* infections (Salama et al. 1997). Complete surgical resection helps with "reducing the pressure effects, reduction of the fungal load and enhancing the response to the antifungal therapy," even though the abscesses might recur (Ajantha et al. 2011).

When complete surgical excision is not possible, surgical debridement and debulking of the abscess should be attempted (Perfect et al. 2003). The physician should be aware that partial decompression might aggravate patient's status, by increasing postoperative edema and swelling (Levin et al. 2004). During surgery, it is imperative to avoid ventricular entry, as fungal contamination of the cerebrospinal fluid (CSF) will often lead to fatal ventriculitis (see Fig. 14.2). Repeated stereotactic aspiration of the cyst abscess to sterilize the lesion leaving the enhancing capsule intact in addition to long-term oral voriconazole and amphotericin B was suggested as a strategy in treating *C. bantiana* (Garzoni et al. 2008).

For the treatment of dematiaceous fungi including *C. bantiana*, there are four potential classes of antifungal medications (Perfect et al. 2003): 1:polyene drugs, such as Amphotericin B, a systemic drug that show moderate in vitro effect; 2:flucytosine, which works better in combination therapies because it develops resistance in single use; 3:azole drugs, such as fluconazole, which inhibit fungal membrane synthesis, which have more efficacy in vitro and safe to use in long-term therapies, and triazoles can be used as first line drugs against phaeohyphomycosis; and 4:echinocandins, such as caspofungin, are newer drugs that inhibit fungal beta-glucan synthase in vitro. However, results of trials using this drug are yet to be reported (Perfect et al. 2003). Theoretically, *C. bantiana* may be resistant to echinocandins, because it doesn't have much glucan in the cell wall (Badali et al. 2010).

In clinical scenarios, *C. bantiana* is resistant to Amphotericin B in vitro, in large part because it cannot diffuse well into the CNS (Badali et al. 2010). Nevertheless, clinical responses to Amphotericin B and its combined use with a triazole, possibly flucytosine (Garzoni et al. 2008), in addition to surgery, were better (Lakshmi et al. 2008; Scheld et al. 2004) than results with Amphotericin B alone. Nephrotoxicity is reduced clinically by using lipid preparations of Amphotericin B (Revankar et al. 2004).

When oral flucytosine and azole drugs are used for a long term, they may cause regression in the lesions that can be observed in the CT (Salama et al. 1997). Although itraconazole penetrates poorly in the CSF, it accumulates in the brain, which makes it efficient (Revankar et al. 2004). New triazoles voriconazole and posaconazole might work better than itraconazole, although there are no randomized studies given the rare nature of this disease. Posaconazole may be better tolerated by the patients since it has low toxicity and less drug-drug interactions, even though its effect is more fungi static than fungicidal (Ajantha et al. 2011). Both newer azole drugs distribute to high volume and can accumulate in tissue, in addition to having good oral bioavailability (Garzoni et al. 2008). The effect of voriconazole is fungicidal and it can infiltrate in the CNS, though it has a high MIC (Ajantha et al. 2011), which in long-term use showed recovery (Ahmad et al. 2017). Unfortunately, fluconazole (Garzoni et al. 2008), ketoconazole, miconazole, and uconazole (Ajantha et al. 2011) are not active against *C. bantiana*.

Combination therapy is more helpful (Perfect et al. 2003) than monotherapy and should be preferred as monotherapy more often resulted in treatment failure in the literature (Ajantha et al. 2011). The most common current recommendations suggest that liposomal amphotericin B should be combined with high-dose azole (Ajantha et al. 2011). Also, in a relatively new case which was published in 2016, post-op oral voriconazole for 6 months after IV amphotericin B and itraconazole administration was clinically successful (Kuan et al. 2016).

In the treatment of *C. bantiana*, importance of the time of diagnosis and starting the appropriate treatment cannot be overlooked, due to their effect on mortality rate (Jayakeerthi et al. 2004). If treatment is delayed, CNS infections of *C. bantiana* can lead to death of the patient in 1–6 months (Ajantha et al. 2011). The side effects of the specific anti-fungal drugs must be considered for each patient. No specific duration is suggested in literature for continuing the treatment; however prolonged therapy and the importance of radiographic follow-up is clear (Ajantha et al. 2011). Any residual abscess remaining after surgery (Levin et al. 2004) can be seen with CT or MRI (Kuan et al. 2016). Follow-up imaging can document progression or resolution of the brain abscess or the development of new lesions. Therefore, imaging every 3–6 months to monitor the infection is required (Garzoni et al. 2008). At this point, it is unclear how long after the termination of antifungal agents one should follow up patients radiographically. Physicians must continue to closely monitor the neurological examinations to identify changes in the examination between radiographic follow-up (Kuan et al. 2016).

14.7 Outcome

Overall survival rates in literature are low for *C. bantiana*, despite advances in surgical therapy, radiographic follow-up, and antifungal therapy. Even so, for most of the cases in literature complete resection have better prognosis. In addition to surgery, combination therapy of amphotericin B, voriconazole, and itraconazole as a long-term treatment were successful clinically. Due to low minimally inhibitory concentrations in vitro, caspofungin and anidulafungin are promising for newer antifungals.

14.8 Conclusion

C. bantiana is a dematiaceous fungus that cause cerebral phaeohyphomycosis and is fatal if left untreated. Therefore, it is important to diagnose it rapidly and accurately, which can be best reached with surgical biopsy, pathological examination, and verification via PCR. Different approaches to *C. bantiana* treatment are still discussed, because it is rare to collect meaningful data and it remains difficult to treat. Aggressive surgical resection is advocated to improve prognosis. Prolonged treatment with anti-fungal medicine, especially when combined with newer antifungals, can give more promising results. Even when complete resection and long-term anti-fungal treatment suggests resolution, infections with *C. bantiana* should be continued for follow-up for 1–2 years after apparent resolution to avoid relapse.

References

Ahmad M, Jacobs D, Wu H, Wolk D, Kazmi S, Jaramillo C, Toms S. Cladophialophora bantiana: a rare intracerebral fungal abscess—case series and review of literature. Surg J. 2017;03(02):e62–8.

Ajantha GS, Raghavendra D, Kulkarni R. Cladophialophora bantiana, the neurotropic fungus – a mini review. J Clin Diagn Res. 2011;5:1301–6.

Badali H, Gueidan C, Najafzadeh MJ, Bonifaz A, van den Ende AH, De Hoog GS. Biodiversity of the genus Cladophialophora. Stud Mycol. 2008;61:175–91.

Badali H, De Hoog GS, Curfs-Breuker I, Klaassen CH, Meis JF. Use of amplified fragment length polymorphism to identify 42 Cladophialophora strains related to cerebral phaeohyphomycosis with in vitro antifungal susceptibility. J Clin Microbiol. 2010;48(07):2350–6.

Chakrabarti A. Epidemiology of central nervous system mycoses. Neurol India. 2007;55:191–7.

De Hoog GS. Black fungi: clinical and pathogenic approaches. Med Mycol. 2000;38:243–50.

van den Ende BG, De Hoog S. Variability and molecular diagnostics of the neurotropic species Cladophialophora bantiana. Stud Mycol. 1999;43:151–62.

Emmens RK, Richardson D, Thomas W, et al. Necrotizing cerebritis in an allogeneic bone marrow transplant recipient due to Cladophialophora bantiana. J Clin Microbiol. 1996;34(05):1330–2.

Garzoni C, Markham L, Bijlenga P, Garbino J. Cladophialophora bantiana: a rare cause of fungal brain abscess. Clinical aspects and new therapeutic options. Med Mycol. 2008;46(05):481–6.

De Hoog SG. History of Medical Mycology, Luciano Polonelli, Department of Biomedical, Biotechnological and Translational Sciences, Unit of Microbiology and Virology, University of Parma, Parma, Italy (from the website of international society for human and animal mycology). 1995

Jayakeerthi SR, Dias M, Nagarathna S, Anandh B, Mahadevan A, Chandramuki A. Brain abscess due to cladophialophora bantiana. Indian J Med Microbiol. 2004;22:193–5.

Kantarcıoğlu AS, De Hoog GS. Infections of the central nervous system by melanized fungi: a review of cases presented between 1999 and 2004. Mycoses. 2004;47:4–13.

Kuan CS, Cham CY, Singh G, Yew SM, Tan Y-C, Chong P-S, et al. Genomic analyses of Cladophialophora bantiana, a major cause of cerebral phaeohyphomycosis provides insight into its lifestyle, virulence and adaption in host. PLoS One. 2016;11(8):e0161008.

Lakshmi V, Padmasri C, Umabala P, Sundaram C, Panigrahi M. Cerebral phaeohyphomycosis due to Cladophialophora bantiana. Indian J Med Microbiol. 2008;26:392–5.

Langfelder K, Streibel M, Jahn B, Haase G, Brakhage AA. Biosynthesis of fungal melanins and their importance for human pathogenic fungi. Fungal Genet Biol. 2003;38:143–58.

Levin TP, Baty DE, Fekete T, Truant AL, Suh B. Cladophialophora bantiana brain abscess in a solid-organ transplant recipient: case report and review of the literature. J Clin Microbiol. 2004;42(09):4374–8.

Moller EM, Bahnweg G, Sandermann H, Geiger HH. Asimpleand efficient protocol for isolation of high molecular weight DNA from filamentous fungi, fruit bodies, and infected plant tissues. Nucleic Acids Res. 1992;20:6115–6.

Perfect J, Schell W, Cox G. Phaeohyphomycosis. In: Dismukes W, Pappas P, Sobel J, editors. Clinical mycology. New York: Oxford University Press; 2003. p. 271–82.

Rantala M, Attia S, Koukila-Kähkölä P, De Hoog S, Anttila M, Katila T. *Cladophialophora bantiana* as an emerging pathogen in animals: case report of equine endometritis and review of the literature. J Clin Microbiol. 2015;53:3047–53.

Revankar SG, Sutton DA. Melanized fungi in human disease. Clin Microbiol Rev. 2010;23(4):884–928.

Revankar SG, Sutton DA, Rinaldi MG. Primary central nervous system phaeohyphomycosis: a review of 101 cases. Clin Infect Dis. 2004;38(02):206–16.

Salama AD, Rogers T, Lord GM, Lechler RI, Mason PD. Multiple Cladosporium brain abscess in a renal transplant patient: aggressive management improves outcome. Transplantation. 1997;63(01):160–2.

Satton DA, Rinaldi MG, Sanche SE. Dematiaceous fungi. In: Anaissie EJ, McGinnis MR, Pfaller MA, editors. Clinical mycology. 2nd ed. Philedelphia, PA: Churchill Livingstone/Elsevier; 2009. p. 329–54.

Scheld MW, Whitley RJ, Marra CM. Infections of the central nervous system. 4th ed. Philadelphia, PA: Lippincott Williams & Wilkins; 2004. p. 719.

Seyedmousavi S, Netea MG, Mouton JW, Melchers WJG, Verweij PE, De Hoog GS. Black yeasts and their filamentous relatives: principles of pathogenesis and host defense. Clin Microbiol Rev. 2014;27(3):527–42.

Trinh JV, Steinbach WJ, Schell WA, Kurtzberg J, Giles SS, Perfect JR. Cerebral phaeohyphomycosis in an immunodeficient child treated medically with combination antifungal therapy. Med Mycol. 2003;41(04):339–45.

15 Cladosporium spp., Fusarium spp., Bipolaris spp., Schizophyllum commune, and Scedosporium apiospermum

A. Serda Kantarcioglu

Abbreviations

ALL	Acute lymphoblastic leukemia
AMB	Amphotericin B
AML	Acute myeloid leukemia
CLSI	Clinical and Laboratory Standards Institute
CNS	Central nervous system
CT	Computed tomography
CSF	Cerebrospinal fluid
ECMM	European Confederation of Medical Mycology
EFISG	European Fungal Infection Study Group
ESCMID	European Society of Clinical Microbiology and Infectious Diseases
EUCAST	European Committee on Antimicrobial Susceptibility
G-CSF	Granulocyte colony-stimulating factor
GM-CSF	Granulocyte-macrophage colony-stimulating factor
GPDH	Glyceraldehyde-3-phosphate dehydrogenase
HSCT	Hematopoietic stem cell transplant recipients
ITS	Internal transcribed spacer
KOH	Potassium hydroxide
MALDI-TOF MS	Matrix-assisted laser desorption/ionization mass spectrometer
MEC	Minimum effective concentration
MIC	Minimum inhibitory concentration
MLST	Multi-locus sequence typing
MRI	Magnetic resonance imaging
PCR	Polymerase chain reaction
SDA	Sabouraud dextrose agar
VRZ	Voriconazole

15.1 *Cladosporium* Species

15.1.1 Introduction

Cladosporium species are among the most common and widespread dematiaceous (dark-pigmented) molds (De Hoog et al. 2000; Bensch et al. 2010, 2012, 2015). Members of *Cladosporium* are commonly isolated from soil and organic matter. They represent the most frequently isolated airborne fungi (Asan et al. 2002, 2003, 2004). *Cladosporium spp* form black spots on foods and have been isolated from cereal grains, peanuts, fruits, and refrigerated meat, particularly beef. *Cladosporium* species, which can grow at low temperatures, can grow under refrigerated storage conditions. In the routine laboratory work, *Cladosporium* species are frequently

A. S. Kantarcioglu (✉)
Division of Mycology, Department of Medical Microbiology, Cerrahpasa Medical Faculty, Istanbul University-Cerrahpasa, Istanbul, Turkey

M. Turgut et al. (eds.), *Fungal Infections of the Central Nervous System*,
https://doi.org/10.1007/978-3-030-06088-6_15

isolated as contaminants, but these species can, though rarely, be pathogenic and toxic to humans, cause allergic reactions, and trigger asthmatic attacks. *Cladosporium* species can rarely be cause of cerebral phaeohyphomycoses.

15.1.2 Taxonomy

The genus *Cladosporium* has been shown to be both morphologically and phylogenetically heterogeneous. The genus has undergone a number of revisions. On the basis of molecular data, the true human-pathogenic species *C. bantiana*, *C. carrionii*, and *C. devriesii*, characterized by their thermotolerance and the absence of conidiophores with pigmented conidial scars, were transferred to *Cladophialophora* (Bensch et al. 2012; De Hoog et al. 2011). Recently, extensive revisions based on polyphasic approaches have demonstrated that *Cladosporium* species associated with human disease, *C. cladosporioides*, *C. herbarum*, and *C. sphaerospermum*, are species complexes encompassing several sibling species that can only be distinguished by phylogenetic analyses (Sandoval-Denis et al. 2015).

15.1.3 Morphology

In the saprophytic phase, species produce olive-green to brown or black colonies and have dark-pigmented conidia that are formed in simple or branching, shorter or longer chains. Colonies are slow growing, suede-like to floccose, often becoming powdery due to the production of abundant conidia (Fig. 15.1a–c). The reverse side of a colony of *Cladosporium* on agar is very dark greenish-black or blue-black. Vegetative hyphae, conidiophores, and conidia are equally pigmented. Conidiophores are more or less distinct from the vegetative hyphae, being erect, straight, or flexuose, unbranched or branched only in the apical region. *Cladosporium* species produce many one-celled conidia, but two- and three-celled forms are also common. Conidia are darkly pigmented, ellipsoid to cylindrical in shape. Conidia are produced in branched acropetal chains, being smooth, verrucose, or echinulate, one to four celled, and have a distinct dark hilum. In the parasitic phase, feoid (brown-pigmented) hyphae can be observed in the tissue. These fungi in the tissue can vary as far as their structure is concerned, ranging from yeast-like to

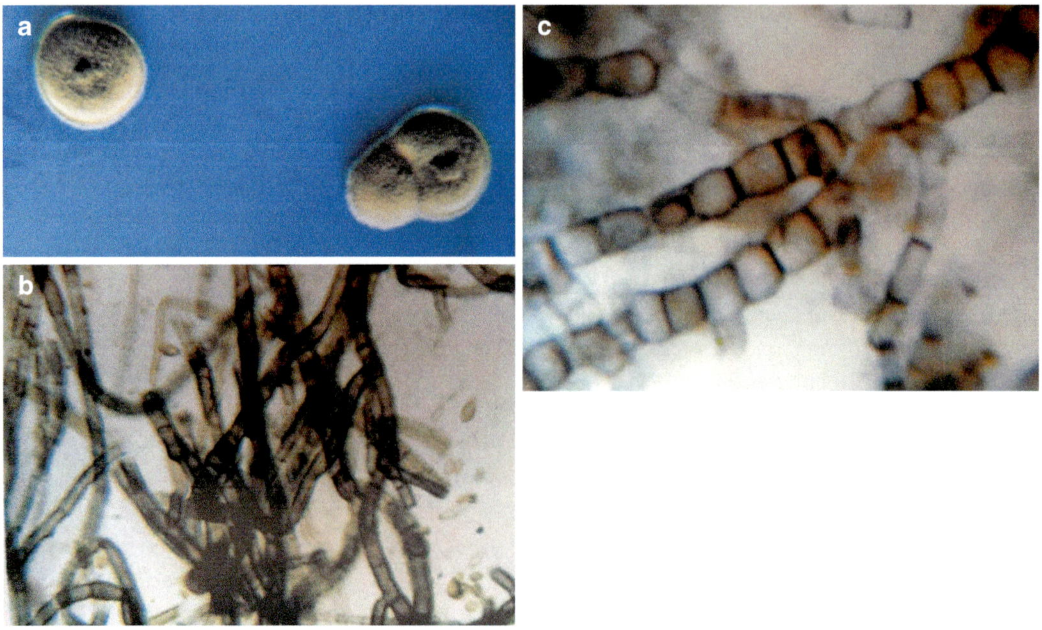

Fig. 15.1 (**a**): Colonies (on SDA) and (**b**) microscopy of *Cladosporium sphaerospermum*, (**c**) microscopy of *Cladosporium macrocarpum* (lactophenol coton blue stain, ×40)

that of long hyphae, or the combination of these may be seen (De Hoog et al. 1995).

15.1.4 Ecology and Epidemiology

Species of *Cladosporium* are widely distributed in the air as well as decayed organic matter, and very often they are food contaminants. These fungi are commonly encountered on plant and other kinds of debris, frequently colonizing lesions of plant pathogenic fungi, and are also isolated from air, soil, food, paint, textiles, and other organic matters as saprobes; they are also common endophytes (Crous et al. 2007). The small conidia of *Cladosporium* species easily spread in large numbers over long distances and represent the most common fungal components isolated from air (Asl et al. 2017). Central nervous system (CNS) infections caused by *Cladosporium* species were rarely reported, from Turkey (Küllü et al. 1985; Kantarcioğlu et al. 2002), Spain (Lalueza et al. 2011), Taiwan (Chen et al. 2013), and Germany (Tauber et al. 2014).

15.1.5 Clinical Presentations

Five cases of culture-proven CNS infections due to *Cladosporium* species have been reported to date, including a posttraumatic cerebral infection in a 30-year-old apparently healthy man due to *Cladosporium cladosporioides* (Kantarcioğlu et al. 2002), acute meningitis in a 73-year-old wood worker due to *Cladosporium sphaerospermum* (Chen et al. 2013), brain abscess in a 45-year-old man due to *Cladosporium macrocarpum* (Lalueza et al. 2011), two mixed fungal encephalitis due to *Cladosporium* spp. in a 47-year-old woman who was receiving chemotherapy, and in a 48-year-old man who had cardiac surgery (Tauber et al. 2014). Two cases were associated with timber puncture (Kantarcioğlu et al. 2002; Chen et al. 2013). Occupational exposure or traumatic inoculation might be important. *C. macrocarpum* could have reached the brain through blood vessels by directly spreading from the upper gastrointestinal tract following celiac plexus neurolysis (Lalueza et al. 2011). The fungus was isolated from cerebrospinal fluid (CSF) and/or brain tissue or abscess martial. Identification of isolated fungi was confirmed by molecular techniques in four of cases (Kantarcioğlu et al. 2002; Chen et al. 2013; Tauber et al. 2014).

The common primary symptom was headache; diplopia was reported in one patient with abscesses in brain stem (Kantarcioğlu et al. 2002), fever in two cases (Lalueza et al. 2011; Chen et al. 2013), and acute urinary retention and right flank pain in one patient with acute meningitis (Chen et al. 2013).

15.1.6 Laboratory Diagnosis

Direct microscopy of a potassium hydroxide (KOH) (10%) preparation of the biopsy or surgical specimen shows the presence of phaeoid (dark colored) septate hyphae. Giemsa-stained preparations of CSF, tissue, or abscess material can show irregularly swollen, septate branched hyphae and/or spherical or oblong, thick-walled conidial chains (Fig. 15.2a–d) (Kantarcioğlu et al. 2002).

Cladosporium spp grows fast on agars (Sabouraud agar with or without addition of antibiotics, without actidione, etc.) forming darkly pigmented (pigmented molds), olive-green to darkly brown colonies of powder-like structure (Fig. 15.1a). The vegetative mycelium is usually dark-colored (Fig. 15.1b, c). The colonies are formed after 5 days. The identification and differentiation of species is possible after cultivation on potato dextrose agar at the temperature of 25 °C. The greatest number of conidia does not multiply at the temperature of 25 °C (De Hoog et al. 1995).

Members of *Cladosporium* are relatively easy to identify to genus and species complex based on their typical conidiogenous structures. However, morphological identification of *Cladosporium* species is difficult given the high morphological similarity between closely related species. It is recommended that phenotypic identifications be confirmed with DNA sequencing. Genus-level identification is usually sufficient, and morphological identification can be confirmed by ITS and D1/D2 sequence

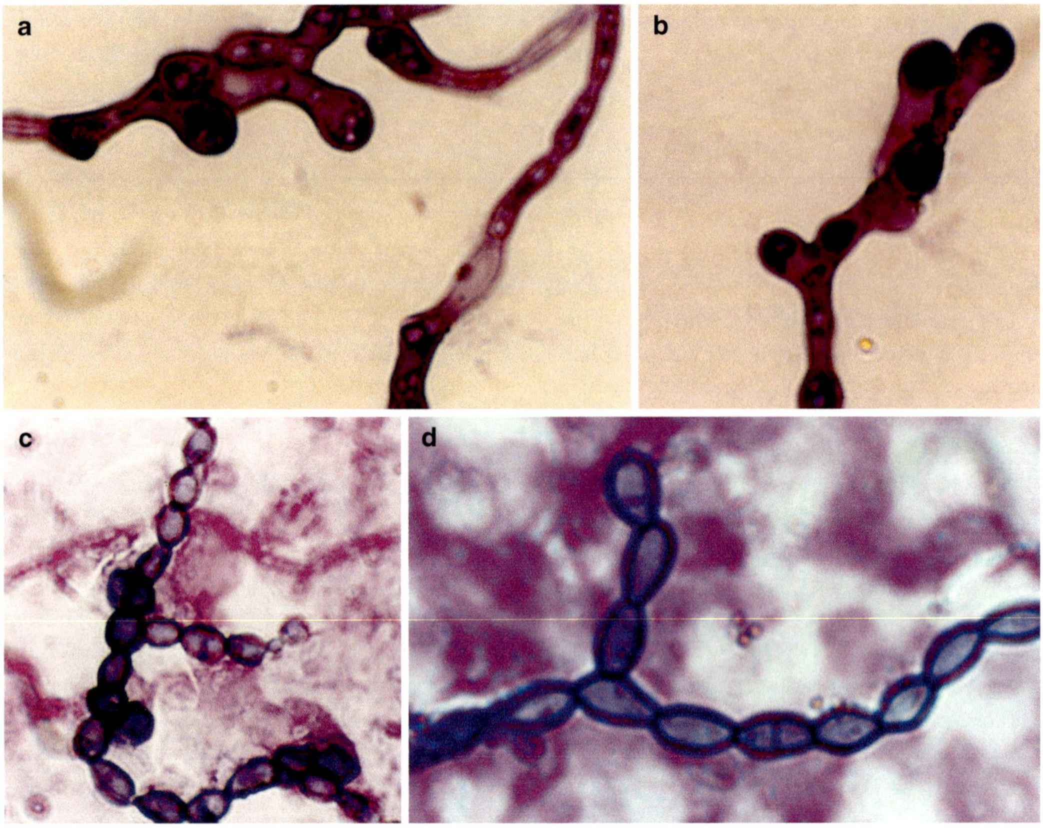

Fig. 15.2 (**a**–**d**) Examples of in vivo fungal elements observed in three subsequent CSF specimens of the patient. (**a**–**c**) Irregularly swollen hyphal elements (stained with Ehrlich–Ziehl–Neelsen); (**d**) chains of swollen cells and septate hyphal element (stained with Giemsa)

analysis. Multilocus gene analysis of the ITS, D1/D2, EF-1α, and actin gene loci is necessary for accurate species identification (Bensch et al. 2012; Asl et al. 2017). This is especially important for members of the *C. cladosporioides* complex, which is demonstrated the greatest species diversity, the highest number of species associated with clinical samples, and also, the greatest number of undescribed species (Sandoval-Denis et al. 2015).

15.1.7 Antifungal Susceptibility, Treatment, and Outcome

Antifungal susceptibility tests of the case isolates were performed using different methodologies. Minimum inhibitory concentrations of the isolates reported in one clinical case (Guarro et al. 1997) and in several in vitro antifungal susceptibility studies (McGinnis and Pasarell 1998; Kantarcioglu and Yucel 2002) were shown in Tables 15.1 and 15.2.

Treatment was done with oral voriconazole (VRZ) (400 mg/day) in one patient (Lalueza et al. 2011) after 30 days he was discharged from hospital on oral VRZ (400 mg/day). Complete excision of the brain abscess combined with antifungal therapy with VRZ or/and amphotericin B (AmB) and flucytosine may be effective in CNS cases.

15.2 *Fusarium* Species

15.2.1 Introduction

Fusarium species are hyaline hyphomycetes widely distributed in nature. They are found in soil, air, and water and can be transported in veg-

Table 15.1 In vitro MICs of non-*bantiana Cladosporium* species mentioned as associated with CNS cases

Reference	Species		MIC (μg/ml)						
			AMB	5-FC	KTZ	FLZ	ITZ	MCZ	TRB
Guarro et al. (1997)[a]	*C. cladosporioides* CBS 171.54	C	1	4	>16	32	0.5	1	
		H	4	64	0.5	>64	2	8	
	C. cladosporioides FMR 5031	C	0.125	0.125	<0.03	16	0.06	0.25	
		H	0.5	0.125	0.5	32	1	4	
	C. cladosporioides IFO 4459	C	0.25	0.25	1		0.5	1	
		H	8	>64	>16		>16	>16	
	C. sphaerospermum CBS 193.54	C	1	4	4	>64	>16	4	
		H	2	4	>16	>64	>16	>16	
	C. sphaerospermum FMR 5030	C	0.5	8	2	>64	0.5	8	
		H	8	>128	4	>64	1	0.5	
SK (2002) case[b]	*C. cladosporioides*		8		<0.03	0.25	0.06	<0.03	0.5

Abbreviations: *MIC* minimal inhibitory concentration, *AMB* amphotericin B, *5-FC* flucytosine, *KTZ* ketoconazole; *FLZ* fluconazol, *ITZ* itraconazol, *MCZ* miconazole, *TRB* terbinafine, *CAS* caspofungin, *MCF* micafungin, *AND* anidulafungin, *C* with conidial inoculum, *H* with hyphal inoculum

[a]A broth method

[b]National Committee for Clinical Laboratory Standards Institute M38-P guidelines

etable tissues. Some are plant pathogens, causing root and stem rot, vascular wilt, or fruit rot. They can be recovered from the deepest roots in soil, and they may occasionally cause infection in animals (Nucci and Anaissie 2007). Several species have emerged as important opportunistic pathogens in humans causing hyalohyphomycosis (especially in burn victims and bone marrow transplant patients) and are documented agents of both superficial and systemic infections in humans. *Fusarium* species are frequently found on cereal grains, where it may cause seedling and head blight and produce mycotoxins and may also cause allergic diseases (sinusitis) in immunocompetent individuals (Nucci and Anaissie 2007; Refai et al. 1969).

15.2.2 Taxonomy

Fusarium genus is a mold of kingdom Fungi, phylum Ascomycota, class Sordariomycetes, order Hypocreales, and family Nectriaceae. The genus *Fusarium* was divided into sections (Nelson et al. 1994), but the current classification scheme replaces the designation "section" with "complex." Currently the genus *Fusarium* comprises at least 300 phylogenetically distinct species, 20 species complexes, and 9 monotypic lineages (Balajee et al. 2009; O'Donnell et al. 2015). Most of the identified opportunistic *Fusarium* pathogens belong to the *F. solani* complex and *F. oxysporum* complex.

15.2.3 Morphology and Biology

Macromorphology. Most *Fusarium* species produce woolly to cottony, flat, spreading colonies. The color of the colony may be white, cream, tan, salmon, cinnamon, yellow, red, violet, pink, or purple; and on the reverse, it may be colorless, tan, red, dark purple, or brown.

Microscopic morphology. Sporodochia consist of masses of branched conidiophores. In culture they build up and are seen macroscopically as light-colored-raised bodies. Macroconidia are borne in sporodochia. They are mostly long, slender, rather pointed at both ends, dorsoventrally curved, sickle-shaped, and septated, and possess a basal foot cell. Microconidia may be formed. Typically they are present on the aerial mycelium of the culture growth, appearing as small, usually one-celled spores, and oval-shaped, tear-drop or pear-shaped and sometimes even spherical. Mesoconidia are the fusoid conidia that are longer than microconidia with three to four septae but shorter than macroconidia with lack of foot-shaped and notched basal cell. The production of both fusoid macroconidia (hyaline, multicellular clusters, macroconidia with foot cells at the base

Table 15.2 MICs and MFCs of non-*bantiana* *Cladosporium* species mentioned as associated with CNS cases from small series

Reference	Species (strain number)	MIC (MFC) parameter	Results for antifungal agents (μg/ml)								
			AMB	5-FC	VRZ	PSZ	ITZ	TRB	CAS	AND	MCF
McGinnis and Pasarell (1998)[a]	*C. cladosporioides* (3)	Range	0.03–2 (0.4)		0.06–1 (0.08)		0.03–0.25 (0.12)				
		GM									
		MIC50									
		MIC90									
	C. sphaerospermum (5)	Range	2–8 (3.48)		0.5–1 (0.87)		0.25–32 (0.76)				
		GM									
		MIC50									
		MIC90									
SK (2002) in vitro[b]	*Cladosporium* sp. (21)	Range	<0.03–>16 (0.06–>16)				<0.03–16 (0.5–>16)	0.125–128 (1–>128)			
		GM	0.9 (2.0)				1.4 (4.1)	3.4 (11.9)			
		MIC50	8 (16)				4 (8)	8–32			
		MIC90									
Sandoval-Denis et al. (2015)[c]	*C. cladosporioides* complex (57)	Range	0.06–2	0.06–>32	0.25–16	<0.03–1	<0.03–2	<0.03–4	0.125–8	0.03–0.5	0.03–0.5
		GM	0.73	1.20	1.65	0.40	0.34	0.12	2.78	0.19	0.11
		MIC50									
		MIC90	1	4	4	0.5	0.5	1	8	0.5	0.25
	C. cladosporioides (3)	Range	0.5–1	1–2	0.5–16	0.25–1	0.25–0.5	0.5–2	1–4	0.125–0.25	0.125
		GM	0.79	1.26	1.59	0.40	0.31	1.00	2.00	0.16	0.13
		MIC50									
		MIC90									
	Cladosporium sp. (29)	Range	0.125–2	0.06–>16	0.25–8	<0.03–1	<0.03–2	<0.03–4	0.125–8	0.03–0.5	0.03–0.5
		GM	0.67	1.10	1.73	0.43	0.36	0.09	2.00	0.18	0.10
		MIC50									

		MIC90	1.00	4.00	4.00	0.50	0.50	1.00	8.00	0.50	0.25
	C. sphaerospermum complex (17)	Range	0.125–2	0.06–4	0.5–16	0.06–4	0.25–>16	<0.03–1	0.06–4	<0.03–1	0.06–1
		GM	1.13	1.13	1.70	0.64	1.13	0.06	1.27	0.15	0.03
		MIC50									
		MIC90	2	2	8	2	32	0.5	4	0.25	0.125
	C. macrocarpum (1)	Range	0.5	2	1	0.25	0.5	0.125	1	0.125	0.5
		GM									
		MIC50									
		MIC90									

Abbreviations: *MIC* minimal inhibitory concentration, *MFC* minimal fungicidal concentration, *AMB* amphotericin B, *5-FC* flucytosine, *KTZ* ketoconazole, *FLZ* fluconazol, *ITZ* itraconazol, *VRZ* voriconazole, *PSZ* posaconazole, *TRB* terbinafine, *CAS* caspofungin, *MCF* micafungin, *AND* anidulafungin, *ND* not determined

In calculating GM values, MICs of ≤0.03 or >16 μg/ml were classed as 0.03, or 32 μg/ml, respectively

50%, MICs (MFCs) at which 50% of isolates are inhibited (killed), respectively

[a]National Committee for Clinical Laboratory Standards M27-A guidelines

[b]National Committee for Clinical Laboratory Standards M38-P guidelines

[c]Clinical Laboratory Standards Institute M38-A2 method

of the macroconidium) and microconidia (hyaline, unicellular, ovoid to cylindrical in slimy head or chains) are characteristic of the genus *Fusarium*. If microconidia are present, the shape and mode of cell formation (chains or false heads) are important in identification. Chlamydoconidia exist in some, but not all *Fusarium* spp. They are sometimes present and appear singly, in clumps or in chains, and their walls may be rough or smooth. Their cytoplasm contains a great deal of nutrients, as is evident by oily globules (Fig. 15.3b–d). *Fusarium* can be distinguished from *Acremonium* by its curved, multicellular macroconidia (Refai et al. 1969; Nucci and Anaissie 2009).

15.2.4 Ecology

Fusarium species are the causal agents of several plant diseases of global importance and cause important diseases in many crops. *Fusarium* spp. cause many different crown, stem, fruit, and root rots, head blights, stalk rots, and vascular wilts of plants important for agriculture. As with other microorganisms, molecular tools are now becoming available to study the ecology of *Fusarium* at various levels. The fungus was isolated from hospital environment and water tanks (Yergeau et al. 2006; Okten and Asan 2012; Edel-Hermann et al. 2016; Anaissie et al. 2001; Chowdhary et al. 2015).

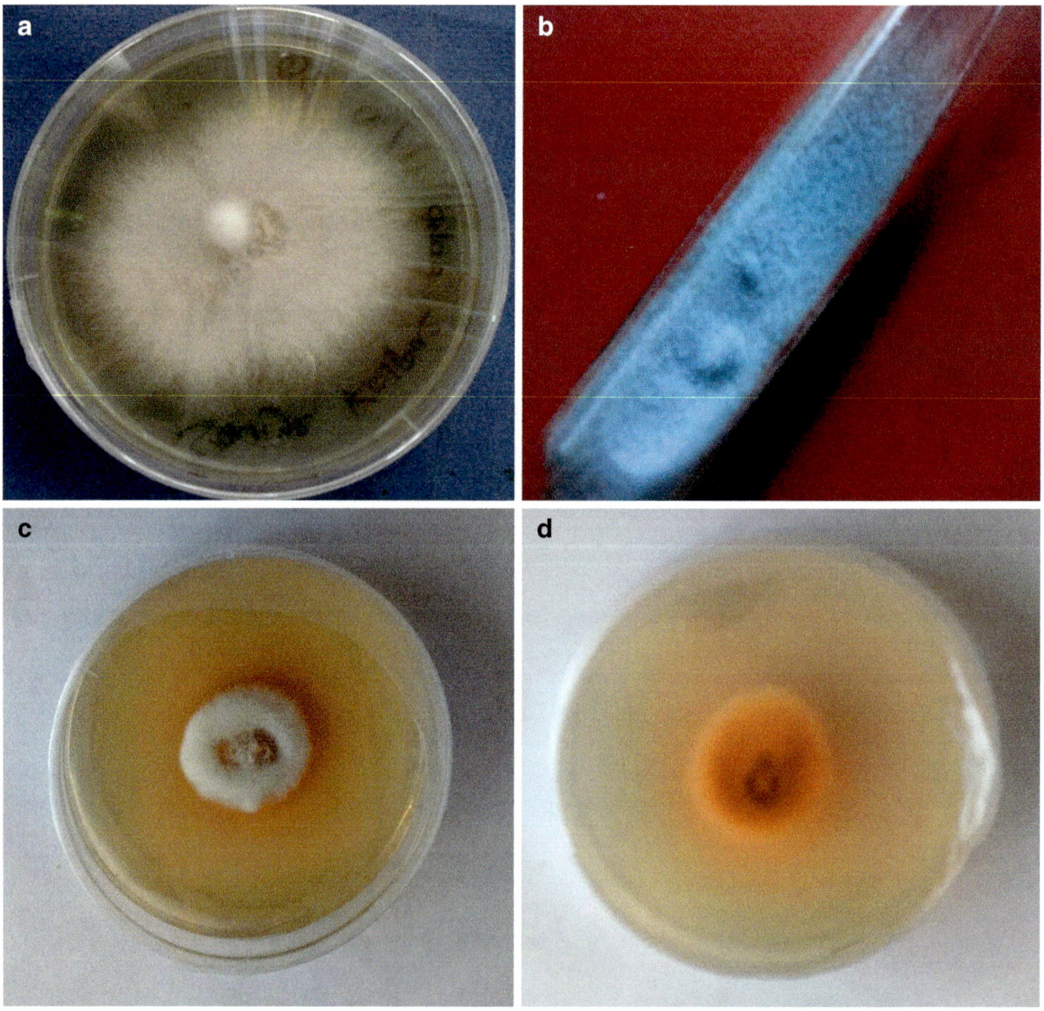

Fig. 15.3 Colonies of (**a**) *F. oxysporum*; (**b**) *F. sporotrichioides*; (**c**) *F. solani*; (**d**) reverse of *F. soloni* (on SDA media)

15.2.5 Epidemiology

Almost all reported CNS infections were in disseminated fusariosis cases. Disseminated disease with *Fusarium* is exceptional and in most cases has occurred in severely immunocompromised patients with hematological malignancies. To our knowledge, disseminated human infection including CNS involvement by the *Fusarium* species was first described in 1973, in a 2 and 1/2-year-old Caucasian boy with a history of acute lymphoblastic leukemia (ALL) (Cho 1973, *F. solani*). *Fusarium solani* was isolated on culture. Another case of Fusarium disseminated infection including brain abscesses in a 2-year-old girl with burns who had also skin and renal abscesses was documented at autopsy (Abramovsky et al. 1974). Another pediatric patient was a 3-year-old boy with a history of ALL. Schwartz et al. (2013) reported a brain abscess due to *F. oxysporum* in a 1-year-old girl with ALL (Antunes et al. 1998), and 4 fatal cases were reported in series of brain abscesses (Lortholary et al. 2010). Agamanolis et al. (1991) described *Fusarium* meningoencephalitis in a child with ALL. A 76-year-old farmer with ALL (Vincent et al. 2003) due to *F. solani*, a 53-year-old woman with acute promyelocytic leukaemia (Anten et al. 2008), a 69-year-old man with acute myeloid leukemia (AML) and an allogeneic stem cell recipient who had basal meningitis and optic nerve involvement (Kapp et al. 2011), and a 50-year old woman with diabetes mellitus and ALL with fatal brain abscesses were reported (Garcia et al. 2015) in the literature. Peterson et al. (2014) described an intracranial *Fusarium* abscess in an immunocompetent Hispanic woman. Other patients were reported in a few case series by Boutati and Anaissie (1997), de Medeiros et al. (2000), and Pagano et al. (2005). Cases were reported from Canada ($n = 1$), Germany ($n = 1$), the Netherlands ($n = 1$), United Kingdom ($n = 1$), France ($n = 4$), and USA ($n = 5$).

Several patients with *Fusarium* brain abscess were reported in a few case series by Lortholary et al. (2010), Boutati and Anaissie (1997), De Medeiros et al. (2000), and Pagano et al. (2005). Cases were reported from Canada ($n = 1$), France ($n = 4$), Germany ($n = 1$), the Netherlands ($n = 1$), and the USA ($n = 8$).

15.2.6 Pathogenesis

15.2.6.1 Virulence and Pathogenic Potential of *Fusarium* Species

Fusarium species possess several virulence factors, including the ability to produce mycotoxins, including trichothecenes, which suppress humoral and cellular immunity, and may also cause tissue breakdown. Angioinvasion by hyphae with consequent necrosis or hemorrhage of surrounding tissue and hematogenous spread up to brain and meninges can be seen in Fusarium infections. In addition, *Fusarium* species have the ability to adhere to prosthetic material and to produce proteases and collagenases. *Fusarium solani* is the most virulent species, as shown in a murine model of fusariosis in immunocompetent animals (Nucci and Anaissie 2007; Garcia et al. 2015).

15.2.6.2 Host Defenses

Although little information is available regarding host defenses against *Fusarium* species, invasive fusariosis shares many features with invasive aspergillosis and other invasive mold infections, including its occurrence in patients receiving high doses of corticosteroids and those with prolonged and profound neutropenia. The importance of immunity in the pathogenesis of fusariosis is supported by in vitro and in vivo experimental studies, the unique susceptibility of severely immunocompromised patients to disseminated fusariosis, and the strong correlation between immune reconstitution and outcome (Nucci and Anaissie 2007).

The innate immunity plays a major role in the defense against mold infections (LeibundGut-Landmann et al. 2012; Romani 2008). Macrophages and neutrophils damage fusarial hyphae, and their effect is primed by gamma interferon, granulocyte colony-stimulating factor (G-CSF), granulocyte-macrophage colony-stimulating factor (GM-CSF) (Gaviria et al. 1999), and interleukin-15 (Winn et al. 2005). The effect of interleukin-15 is mediated by the release of interleukin-8 and by direct stimulation of hyphal damage. More recently, the role of

Toll-like receptors in the innate immune recognition of fungi has been recognized (Romani 2004, 2008; Verma et al. 2015), and although little is known about fusariosis and Toll-like receptors, this system is likely important in invasive fusariosis as well.

The importance of T-cell defenses against *Fusarium* is illustrated by the occurrence of disseminated fusariosis in nonneutropenic hematopoietic stem cell transplant recipients (HSCT) (Nucci et al. 2004). These patients have severe T-cell immunodeficiency caused by multiple therapies for their underlying disease and for graft-versus-host disease. Further supporting the importance of T-cell immunity and phagocytes is the major impact of corticosteroid therapy on the outcome of fusariosis, as shown by the much higher death rate among recipients of such therapy than among patients who were not receiving corticosteroids (Nucci et al. 2003).

15.2.7 Portal of Entry and Routes of Infection

Given the ubiquity of *Fusarium* species in the environment, fusariosis may potentially be acquired in the community, as suggested by the presence of airborne fusarial conidia in outdoor air samples. Showering and other water-related activities appeared to be an efficient mechanism for the dispersion of airborne fusarial conidia and transmission to the immunocompromised host, as shown by the close molecular relatedness between water and patient isolates (Anaissie et al. 2001; Boutati and Anaissie 1997; Raad et al. 2002).

15.2.8 Signs and Symptoms

Symptoms of CNS fusariosis are nonspecific, involving severe headache, altered mental status, confusion, fever, nausea, vomiting, and neck stiffness in meningitis cases.

15.2.9 Clinical Presentations

Immunocompromised patients at high risk for fusariosis are those with prolonged and profound neutropenia and/or severe T-cell immunodeficiency (Table 15.3). Brain abscess was the main clinical presentation (Cho et al. 1973; Abramovsky et al. 1974; Antunes et al. 1998; Agamanolis et al. 1991; Vincent et al. 2003; Kapp et al. 2011; Garcia et al. 2015; Peterson et al. 2014; Steinberg et al. 1983; Schwartz et al. 2013).

The principal portal of entry for *Fusarium* spp. is the airways, followed by the skin at site of tissue breakdown and possibly the mucosal membranes (Nucci and Anaissie 2007). Nasal route was the presumed mode of entry of the fungus into the cerebrum in one patient (Garcia et al. 2015). Brain abscess and/or meningitis and ventriculitis were reported, and concomitant endophthalmitis were reported in one patient (Kapp et al. 2011).

Disseminated disease is the most frequent and challenging clinical form of fusariosis in immunocompromised patients, accounting for approximately 70% of fusariosis in this population. Patients at risk for disseminated fusariosis include those with acute leukemia and prolonged and profound neutropenia and patients undergoing HSCT.

15.2.10 Histopathology

Pathologic examination of necrotic purulent abscess and biopsy materials with slides stained with hematoxylin and eosin showed inflamatory cells, branched septate hyphae invading the walls of the blood vessels (Peterson et al. 2014; Steinberg et al. 1983), and Gomori methenamine silver staining showed septated hyphae with acute angled branching in reported cases (Peterson et al. 2014).

In tissue, the hyphae can be similar to those of *Aspergillus* species, with hyaline and septate filaments that typically dichotomize in acute and right angles. However, adventitious sporulation may be present in tissue, and the finding of hyphae and yeast-like structures together is highly suggestive of fusariosis in the high-risk population. In the absence of microbial growth, distinguishing fusariosis from other hyalohyphomycoses may be difficult and requires the use of in situ hybridization in paraffin-embedded tissue specimens (Hayden et al. 2003).

Table 15.3 CNS infections by *Fusarium* species

Reference	Pathogen	Age/sex/race/geography	Risk factor/underlying disease	Clinical syndrome	Therapy	Outcome
Cho et al. (1973)	*F. solani*	2[illegible]/M/C/USA	ALL	Disseminated		
Abramovsky et al. (1974)	*Fusarium* sp.	2/F/B/USA	Burned	Brain, renal abscess		
Steinberg et al. (1983)	*Fusarium* sp.	17/F/W/USA	Infectious mononucleous	Brain abscess	AmB	Died
Agamanolis et al. (1991)	*Fusarium* sp.	15/M/USA	ALL, contaminated skin wound	Meningoencephalitis	MCZ, 5-FC, AmB	Died
Antunes et al. (1998)	*Fusarium* sp.	[illegible]/USA	ALL	Brain abscess (M)	Surgery	Survived
Kapp et al. (2011)	*Fusarium* sp.	69/M/Germany	AML	Meningitis, endophthalmitis	AmB	Died
Vincent et al. (2003)	*Fusarium* sp.	76/M/USA	AML, N	Disseminated	L-AmB, ITZ, VRZ	Died
Schwartz et al. (2013)	*F. oxysporum*	1/F/Canada	AA, HSCT, N	Brain abscess, lung, blood	L-AmB, VRZ, granulocytes	Died
	F. solani	15/F/Canada	AML, HSCT, N	Brain abscess, lung	L-AmB, VRZ	Died
Peterson et al. (2014)	*Fusarium* sp.	33/F/H/USA	none	Brain abscess	Surgery, VRZ, TRB, AmB	
Garcia et al. (2015)	*F. solani*	50/F/USA	DM, ALL, APST, N	Brain abscess	VRZ, L-AmB, G-CSF	

Abbreviations: *ALL* acute lymphocytic leukemia, *AML* acute myeloid leukemia, *N* neutropenia, *AA* aplastic anemia, *HSCT* hematopoietic stem cell transplant, *DM* diabetes mellitus, *APST* autologous peripheral stem cell transplant, *B* black, *C* Caucasian, *H* Hispanic, *W* white, *M* multiple, *5-FC* flucytosine, *AMB* amphotericin B deoxycholate, *L-AMB* liposomal amphotericin B, *KTZ* ketoconazole, *ITZ* itraconazole, *MCZ* miconazole, *VRZ* voriconazole, *TRB* terbinafine, *G-CSF* granulocyte colony-stimulating factor, *w* week(s), *m* month(s)

15.2.11 Laboratory Diagnosis

Microbiologically examined specimens reported were usually brain biopsy or aspirated abscess contents and only occasionally CSF. Direct microscopy of a KOH (10%) preparation of the biopsy or surgical specimen showed the presence of hyaline septate hyphae. Giemsa stained imprinted preparations can show septate branched hyphal elements. They typically branch at acute and usually at right angles. The hyphae of *Fusarium* in tissue resemble those of *Aspergillus* spp.; the filaments are hyaline, septate, and 3–8 µm in diameter (Fig. 15.4a).

Fusarium spp is a hyaline fungus; however, darkly pigmented hyphae have also been reported from infected humans (Segal et al. 1998; Kantarcioglu et al. 2010) and rat tissue (Sugiura et al. 2003).

Some portions of tissue samples can be inoculated both on multipoints of Sabouraud Dextrose Agar (SDA) supplemented with chloramphenicol (0.5 µg/ml), or containing gentamycin, and on Brain Heart Infusion Agar and can be incubated at 30 °C for 4–10 days. Contrary to aspergillosis, 50–70% of cases with disseminated fusariosis have positive blood cultures. Growth on SDA can be rapid, cottony, whitish, and raised in center (Fig. 15.3a–c). Colonies can become slightly powdery and pale buff or tan having a pale brown reverse after 2 weeks at 25 °C (Fig. 15.3d). It may produce a strong disagreeable odor. Cycloheximide inhibits the growth on SDA. On potato dextrose agar, *Fusarium* spp. produce white-, lavender-, pink-, salmon-, or gray-colored colonies (which readily change in color) with velvety to cottony surfaces. Dark buff mycelial colonies can grow from tissue and abscess samples and should be examined using unstained wet mounts with physiological.

saline that may reveal darkly pigmented *Fusarium* strains (Kantarcioglu et al. 2010). Microscopic morphology of the isolate should be examined by staining with lactophenol cotton blue (Fig. 15.4b–d).

Phenotypical identification of *Fusarium* to the genus or species complex level is possible in the clinical microbiology laboratories relying mainly on morphology-based identification by recognizing macroscopic (colony appearance, texture/structure, pigmentation, and color of exudates) and microscopic (conidiogenous cells (type and size of conidia) and type of conidiogenesis) (Al-Hatmi et al. 2017). *Fusarium* species grow easily and rapidly in most media without cycloheximide. Although the genus *Fusarium* can be identified by the production of hyaline, banana-shaped, multicellular macroconidia with a foot cell at the base, species identification is difficult and may require molecular methods. *Fusarium* spp. may be confirmed DNA polymerase chain reaction genetic analysis.

Many species within the genus *Fusarium* that were recognized based on morphological characters proved to be species complexes, with little to no morphological differences, rather than single species. For their recognition, often multi-locus sequence typing (MLST) is required. Multi-locus sequence analysis of EF-1α, β-tubulin, calmodulin, and RPB2 has revealed the presence of multiple cryptic species within each "morphospecies" of medically important fusaria (Balajee et al. 2009; van Diepeningen et al. 2015). For instance, *Fusarium solani* represents a complex (i.e., *F. solani* complex) of over 45 phylogenetically distinct species of which at least 20 are associated with human infections. Similarly, members of the *Fusarium oxysporum* complex are phylogenetically diverse, as are members of the *Fusarium incarnatum-equiseti* complex and *Fusarium chlamydosporum* complex (Balajee et al. 2009; Tortorano et al. 2014; Salah et al. 2015).

The clinician and the microbiologist must be cautious, because *Fusarium* species may contaminate laboratory specimens and pseudo-outbreaks of fusariosis may occur. In support of infection is the isolation of several colonies from the same specimen or of the same fungus from different specimens (as opposed to isolating a single colony from only one biological sample), a positive direct examination of the biological material, and, most importantly, the site of isolation and the host (Nucci and Anaissie 2007).

The 1,3-β-D-glucan test is usually positive in invasive fusarial infections but cannot distinguish

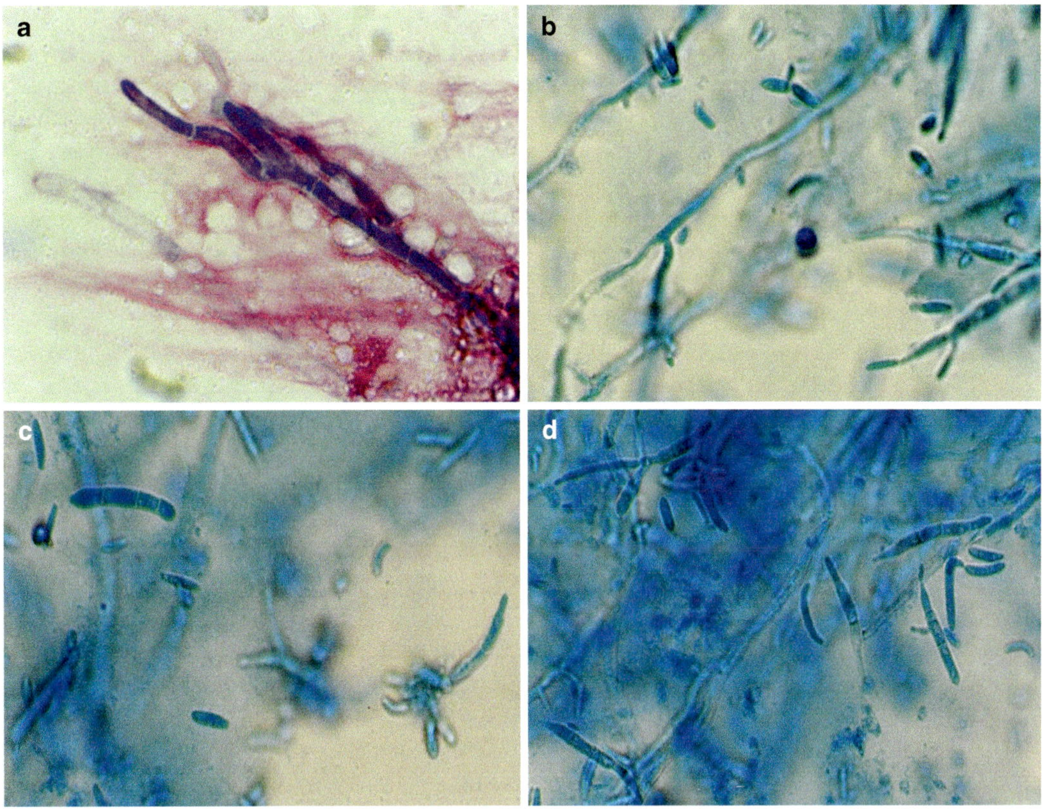

Fig. 15.4 (**a**) The hyphae of *Fusarium* in tissue resemble those of *Aspergillus* spp. (Giemsa-stained imprint slide preparation, ×100); (**b**) mesoconidia and single, smooth-walled chlamydoconidia, (**c**) macroconidia, (**d**): acute- and right-angled branching hyphae with meso- and macroconidia (lactophenol cotton blue stained, ×40)

Fusarium from other fungal infections (*Candida*, *Aspergillus*, *Trichosporon*, and others) which are also detected by the assay (Wright et al. 2011; Lamoth 2016). However, a positive 1,3-β-D-glucan test and a negative galactomannan test in a high-risk patient with mold infection are highly suggestive of fusariosis.

Fusarium spp. was identified using MALDI-TOF mass spectrometry, and identifications were confirmed via DNA sequence analysis (Triest et al. 2015; Marinach-Patrice et al. 2009). Results from mass spectrometry and molecular identification agreed in five of the six cases in which results from morphological and molecular identification were not in agreement. MALDI-TOF yielded results within 1 h, making it a valuable tool for identifying clinical *Fusarium* isolates at the species level (van Diepeningen et al. 2015; Marinach-Patrice et al. 2009).

15.2.12 Antifungal Susceptibility, Treatment, and Outcome

In vitro susceptibility testing of *Fusarium* is becoming important because resistance profiles are species-specific. Reference methods for in vitro antifungal susceptibility testing are those of Clinical and Laboratory Standards Institute (CLSI) and European Committee on Antimicrobial Susceptibility (EUCAST), but breakpoints have not yet been established. Epidemiological cut-off values for some *Fusarium* species have been determined in order to differentiate wild-type from non-wild-type isolates (Al-Hatmi et al. 2017). *Fusarium* species do not have a normal minimum inhibitory concentration (MIC) and minimum effective concentration (MEC) distribution (Alastruey-Izquierdo et al. 2008; Al-Hatmi et al. 2014), and therefore prediction of antifungal susceptibility of a single strain is difficult. However, at least the species show different tendencies in their susceptibility against various antifungal compounds (Al-Hatmi et al. 2014).

Fusarium strains have high levels of intrinsic antifungal resistance. Recently, diagnostic guidelines recommend AmB and VRZ as the preferred drugs of choice for treatment of deep and disseminated infections (Tortorano et al. 2014). Although AMB and VRZ are sufficient for the treatment of the majority of *Fusarium* infections, some *Fusarium* species are not susceptible to AmB and VRZ or posaconazole (Al-Hatmi et al. 2014). However, both drugs may be preferred because of good CNS penetration.

In vitro antifungal susceptibility profiles of *Fusarium* species demonstrate high MICs to most antifungal agents. Notably, some species may exhibit different patterns of susceptibility: *F. solani* species complex are usually resistant to azoles and exhibit higher AmB MIC values than other species, whereas *F. oxysporum* and *F. verticilloides* may be susceptible to VRZ and posaconazole. The echinocandins are not active against *Fusarium* spp. and lack CNS penetration (Nucci and Anaissie 2007; Al-Hatmi et al. 2014, 2017; Alastruey-Izquierdo et al. 2008).

Multiresistance to antifungals, observed in all *Fusarium* species, is intrinsic; therefore these fungi are notoriously difficult to treat. The executive board of the European Fungal Infection Study Group (EFISG) of the European Society of Clinical Microbiology and Infectious Diseases (ESCMID) and the European Confederation of Medical Mycology (ECMM) decided to proceed with a pan-European guideline for the diagnosis and management of hyalohyphomycosis caused by Fusarium and other nonmelanized fungi (Tortorano et al. 2014). Due to the lack of clinical trials and the critical role of immune reconstitution in the outcome of fusariosis, the optimal treatment strategy for patients with severe *Fusarium* infection remains unclear. Reversal of immunosuppression is recommended whenever possible. In immunocompromised patients, VRZ, AmB deoxycholate, lipid-based AmB (L-AmB) formulations, and various combinations have been reported with varying success. Based on the data available, ESCMID and ECMM joint guideline recommend VRZ and lipid-based AmB formulations. Lipid-based AmB preparations exhibit fewer side effects when compared with AmB deoxycholate and should be favored. The response rate to a lipid formulation of AmB appeared superior to that of conventional AmB. In addition to antifungal treatment, the optimal management of patients with fusariosis includes surgical debridement of infected tissues, removal of venous catheters in confirmed catheter-related fusariosis, and reversal of the immunocompromised state (Tortorano et al. 2014).

Fusarium CNS infection in patients with prolonged neutropenia carries a poor prognosis (Vincent et al. 2003). The prognosis of fusariosis in the immunocompromised host is directly related to the immune status of the patient, with high death rates in patients with persistent immunodeficiency. In general, patients with localized CNS infection are likely to benefit from surgical debridement, while disseminated infection requires the use of systemic agents and immunotherapy, when possible (Vincent et al. 2003; Tortorano et al. 2014).

15.3 *Bipolaris* spp.

15.3.1 Introduction

Bipolaris is a large genus of dematiaceous hyphomycetes with more than 100 species, most of them being saprobes in soil and pathogens of plants, while some of the saprobic species are potentially able to infect humans and animals. Hyphomycetes are a form classification of Fungi, and dematiaceous or phaeoid (Pappagianis and Ajello 1994) fungi include a large group of organisms darkly pigmented (dark brown, olivaceous, or black). In most cases the pigment is melanin (Dixon and Polak-Wyss 1991). These fungi are alternately called phaeoid, dematiaceous, dark, or black molds. Phaeohyphomycosis, a term introduced by Ajello et al. in 1974, literally means "infection caused by dark-walled fungi" (Ajello et al. 1974; Revankar and Sutton

2010). Most species belonging to the genus *Bipolaris* are saprobes in nature, found in wood and decomposing plants. The prevalent clinically significant saprobes are *Bipolaris australiensis*, *Bipolaris hawaiiensis*, and *Bipolaris spicifera*. *Bipolaris hawaiiensis* is particularly associated with CNS infections (Chowdhary et al. 2015; Da Cunha et al. 2012). These fungi are able to infect both immunocompetent and immunosuppressed patients, mainly in tropical and subtropical areas (Da Cunha et al. 2012).

A computerized search of the MEDLINE database (National Library of Medicine, Bethesda, MD, USA) was performed for cases reported in the literature, with (by cross-referencing) the terms "*Helminthosporium*," "*Drechslera*," "*Bipolaris*," "*Bipolaris hawaiiensis*," "*Bipolaris spicifera*," "cerebral," "brain abscess," "meningitis," "central nervous system infection," "rhinocerebral infection," "rhino-orbito-cerebral infection," "allergic fungal sinusitis," "disseminated," "immunocompetent," and "otherwise healthy." These keywords were used alone and/or in combination with an "and" statement. Additional cases were obtained by scanning the references cited in the original articles. Original full texts of all the relevant articles were obtained via MEDLINE, TUBITAK-ULAKBIM (Turkish Academic Network and Information Center), and other international libraries and were used for the analysis.

15.3.2 Taxonomy

Traditionally, darkly pigmented fungi have been collectively indicated under umbrella terms, such as "dematiaceous" or "phaeoid" fungi, referring to the presence of brown hyphae or yeast cells. Today, the leading principle of fungal classification is molecular phylogeny. Species in *Bipolaris* were initially described in the genus *Helminthosporium*; after several taxonomic refinements, *Helminthosporium* were segregated into several genera including *Bipolaris*, *Curvularia*, *Drechslera*, and *Exserohilum* (Sivanesan 1987). The genera *Drechslera*, *Bipolaris*, *Curvularia*, and *Exserohilum* are all closely related. In the past, morphological differentiation of the genera relied upon a combination of characters including conidial shape, the presence or absence of a protruding hilum, the contour of the basal portion of the conidium and its hilum, the point at which the germ tube originates from the basal cell, and, to a lesser degree, the sequence and location of the first three conidial septa. *Drechslera* can be differentiated from all other helminthosporoid genera by its ability to develop a germ tube from any of the cells in the conidia.

Molecular phylogenetic analysis based on ITS (internal transcribed spacers and intervening 5.8S nrDNA) and GPDH (partial glyceraldehyde-3-phosphate dehydrogenase) genes (Berbee 2001) showed *Drechslera* and *Bipolaris* to be two distinct genera. *Bipolaris* and *Curvularia* share many morphological similarities, and both genera have sexual morphs in *Cochliobolus*. According to molecular analyses of ITS and GPDH sequence data, some *Bipolaris* species clustered with *Curvularia*. Manamgoda et al. (Manamgoda et al. 2012) have found that glyceraldehyde-3-phosphate dehydrogenase (GPDH) gene is the best single marker for species of *Bipolaris*. Generic boundaries between *Bipolaris* and *Curvularia* are revised and presented in an updated combined ITS and GPDH phylogenetic tree. The genus *Bipolaris* belongs to *Ascomycota*, *Dothideomycetes*, *Pleosporales*, and *Pleosporaceae*. Its sexual morph, the genus *Cochliobolus*, is not common in nature, but it is occasionally produced under laboratory conditions (Manamgoda et al. 2014).

15.3.3 Morphology

Macroscopic morphology: Rapidly growing dark colonies on SDA are hairy and expanding, effuse, grey to blackish brown, woolly, suede-like to floccose with a black reverse. Colonies on potato dextrose agar at 25 °C are initially white, soon becoming dark gray to black with a black reverse.

Microscopic morphology: Hyphae are septate and dark. Conidiophores are brown, erect, multicelled, producing ellipsoidal, straight, or curved conidia with dark-brown, flat conidial scars. Conidia germinate from both poles. Conidia mostly curved, canoe-shaped, fusoid or obclavate, rarely straight, 2–14 pseudoseptate (usually more than 6), germinating only from the ends (bipolar). The conidia of *B. hawaiiensis* have a more overall delicate look and are generally somewhat narrower than either *B. spicifera* or *B. australiensis*. Been developed for the direct detection of *Bipolaris* species (Chowdhary et al. 2015; Shin et al. 2003; El-Morsy et al. 2010) (Fig. 15.5).

15.3.4 Virulence Factors

Bipolaris is a melanized fungus. Melanin is believed to be a major virulence factor-enhancing opportunism (Jacobson 2000; Nosanchuk and Casadevall 2003). The function of melanin in their natural habitat mostly is protection against solar irradiation because of growth on exposed surfaces, such as natural rock, or against factors prevalent under conditions of stress. Melanin is believed to contribute to microbial virulence by reducing a pathogen's susceptibility to killing by host antimicrobial mechanisms and by influencing the host immune response to infection. Melanin has been shown to interfere with numerous host defense mechanisms. Melanin is an important mechanism to decrease phagocytosis and escape the oxidative burst of macrophages, capable to alter cytokine responses (Nosanchuk and Casadevall 2003, 2006; Gómez and Nosanchuk 2003; Nosanchuk et al. 2015). Melanized cells are less susceptible to killing by oxygen- and nitrogen-derived radicals. *B. hawaiiensis* is a neurotropic fungus and may

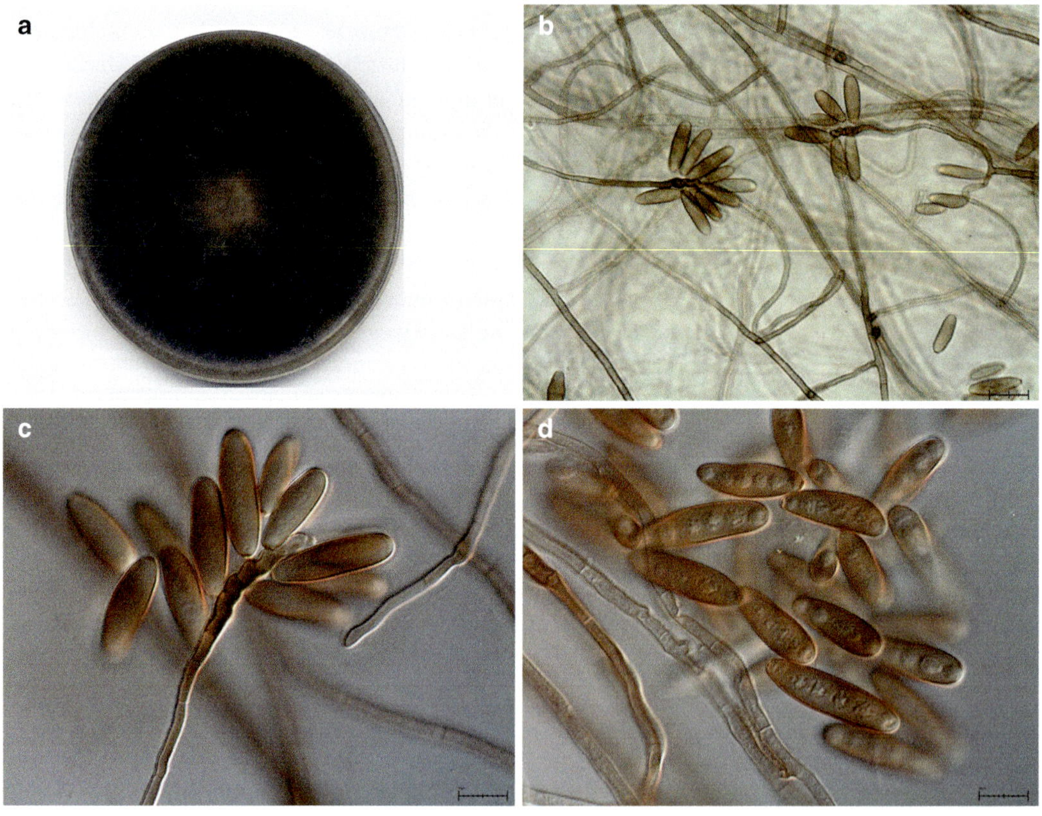

Fig. 15.5 (**a**): Colony of *B. hawaiiensis* (10 days); (**b**) conidiophores (40×, lactic acid preparation); (**c**) conidiophores (100×, lactic acid preparation); (**d**) conidia nomarsky-8 (100×, lactic acid preparation). (Courtesy of Josep Guarro, Prof., MD, Unitat de Microbiologia, Facultat de Medicina i Ciencies de la Salut, University of Rovira i Virgilli, Reus, Spain)

probably utilize catecholamines in the brain to produce melanin and may be protected from oxidative damage by scavenging free radicals.

Melanin production provides survival advantages to fungi in the environment and during infection of diverse hosts. There is conclusive evidence that many types of drugs, including antimicrobial drugs, bind to melanin. In particular, the melanization of certain fungi is associated with reduced susceptibilities to polyene and echinocandin-type drugs in vitro. In contrast, melanization has not been associated with reduced susceptibilities to azole-type drugs, except at high concentrations. Interestingly, the drug-binding properties of both host and microbial melanins could influence the outcome of antimicrobial therapy (Nosanchuk and Casadevall 2006; Nosanchuk et al. 2015).

15.3.5 Epidemiology

The prevalence of the different species of *Bipolaris* in human infections is poorly known since only a few studies involving this genus have been published and the isolates were usually identified only by morphological criteria (Revankar and Sutton 2010; Da Cunha et al. 2012; El Khizzi et al. 2010).

Overall, the reported human infections (n = 15) were from the USA and encountered in areas where a hot climate is predominant. Four patients were African-Americans.

15.3.6 Clinical Presentations

Species recognition in the genus has been uncertain due to the lack of molecular data as well as overlapping morphological characteristics. Considering the similarity among the species of *Bipolaris* and the fact that the separation of species is based on subtle characters, some published identifications are doubtful or remain unresolved (Da Cunha et al. 2012; Manamgoda et al. 2014). Therefore, reported CNS infections by *Bipolaris species* were outlined in Table 15.4 (Fuste et al. 1973; Yoshimori et al. 1982; Adam et al. 1986; Biggs et al. 1986; Morton et al. 1986; McGinnis et al. 1992; Latham 2000; Moore et al. 2001; Filizzola et al. 2003; Viola and Sutton 2010; Rosow et al. 2011; Patel et al. 2012; Jelinek et al. 2014; Teran et al. 2014; Frank et al. 2016). Two cases were due to *B. hawaiiensis*, eight were *B. spicifera*, one is with *B. australiensis*, and the remaining were reported due to *Bipolaris* spp. Seven patients died; outcome was not reported in one case.

15.3.7 Signs and Symptoms

Symptoms of CNS infection due to *Bipolaris* species are nonspecific, involving headache, fascial pain, fever, neck stiffness, and vomiting.

15.3.8 Laboratory Diagnosis

Fontana-Mason stain, specific for melanin, usually confirms the diagnosis of phaeohyphomycosis. Histopathologic examination of clinical specimens is significant. Hematoxylin and eosin stain shows dark-colored hyphae. Phaeoid hyphae of *Cladosporium* may be seen even on unstained sections of the abscess.

Molecular identification can be done using ITS sequencing. GPDH has been determined to be the best single phylogenetic marker of *Bipolaris* species (Da Cunha et al. 2012; Manamgoda et al. 2012, 2014). A specific polymerase chain reaction (PCR) has been developed for the direct detection of Bipolaris species (Chowdhary et al. 2015; Shin et al. 2003; El-Morsy et al. 2010).

15.3.9 Treatment

There are no standardized therapies, but VRZ and ITZ demonstrate the most consistent in vitro activity against dematiaceous fungi. VRZ penetrates into brain tissue effectively (Chowdhary et al. 2014). The treatments reported in CNS infections by *Bipolaris* species include surgical debridement, antifungal therapy with AmB, ketoconazole, ITZ, VRZ, or combination with

Table 15.4 CNS infections by *Bipolaris* (*Drechslera*) species

Reference	Pathogen	Age/sex/race/ geography	Risk factor/underlying disease	Clinical syndrome	Therapy	Outcome
Fuste et al. (1973)	*B. hawaiiensis*	31/F/	Metastatic lymphosarcoma	Meningitis	None	Died
Yoshimori et al. (1982)	*B. spicifera*	21/F/USA	None	Cerebral abscess	AmB, 5-FC	Survived (4 m follow-up)
Adam et al. (1986)	*B. spicifera*	49/F/USA	Metastatic breast carcinoma	Meningitis	None	Died
Biggs et al. (1986)	*B. spicifera*	21/F/USA	Head trauma	Encephalitis	Partial excision	Died
Morton et al. (1986)	*B. hawaiiensis*	18/M/USA		Cerebral abscess	AmB, 5-FC, excision	Survived (2 m follow-up)
McGinnis et al. (1992)	*B. spicifera*	26/F/USA		Cerebral abscess, sinusitis	AmB, KTZ	Survived
Latham (2000)	*B. spicifera*	18/M/USA	Neurosurgery	Meningitis	AmB, ITZ	Survived
Moore et al. (2001)	*B. spicifera*	0/USA	Neonate	Disseminated	L-AmB (5 mg/kg/d), ITZ (7.5 mg/kg/d), surgery	Died
Filizzola et al. (2003)	*Bipolaris* sp.	28/M/black/USA	None	Cerebral abscess	ITZ + AmB, L-AmB, VRZ	Died
Viola and Sutton (2010)	*B. australiensis*	35/F/black/USA	None	Cerebral abscess, sinusitis	Surgery, AmB	Died
Rosow et al. (2011)	*B. spicifera*	55/M/USA	Heart transplant	Cerebral abscess	L-AmB (400 mg/d), VRZ (200 mg twice daily)	Survived (12 m follow-up)
Patel et al. (2012)	*Bipolaris* sp.	35/M/black/USA	Steroids	Cerebral abscess	VRZ, L-AmB, abscess drainage	Survived
Jelinek et al. (2014)	*Bipolaris* sp.	22/M/black/USA	None	Meningoencephalitis	AmB + VRZ	Died
Teran et al. (2014)	*B. spicifera*	20 m/M/USA	Heart transplant	Skin and cerebral abscess (possible)	AmB	Died
Frank et al. (2016)	*Bipolaris* sp.		none	Disseminated		

Abbreviations: *AMB* amphotericin B deoxycholate, *L-AMB* liposomal amphotericin B, *KTZ* ketoconazole, *ITZ* itraconazole, *VRZ* voriconazole, *d* day, *w* week(s), *m* month(s)

AmB and 5-FC or ITZ, and the prognosis reported was poor.

15.4 *Schizophyllum commune*

15.4.1 Introduction

Schizophyllum commune is a mold of phylum Basidiomycota, subphylum Agaricomycotina, order Agaricales, and family Schizophyllaceae, with worldwide distribution that colonizes diverse trees and rotting wood. The distinctive feature of these fungi is the formation of a macroscopic fructification, the basidiocarp, that contains basidiospores (sexual spores) developing on the outside of a club-shaped or elongate structure called the basidium (De Hoog et al. 2000). *S. commune* is one of the most commonly found mushroom-forming fungus (teleomorphic state) and contains genes that encode enzymes for degrading woody cell wall components (Schmidt and Liese 1980).

15.4.2 Morphology and Biology

S. commune, like most basidiomycete fungi, have dikaryotic (binucleate condition) or monokaryotic stages in their life cycle. In the life cycle of *S. commune* (Wösten and Wessels 2006), meiospores germinate to form a sterile monokaryotic mycelium, in which each hyphal compartment contains one nucleus. Initial growth of this mycelium occurs beneath the surface of the substrate, with formation of aerial hyphae a few days after germination. Monokaryons that encounter each other fuse, and a fertile dikaryon forms when the alleles of the mating-type loci *matA* and *matB* of the partners differ. A short exposure to light is essential for fruiting, whereas a high concentration of carbon dioxide and high temperatures (30–37 °C) are inhibitory. Mushroom formation is initiated with the aggregation of aerial dikaryotic hyphae. These aggregates form fruiting body primordia, which further develop into mature fruiting bodies. Karyogamy and meiosis occur in the basidia within the mature fruiting body, and the resulting basidiospores can give rise to new monokaryotic mycelia (Ohm et al. 2010).

Dikaryotic isolates of *S. commune* were characterized by clamp connections, hyphal spicules, and formation of basidiocarps (mushroom) with basidiospores. A monokaryon generates septate sterile aerial hyphae that form a fluffy white layer on top of the vegetative mycelium (Sigler et al. 1995).

15.4.3 Ecology

S. commune is one of the most commonly found fungi and can be isolated from all continents, except for Antarctica. *S. commune* has been reported to be a pathogen of humans and trees, but it mainly adopts a saprobic lifestyle by causing white rot (Schmidt and Liese 1980). It is predominantly found on fallen branches and timber of deciduous trees (Ohm et al. 2010). *Schizophyllum* basidiospores are readily airborne and dispersed over long distances (James and Vilgalys 2001; O'Gorman and Fuller 2008).

The fungus is found so abundantly in some parts of the world that in Hong Kong and Indonesia, it is used as a substitute for chewing gum; in Peru, the Congo, and Thailand, it is cooked and eaten (Greer 1978).

15.4.4 Epidemiology

CNS infection by the *S. commune* was first reported in 1955 by Batista from Brazil (Batista et al. 1955), who repeatedly isolated it from cerebral spinal fluid of a patient with meningeal symptoms (basidioneuromycosis). Other cases were reported from the USA (Rihs et al. 1996), Austria (Hoenigl et al. 2013), and Japan (Tone et al. 2018). Currently, there is no information on the isolation of *S. commune* from any clinical material in the African continent (Chowdhary et al. 2013a).

15.4.5 Clinical Presentations

Infective propagules in this fungus are air transported (De Hoog et al. 2000). Although the worldwide distribution of *S. commune*, infections originating from this fungus other than chronic or allergic sinusitis have been rarely reported in humans. Four cases of CNS infections have been reported to date, including atypical meningitis (basidioneuromycosis) (Batista et al. 1955), epidural (Tone et al. 2018) and cerebral abscesses extended from sinusitis (Hoenigl et al. 2013), and a disseminated case from pulmonary infection to the brain (Rihs et al. 1996) in immunocompetent and immunocompromised individuals (by diabetes mellitus or corticosteroid therapy). All cases involved men.

The four cases with central nervous system involvement available in English literature are summarized below with diagnosis and treatment processes.

Case 1: The patient was a 24-year-old Brazilian man who suffered from a disorder of the central nervous system marked by mental dullness and signs and symptoms indicating increased intracranial pressure without any focalizing sign. An electroencephalogram seemed to point to a diffuse lesion in the anterior part of the brain. A *basidiomycetes* fungus of the genus *Schizophyllum* was repeatedly isolated it from cerebral spinal fluid samples (Batista et al. 1955). This was the first reported case.

Case 2: The patient was a 58-year-old American man with progressive muscle weakness and multiple lung and brain lesions but had no respiratory tract symptoms. A magnetic resonance imaging scan (MRI) revealed an enhancing mass in the left pons. An empiric trial dexamethasone was begun and continued 5 weeks (total dose 330 mg). Computed tomographic examination of the head showed a new ring-enhancing lesion within the right frontal lobe. A wedge resection of a lung mass revealed necrotizing granulomatous inflammation with hyphae consistent with an *Aspergillus* spp. Treatment of AMB and itraconazole was begun. An MRI of the brain showed increase in size and number of the frontal brain lesions. A stereotactic biopsy was performed and the fluid showed fungal elements suggestive of *Aspergillus* spp. on frozen section. Histologic examination of biopsy tissue from lungs and brain showed numerous septate, hyaline, hyphal elements of various widths, measuring 2.5–5.5 μm in diameter with hematoxylin and eosin and Gomori methenamine silver stains. Many hyphae branched at acute as well as right angles but did not exhibit dichotomous branching. Many hyphal elements seen in the tissue slides of both the lung and brain showed clamp connections. Isolated fungus was identified by characteristic phenotypical features. According to the in vitro antifungal susceptibility results, fluconazole (600 mg twice daily) was substituted for itraconazole. After the patient had received 1.754 mg of AMB over 36 days, he died developing respiratory failure and sepsis.

Case 3: A 59-year-old Australian man with diabetes mellitus and severe headache was diagnosed as sinusitis. A MRI revealed three abscess formations in the right frontal lobe of brain. Functional endoscopic sinus surgery was performed. Histology of sinus tissue revealed multiple branched and septate fungal hyphae. Culture of brain abscess drainage grew *S. commune*. L-AMB (3 mg kg^{-1} body weight) was administered for total of 5 weeks. Control MRI showed complete resolution of cerebral abscess formation. Therapy was changed to oral posaconazole 400 mg twice daily for 4. The patient was released in good clinical condition and without any residual symptoms.

Case 4: A 53-year-old Japanese man with history of bronchial asthma and pollen allergy and no prior treatment, presented with headache and was diagnosed with ethmoid and sphenoid sinusitis by computed tomography (CT) of the cranium (Tone et al. 2018). He developed an epidural abscess after antibiotic treatment. Samples were obtained from epidural abscess and from sinuses by endoscopic sinus fenestration. Direct microscopical examination of the epidural abscess material showed filamentous fungal elements. Microscopic examination of slide cultures showed white cottony sterile mycelia without clamp connections. The isolated fungus was identified by sequence analysis of the ITS of ribosomal DNA (rDNA) and D1/D2 domain of 285 rDNA. Antifungal susceptibility tests were done using E test strips, and he was treated with liposomal amphotericin B (L-AMB, 300 mg/day, titrated from 0.2 to 5 mg/kg/day). He was discharged from the hospital on day 25, and no recurrence has been observed for over 2 years.

15.4.6 Histopathology

The biopsied tissue or surgical specimen should be submitted to laboratory for mycological as well as histopathological examination. Histological examination may be performed using conventional hematoxylin-eosin, Gomori methenamine silver and periodic acid-Schiff stains and may reveal an inflammation consisting of mixed inflammatory cells and hyphae in the involved tissue. No angioinvasion was reported by this fungus.

The fungus was characterized by clamp connections, hyphal spicules, and formation of basidiocarps with basidiospores (Sigler et al. 1995; Chowdhary et al. 2013a). In tissue sections, the hyphae may not always exhibit clamp connections. Their differentiation from hyphal elements of *Aspergillus* spp. could be readily achieved by the use of serologic tests for the detection of *Aspergillus* antibodies and antigens (Rihs et al. 1996).

15.4.7 Laboratory Diagnosis

Direct microscopy of a KOH (10%) preparation of the biopsy or surgical specimen showed the presence of hyaline septate hyphae. Giemsa stained preparations can show septate branched hyphae.

Some portions of tissue samples can be inoculated both on multipoints of SDA supplemented with chloramphenicol (0.5 μg/ml), or containing gentamycin, and on Brain Heart Infusion Agar and can be incubated at 30 °C for 4–10 days. Growth on SDA can be rapid, cottony, and whitish and raised in center. Colonies can become slightly powdery and pale buff or tan having a pale brown reverse after 2 weeks at 25 °C. It produces a strong disagreeable odor. Cycloheximide inhibits the growth on SDA.

Microscopic examination of the mold showed hyphae of various widths. Lactophenol cotton blue mount of the cultured fungus can reveal hyaline septate hyphae, often with clamp connections or lateral pegs (O'Gorman and Fuller 2008).

Most isolates readily produce basidiocarps and clamp connections on Czapek's, potato dextrose, or corn meal agars and lateral tubercles on their hyphae (Rihs et al. 1996). Slide cultures showed hyaline, septate, branched hyphae of 2.0–4.5 mm in diameter with clamp connections. Many hyphae developed lateral, short, thin, truncate tubercles diagnostic of *S. commune*.

Due to the presence of sterile filaments and lack of specific structures in early stage of identification, for induction of sporulation, inoculated Petri dishes containing malt extract agar, malt yeast glucose agar may be incubated at 25 °C, Czapek Dox agar at 28 °C, and potato dextrose agar at 30 °C for 4–20 days in different environmental condition (dark, light, and UV exposure) for further examinations (O'Gorman and Fuller 2008).

Because monokaryotic isolates of *S. commune* are difficult to identify, techniques such as mating (vegetative compatibility) tests or gene sequencing may be required to identify *S. commune*. However, the mating test is not easy to perform in a conventional laboratory and may require prolonged time for identification of the pathogen in most cases. Instead, a few studies have shown that gene sequencing is an attractive method to identify this fungus. Won et al. (2012) recommended that gene sequencing of the ITS region and D1/D2 regions of the 26S ribosomal DNA was very helpful for accurate identification of this fungus. In fact, given the excellent specificity of this technique, gene sequencing has been recognized as the gold standard for fungal identification. However, for accurate identification of rare molds such as *S. commune*, morphological findings and molecular data should be compared to ensure consistency (Balajee et al. 2007, 2009).

The characteristic phenotypical features that were indicative of *S. commune* were as follows:

(a) It grew well at 37 °C.
(b) It is easy to culture on media commonly used in clinical laboratories and formed rapidly growing, woolly colonies with septate hyaline, branching hyphae of two widths.
(c) It is susceptible to cycloheximide (400 μg/ml).
(d) It tolerates to 2–10 mg of benomyl per ml.
(e) It forms a dense, tough (i.e., difficult to cut), woolly colony.
(f) It has a tart and pronounced odor (Won et al. 2012; Premamalini et al. 2011).

Matrix-assisted laser desorption/ionization mass spectrometer (MALDI-TOF MS) makes it possible to identify fungi whose macroscopic and microscopic morphological features are usually uninformative. *S. commune* was identified using MALDI-TOF MS, and identifications were confirmed via DNA sequence analysis (Chowdhary et al. 2013a; Michel et al. 2015).

15.4.8 Antifungal Susceptibility, Treatment, and Outcome

Although the interpretive MIC breakpoints have not yet been defined for *S. commune* and the correlations between clinical response and MIC values for a given strain are uncertain, MICs of the isolates, treatment, and outcome reported in different clinical cases and in an in vitro antifungal susceptibility study were shown in Tables 15.4 (Rihs et al. 1996; Hoenigl et al. 2013; Tone et al. 2018) and 15.5 (Chowdhary et al. 2013b). Delay in initiation of appropriate antifungal treatment and the use of corticosteroids was associated with treatment failure.

The occurrence of *S. commune* as a human pathogenic fungus may be much more frequent than previously assumed. Improved mycological identification methods may have given rise to a larger number of *S. commune* rhinocerebral cases. Those cases would probably have been misdiagnosed in the past because of the close clinical and histological similarity with *Aspergillus* infections and of the difficult identification of the isolated fungus with sterile mycelia.

15.5 *Scedosporium apiospermum*

15.5.1 Introduction

The fungus *Scedosporium apiospermum*, initially considered the anamorph or asexual state of ascomycetous fungus *Pseudallescheria boydii*, is a filamentous fungus that can be commonly found as a saprophyte in soil, sewage, mud, and the polluted waters of streams and ponds with still water (de Hoog et al. 1994). Recent molecular studies have demonstrated that *P. boydii* is a complex that includes several phylogenetic species (Gilgado et al. 2005; Chen et al. 2016).

As a result of fundamental changes in the International Code of Nomenclature on the use of separate names for sexual and asexual stages of fungi, generic names of many groups should be reconsidered. Members of the ECMM/ISHAM working group on *Pseudallescheria/Scedosporium* infections proposed a novel nomenclature for genera and species in *Pseudallescheria*, *Scedosporium*, and allied taxa (Lackner et al. 2014).

The *Scedosporium apiospermum* species complex, comprising five filamentous fungal species *S. apiospermum* sensu stricto, *S. boydii* (= *Pseudallescheria boydii*, *P. angusta*), *S. aurantiacum*, *S. dehoogii*, and *S. minutispora*, are important pathogens that cause a wide variety of infections (Giraud and Bouchara 2014). The species of genus *Scedosporium* can be distinguished with the primary fungal DNA barcode, the ITS1/2 region of the rDNA gene cluster (Chen et al. 2016). Chen et al. (2016) stated that for reasons of absence of genetic separation, as well as absence of clinical relevance of individual lineages, the species *S. apiospermum*, *P. angusta*, and *S. boydii* should be referred to as the "*S. apiospermum* species complex." Because of the degree of involvement of each individual species in human infections has not been determined, the present chapter

Table 15.5 Antifungal susceptibility test results of *S. Commune* case isolates reported

Reference	MIC (μg/ml)						Antifungal therapy	Outcome
	AMB	FLZ	ITZ	VRZ	PSZ	CAS		
Rihs et al. (1996)[a]	<0.03	8	ND	ND	ND	ND	AMB + ITZ (4 d), AMB (over 36 d) + FLZ (600 mg twice daily)	Died
Hoenigl et al. (2013)[b]	0.25	12	>32	0.125	0.25	>32	L-AMB (5 w), PSZ (400 mg twice daily)	Survived
Tone et al. (2018)[b]	0.75	ND	1	ND	ND	>32	L-AMB (300 mg/d, titrated from 0.2 to 5 mg/kg/d, 3 w)	Survived (2 y follow-up, no recurrence)

Abbreviations: *MIC* minimal inhibitory concentration, *AMB* amphotericin B, *FLZ* fluconazol, *ITZ* itraconazol, *VRZ* voriconazole, *PSZ* posaconazole, *CAS* caspofungin, *L-AMB* liposomal AMB, *ND* not determined, *d* day, *w* weeks, *y* years

[a]Method unknown

[b]E test

will maintain the name *S. apiospermum* in all disease entities.

A computerized search of the MEDLINE database (National Library of Medicine, Bethesda, MD, USA) was performed for cases reported in the literature between 1948 and mid-2006, with (by cross-referencing) the terms "*Pseudallescheria boydii*" and "*Scedosporium apiospermum*," "*Scedosporium apiospermum* species complex," "*Pseudallescheria boydii/Scedosporium species* complex," "cerebral," "brain abscess," "meningitis," "central nervous system infection," "disseminated," and "near-drowning." Additional search terms included were "*Allescheria boydii*," "*Monosporium apiospermum*," and "*Petriellidium boydii*" as referring to prior or other nomenclature for this fungus. These keywords were used alone and/or in combination with an "and" statement. Additional cases were obtained by scanning the references cited in the original articles. Original full texts of all the relevant articles were obtained via MEDLINE, TUBITAK-ULAKBIM (Turkish Academic Network and Information Center), or personal communication of the authors and/or other international libraries and were used for the analysis.

15.5.2 Epidemiology

This fungus shows a particular tropism for the CNS in both healthy and immunocompromised patients. The first report of *S. apiospermum* CNS infection was by Benham et al. in 1948. The majority of the CNS infections by *S. apiospermum* were reported from the USA, Germany, France, and Canada, and sporadic cases were reported in other countries around the world (Kantarcioglu et al. 2008).

15.5.3 Predisposing Factors, Underlying Conditions

In a recent review of 99 patients with *Pseudallescheria* CNS infection, the majority of patients (44%) were previously healthy, and the others had one or more underlying diseases and/or predisposing factors. Twenty-four of the previously healthy patients (55%) had a history of aspiration of polluted water in association with near drowning. Nine of the previously healthy patients were posttraumatic cases. A majority of patients with underlying disease and/or predisposing factor were transplant recipients. Apparent major risk factors for CNS infection were aspiration of polluted water in near drowning episodes in immunologically intact patients and medical immunosuppression in the remaining patient groups (Kantarcioglu et al. 2008). The overall fatality rate was very high (76%).

15.5.4 Portal of Entry and Routes of Infection

S. apiospermum shows a marked neurotropism and a high propensity to cause CNS infections. In most of the CNS associated disseminated cases, particularly the vascular organs such as the kidney, the thyroid and heart have been also involved probably due to the particular tropism for blood vessels and hematogenous spread of this fungus. The usual portal of entry of CNS infection by *S. apiospermum* was presumed to be the respiratory tract with hematogenous spread to the brain. However, isolation of *S. apiospermum* from outside and indoor air was extremely infrequent. Remarkably, direct entry by aspiration of contaminated water from the pharynx, through sinuses close to the brain and ethmoid bone, seemed the most frequent portal of entry regarding the 16 near-drowned cases in whom no pulmonary involvement was observed (Kantarcioglu et al. 2008).

15.5.5 Signs and Symptoms

The predominantly reported symptoms were headache, altered mental status, seizures, hydrocephalus, infarcts, eye pain, arm and leg weakness, vomiting, vision loss and back pain, neck stiffness, hemiparesis, general convulsions, lethargy and confusion, and dizziness, facial paresis, nausea, skin rash, photophobia, and abnormal behavior. Fifteen percent of the patients had coma on admission, and 12% had no complaints and/or had no abnormal neurological signs (Kantarcioglu et al. 2008).

15.5.6 Clinical Presentations

Main clinical types were brain abscess, coinfection of brain tissue, and/or spinal cord with meninges and meningitis. The mortality rate was of 74% regardless of the patient's immune status or the infection type and/or location (Kantarcioglu et al. 2008).

15.5.7 Histology

The most characteristic histological findings in the brain tissue of patients infected by *S. apiospermum* were the presence of a neutrophilic inflammatory infiltrate, granulomatous inflammation with multinucleated giant cells and microabscesses with hyphae invading cerebellar blood vessels. Hyphae of *S. apiospermum* are usually well stained with the routine histological stains such as hematoxylin and eosin (H-E), Gomori methenamine silver, periodic acid-Schiff (PAS), or even with potassium hydroxide (Kantarcioglu et al. 2008).

15.5.8 Laboratory Diagnosis

Morphological identification of *Scedosporium* species has become increasingly unreliable. The conidial states of *S. apiospermum* and *S. boydii* are morphologically indistinguishable, although the latter is homothallic and produces ascocarps. *S. aurantiacum* also exhibits similar conidial morphology, but most strains produce a pale to bright yellow diffusible pigment on potato dextrose agar. Therefore, molecular identification methods are now recommended.

Because antifungal susceptibilities differ among *S. apiospermum* complex members (Lackner et al. 2012; Gilgado et al. 2006, 2008), species identification is important. In addition to morphological and physiological observations, molecular techniques involving genes such as β-tubulin and calmodulin and ITS regions 1 and 2 had been recommended for species identification (Lackner et al. 2012; Gilgado et al. 2008; Lu et al. 2011).

MALDI-TOF MS can be used in the routine clinical laboratory in the identification of members of the complex provided that valid spectra libraries are developed. Species identification appears feasible with MALDI-TOF MS (Coulibaly et al. 2011).

15.5.9 Treatment and Outcome

In a recent review (Kantarcioglu et al. 2008), the overall death rate in these patients was 74%, while the predictors of outcome were largely unknown, and 64% of the survivors were previously healthy patients. Since numerous therapeutic approaches have been used, both monotherapies and combinations, with variable results, a general consensus for the treatment of these infections does not yet exist. CNS infection caused by *S. apiospermum* has a poor prognosis. According to the analyzed data, mortality rates were high regardless of the patient's immune status, or the infection type and/or location, but likely affected by infection route and inoculum size (Kantarcioglu et al. 2008).

S. apiospermum is resistant to conventional antifungal drugs, including AmB (Tortorano et al. 2014; Kantarcioglu et al. 2008). The executive board of the European Fungal Infection Study Group (EFISG) of the European Society of Clinical Microbiology and Infectious Diseases (ESCMID) and the European Confederation of Medical Mycology (ECMM) proposed with a pan-European guideline for the diagnosis and management of hyalohyphomycosis including *Scedosporium* spp. infections. VRZ represents the first-line treatment of infections due to members of the genus *Scedosporium* because of its efficacy and possible good CNS penetration. Surgery, if possible, and VRZ are the strongly recommended as therapeutic strategies for CNS infections by *Scedosporium* genus (Tortorano et al. 2014).

15.6 Conclusion

CNS involvement by dematiaceous fungi (*Cladosporium spp, Bipolaris spp, Schizophyllum spp*) is uncommon. These fungi are neurotropic and can cause disease both in healthy and immunocompromised patients. CNS involvement by *Fusarium spp* is almost always as part of disseminated disease and associated with high morbidity and mortality. The antifungal susceptibility of these rare fungi is species/strain dependent and hence optimal management includes surgical debridement and broad spectrum antifungals.

References

Abramovsky C, et al. Systemic infection by Fusarium in a burned child. J Pediatr. 1974;84:561–4.

Adam RD, et al. Phaeohyphomycosis caused by the fungal genera Bipolaris and Exserohilum. A report of 9 cases and review of the literature. Medicine. 1986;65(4):203–17.

Agamanolis D, et al. Fusarium meningoencephalitis in a child with acute leukemia. Neuropediatrics. 1991;22(02):110–2.

Ajello L, et al. A case of phaeohyphomycosis caused by a new species of Phialophora. Mycologia. 1974;66:490–8.

Alastruey-Izquierdo A, et al. Antifungal susceptibility profile of clinical Fusarium spp. isolates identified by molecular methods. J Antimicrob Chemother. 2008;61(4):805–9.

Al-Hatmi AM, et al. Specific antifungal susceptibility profiles of opportunists in the Fusarium fujikuroi complex. J Antimicrob Chemother. 2014;70(4):1068–71.

Al-Hatmi A, et al. Antifungal susceptibility testing of Fusarium: a practical approach. J Fungi. 2017;3(2):19.

Anaissie EJ, et al. Fusariosis associated with pathogenic Fusarium species colonization of a hospital water system: a new paradigm for the epidemiology of opportunistic mold infections. Clin Infect Dis. 2001;33(11):1871–8.

Anten S, et al. Cerebral fungal abscess in a patient with acute promyelocytic leukaemia. Br J Haematol. 2008;140(3):253.

Antunes NL, Hariharan S, DeAngelis LM. Brain abscesses in children with cancer. Med Pediatr Oncol. 1998;31(1):19–21.

Asan A, Sen B, Sarica S. Airborne fungi in urban air of Edirne city (Turkey). Biologia Bratislava. 2002;57:59–68.

Asan A, et al. Isolation, identification and seasonal distrubution of airborne and waterborne fungi in Terkos Lake (Istanbul—Turkey). J Basic Microbiol. 2003;43(2):83–95.

Asan A, et al. Airborne fungi and actinomycetes concentrations in the air of Eskisehir City (Turkey). Indoor Built Environ. 2004;13(1):63–74.

Asl IG, et al. Molecular characterization of environmental Cladosporium species isolated from Iran. Curr Med Mycol. 2017;3(1):1.

Balajee SA, Sigler L, Brandt ME. DNA and the classical way: identification of medically important molds in the 21st century. Med Mycol. 2007;45(6):475–90.

Balajee S, et al. Sequence-based identification of Aspergillus, Fusarium, and Mucorales species in the clinical mycology laboratory: where are we and where should we go from here? J Clin Microbiol. 2009;47(4):877–84.

Batista A, Maia J, Singer B. Basidioneuromycosis on man. An Soc Biol Pernambwco. 1955;13(2):52–60.

Bensch K, et al. Species and ecological diversity within the Cladosporium cladosporioides complex (Davidiellaceae, Capnodiales). Stud Mycol. 2010;67:1–94.

Bensch K, et al. The genus cladosporium. Stud Mycol. 2012;72:1–401.

Bensch K, et al. Common but different: the expanding realm of Cladosporium. Stud Mycol. 2015;82:23–74.

Berbee ML. The phylogeny of plant and animal pathogens in the Ascomycota. Physiol Mol Plant Pathol. 2001;59(4):165–87.

Biggs PJ, et al. Phaeohyphomycosis complicating compound skull fracture. Surg Neurol. 1986;25(4):393–6.

Boutati EI, Anaissie EJ. Fusarium, a significant emerging pathogen in patients with hematologic malignancy: ten years' experience at a cancer center and implications for management. Blood. 1997;90(3):999–1008.

Chen CY, et al. Acute meningitis caused by Cladosporium sphaerospermum. Am J Med Sci. 2013;346(6):523–5.

Chen M, et al. The 'species complex' issue in clinically relevant fungi: a case study in Scedosporium apiospermum. Fungal Biol. 2016;120(2):137–46.

Cho CT, et al. Fusarium solani infection during treatment for acute leukemia. J Pediatr. 1973;83(6):1028–31.

Chowdhary A, et al. Schizophyllum commune as an emerging fungal pathogen: a review and report of two cases. Mycoses. 2013a;56(1):1–10.

Chowdhary A, et al. Molecular characterization and in vitro antifungal susceptibility profile of Schizophyllum commune, an emerging basidiomycete in bronchopulmonary mycoses. Antimicrob Agents Chemother. 2013b;57(6):2845–8.

Chowdhary A, et al. ESCMID and ECMM joint clinical guidelines for the diagnosis and management of systemic phaeohyphomycosis: diseases caused by black fungi. Clin Microbiol Infect. 2014;20:47–75.

Chowdhary A, Perfect J, de Hoog GS. Black molds and melanized yeasts pathogenic to humans. Cold Spring Harb Perspect Med. 2015;5(8):a019570.

Coulibaly O, et al. Pseudallescheria/Scedosporium complex species identification by matrix-assisted laser desorption ionization time-of-flight mass spectrometry. Med Mycol. 2011;49(6):621–6.

Crous PW, et al. The genus Cladosporium and similar dematiaceous hyphomycetes. Utrecht, The Netherlands: Centralbureau voor Schimmelcultures; 2007.

Da Cunha K, et al. Diversity of Bipolaris species in clinical samples in the United States and their antifungal susceptibility profiles. J Clin Microbiol. 2012;50(12):4061–6.

De Hoog G, et al. Nutritional physiology and taxonomy of human-pathogenic Cladosporium-Xylohypha species. J Med Vet Mycol. 1995;33(5):339–47.

De Hoog G, et al. Atlas of clinical fungi. 2nd ed. Utrecht: Centraalbureau voor Schimmelcultures; 2000.

De Hoog G, Guarro J, Figueras M. Atlas of clinical fungi. Utrecht, The Netherlands: CBS-KNAW Fungal Biodiversity Centre; 2011.

De Medeiros BC, et al. Central nervous system infections following bone marrow transplantation: an autopsy report of 27 cases. J Hematother Stem Cell Res. 2000;9(4):535–40.

van Diepeningen AD, et al. Diagnosis of Fusarium infections: approaches to identification by the clinical mycology laboratory. Curr Fungal Infect Rep. 2015;9(3):135–43.

Dixon D, Polak-Wyss A. The medically important dematiaceous fungi and their identification. Mycoses. 1991;34(1–2):1–18.

Edel-Hermann V, et al. A clonal lineage of Fusarium oxysporum circulates in the tap water of different French hospitals. Appl Environ Microbiol. 2016;82(21):6483–9.

El Khizzi N, Bakheshwain S, Parvez S. Bipolaris: a plant pathogen causing human infections: an emerging problem in Saudi Arabia. Res J Microbiol. 2010;5(3):212–7.

El-Morsy S, Khafagy Y, El-Naggar M. Allergic fungal rhinosinusitis: detection of fungal DNA in sinus aspirate using polymerase chain reaction. J Laryngol Otol. 2010;124(2):152–60.

Filizzola MJ, Martinez F, Rauf SJ. Phaeohyphomycosis of the central nervous system in immunocompetent hosts: report of a case and review of the literature. Int J Infect Dis. 2003;7(4):282–6.

Frank T, et al. Disseminated phaeohyphomycosis with brain abscess and biliary invasion due to Bipolaris spp. in an immunocompetent patient. Ann Clin Lab Sci. 2016;46(4):439–42.

Fuste F, et al. Drechslera hawaiiensis: causative agent of a fatal fungal meningo-encephalitis. Sabouraudia. 1973;11(1):59–63.

Garcia RR, et al. Fusarium brain abscess: case report and literature review. Mycoses. 2015;58(1):22–6.

Gaviria JM, et al. Comparison of interferon-γ, granulocyte colony-stimulating factor, and granulocyte-macrophage colony-stimulating factor for priming leukocyte-mediated hyphal damage of opportunistic fungal pathogens. J Infect Dis. 1999;179(4):1038–41.

Gilgado F, et al. Molecular phylogeny of the Pseudallescheria boydii species complex: proposal of two new species. J Clin Microbiol. 2005;43(10):4930–42.

Gilgado F, et al. Antifungal susceptibilities of the species of the Pseudallescheria boydii complex. Antimicrob Agents Chemother. 2006;50(12):4211–3.

Gilgado F, et al. Molecular and phenotypic data supporting distinct species statuses for Scedosporium apiospermum and Pseudallescheria boydii and the proposed new species Scedosporium dehoogii. J Clin Microbiol. 2008;46(2):766–71.

Giraud S, Bouchara J-P. Scedosporium apiospermum complex: diagnosis and species identification. Curr Fungal Infect Rep. 2014;8(3):211–9.

Gómez BL, Nosanchuk JD. Melanin and fungi. Curr Opin Infect Dis. 2003;16(2):91–6.

Greer DL. Basidiomycetes as agents of human infections: a review. Mycopathologia. 1978;65(1–3):133–9.

Guarro J, et al. Comparison of in vitro antifungal susceptibilities of conidia and hyphae of filamentous fungi. Antimicrob Agents Chemother. 1997;41(12):2760–2.

Hayden R, et al. In situ hybridization for the differentiation of Aspergillus, Fusarium, and Pseudallescheria species in tissue section. Diagn Mol Pathol. 2003;12(1):21–6.

Hoenigl M, et al. Sinusitis and frontal brain abscess in a diabetic patient caused by the basidiomycete Schizophyllum commune: case report and review of the literature. Mycoses. 2013;56(3):389–93.

de Hoog G, et al. Ecology and physiology of the emerging opportunistic fungi Pseudallescheria boydii and Scedosporium prolificans. Mycoses. 1994;37(3–4):71–8.

Jacobson ES. Pathogenic roles for fungal melanins. Clin Microbiol Rev. 2000;13(4):708–17.

James TY, Vilgalys R. Abundance and diversity of Schizophyllum commune spore clouds in the Caribbean detected by selective sampling. Mol Ecol. 2001;10(2):471–9.

Jelinek AG, et al. Headaches and hemiparesis in an immunocompetent inmate. Neuropathology. 2014;34(3):314–7.

Kantarcioglu A, Yucel A. In-vitro activities of terbinafine, itraconazole and amphotericin B against Aspergillus and Cladosporium species. J Chemother. 2002;14(6):562–7.

Kantarcioğlu A, Yücel A, Hoog GD. Case report. Isolation of Cladosporium cladosporioides from cerebrospinal fluid. Mycoses. 2002;45(11–12):500–3.

Kantarcioglu AS, Guarro J, De Hoog G. Central nervous system infections by members of the Pseudallescheria boydii species complex in healthy and immunocompromised hosts: epidemiology, clinical characteristics and outcome. Mycoses. 2008;51(4):275–90.

Kantarcioglu AS, et al. A dark strain in the Fusarium solani species complex isolated from primary subcutaneous sporotrichioid lesions associated with traumatic inoculation via a rose bush thorn. Med Mycol. 2010;48(1):103–9.

Kapp M, et al. Endophthalmitis as primary clinical manifestation of fatal fusariosis in an allogeneic stem cell recipient. Transpl Infect Dis. 2011;13(4):374–9.

Küllü S, et al. Cerebral cladosporiosis. Surg Neurol. 1985;24(4):437–40.

Lackner M, et al. Rapid identification of Pseudallescheria and Scedosporium strains by using rolling circle amplification. Appl Environ Microbiol. 2012;78(1):126–33.

Lackner M, et al. Proposed nomenclature for Pseudallescheria, Scedosporium and related genera. Fungal Divers. 2014;67(1):1–10.

Lalueza A, et al. Cladosporium macrocarpum brain abscess after endoscopic ultrasound-guided celiac plexus block. Endoscopy. 2011;43(Suppl 2):E9–E10.

Lamoth F. Galactomannan and 1, 3-β-d-glucan testing for the diagnosis of invasive aspergillosis. J Fungi. 2016;2(3):22.

Latham RH. Bipolaris spicifera meningitis complicating a neurosurgerical procedure. Scand J Infect Dis. 2000;32(1):102–3.

LeibundGut-Landmann S, Wüthrich M, Hohl TM. Immunity to fungi. Curr Opin Immunol. 2012;24(4):449–58.

Lortholary O, et al. International retrospective analysis of 73 cases of invasive fusariosis treated with voriconazole. Antimicrob Agents Chemother. 2010;54(10):4446–50.

Lu Q, et al. Identification of Pseudallescheria and Scedosporium species by three molecular methods. J Clin Microbiol. 2011;49(3):960–7.

Manamgoda DS, et al. A phylogenetic and taxonomic re-evaluation of the Bipolaris-Cochliobolus-Curvularia complex. Fungal Divers. 2012;56(1):131–44.

Manamgoda D, et al. The genus bipolaris. Stud Mycol. 2014;79:221–88.

Marinach-Patrice C, et al. Use of mass spectrometry to identify clinical Fusarium isolates. Clin Microbiol Infect. 2009;15(7):634–42.

McGinnis MR, Pasarell L. In vitro testing of susceptibilities of filamentous ascomycetes to voriconazole, itraconazole, and amphotericin B, with consideration of phylogenetic implications. J Clin Microbiol. 1998;36(8):2353–5.

McGinnis M, et al. Phaeohyphomycosis caused by Bipolaris spicifera: an informative case. Eur J Epidemiol. 1992;8(3):383–6.

Michel J, et al. Schizophyllum commune: an emergent or misdiagnosed fungal pathogen in rhinology? Sabouraudia. 2015;54(3):301–9.

Moore ML, et al. Disseminated Bipolaris spicifera in a neonate. J Perinatol. 2001;21(6):399.

Morton S, Midthun K, Merz W. Granulomatous encephalitis caused by Bipolaris hawaiiensis. Arch Pathol Lab Med. 1986;110(12):1183–5.

Nelson PE, Dignani MC, Anaissie EJ. Taxonomy, biology, and clinical aspects of Fusarium species. Clin Microbiol Rev. 1994;7(4):479–504.

Nosanchuk JD, Casadevall A. The contribution of melanin to microbial pathogenesis. Cell Microbiol. 2003;5(4):203–23.

Nosanchuk JD, Casadevall A. Impact of melanin on microbial virulence and clinical resistance to antimicrobial compounds. Antimicrob Agents Chemother. 2006;50(11):3519–28.

Nosanchuk JD, Stark RE, Casadevall A. Fungal melanin: what do we know about structure? Front Microbiol. 2015;6:1463.

Nucci M, Anaissie E. Fusarium infections in immunocompromised patients. Clin Microbiol Rev. 2007;20(4):695–704.

Nucci M, Anaissie EJ. Hyalohyphomycosis. In: Clinical mycology. 2nd ed. London: Elsevier; 2009. p. 309–27.

Nucci M, et al. Outcome predictors of 84 patients with hematologic malignancies and Fusarium infection. Cancer. 2003;98(2):315–9.

Nucci M, et al. Fusarium infection in hematopoietic stem cell transplant recipients. Clin Infect Dis. 2004;38(9):1237–42.

O'Donnell K, et al. Discordant phylogenies suggest repeated host shifts in the Fusarium–Euwallacea ambrosia beetle mutualism. Fungal Genet Biol. 2015;82:277–90.

O'Gorman CM, Fuller HT. Prevalence of culturable airborne spores of selected allergenic and pathogenic fungi in outdoor air. Atmos Environ. 2008;42(18):4355–68.

Ohm RA, et al. Genome sequence of the model mushroom Schizophyllum commune. Nat Biotechnol. 2010;28(9):957.

Okten S, Asan A. Airborne fungi and bacteria in indoor and outdoor environment of the Pediatric Unit of Edirne Government Hospital. Environ Monit Assess. 2012;184(3):1739–51.

Pagano L, et al. Fungal CNS infections in patients with hematologic malignancy. Expert Rev Anti Infect Ther. 2005;3(5):775–85.

Pappagianis D, Ajello L. Dematiaceous—a mycologic misnomer? J Med Vet Mycol. 1994;32(4):319–21.

Patel M, et al. Bipolaris brain abscess in a patient treated with steroids for neurosarcoidosis. Chest. 2012;142(4):259A.

Peterson A, et al. Intracranial Fusarium fungal abscess in an immunocompetent patient: case report and review of the literature. J Neurol Surg Rep. 2014;75(2):e241.

Premamalini T, et al. Schizophyllum commune a causative agent of fungal sinusitis: a case report. Case Rep Infect Dis. 2011;2011:821259.

Raad I, et al. Epidemiology, molecular mycology, and environmental sources of Fusarium infection in patients with cancer. Infect Control Hosp Epidemiol. 2002;23(9):532–7.

Refai M, Gobba A, Rieth H. Monograph on yeasts. Diagnosis, diseases, and treatment. Vet Med J. 1969;16(17):255–316.

Revankar SG, Sutton DA. Melanized fungi in human disease. Clin Microbiol Rev. 2010;23(4):884–928.
Rihs JD, Padhye AA, Good CB. Brain abscess caused by Schizophyllum commune: an emerging basidiomycete pathogen. J Clin Microbiol. 1996;34(7):1628–32.
Romani L. Immunity to fungal infections. Nat Rev Immunol. 2004;4(1):11.
Romani L. Cell mediated immunity to fungi: a reassessment. Sabouraudia. 2008;46(6):515–29.
Rosow L, et al. Cerebral phaeohyphomycosis caused by Bipolaris spicifera after heart transplantation. Transpl Infect Dis. 2011;13(4):419–23.
Salah H, et al. Phylogenetic diversity of human pathogenic Fusarium and emergence of uncommon virulent species. J Infect. 2015;71(6):658–66.
Sandoval-Denis M, et al. Cladosporium species recovered from clinical samples in the United States. J Clin Microbiol. 2015;53(9):2990–3000. https://doi.org/10.1128/JCM.01482-15.
Schmidt O, Liese W. Variability of wood degrading enzymes of Schizophyllum commune. Holzforschung. 1980;34(2):67–72.
Schwartz KL, et al. Invasive fusariosis: a single pediatric center 15-year experience. J Pediatr Infect Dis Soc. 2013;4(2):163–70.
Segal BH, et al. Invasive infection with Fusarium chlamydosporum in a patient with aplastic anemia. J Clin Microbiol. 1998;36(6):1772–6.
Shin EJ, et al. Screening of middle ear effusion for the common sinus pathogen Bipolaris. Eur Arch Otorhinolaryngol. 2003;260(2):78–80.
Sigler L, et al. Diagnostic difficulties caused by a nonclamped Schizophyllum commune isolate in a case of fungus ball of the lung. J Clin Microbiol. 1995;33(8):1979–83.
Sivanesan A. Graminicolous species of Bipolaris, Curvularia, Drechslera, Exserohilum and their teleomorphs. UK: CAB International; 1987.
Steinberg GK, et al. Fusarium brain abscess: case report. J Neurosurg. 1983;58(4):598–601.
Sugiura Y, et al. Experimental murine hyalohyphomycosis with soil-derived isolates of Fusarium solani. Med Mycol. 2003;41(3):241–7.
Tauber SC, et al. Fungal encephalitis in human autopsy cases is associated with extensive neuronal damage but only minimal repair. Neuropathol Appl Neurobiol. 2014;40(5):610–27.
Teran CG, Downes K, Medows M. Fatal Bipolaris spicifera infection in an immunosuppressed child. BMJ Case Rep. 2014;2014:bcr2013009703.
Tone K, et al. Epidural abscess caused by Schizophyllum commune: a rare case of rhinogenic cranial complication by a filamentous basidiomycete. Mycoses. 2018;61(3):213–7.
Tortorano A, et al. ESCMID and ECMM joint guidelines on diagnosis and management of hyalohyphomycosis: Fusarium spp., Scedosporium spp. and others. Clin Microbiol Infect. 2014;20(s3):27–46.
Triest D, et al. Use of matrix-assisted laser desorption ionization–time of flight mass spectrometry for identification of molds of the Fusarium genus. J Clin Microbiol. 2015;53(2):465–76.
Verma A, et al. Adaptive immunity to fungi. Cold Spring Harb Perspect Med. 2015;5(3):a019612.
Vincent AL, et al. Successful voriconazole therapy of disseminated Fusarium solani in the brain of a neutropenic cancer patient. Cancer Control. 2003;10(5):414–9.
Viola GM, Sutton R. Allergic fungal sinusitis complicated by fungal brain mass. Int J Infect Dis. 2010;14:e299–301.
Winn RM, et al. Effects of interleukin-15 on antifungal responses of human polymorphonuclear leukocytes against Fusarium spp. and Scedosporium spp. Cytokine. 2005;31(1):1–8.
Won EJ, et al. Molecular identification of Schizophyllum commune as a cause of allergic fungal sinusitis. Ann Lab Med. 2012;32(5):375–9.
Wösten H, Wessels J. The emergence of fruiting bodies in basidiomycetes. In: Growth, differentiation and sexuality. Berlin: Springer; 2006. p. 393–414.
Wright WF, Overman SB, Ribes JA. (1–3)-β-D-Glucan assay: a review of its laboratory and clinical application. Lab Med. 2011;42(11):679–85.
Yergeau E, et al. Relationships between Fusarium population structure, soil nutrient status and disease incidence in field-grown asparagus. FEMS Microbiol Ecol. 2006;58(3):394–403.
Yoshimori RN, et al. Phaeohyphomycosis of brain: granulomatous encephalitis caused by Drechslera spicifera. Am J Clin Pathol. 1982;77(3):363–70.

Part III

Clinical Syndromes of Fungal Infections Involving Central Nervous System and Its Coverings

16 Cranial Vault Lesions

Ali Akhaddar

Abbreviation

CVM Cranial vault mycosis

16.1 Introduction

The skull is an uncommon location of fungal infections which are often described in the skull base (Blyth et al. 2011). The cranial vault (calvaria) has significant proximity with extracranial tissues, paranasal sinuses, orbits, skull base, and intracranial structures which largely explain the location of infection and its extension. Although still uncommon in our daily practice, it is important to be attentive of cranial vault mycosis (CVM) and to consider them in the differential diagnosis of appropriate presentations. The infection has a spectrum of presenting features, and most patients are immunocompromised hosts, although immunocompetent subjects can also be affected (Corral et al. 2011; Kong et al. 2013; Letscher et al. 1997; Rodríguez-Hernández et al. 2001; Wolkow et al. 2017). Fungal cranial vault bony infections are often misdiagnosed and frequently considered only following failure of antibacterial therapy resulting in high rate of morbidity and intracranial complications. Although there is a paucity of publication in the current literature regarding mycosis involving the cranial vault, we will provide in this chapter a practical review regarding these dangerous and neglected diseases and their management strategies.

A. Akhaddar (✉)
Department of Neurosurgery, Avicenne Military Hospital of Marrakech, Mohammed V University of Rabat, Rabat, Morocco

16.2 Epidemiology

Cranial mycosis is a rare disease. Often located in the skull base, few cases of cranial vault involvement have been reported in fungal infections (less than 100 cases). Among 180 cases of *Aspergillus* osteomyelitis reported in the literature as on 2014, 41 (23%) were located in the skull, often in the skull base with male predominance (71%) (Gamaletsou et al. 2014). Cranial cryptococcosis is also rare; to date less than 20 cases have been reported in the literature representing about 20% of all cryptococcal infections with bone involvement (Agadi et al. 2010; Amit et al. 2008; Corral et al. 2011; Kong et al. 2013; Pudipeddi et al. 2016; Rerolle et al. 2005; Rootjes et al. 2016; Wood and Miedzinski 1996). Coccidioidomycosis osteomyelitis of the cranium has only been reported on five previous occasions, three of them in the cranial vault (Antony et al. 2015; Arnold et al. 2004; Baddley et al. 2004). Only three cases of cranial vault maduromycosis were previously described (Beeram et al. 2008; Goel et al. 2012; Hickey

M. Turgut et al. (eds.), *Fungal Infections of the Central Nervous System*,
https://doi.org/10.1007/978-3-030-06088-6_16

1950). Mucormycosis is habitually a skull base infection. However, two cases of mucormycosis were reported in the calvaria following rhinocerebral invasion (Fortún et al. 1995; Honeybul and Morrison 2012; Taj-Aldeen et al. 2017). Other fungi have been described involving the cranial vault, but often much less frequently. The majority of cases of calvarial mycosis are reported from developing countries. However, changes in the socioeconomic status and advances in medicine are responsible for a relative increasing number of infections secondary to fungi especially in immunocompromised subjects and those with fungal paranasal sinusitis and orbital sepsis (Patel et al. 2011). In the calvaria, parietal and frontal bones are more usually affected than occipital and temporal which are less vascularized. CVM are less commonly described in infants than in adults without apparent sex predominance. Nevertheless, Rosanova et al. reported 3 children with CVM in a recent series of 12 children with burns and osteomyelitis. The youngest child described was only 18 months old (Wright et al. 1993). Unlike skull base osteomyelitis, CVM arises mostly from disseminated infection and skull trauma (Fortún et al. 1995; Honeybul and Morrison 2012; Rodríguez-Hernández et al. 2001; Rosanova et al. 2018). One case of cranial *Aspergillus fumigatus* infection with intracranial epidural abscess following craniotomy was previously reported in an immunocompetent young patient (Letscher et al. 1997).

16.3 Pathogenesis and Pathology

Traditionally, cranial osteomyelitis is usually related to three main sources of infection: (1) direct extension from contiguous site of infection, (2) postsurgical or post-traumatic direct inoculation (from a contaminated wound), and (3) hematogenous dissemination from remote source of infection. In developed countries, postsurgical craniotomy infections remain the most common cause of cranial osteomyelitis, while in developing nations, paranasal sinusitis and scalp infections have become the predominant sources (Akhaddar 2016).

The cranial vault has important and complex anatomic relationships with extracranial and intracranial structures. So, the problem of this disease is likely to get worse when intracranial invasion occurs with their potentially life-threatening consequences (Akhaddar 2017a).

In general, the fungal agent reaches the skull vault by the outer table (local invasion) or through the diploe (hematogenously). Unlike fungal skull base osteomyelitis, direct extension from paranasal sinusitis or orbital infections is rare (Panda and Ekambar Eshwara Reddy 2005; Patel et al. 2011; Wolkow et al. 2017). CVM may be very invasive, involving both tables, and in extreme cases may destroy the galea, scalp, and dura with subdural and brain invasion (Fig. 16.1).

Some comorbidities or patient-predisposing risk factors should be taken into consideration. These include vulnerability due to metabolic states, compromised immune function, malignancy, and advanced age (Agadi et al. 2010; Amit et al. 2008; Effat et al. 2005; Pudipeddi et al. 2016; Qiu et al. 2015; Rerolle et al. 2005; Rootjes et al. 2016; Wolkow et al. 2017; Wright et al. 1993). The use of broad-spectrum antibiotics is known to be one major risk factor for fungal infections (Akhaddar 2017b).

The cranial vault may be infected by various fungal pathogens, mostly from *Aspergillus* species which are ubiquitous in the environment and usually noninvasive. Several species have been reported as pathogens especially *A. fumigatus* and *A. flavus*. Apart from *Aspergillus spp, Cryptococci, Coccidioidomycetes and Mucorales (Zygomycetes)* are the most common pathogens involved. Other reported fungi causing CVM include *Blastomyces*, *Candida* species, *Trichosporon asahii*, *Penicillium marneffei*, *Pseudallescheria boydii*, *Apophysomyces variabilis*, and *Streptomyces somaliensis* (Fernández-Guerrero et al. 1987; Mateev et al. 1993;

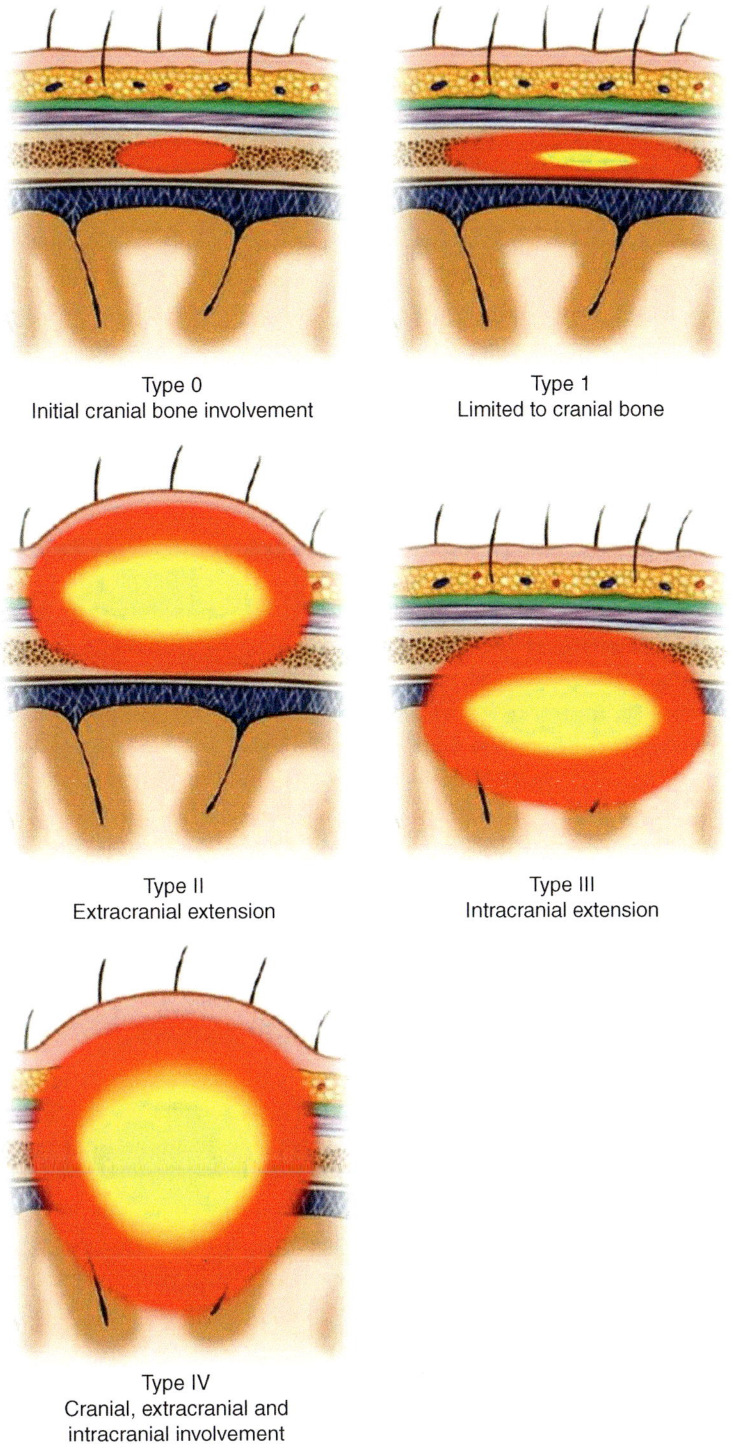

Fig. 16.1 Staging system for skull osteomyelitis (3SO). Five main types of cranial osteomyelitis based on the location of infection and its extension (Reproduced from Akhaddar A (ed) Cranial osteomyelitis (2016); with permission)

Naim-Ur-Rahman et al. 1987; Patel et al. 2011; Qiu et al. 2015; Rosanova et al. 2018; Wolkow et al. 2017; Yocum and Seligson 1991).

16.4 Clinical Features

Clinical features of CVM may vary greatly according to many factors such as age of onset, duration of disease, route of infection, underlying etiologies, type of fungi, comorbidities, and anatomic location of infection and its extension. Generally, the most usually described clinical presentations are not too different from those with bacterial cranial vault osteomyelitis: mainly local signs of inflammation and/or infection (soft tissue swelling, pain, purulent discharge, and exposed bone) (Patel et al. 2011). Fever was not a common feature in CVM (Akhaddar 2016; Agadi et al. 2010). However, many patients presented skin tenderness and more rarely a draining fistulous tract (Mateev et al. 1993; Yocum and Seligson 1991). When the infection spreads into the epidural space, headache worsens. In advanced conditions if the lesion increases in size, altered mental status and occasionally focal neurologic signs develop with or without signs of raised intracranial pressure (Letscher et al. 1997; Naim-Ur-Rahman et al. 1987). Focal neurologic deficits are according to the site of the lesion in the cranial vault such as hemiparesis, hemisensory deficit, cognitive disorder, visual deficit, seizures, and meningismus. Rarely, more severe cerebral complications may arise with rapid neurologic deterioration, respiratory failure, hemodynamic instability, loss of consciousness, and death (Reining et al. 1984; Wright et al. 1993). When the duration of symptoms is less than one month, the cranial bone infection is considered acute. In chronic infections, the duration of symptoms is several months (Akhaddar 2016).

Four cases of CVM were previously reported with frontal sinusitis and forehead swelling mimicking a Pott's puffy tumor (Effat et al. 2005; Panda and Ekambar Eshwara Reddy 2005; Patel et al. 2011). This is named after Sir Percival Pott who described the association of forehead localized swelling with overlying subperiosteal abscess and underlying frontal bone osteomyelitis of frontal bone (Akhaddar 2016).

In more chronic forms, the onset of symptoms is more insidious and the clinical course more prolonged, masked in part by the primary illness. In fact, more immunocompromised patients are less likely to exhibit florid systemic signs of infections. It is important to pay attention to multifocal lesion in the body. Routine general systemic examination should be performed to identify apparent anomalies and possible other distal source of fungal infection (Mateev et al. 1993; Qiu et al. 2015; Rerolle et al. 2005).

Clinically, some patients with cranial vault osteomyelitis can present with signs and symptoms that imitate other calvarial and scalp pathologies (especially its tumoral or pseudocystic presentations) such as many inflammatory cutaneous lesions, vascular malformations, infected hematoma or scalp tumors, folliculitis, sebaceous cysts, skin and scalp abscesses, cellulitis, dermoid and epidermoid cysts, encephaloceles fibrous dysplasia, and different benign and malignant tumors (Akhaddar 2016).

Any nonhealing ulcerations, spontaneous scalp infections, and/or chronic sinus tracts should raise a suspicion of a fungal infection (Beeram et al. 2008; Mateev et al. 1993).

16.5 Diagnosis

Diagnosis is often delayed and frequently considered only following failure of antibacterial therapy (Effat et al. 2005). A detailed history, clinical evaluation, laboratory investigations, culture, and imaging explorations help the diagnosis. However, the most significant finding for diagnosis should be made by histopathological examination and culture of specimens obtained at surgery (direct biopsy or surgical debridement).

Neuroimaging data are usually indicative of osteomyelitis but are not specific for cranial vault mycosis. The diagnostic imaging features of osteolysis (irregular and well-defined lytic lesion), bone destruction, sometimes showing sequestrum (Fig. 16.2), and increased T2-weighted image on magnetic resonance

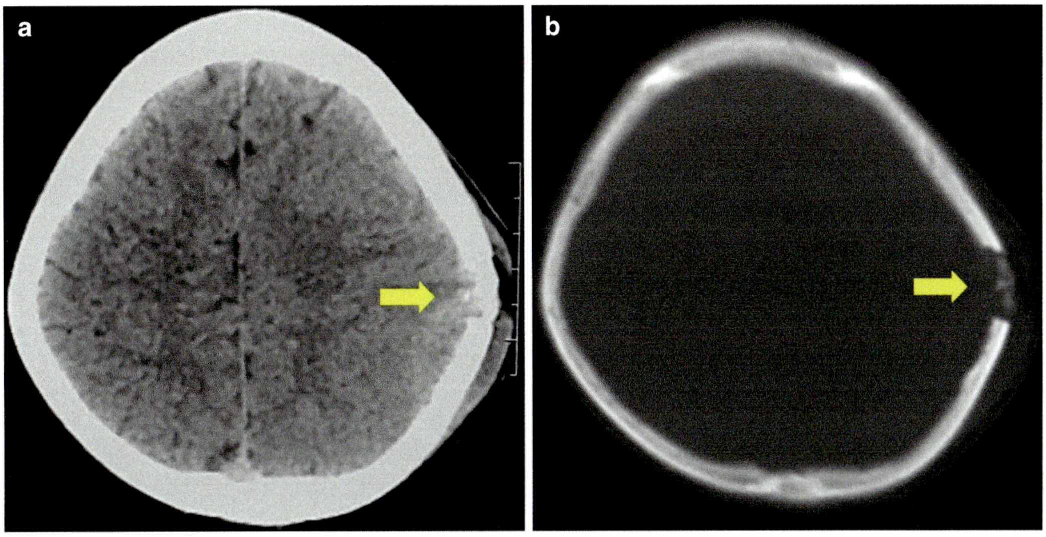

Fig. 16.2 Chronic skull bone osteomyelitis with sequestrum. Axial CT scan of the skull in parenchymal (**a**) and bone windows (**b**) showing isodense parietal bone lesion (arrows) with extracranial extension

imaging are compatible with any osseous infection but without specificity for fungal pathogens. Dura matter involvement after contrast enhancement is not rare. In developing countries, tuberculosis should be considered as differential diagnosis (Amit et al. 2008). Besides computed tomography scan and magnetic resonance imaging, nuclear medicine techniques are very sensitive for skull infection and are an excellent positive indicator (Wood and Miedzinski 1996).

The results of routine laboratory investigations are usually within normal limits.

In aspergillosis, histopathologic study shows vascular thrombosis that is surrounded by extensive coagulative necrosis and hemorrhage. Granulomatous inflammation with septate hyphae branching at acute angle or dichotomously at irregular intervals is highly suggestive of the diagnosis. On the contrary, mucormycosis is characterized by irregular hyphae without septae, branching at right-angle (90°). Histologic features of cryptococcal infections correspond to chronic granulomatous inflammation and the presence of numerous yeast-like organisms using hematoxylin and eosin, periodic acid Schiff, Gomori methenamine silver and alcian blue stains (Wood and Miedzinski 1996). However, in some difficult cases, definitive diagnosis requires culture on enriched agars. The role of a histopathology is also to differentiate mycosis from tuberculosis and malignant tumors (Akhaddar 2016).

Morphologic and molecular diagnosis of fungal infections of the central nervous system is discussed in the other chapters of the book.

16.6 Treatment Options and Outcomes

There are no specific treatment recommendations for cranial bone osteomyelitis. Old publications have stressed the importance of radical surgery in combination with an antifungal agent in treating most osseous mycosis. Data on patient survival is available only from case reports and small case series.

The antifungal agents of choice have changed over the past two decades. For aspergillosis, voriconazole now represents the first-line treatment for invasive aspergillosis and especially for bony invasion (Gamaletsou et al. 2014). Recent cases with cryptococcal cranial vault were treated successfully with intravenous amphotericin B and oral fluconazole. Coccidioidomycosis involving the skull is also treated with a combination of lipid amphotericin B and long-term fluconazole (Antony et al. 2015). Currently, itraconazole and ketoconazole are the best treatment options for bone mycetoma. Amphotericin B is the antifungal drugs of choice for mucormycosis. Alternatively, posaconazole can be considered. Treatment duration depends on the condition of the patients, the presence of complications, and the precocity of diagnosis. A minimum of 3 months is necessary to avoid recurrences. Some authors, suggest that treatment duration of 6 months is mandatory (Rodríguez-Hernández et al. 2001). More details concerning chemotherapy for fungal infections are discussed in another chapter of the book.

Patients with partial extracranial soft tissue infection with mild cranial osteomyelitis can be treated with antifungal drugs alone. Sometimes, simple cutaneous drainage or limited scalp incision are sufficient and may be used to collect specimens for diagnosis. Surgical debridement remains critical to eliminate areas of necrosis and sequestrum. Infected bone with evidence of necrosis should be removed (more or less extensive craniectomy), followed by cranioplasty on a second intervention (using methyl methacrylate or titanium plate) (Antony et al. 2015). An extradural closed drainage system can be used. Management of associated intracranial complications should be taken into consideration. Treatment of concomitant fungal infections is needed for some patients to eliminate the primary source of infection.

Some authors suggest that hyperbaric oxygen therapy should be considered postoperatively for some refractory cases of skull base mycosis (Blyth et al. 2011).

The spread of infection could be disastrous, not only locally and regionally but possibly even systemically. Sadly, there is always a chance of lethal complication from calvarial fungal osteomyelitis. Successful patient outcome depends on high index of clinical suspicion, adequate and appropriate sinus biopsies and rapid microbiological, pathological, and radiological diagnosis, followed by prompt aggressive and concomitant surgical debridement, antifungal treatment, and management of the underlying or predisposing metabolic or other systemic disorders.

In some patients on antifungal therapy, disease may progress slowly and intermittently, requiring multiple courses of antifungal drugs (Wolkow et al. 2017).

Immunocompetent patients tend to have better outcomes as compared to those who are immunocompromised. Patients with intradural disease carry the worst prognosis (Wright et al. 1993).

16.7 Conclusion

Cranial vault fungal infection is a rare disease, infrequently encountered, and not always considered as a first differential diagnosis. Pathology plays an important role for confirming the definitive diagnosis of CVM, especially if clinical findings, laboratory studies, and diagnostic imaging investigations are not conclusive.

The diagnosis should be considered in any insidious growing soft tissue mass or scalp abscess of unertain origin in addition to any osteolytic calvarial lesion with granulomatous reaction.

References

Agadi JB, Madni NA, Nanjappa V, Govindaiah HK. Cryptococcal osteomyelitis of the skull in a patient with transient lymphopenia. Neurol India. 2010;58(2):300–2. https://doi.org/10.4103/0028-3886.63798.

Akhaddar A. Cranial osteomyelitis. Diagnosis and treatment. 1st ed. Switzerland: Springer International Publishing; 2016. https://doi.org/10.1007/978-3-319-30268-3.

Akhaddar A. Cranial osteomyelitis. In: Atlas of infections in neurosurgery and spinal surgery. 1st ed. Switzerland: Springer International Publishing; 2017a. p. 33–42. https://doi.org/10.1007/978-3-319-60086-4_4.

Akhaddar A. Fungal infections of the central nervous system. In: Atlas of infections in neurosurgery and spinal surgery. 1st ed. Switzerland: Springer International Publishing; 2017b. p. 317–3. https://doi.org/10.1007/978-3-319-60086-4_29.

Amit A, Sudish K, Pople IK. Primary calvarial cryptococcal osteomyelitis in a patient with idiopathic lymphopenia. Acta Neurochir (Wien). 2008;150(7):713–4. https://doi.org/10.1007/s00701-008-1608-8.

Antony SJ, Parikh MS, Friedman G. Coccidioidomycosis involving the cranium: a case report and review of current literature. Infect Disord Drug Targets. 2015;15(3):202–6.

Arnold MG, Arnold JC, Bloom DC, Brewster DF, Thiringer JK. Head and neck manifestations of disseminated coccidioidomycosis. Laryngoscope. 2004;114(4):747–52.
Baddley JW, Cobbs CS, Pappas PG. Surgical treatment of multiple skull abscesses associated with coccidioidomycosis. Mycoses. 2004;47(1–2):69–71.
Beeram V, Challa S, Vannemreddy P. Cerebral mycetoma with cranial osteomyelitis. J Neurosurg Pediatr. 2008;1(6):493–5. https://doi.org/10.3171/PED/2008/1/6/493.
Blyth CC, Gomes L, Sorrell TC, da Cruz M, Sud A, Chen SC. Skull-base osteomyelitis: fungal vs. bacterial infection. Clin Microbiol Infect. 2011;17(2):306–11. https://doi.org/10.1111/j.1469-0691.2010.03231.x.
Corral JE, Lima S, Quezada J, Samayoa B, Arathoon E. Cryptococcal osteomyelitis of the skull. Med Mycol. 2011;49:667–71. https://doi.org/10.3109/13693786.2011.558124.
Effat KG, Karam M, El-Kabani A. Pott's puffy tumour caused by mucormycosis. J Laryngol Otol. 2005;119(8):643–5.
Fernández-Guerrero ML, Ruiz Barnés P, Alés JM. Postcraniotomy mycetoma of the scalp and osteomyelitis due to Pseudallescheria boydii. J Infect Dis. 1987;156(5):855.
Fortún J, Cobo J, Cañal J, Martínez-San Millán J. Posttraumatic cranial mucormycosis in an immunocompetent patient. J Oral Maxillofac Surg. 1995;53(9):1099–102.
Gamaletsou MN, Rammaert B, Bueno MA, Moriyama B, Sipsas NV, Kontoyiannis DP, et al. Aspergillus osteomyelitis: epidemiology, clinical manifestations, management, and outcome. J Infect. 2014;68(5):478–93. https://doi.org/10.1016/j.jinf.2013.12.008.
Goel RS, Kataria R, Sinha VD, Gupta A, Singh S, Jain A. Craniocerebral maduromycosis. J Neurosurg Pediatr. 2012;10(1):67–70. https://doi.org/10.3171/2012.3.PEDS1252.
Hickey BB. Cranial maduromycosis. Trans R Soc Trop Med Hyg. 1950;50:393–6.
Honeybul S, Morrison DA. Skull vault destruction after rhinocerebral mucormycosis. World Neurosurg. 2012;78(5):553.e1–4. https://doi.org/10.1016/j.wneu.2011.12.009.
Kong QT, Zhou WQ, Feng J, Sang H, Deng DQ, Wang Z, et al. Isolated skull cryptococcosis in an immunocompetent patient. Mycopathologia. 2013;175(1–2):187–91. https://doi.org/10.1007/s11046-012-9609-9.
Letscher V, Herbrecht R, Gaudias J, Taglang G, Koenig H, Dupuis MG, et al. Post-traumatic intracranial epidural Aspergillus fumigatus abscess. J Med Vet Mycol. 1997;35(4):279–82.
Mateev G, Kantardjiev T, Vassileva S, Tsankov N. Chronic mucocutaneous candidosis with osteolysis of the frontal bone. Int J Dermatol. 1993;32(12):888–9.
Naim-Ur-Rahman, Abdullah AK, Hawass NE, Sadiq S, el-Nageeb S, Akhtar-Uz-Zaman. Cranial and epidural mycetoma caused by streptomyces somaliensis. Neuroradiology. 1987;29(1):95–7.
Panda NK, Ekambar Eshwara Reddy C. Primary frontal sinus aspergillosis: an uncommon occurrence. Mycoses. 2005;48(4):235–7.
Patel SA, Chatterjee A, Simonsen K. Recurrent midline frontal mass in a patient with sinusitis. Clin Pediatr (Phila). 2011;50(3):266–8. https://doi.org/10.1177/0009922809352680.
Pudipeddi AV, Liu K, Watson GF, Davis RJ, Strasser SI. Cryptococcal osteomyelitis of the skull in a liver transplant patient. Transpl Infect Dis. 2016;18(6):954–6. https://doi.org/10.1111/tid.12602.
Qiu Y, Zhang J, Liu G, Zhong X, Deng J, He Z, et al. Retrospective analysis of 14 cases of disseminated Penicillium marneffei infection with osteolytic lesions. BMC Infect Dis. 2015;15:47. https://doi.org/10.1186/s12879-015-0782-6.
Reining JW, Hungerford GD, Mohrmann ME, Vera CL. Case report 268. Skelet Radiol. 1984;11:221–3.
Rerolle JP, Szelag JC, Diaconita M, Paraf F, Aldigier JC, Le Meur Y. Intracranial granuloma and skull osteolysis: complication of a primary cutaneous cryptococcosis in a kidney transplant recipient. Am J Kidney Dis. 2005;46(6):e113–7.
Rodríguez-Hernández MJ, Jiménez-Mejías ME, Montero JM, Regordan C, Ferreras G. Aspergillus fumigatus cranial infection after accidental traumatism. Eur J Clin Microbiol Infect Dis. 2001;20(9):655–6.
Rootjes PA, Rozemeijer W, Dutilh JC. A patient with sarcoidosis and a cryptococcal infection of the skull. Med J Aust. 2016;204(9):353.
Rosanova MT, Voto C, Carnovale S, Tramonti N, Lema J, Pinheiro JL, et al. Osteomyelitis in burn children: ten years of experience. Arch Argent Pediatr. 2018;116(1):59–61. https://doi.org/10.5546/aap.2018.eng.59.
Taj-Aldeen SJ, Gamaletsou MN, Rammaert B, Sipsas NV, Zeller V, Roilides E, et al. Bone and joint infections caused by mucormycetes: a challenging osteoarticular mycosis of the twenty-first century. Med Mycol. 2017;55(7):691–704. https://doi.org/10.1093/mmy/myw136.
Wolkow N, Jakobiec FA, Stagner AM, Cunnane ME, Piantadosi AL, Basgoz N, et al. Chronic orbital and calvarial fungal infection with Apophysomyces variabilis in an immunocompetent patient. Surv Ophthalmol. 2017;62(1):70–82. https://doi.org/10.1016/j.survophthal.2016.05.006.
Wood L, Miedzinski L. Skeletal cryptococcosis: case report and review of the literature. Can J Infect Dis. 1996;7(2):125–32.
Wright M, Fikrig S, Haller JO. Aspergillosis in children with acquired immune deficiency. Pediatr Radiol. 1993;23(6):492–4.
Yocum J, Seligson D. Blastomycosis of the knee and skull after arthroscopy. Am J Sports Med. 1991;19(6):670–2.

Meningitis and Meningoencephalitis

17

Alexa Bodman and Walter A. Hall

Abbreviations

AIDS	Acquired immunodeficiency syndrome
CNS	Central nervous system
CSF	Cerebrospinal fluid
HIV	Human immunodeficiency virus
ICU	Intensive care unit

17.1 Introduction

Meningitis and meningoencephalitis resulting from fungal organisms, though uncommon, are serious conditions associated with significant neurological morbidity and mortality. Fungal meningitis accounts for 2.7% of all meningoencephalitis cases in the United States with a mortality rate of 8.2% (Hasbun et al. 2017). The length of hospital stay in fungal meningitis is longer than for other forms of meningitis with a median stay of 13 days (Hasbun et al. 2017). The prompt recognition and treatment of this entity can aid in curbing the significant morbidity and mortality associated with fungal meningitis.

As fungal meningitis is an unusual diagnosis, its recognition is often delayed. Neuroimaging and lumbar puncture may aid in making the diagnosis. Only 50% of patients with the diagnosis of meningitis have accompanying changes on radiographic imaging (Gavito-Higuera 2016). Enhancement patterns of the leptomeninges from a fungal infection are highly variable, where the enhancement may be thick, irregular, continuous, asymmetric, or smooth with extension into the base of the sulci (Gavito-Higuera 2016). (1–3)-β-D-Glucan, a polysaccharide from the fungal cell wall, is found in the serum and can aid in the detection of invasive fungal disease (Lyons et al. 2014). This carbohydrate can also be measured in the cerebrospinal fluid (CSF) and can aid in the diagnosis of central nervous system (CNS) fungal disease (Lyons et al. 2014). In this chapter we will review the common etiologies of fungal meningitis and meningoencephalitis that include *Candida* spp., *Cryptococcus* spp., *Aspergillus* spp., *Coccidioides immitis*, *Histoplasma capsulatum*, *Blastomyces dermatitidis*, and *Mucorales*, as well as rare causes of fungal meningitis.

17.2 Candidiasis

Candidiasis is the most common invasive fungal infection globally (Bongomin et al. 2017). *Candida* spp. causing CNS infections are frequently nosocomial (Hall and Kim 2013). *Candida albicans* is the most common pathogen, but infections with *C. glabrata*, *C. parap-*

A. Bodman · W. A. Hall (✉)
Department of Neurosurgery, SUNY Upstate Medical University, Syracuse, NY, USA
e-mail: hallw@upstate.edu

M. Turgut et al. (eds.), *Fungal Infections of the Central Nervous System*,
https://doi.org/10.1007/978-3-030-06088-6_17

silosis, *C. tropicalis*, *C. krusei*, and *C. auris* have been increasing in frequency (Bongomin et al. 2017). Risk factors for a nosocomial invasive infection with *Candida* spp. include central lines, abdominal surgery, long hospital stay, use of total parenteral nutrition, and antibiotic use (Patterson 2005). Genetic factors can increase a patient's risk for developing a CNS infection with *Candida* spp. Inherited CARD9 deficiency has been associated with an increased risk for *Candida* meningoencephalitis (Lanternier et al. 2015). Infection of the CNS with this species can also lead to the development of vasculitis, mycotic aneurysms, and intraventricular fungal balls (Hall and Kim 2013). In premature infants, *Candida* is an important cause of late-onset neonatal sepsis and meningitis. In one large multicenter study, 4.2% of extremely low birth weight infants with sepsis developed meningitis with positive CSF cultures for *Candida*, most commonly *C. albicans* (Adams-Chapman et al. 2013). Invasive candidiasis is associated with a significant mortality rate (Bongomin et al. 2017). The mortality rate associated with *Candida* sepsis/meningitis in one study of premature infants was as high as 41% in those who survived with rates of neurodevelopmental impairment being significantly greater than in uninfected infants with no history of sepsis (Adams-Chapman et al. 2013). Nosocomial infection also occurs after neurosurgical procedures. Though this occurrence is rare, *Candida* is the most common postoperative fungal infection in neurosurgery. In one retrospective review, external ventricular drain placement was the most common neurosurgical procedure associated with *Candida* meningitis with a mortality rate of 27% (O'Brien et al. 2011). Broad-spectrum antibiotics are often administered prior to the development of a *Candida* infection in post-neurosurgical patients (O'Brien et al. 2011). Brown heroin use has also been associated with *Candida* meningitis (Melnychuk and Sole 2017). Once suspected, antifungal treatment should be started empirically. *C. albicans* is typically susceptible to a wide range of antifungal agents that include the echinocandins and amphotericin B (Patterson 2005). Resistance to fluconazole is prevalent in intensive care unit (ICU) patients with candidiasis (Modrzewska et al. 2017). In neonates, amphotericin B is recommended for CNS candidiasis with fluconazole being an acceptable alternative (Pappas et al. 2016). In adults, liposomal amphotericin B is recommended for the initial treatment with a transition to fluconazole being planned after an initial response to therapy (Pappas et al. 2016).

17.3 Cryptococcal Meningitis

In patients with the human immunodeficiency virus (HIV), *Cryptococcus neoformans* is the most common cause of fungal meningitis (Murthy and Sundaram 2014). This disease became prevalent at the beginning of the acquired immune deficiency syndrome (AIDS) epidemic, and then following the discovery of anti-retroviral therapy, its incidence has been decreasing (Pukkila-Worley and Mylonakis 2008). In immunocompetent patients with cryptococcal meningitis, *Cryptococcus gattii* is often the causative fungus (Pukkila-Worley and Mylonakis 2008). The clinical presentation of cryptococcal meningitis often includes a severe headache and malaise of a more chronic nature, which may be related to raised intracranial pressure and hydrocephalus (Chen et al. 2012). Diplopia, blindness, and other visual symptoms are also common (Zunt and Baldwin 2012). Increased intracranial pressures with hydrocephalus may not show enlargement of the ventricular system in cryptococcal meningitis, and treatment with lumbar drainage, serial lumbar punctures, external ventricular drainage and possible permanent CSF diversion may be necessary (Cherian et al. 2015). CSF analysis in cryptococcal meningitis can show an elevated or normal white blood cell count with predominantly mononuclear cells, a decrease in glucose level, and an increase in protein level (Zunt and Baldwin 2012). India ink staining and fungal culture may demonstrate the organism (Zunt and Baldwin 2012).

The recommended treatment for cryptococcal meningitis is with amphotericin B and flucytosine. At least 2 weeks of intravenous amphotericin B should be used prior to a transition to oral fluconazole therapy for a minimum of 8 weeks (Murthy and Sundaram 2014; Franco-Paredes et al. 2015). Patients with HIV should be placed on maintenance therapy to prevent relapse, which is typically oral fluconazole 200 mg/day (Pukkila-Worley and Mylonakis 2008). One should be wary of immune reconstitution inflammatory syndrome after the initiation of anti-retroviral therapy for cryptococcal meningitis (Pukkila-Worley and Mylonakis 2008). In limited access regions, mortality rates for cryptococcal meningitis associated with AIDS can approach 100% (Mwaba et al. 2001). Even in those that are able to obtain care in areas with limited resources, the prognosis continues to be poor with a mortality rate of approximately 70% (Rajasingham et al. 2017). In patients that are HIV positive in countries that are considered middle-income, the 1-year mortality rate associated with cryptococcal meningitis is 60% in those that are not on anti-retroviral therapy and 40% in those being treated. In Europe and North America, patients on anti-retroviral therapy that have cryptococcal meningitis are 20–30% (Rajasingham et al. 2017). Access to effective therapies and long-term anti-retroviral therapy in patients with HIV reduces the mortality associated with cryptococcal meningitis significantly. In patients with HIV, early clearance of their cryptococcal meningitis is acheived with combination therapy using amphotericin B and fluconazole (Concha-Velasco et al. 2017). High fungal burden and severely elevated intracranial pressure are associated with delayed fungal clearance (Concha-Velasco et al. 2017). CSF cultures can be used to monitor the response to therapy with patients having persistent positive cultures having a worse clinical outcome (Pukkila-Worley and Mylonakis 2008; van der Horst et al. 1997). Dexamethasone should not be used in the treatment of cryptococcal meningitis in patients with HIV because a randomized controlled trial showed that dexamethasone therapy increased the likelihood of adverse outcomes such as cardiac events and renal failure and was associated with a higher degree of disability at 10 weeks (Beardsley et al. 2016).

17.4 Aspergillosis

Aspergillosis is the most common CNS fungal infection to develop after solid organ transplantation (Şahintürk et al. 2018). This species is ubiquitous in the soil, and daily exposure through environmental sources is common (Zunt and Baldwin 2012). CNS aspergillosis is commonly found in patients following bone marrow transplantation, with hematologic malignancies, aplastic anemia, chronic asthma, chronic steroid use, and AIDS (Kleinschmidt-DeMasters 2002). Fever, headaches, and neck stiffness are the most common clinical presentation for *Aspergillus* meningoencephalitis (Antinori et al. 2013). The most common species to infect humans is *Aspergillus fumigatus* (Kleinschmidt-DeMasters 2002). Hematogenous spread or direct extension from the nasopharynx can result in aspergillosis. If originating from the nasal sinuses, ethmoidal involvement can extend into the cavernous sinus resulting in thrombosis. In this event, patients may present with ophthalmoplegia (Zunt and Baldwin 2012). CSF analysis will show a lymphocyte predominance, an elevated white blood cell count, an increased protein level, and a decreased glucose level (Zunt and Baldwin 2012). Galactomannan detection in the CSF can be useful in the diagnosis of *Aspergillus* meningitis (Ullmann et al. 2018). Growth from cultures is positive in only 31% of cases and results improved with repeat lumbar punctures. It is not uncommon for the diagnosis to be made on post-mortem examination (Antinori et al. 2013).

In patients that have had a solid organ transplant who develop CNS aspergillosis, 86% will have a concomitant severe infection that is either bacterial or due to a different fungus (Torre-Cisneros et al. 1993). Another study confirmed that there is a high rate of coinfection with another bacterial or fungal species in patients with CNS aspergillosis where 74% of patients had positive cultures for another species (Kleinschmidt-DeMasters 2002). Rejection of a transplanted organ with the subsequent need for increased immunosuppression often occurred prior to the development of CNS aspergillosis (Kleinschmidt-DeMasters 2002; Torre-Cisneros et al. 1993).

Infection with *Aspergillus* spp. in the CNS can result in devastating neurological consequences. *Aspergillus* spp. gather near leptomeningeal vessels, forming fungal thrombi that can lead to cerebral infarction (Kleinschmidt-DeMasters 2002). CNS aspergillosis is associated with a poor prognosis and low survival rate (Hall and Kim 2013). One study showed a mortality rate of 57.5% in hematopoietic stem cell transplantation patients that had invasive aspergillosis (Baddley et al. 2010). Susceptibility testing to antifungal agents may be useful in guiding treatment (Ullmann et al. 2018). Voriconazole and isavuconazole are recommended for the treatment of CNS aspergillosis where in those cases that are resistant to azoles, liposomal amphotericin B can be used (Ullmann et al. 2018).

17.5 Coccidioidomycosis

Coccidioides immitis is a fungal species endemic to the southwestern United States that is resistant to extremes of climate and multiplies after rainfalls (Zunt and Baldwin 2012). Once inhaled, a respiratory infection may develop that is known as valley fever with disseminated disease which typically only occurs in immunocompromised patients (Zunt and Baldwin 2012). Meningitis occurs in roughly one-half to one-third of patients with disseminated *C. immitis* (Zunt and Baldwin 2012). Males of an African American or Asian descent, specifically Pacific Islanders, are at higher risk for spread to the CNS (Drake and Adam 2009). Clinical manifestations include headache, altered mental status, nausea, vomiting, nuchal rigidity, and focal neurologic deficits (Zunt and Baldwin 2012; Drake and Adam 2009). Vasculitis, cerebral infarction, and hydrocephalus are common complications of *C. immitis* meningitis (Zunt and Baldwin 2012; Arsura et al. 2005). The presence of hydrocephalus was found in 51.6% of patients that had radiographic imaging and was associated with a mortality increase of 12.5-fold (Arsura et al. 2005). Ventriculoperitoneal shunt placement may be necessary to treat hydrocephalus in the setting of coccidioidal meningitis (Galgiani et al. 2016). The blood or CSF in coccidioidal meningitis will often show eosinophilia (Hall and Kim 2013). CSF analysis in coccidioidal meningitis can show an elevated white blood cell count with a predominance of lymphocytes and eosinophils, a decreased or normal glucose level, and a normal or elevated protein level (Zunt and Baldwin 2012). Cultures of CSF will only demonstrate growth in 15% of coccidioides infections (Zunt and Baldwin 2012). Prior to the advent of antifungal agents, the mortality for this disease approached 100% (Drake and Adam 2009). Coccidioidal meningitis should be managed with oral fluconazole initially with doses of 400–1200 mg daily followed by lifelong maintenance therapy (Galgiani et al. 2016). If patients fail management with an azole, intravenous amphotericin B can be used (Johnson and Einstein 2007). Coccidioidal meningitis can cause a vasculitis which can result in vascular occlusion and stroke (Williams et al. 1992). In patients who develop a stroke due to coccidioidal meningitis, corticosteroids may reduce the incidence of experiencing a second adverse event (Thompson III et al. 2017).

17.6 Histoplasmosis

Disseminated disease from *Histoplasma capsulatum* is usually associated with an immunocompromised state and spreads to the CNS in 10–20% of cases (Hall and Kim 2013). This disease is endemic to the Mississippi and Ohio river valleys in the United States (Zunt and Baldwin 2012). Leptomeningeal involvement is usually basilar in nature presenting with headaches and altered mental status but can also present with multiple cranial neuropathies, hydrocephalus, and seizures (Hall and Kim 2013). CSF analysis shows a predominantly elevated mononuclear white blood cell count with elevated protein levels and decreased glucose levels (Zunt and Baldwin 2012). Histoplasmosis in the CNS should be treated with 4–6 weeks of liposomal amphotericin B followed by itraconazole for 1 year. *Histoplasma* antigen levels can be followed to monitor the response to treatment (Wheat et al. 2007).

17.7 Blastomycosis

Blastomycosis occurs after the inhalation of spores which multiply in the lungs and then spread hematogenously (Zunt and Baldwin 2012). Sixty percent of patients have cutaneous involvement with blastomycosis (McKinnell and Pappas 2009). *Blastomyces dermatitidis* infection of the CNS occurs in less than 10% of patients with disseminated disease and can present as acute or chronic meningitis (Zunt and Baldwin 2012). Though typically preceded by a primary pulmonary infection, solitary *B. dermatitidis* infection to the CNS has been reported (Dobre et al. 2011). Hydrocephalus can develop in the setting of chronic blastomycosis meningitis (Kravitz et al. 1981). CSF analysis will show a predominantly lymphocytic elevated white blood cell count with an increased protein level and decreased glucose level (Zunt and Baldwin 2012). Treatment should consist of amphotericin B administered intravenously in its lipid formulation over 4–6 weeks followed by oral fluconazole, itraconazole, or voriconazole for 12 months (Chapman et al. 2008).

17.8 Mucormycosis

Mucormycosis is an aggressive fungal infection that results from infection with species from *Rhizopus*, *Absidia*, and *Mucor* genera (Hall and Kim 2013). Patients with uncontrolled type 2 diabetes mellitus are most at risk for the development of this disease where one retrospective series showed that 86.7% of patients with rhino-orbital-cerebral mucormycosis had uncontrolled diabetes mellitus (Abdollahi et al. 2016). Patients who are on renal dialysis or receive treatment with deferoxamine are also at risk for developing mucormycosis (Boelaert et al. 1991). CNS infection most often occurs through direct extension from the nasopharynx or the face (Hall and Kim 2013). Patients with impaired phagocyte function are more vulnerable to infection from *Mucor* spp. (Riley et al. 2016). When cultures are obtained, this fungus typically grows rapidly (Riley et al. 2016). Rhino-orbital-cerebral mucormycosis often presents with sinusitis, eye/face pain, changes in vision, orbital edema, and headache (Riley et al. 2016). This disease is associated with a high mortality rate, especially in patients who are severely immunocompromised (Riley et al. 2016). In patients on dialysis or receiving iron chelating therapy, mucormycosis is associated with a mortality rate of 86% (Boelaert et al. 1991). Treatment should include surgical debridement of the sinuses and intravenous amphotericin B (Riley et al. 2016).

17.9 Rare Fungal Meningitis

Outbreaks of rare species of fungal meningitis have been associated with contaminated epidural injections of methylprednisolone. In 2012, *Exserohilum rostratum* was grown from the CSF of patients who received contaminated steroid injections (Kainer et al. 2012). The median time to symptom presentation from the last injection was 18 days (Kainer et al. 2012). In a study of the infected patients in Tennessee, approximately 20% of the patients had a stroke, 7 of whom subsequently died (Kainer et al. 2012). Across all states, 751 patients were reported to have fungal meningitis associated with contaminated epidural steroid injections with an associated 8.5% mortality rate and a 5% stroke rate, almost all involving the posterior circulation of the brain (Kauffman and Malani 2016). Treatment with voriconazole was recommended for these patients (Kauffman and Malani 2016). This large outbreak brought awareness to the possibility of the development of fungal meningitis after epidural steroid injections.

Another rare cause of fungal meningoencephalitis is *Cladophialophora bantiana*. This fungus is rare outside the human CNS and typically presents as a brain abscess but can present as meningitis alone (Kantarcioglu et al. 2016). Patients may present with headache, seizures, altered mentation, speech difficulty, difficulty ambulating, nausea and/or vomiting, neck stiffness, hydrocephalus, and hemiparesis. Diagnosis is made by CSF culture or brain biopsy. Amphotericin B is the most commonly used anti-

Table 17.1 The common causative of fungal meningitis and meningoencephalitis in humans

Common causative agents of fungal meningitis
Aspergillus fumigatus
Blastomyces dermatitidis
Candida albicans
Coccidioides immitis
Cryptococcus gattii
Cryptococcus neoformans
Histoplasma capsulatum

fungal agent for *C. bantiana*. This fungal infection is associated with a 65% mortality rate (Kantarcioglu et al. 2016).

17.10 Conclusion

Fungal meningitis and meningoencephalitis often have a subacute or chronic presentation delaying their diagnosis (Zunt and Baldwin 2012). Cultures can be slow to grow and may be negative. Recognition of fungal meningitis and the subsequent initiation of appropriate therapies is the key to decreasing the significant neurological morbidity and mortality associated with this disease (Table 17.1).

References

Abdollahi A, Shokohi T, et al. Clinical features, diagnosis, and outcomes of rhino-orbito-cerebral mucormycosis: a retrospective analysis. Curr Med Mycol. 2016;2:15–23.

Adams-Chapman I, Bann CM, Das A, et al. Neurodevelopmental outcome of extremely low birth weight infants with Candida infection. J Pediatr. 2013;163:961–967.e3.

Antinori S, Corbellino M, Meroni L, et al. Aspergillus meningitis: a rare clinical manifestation of central nervous system aspergillosis. Case report and review of 92 cases. J Infect. 2013;66:218–38.

Arsura EL, Johnson R, Penrose J, Stewart K, Kilgore W, Reddy CM, Bobba RK. Neuroimaging as a guide to predict outcomes for patients with coccidioidal meningitis. Clin Infect Dis. 2005;40:624–7.

Baddley JW, Andes DR, Marr KA, et al. Factors associated with mortality in transplant patients with invasive aspergillosis. Clin Infect Dis. 2010;50:1559–67.

Beardsley J, Wolbers M, Kibengo FM, et al. Adjunctive dexamethasone in HIV-associated Cryptococcal meningitis. N Engl J Med. 2016;374:542–54.

Boelaert JR, Fenves AZ, Coburn JW. Deferoxamine therapy and mucormycosis in dialysis patients: report of an international registry. Am J Kidney Dis. 1991;18:660–7.

Bongomin F, Gago S, Oladele R, Denning D. Global and multi-national prevalence of fungal diseases—estimate precision. J Fungi (Basel). 2017;3 https://doi.org/10.3390/jof3040057.

Chapman SW, Dismukes WE, Proia LA, Bradsher RW, Pappas PG, Threlkeld MG, Kauffman CA. Clinical practice guidelines for the management of blastomycosis: 2008 update by the Infectious Diseases Society of America. Clin Infect Dis. 2008;46:1801–12.

Chen SCA, Slavin MA, Heath CH, et al. Clinical manifestations of Cryptococcus gattii infection: determinants of neurological sequelae and death. Clin Infect Dis. 2012;55:789–98.

Cherian J, Atmar RL, Gopinath SP. Shunting in cryptococcal meningitis. J Neurosurg. 2015;125(1):177–86.

Concha-Velasco F, González-Lagos E, Seas C, Bustamante B. Factors associated with early mycological clearance in HIV-associated cryptococcal meningitis. PLoS One. 2017;12:e0174459–12.

van der Horst CM, Saag MS, Cloud GA, et al. Treatment of Cryptococcal meningitis associated with the acquired immunodeficiency syndrome. N Engl J Med. 1997;337:15–21.

Dobre MC, Smoker WRK, Kirby P. A case of solitary Blastomyces dermatitidis meningitis. Clin Neurol Neurosurg. 2011;113:665–7.

Drake KW, Adam RD. Coccidioidal meningitis and brain abscesses: analysis of 71 cases at a referral center. Neurology. 2009;73:1780–6.

Franco-Paredes C, Womack T, Bohlmeyer T, Sellers B, Hays A, Patel K, Lizarazo J, Lockhart SR, Siddiqui W, Marr KA. Management of Cryptococcus gattii meningoencephalitis. Lancet Infect Dis. 2015;15:348–55.

Galgiani JN, Ampel NM, Blair JE, et al. Executive summary: 2016 Infectious Diseases Society of America (IDSA) clinical practice guideline for the treatment of coccidioidomycosis. Clin Infect Dis. 2016;63:717–22.

Gavito-Higuera. Fungal infections of the central nervous system: a pictorial review. J Clin Imaging Sci. 2016;6:24.

Hall WA, Kim P. Fungal infections of the nervous system. In: Hall WA, Kim P, editors. Neurosurgical infectious disease. New York, Stuttgart: Georg Thieme Verlag; 2013. p. 68–80.

Hasbun R, Rosenthal N, Balada-Llasat JM, Chung J, Duff S, Bozzette S, Zimmer L, Ginocchio CC. Epidemiology of meningitis and encephalitis in the United States, 2011–2014. Clin Infect Dis. 2017;65:359–63.

Johnson RH, Einstein HE. Amphotericin B and coccidioidomycosis. Ann N Y Acad Sci. 2007;1111:434–41.

Kainer MA, Reagan DR, Nguyen DB, et al. Fungal infections associated with contaminated methylprednisolone in Tennessee. N Engl J Med. 2012;367:2194–203.

Kantarcioglu AS, Guarro J, De Hoog S, Apaydin H, Kiraz N. An updated comprehensive systematic review of Cladophialophora bantiana and analysis of epidemiol-

ogy, clinical characteristics, and outcome of cerebral cases. Med Mycol. 2016;23:579–604.
Kauffman CA, Malani AN. Fungal infections associated with contaminated steroid injections. In: Emerging infections 10. Washington, DC: American Society of Microbiology; 2016. p. 359–74.
Kleinschmidt-DeMasters BK. Central nervous system aspergillosis: a 20-year retrospective series. Hum Pathol. 2002;33:116–24.
Kravitz GR, Davies SF, Eckman MR, Sarosi GA. Chronic blastomycotic meningitis. Am J Med. 1981;71:501–5.
Lanternier F, Mahdaviani SA, Barbati E, et al. Inherited CARD9 deficiency in otherwise healthy children and adults with Candida species-induced meningoencephalitis, colitis, or both. J Allergy Clin Immunol. 2015;135:1558–1568.e2.
Lyons JL, Thakur KT, Lee R, et al. Utility of measuring (1,3)-β-d-glucan in cerebrospinal fluid for diagnosis of fungal central nervous system infection: Table 1. J Clin Microbiol. 2014;53:319–22.
McKinnell JA, Pappas PG. Blastomycosis: new insights into diagnosis, prevention, and treatment. Clin Chest Med. 2009;30:227–39.
Melnychuk EM, Sole DP. A rare central nervous system fungal infection resulting from brown heroin use. J Emerg Med. 2017;52:314–7.
Modrzewska BD, Kurnatowska AJ, Khalid K. Drug susceptibility of fungi isolated from ICU patients. Ann Parasitol. 2017;63:189–98.
Murthy JMK, Sundaram C. Fungal infections of the central nervous system. In: Neurologic aspects of systemic disease, part III, vol. 121. 1st ed. Amsterdam: Elsevier; 2014. p. 1383–401.
Mwaba P, Mwansa J, Chintu C, Pobee J, Scarborough M, Portsmouth S, Zumla A. Clinical presentation, natural history, and cumulative death rates of 230 adults with primary cryptococcal meningitis in Zambian AIDS patients treated under local conditions. Postgrad Med J. 2001;77:769–73.
O'Brien D, Stevens NT, Lim CH, O'Brien DF, Smyth E, Fitzpatrick F, Humphreys H. Candida infection of the central nervous system following neurosurgery: a 12-year review. Acta Neurochir. 2011;153:1347–50.
Pappas PG, Kauffman CA, Andes DR, et al. Executive summary: clinical practice guideline for the management of candidiasis: 2016 update by the Infectious Diseases Society of America. Clin Infect Dis. 2016;62:409–17.
Patterson TF. Advances and challenges in management of invasive mycoses. Lancet. 2005;366:1013–25.
Pukkila-Worley R, Mylonakis E. Epidemiology and management of cryptococcal meningitis: developments and challenges. Expert Opin Pharmacother. 2008;9:551–60.
Rajasingham R, Smith RM, Park BJ, Jarvis JN, Govender NP, Chiller TM, Denning DW, Loyse A, Boulware DR. Global burden of disease of HIV-associated cryptococcal meningitis: an updated analysis. Lancet Infect Dis. 2017;17:873–81.
Riley TT, Muzny CA, Swiatlo E, Legendre DP. Breaking the mold. Ann Pharmacother. 2016;50:747–57.
Şahintürk F, Demirkaya H, Dere ÜA, Sönmez E, Altınörs N, Moray G, Haberal M. Intracranial fungal infection after solid-organ transplant. Exp Clin Transplant. 2018;16:179–82.
Thompson GR III, Blair JE, Wang S, et al. Adjunctive corticosteroid therapy in the treatment of coccidioidal meningitis. Clin Infect Dis. 2017;65:338–41.
Torre-Cisneros J, Lopez OL, Kusne S, Martinez AJ, Starzl TE, Simmons RL, Martin M. CNS aspergillosis in organ transplantation: a clinicopathological study. J Neurol Neurosurg Psychiatry. 1993;56:188–93.
Ullmann AJ, Aguado JM, Arikan-Akdagli S, et al. Diagnosis and management of Aspergillus diseases: executive summary of the 2017 ESCMID-ECMM-ERS guideline. Clin Microbiol Infect. 2018;24(Suppl 1):e1–e38.
Wheat LJ, Freifeld AG, Kleiman MB, Baddley JW, McKinsey DS, Loyd JE, Kauffman CA. Clinical practice guidelines for the management of patients with histoplasmosis: 2007 update by the Infectious Diseases Society of America. Clin Infect Dis. 2007;45:807–25.
Williams PL, Johnson R, Pappagianis D, Einstein H, Slager U, Koster FT, Eron JJ, Morrison J, Aguet J, River ME. Vasculitic and encephalitic complications associated with *Coccidioides immitis* infection of the central nervous system in humans: report of 10 cases and review. Clin Infect Dis. 1992;14:673–82.
Zunt JR, Baldwin KJ. Chronic and subacute meningitis. Continuum (Minneap Minn). 2012;18:1290–318.

18 Raised Intracranial Pressure

Hasan Emre Aydın and Ismail Kaya

Abbreviations

CNS	Central nervous system
CSF	Cerebrospinal fluid
EVD	Extraventricular drainage
ICP	Intracranial pressure
ONS	Optic nerve sheath
PI	Pulsatility index
VA	Ventriculoatrial
VP	Ventriculoperitoneal

Fungal infections of the central nervous system (CNS) are widely observed in healthy hosts (*Cryptococcus*, *Coccidioides*, *Histoplasma*, *Blastomyces*, and *Sporothrix*) or in immunocompromised hosts by opportunistic pathogens (*Candida*, *Aspergillus*, *Zygomycetes*, and *Trichosporon*) (Redmond et al. 2007). Chronic meningitis or meningoencephalitis syndrome, brain abscess, rhino-cerebral syndrome, and rare fungal ventriculitis are among the clinical syndromes of CNS fungal infections and are frequently observed among children in clinical practice. CNS fungal infections should be considered in patients who have serous nasal flow, orbital pain, seizures, increased intracranial pressure, and meningitis with or without chronic febrile encephalitis. Initial characteristics of these CNS fungal infections are usually non-specific symptoms such as general fatigue, chronic fever, headache, subacute dementia, episodes, and neurologic deficits (Teive et al. 2008). Increased intracranial pressure (ICP) is responsible for both early mortality and auditory, visual, and cognitive symptoms of meningitis caused by fungal infections (Sun et al. 2004).

H. E. Aydın (✉) · I. Kaya
Department of Neurosurgery, Kutahya Health Sciences University, Kütahya, Turkey

18.1 Increased ICP

When cerebral autoregulation is impaired, pressure values increase due to increased autoregulation and cause hyperaemia and cerebral oedema. Increased ICP can in time cause irreversible brain damage and mortality due to herniation. Medical and surgical treatments used to decrease ICP should be performed in case ICP is 15–20 mmHg. On the other hand, in decreased autoregulation, oedema due to cerebral ischaemia and poor patient prognosis will develop. Moreover, vasomotor paralysis may occur as a result of the impairment of autoregulation in the brain (Gjerris and Brennum 2004). It is possible to examine factors causing increased ICP in five groups. These include increase in (i). brain volume, (ii). cerebrospinal fluid (CSF) volume, (iii). brain blood volume, (iv). craniosynostosis and (v). pseudotumor cerebri (Akopian et al. 2007).

M. Turgut et al. (eds.), *Fungal Infections of the Central Nervous System*,
https://doi.org/10.1007/978-3-030-06088-6_18

18.2 Increased ICP: Clinical features

Despite all the current advances, preventing ICP increase is of great importance in terms of saving patient lives. The signs and symptoms associated with increased ICP may vary by the location and pathologic characteristics of the lesion. The signs and symptoms associated with increased ICP can be divided into two groups. The main symptoms include headache, nausea/vomiting, papilloedema, and changes in consciousness. Other symptoms are due to brain stem involvement (Cushing response), VI nerve paresis, and mental or endocrinological changes.

One of the most important complications of increased ICP is cerebral herniation. The dura protects the brain and limits the inside movement. It is a rigid structure and divides the cranium into compartments. The two most fundamental folds are falx cerebri and tentorium cerebelli. The falx cerebri is in the centre of the two cerebral hemispheres and divides the cerebrum into two. The tentorium cerebelli is shaped like a tent and separates the occipital lobes. According to the localization and size of the lesion, some parts of the brain are pushed outward and herniated from the sides of the dural folds or foramen magnum. During the herniation, brain parenchyma, cerebral veins, and cranial nerves come under pressure, and increase in ICP is observed (Altunbaşak 2008).

18.3 ICP Measurement

ICP can be measured invasively or non-invasively.

18.4 Invasive Methods of ICP Measurement

Depending on the technique, ICP can be measured using different methods from different anatomic points like intraventricular, intraparenchymal, epidural, subdural and subarachnoidal sites (Speck et al. 2011).

External ventricular drainage (EVD): In this method of invasive monitoring, the catheter is placed in the third ventricle via a burr hole. This method is accepted as the gold standard (Steiner and Andrews 2006). This method can also be used in occipital–parietal, posterior–parietal, and occipital areas. This method is used not only for monitoring ICP but also for CNS drainage and intrathecal administration. There may be ventricular system pressure due to progressive oedema developing in prolonged CNS drainage via EVD. This may obstruct EVD.

Microtransducer ICP monitoring tools: The invasive ICP monitoring tools in this group are strain gauge devices, fibre optic devices, and pneumatic sensors. The measurement is carried out using the catheter placed into the intraventricular, intraparenchymal, epidural, subdural, or subarachnoid compartments. The catheter is usually placed 2 cm deep in the right frontal area. However, its location can be changed and modified depending on the known or suspected pressure gradients through intracranial compartments.

18.5 Non-invasive Methods of ICP Measurement

Although many non-invasive methods have been defined, most of these did not go beyond a few studies. Thus, only methods with clinical use will be presented. Non-invasive methods used for ICP measurement can eliminate risks such as haemorrhage and infection (Albeck et al. 1991).

Transcranial doppler ultrasonography: With this method, the ratio of the difference between systolic and diastolic blood flow rates in the middle cerebral artery is stated as pulsatility index (PI). It was shown that this measured PI value has a correlation with invasively measured ICP value, and only very slight deviations can be tolerated (Bellner et al. 2004).

Tympanic membrane shift: This is based on the idea of quantitatively measuring the movement formed by the tympanic membrane, which is flexible as a result of the stimulation of stapedial reflex. This measured value has a correlation with ICP.

Optic nerve sheath (ONS) diameter: In the study on monkeys by Hayreh in 1968, subjects with high ICP were shown to have ONS dilation. With the development of ultrasonography and following the non-invasive evaluation of ICP through the ONS diameter method, ONS diameter has been started to be evaluated with ultrasonography in many pathologies, which may have increased ICP (Sekhon et al. 2014). The optic nerve is surrounded by the dural sheath, which is a part of the CNS, and there is an area between the sheath and the white matter related to the subarachnoid space. In cases of increased ICP, this sheath widening was shown to be correlated with ICP.

Involvement of brain parenchyma and meninges, observed in 40–86% of the patients, is specific to CNS fungal infections and the predisposition of these areas to infection cannot be explained. It may be acute or chronic. Headache, fever, and neck stiffness, which indicate meningeal irritation, manifest as acute (<3 days) or chronic (>30 days) symptoms. However, in human immunodeficiency virus (HIV)-infected patients, headache and fever are not always observed. Instead, there may be lethargy, stupor, coma, and even dementia in these patients. Clinical symptoms are not adequate in determining the etiology of meningitis. Although papilloedema is observed, focal neurologic symptoms such as paralysis of cranial nerves are not observed. Intracerebral, cerebellar, and spinal cord lesions are rarely reported. Complications of CNS fungal infections are related to hydrocephalus, focal motor disorders, mental changes, and increased ICP.

Increased ICP is a prevalent complication of fungal meningitis. It has been suggested that the reason for this is block in the outflow because of accumulation of fungal polysaccharide residues in the arachnoid villus and subarachnoid spaces; thus, CSF canals could be blocked (Bellner et al. 2004; Lee et al. 1996). Another important factor may be cytokine-induced inflammation and cerebral oedema, possibly due to the osmotic effect of the fungal origin of mannitol (Denning et al. 1991).

Increased CSF pressure is commonly observed among these patients. If the high CSF pressure is inadequately managed, a significant neurologic deficit may occur.

In this context, various treatment strategies have been defined for intracranial hypertension. Among these are medical treatment, series of lumbar punctures and placing external lumbar and ventricular drains. The literature is not clear regarding which approach is indicated and when and how often the patients need neurosurgical intervention. The importance of early diagnosis and adequate treatment of cryptococcal meningitis and severe intracranial hypertension are emphasized (Cherian et al. 2016).

A recently conducted autopsy study showed that there was a correlation between high concentration of live and dead organisms in arachnoid granulations and increased CSF pressure. Prevention of CSF resorption was suggested as a cause for increased pressure and development of hydrocephalus (Loyse et al. 2010). Cerebral herniation and brain death due to cryptococcal meningoencephalitis have been reported to be rare. Many studies have shown that high CSF fungal load (stated with high cryptococcal antigen titres) alters mental state, increases spread of infection (with the manifestation of fungaemia), and symptomatically increases ICP. Moreover, the low number of CSF leukocytes is a factor associated with poor outcome of acquired immunodeficiency syndrome (AIDS)-related cryptococcal meningoencephalitis (Jarvis et al. 2014).

In most recent studies, non-invasive ICP monitoring methods have been shown to be systems that provide ICP diagnostic findings, results of interventional operations, and simultaneous monitoring of ICP. Currently, ICP monitoring is carried out by placing invasive sensors inside the skull to detect pressure over time and its variation. Invasiveness and high cost of this method limit its use for most patients. Monitoring of ICP with non-invasive methods is being developed by various groups around the world using technologies such as transcranial doppler and imaging (Alperin et al. 2015). Non-invasive ICP sensors can monitor the pulses of ICP, which shows the morphologic changes consistent with the patient clinical state. Severe intracranial hypertension can develop in patients with neuroinfection and even cause decrease in the cerebral perfusion pressure connected to intracranial hypertension in patients with a normal opening pressure. Monitoring of ICP and cerebral perfusion pressure may be performed in patients with neuroinfection and can be used in estimating cerebral hemodynamic changes.

Intracranial hypertension is prevalent in fungal meningitis and is related to increased mortality rates. CSF opening pressure in 60–75% of patients is >20 cmH_2O. The effect of CSF hypertension on morbidity and mortality related to this disease supports current suggestions with routine and frequent ICP measurement using spinal needle manometry. When CSF opening pressure is >25 cmH_2O, it is recommended for the CSF drainage to be conducted with daily spinal needles and the opening pressure to be lowered to <20 cmH_2O or to 50% of the starting value. Usually there is a high level of uncertainty, and the basis of clinical decisions regarding ICP hypertension tends to be based on clinical symptoms (headache, nausea, and vomiting), low Glasgow Coma Scale score, and/or fundoscopic papilloedema. Inadequate management of high CSF pressure can result in neurologic decline (Bolela et al. 2017).

Optimal medical treatment consists of a combination of amphotericin-B and 5-flucytosine for 2 weeks, which is known as the fungal meningoencephalitis induction phase. Consolidation phase is 8-week-long treatment period monitored with fluconazole and is followed by care phase or secondary prophylaxis to prevent relapses. Despite severe toxicity, triple treatment in acceptable doses is a superior treatment method in cryptococcal meningitis related and unrelated to HIV (Xu et al. 2018). The management of increased ICP without hydrocephalus in patients with fungal meningitis consists of CSF drainage with lumbar puncture with or without temporary percutaneous lumbar drains in patients who require repeated daily lumbar punctures. However, although daily lumbar punctures provide quick relief from headache, they may increase the risk of brain herniation (Jarvis et al. 2014; Antinori et al. 2000).

Different studies put forth that opening pressure must be measured as the first step in all patients with suspected fungal meningitis. Additional lumbar punctures including daily lumbar punctures should be performed until the pressure is adequately controlled for patients with high ICP (Day et al. 2013). Pharmacologic agents such as mannitol and corticosteroids are avoided, and neurologic interventions including ventriculoperitoneal (VP) or ventriculoatrial (VA) shunt placements are usually avoided or delayed. The most appropriate time to implant a permanent shunt (VP or VA) in patients with uncontrollable ICP is controversial, but usually the device should be placed after starting the optimal antifungal treatment (Pappas 2005).

A series of lumbar punctures is a prevalent application among clinicians for the treatment of these patients. As a secondary choice, some clinicians prefer placing lumbar drainage, which has a high risk of infections or complications. Permanent VP shunting is required after 4 weeks of appropriate antifungal treatment in patients who need a series of lumbar punctures (Corti et al. 2010).

ICP is associated with severe complications in patients with cryptococcal meningitis, and placing a VP shunt can ensure adequate treatment even in cases wherein neurologic imaging studies show no hydrocephalus or permanent CSF cryptococcus infection. Although medical treatment of ICP among these patients is being discussed, placing a VP shunt should be the first therapeutic alternative. However, post-operative meningitis and ventriculitis after shunt infection are well-documented complications among these patients. Both complications frequently occur in post-operative early period and are secondary to wound infection or intraoperative contamination. Moreover, clinical status and potential or established complications can still be considered for device implantation. In a harm–benefit evaluation, VP shunts can be beneficial in patients who are independently selected from the permanence of cryptococcus infection to prevent sequels and to optimise the management of ICP (Perfect et al. 2010).

18.6 Conclusion

In sum, patients who do not benefit from antifungal treatment alone have high CSF pressure, and those who continue neurologic symptoms despite the frequent lumbar punctures should be considered for VP shunt placement. Early diagnosis and shunt placement are important to improve the low survival rate and neurologic functions in these critical patients.

References

Akopian G, Gaspard DJ, Alexander M. Outcomes of blunt head trauma without intracranial pressure monitoring. Am Surg. 2007;73(5):447–50.

Albeck MJ, Børgesen SE, Gjerris F, Schmidt JF, Sørensen PS. Intracranial pressure and cerebrospinal fluid outflow conductance in healthy subjects. J Neurosurg. 1991;74(4):597–600.

Alperin N, Lee SH, Bagci AM. MRI measurements of intracranial pressure in the upright posture: the effect of the hydrostatic pressure gradient. J Magn Reson Imaging. 2015;42:1158–63. https://doi.org/10.1002/jmri.24882.

Altunbaşak Ş. Şuuru Kapalı Hastaya Yaklaşım ve Kafa İçi Basınç Artışı Sendromu (KİBAS) Türkiye Klinikleri. J Pediatr. 2008;4(4):55–66.

Antinori S, Ridolfo AL, Gianelli E, Piazza M, Gervasoni C, Monforte AA. The role of lumbar puncture in the management of elevated intracranial pressure in patients with AIDS associated cryptococcal meningitis. Clin Infect Dis. 2000;31:130910.

Bellner J, Romner B, Reinstrup P, Kristiansson K-A, Ryding E, Brandt L. Transcranial Doppler sonography pulsatility index (PI) reflects intracranial pressure (ICP). Surg Neurol. 2004;62(1):45–51.

Bolela VR, Frigieri G, Vilar FC, Spaiveri DL, Tallarico FJ, Tallaico GM, et al. Noninvasive intracranial pressure monitoring for HIV-associated cryptococcal meningitis. Braz J Med Biol Res. 2017;50(9):e6392.

Cherian J, Atmar RL, Gopinath SP. Shunting in cryptococcal meningitis. J Neurosurg. 2016;125:177–86. https://doi.org/10.3171/2015.4.JNS15255.

Corti M, Solari R, Cangelosi D, Dominguez C, Yampolsky C, Negroni R, et al. Sudden blindness due to bilateral optic neuropathy associated with cryptococcal meningitis in an AIDS patient. Rev Iberoam Micol. 2010;27:207–9.

Day JN, Chau TT, Wolbers M, Mai PP, Dung NT, Mai NH, et al. Combination antifungal therapy for cryptococcal meningitis. N Engl J Med. 2013;368:1291–302.

Denning DW, Armstrong RW, Lewis BH, Stevens DA. Elevated cerebrospinal fluid pressures in patients with cryptococcal meningitis and acquired immunodeficiency syndrome. Am J Med. 1991;91:26772.

Gjerris F, Brennum J. The cerebrospinal fluid, intracranial pressure and herniation of the brain. In: Paulson OB, Gjerris F, Sorensen PS, editors. Clinical neurology and neurosurgery. Copenhagen, Denmark: FADL's Forlag Aktieselskab; 2004. p. 179–96.

Jarvis JN, Bicanic T, Loyse A, Namarika D, Jackson A, Nussbaum JC, et al. Determinants of mortality in a combined cohort of 501 patients with HIV-associated cryptococcal meningitis: implications for improving outcomes. Clin Infect Dis. 2014;58:73645.

Lee SC, Dickson DW, Casadevall A. Pathology of cryptococcal meningoencephalitis: analysis of 27 patients with pathogenetic implications. Hum Pathol. 1996;27:83947.

Loyse A, Wainwright H, Jarvis JN, Bicanic T, Rebe K, Meintjes G, et al. Histopathology of the arachnoid granulations and brain in HIV-associated cryptococcal meningitis: correlation with cerebrospinal fluid pressure. AIDS. 2010;24:40510.

Pappas PG. Management cryptococcal meningitis is about handling the pressure. Clin Infect Dis. 2005;40:480–2.

Perfect JR, Dismukes WE, Dromer F, Graybill JR, Hamill RJ, Harrison TS, et al. Clinical practice guidelines for the management of cryptococcal disease: 2010 update by the Infectious Disease Society of America. Clin Infect Dis. 2010;50:291–322.

Redmond A, Dancer C, Woods ML. Fungal infections of the central nervous system: a review of fungal pathogens and treatment. Neurol India. 2007;55:251–9.

Sekhon MS, McBeth P, Zou J, Qiao L, Kolmodin L, Henderson WR, et al. Association between optic nerve sheath diameter and mortality in patients with severe traumatic brain injury. Neurocrit Care. 2014;21(2):245–52.

Speck V, Staykov D, Huttner HB, Sauer R, Schwab S, Bardutzky J. Lumbar catheter for monitoring of intracranial pressure in patients with post-hemorrhagic communicating hydrocephalus. Neurocrit Care. 2011;14(2):208–15.

Steiner L, Andrews P. Monitoring the injured brain: ICP and CBF. Br J Anaesth. 2006;97(1):26–38.

Sun HY, Hung CC, Chang SC. Management of cryptococcal meningitis with extremely high intracranial pressure in HIV-infected patients. Clin Infect Dis. 2004;38(12):1790–2. https://doi.org/10.1086/421272.

Teive H, Carsten AL, Iwamoto FM, Almedia SM, Munhoz RP, Werneck LC, et al. Fungal encephalitis following bone marrow transplantation: clinical findings and prognosis. J Postgrad Med. 2008;54:203–5.

Xu L, Liu J, Zhang Q, Li M, Liao J, Kuang W, et al. Triple therapy versus amphotericin B plus flucytosine for the treatment of non-HIV- and nontransplant-associated cryptococcal meningitis: retrospective cohort study. Neurol Res. 2018. https://doi.org/10.1080/01616412.2018.1447319.

Hydrocephalus

19

Manish Jaiswal

Abbreviations

ABCD	Amphotericin B colloidal dispersion
ABLC	Amphotericin B lipid complex
AIDS	Acquired immune deficiency syndrome
CNS	Central nervous system
CSF	Cerebrospinal fluid
CT	Computed tomography
FLAIR	Fluid-attenuated inversion recovery
GCS	Glasgow Coma Scale
HIV	Human immunodeficiency virus
ICU	Intensive care unit
MRI	Magnetic resonance imaging
VP shunt	Ventriculoperitoneal shunt

19.1 Introduction

Under the microscope after staining with various reagents, the look of fungi is as mesmerizing as modern art on canvas, but these organisms are as lethal as these could be, if the central nervous system is infected. Fungal meningitis is the most common life-threatening opportunistic central nervous system (CNS) fungal infection (Jellinger et al. 2000; Baddley et al. 2002; Treseler and Sugar 1990). Despite the advent of new antifungal drugs and modern imaging techniques, mortality and morbidity rates for fungal meningitis remain high (Baddley et al. 2002; Treseler and Sugar 1990; Zarrin et al. 2010; Ito-Kuwa et al. 2008; Speed and Dunt 1995). Hydrocephalus is an occasional complication of fungal meningitis (Treseler and Sugar 1990; Ito-Kuwa et al. 2008; Nakouzi et al. 2009; Levitz 1991; Kovoor et al. 2002; Fessler et al. 1998). Delays in the diagnosis and treatment of hydrocephalus are directly related to poor outcome, including various degrees of residual neurological consequences.

19.2 Epidemiology and Classification

CNS fungal infections are becoming increasingly common. Reasons for increasing frequency of CNS fungal infection are the following (Baddley et al. 2002; Treseler and Sugar 1990; Zarrin et al. 2010; Ito-Kuwa et al. 2008; Speed and Dunt 1995; Nakouzi et al. 2009; Levitz 1991):

1. Epidemic outbreaks due to intrathecal administration of contaminated medication.
2. Increase in prevalence of diabetes mellitus, renal failure, malnutrition.
3. Increase in solid organ transplantation with the use of immune suppression.

M. Jaiswal (✉)
Department of Neurosurgery, King George's Medical University, Lucknow, Uttar Pradesh, India
e-mail: manishjaiswal@kgmcindia.edu

M. Turgut et al. (eds.), *Fungal Infections of the Central Nervous System*,
https://doi.org/10.1007/978-3-030-06088-6_19

4. Increase in haemopoietic stem cell transplantation with the use of immunosuppressant.
5. Increase in immune-suppressed states like human immunodeficiency virus (HIV)-associated acquired immune deficiency syndrome (AIDS).
6. Prolonged use of broad-spectrum antibiotics and the use of antimetabolites and steroids.
7. Social evils such as drug addiction and substance abuse.
8. Increase in international travel with the risk of environmental exposure.
9. Longer survival of patients with lymphoproliferative malignancies.
10. Larger ageing population.

Fungal infections are not notifiable diseases, and precise information on their prevalence throughout the world is not available. Although, in general, fungi are cited to be ubiquitous, some forms have a more restricted geographical distribution than others. More than 100 thousand fungal species are recognized by now, and only a couple of hundreds are found to be pathogenic to humans. Fortunately, only about 10–15% of pathologenic fungi usually produce systemic/CNS mycosis (Levitz 1991; Kovoor et al. 2002; Fessler et al. 1998; Wright et al. 1997).

True pathogenic fungi (having a restricted geographic distribution, mostly in United States of America) are *Blastomycetes*, *Coccidioides*, *Paracoccidioides*, *Histoplasma*, *Sporothrix*, etc. They produce clinical disease in normal individuals and then provide long-term immunity to the patients recovered from the active infections. On the other hand, the opportunistic fungi (having ubiquitous distribution) are *Aspergillus fumigatus*, *Candida albicans*, *Cryptococcus neoformans*, *Rhizopus arrhizus*, etc. and provide no long-term immunity to the patients, and hence relapses are noted (Kovoor et al. 2002; Fessler et al. 1998; Wright et al. 1997; Borha et al. 2009).

Fungi present mainly into three forms: molds (colonies of branching hyphae-mycelium), yeasts (colonies of single cells), and intermediate forms. Some fungi are thermodimorphic changing their forms from mould to yeast under different environmental conditions. Clinically important true pathogenic dimorphic fungi are *Blastomycetes*, *Coccidioides*, *Histoplasma*, *Sporotrichum*, and *Paracoccidioides*. *Cryptococcus* remains as an encapsulated yeast in all environmental conditions (Dupont 2003; Nguyen and Yu 1995; Zarrin and Zarei Mahmoudabadi 2009; Chimelli and Mahler-Araujo 1997; Zarrin et al. 2009; Kedziora et al. 2008).

Fungi are broadly classified in three major groups as follows (Baddley et al. 2002; Ito-Kuwa et al. 2008; Levitz 1991; Fessler et al. 1998; Nguyen and Yu 1995; Zarrin and Zarei Mahmoudabadi 2009; Chimelli and Mahler-Araujo 1997; Zarrin et al. 2009; Kedziora et al. 2008; Dotis et al. 2007):

1. Pseudomycetes/yeast: *Blastomycetes*, *Candida*, *Coccidioides*, *Cryptococcus*, *Histoplasma*, *Paracoccidioides*, *Sporotrichum*
2. Septate mycetes: *Aspergillus*, *Cephalosporium*, *Cladosporium*, *Diplorhinotrichum*, *Hormodendrum*, *Paecilomyces*, *Penicillium*
3. Non-septate mycetes: *Absidia*, *Basidiobolus*, *Cunninghamella*, *Mucor*, *Rhizopus*

Usually, the inhaled aerosolized fungi initiate a primary mycotic infection in the lungs and/or paranasal sinuses which is usually self-limiting but may spread to other organs. The routes of infection to the CNS are thought to be as follows: directly, most frequently the paranasal sinus but also through the orbit and middle ear; haematogenous infection, usually originating in the lung but some times in the intestine; and trauma or operation, contamination of intracranial devices (Chakrabarti and Sharma 2000; Moore et al. 2000; Ribaud et al. 1999; Dubey et al. 2005; Chakrabarti et al. 2006). Identifying the etiological agents as fungi and not bacteria is vital since antibacterial therapy is not effective against fungi and CNS mycoses lead to high morbidity and mortality.

19.3 Clinical Syndrome and Hydrocephalus

The CNS fungal infections may present with various clinical syndromes which may be specific for certain fungi. Among these, common syndromes are basal meningitis, hydrocephalus, space-occupying lesions (such as cerebral abscesses, granulomas, etc.), stroke syndromes (aspergillosis, zygomycosis), and spinal infections. In general, symptomatic CNS fungal infection carries higher risks of morbidities and mortality as compared to viral, bacterial, or parasitic CNS disorders (Pagano et al. 1997; Verma et al. 2006; Kantarcioglu and de Hoog 2004; Revankar et al. 2004; Casadevall et al. 2000; Feng et al. 2001; Middleton et al. 1976). Early recognition and appropriate medical and surgical management strategies are therefore of paramount importance in improving the overall prognosis in CNS mycosis. Clinical picture may mimic tubercular meningitis and, therefore, needs careful evaluation.

19.3.1 Pathophysiology of Hydrocephalus in CNS Fungal Infection

The cause of the hydrocephalus is thought to be blockage of the CSF route, increased production of CSF, and disturbed absorption of CSF induced by fungal meningitis. Fungal infection of the CNS tends to localize in the base of the brain. The inflammatory response may result in hydrocephalus with involvement of the aqueduct of Sylvius and obstruction of the subarachnoid space and spinal fluid channels (Singh and Husain 2001; Wheat et al. 1990; Venger et al. 1987; Pappas et al. 1992; Guarro and Gene 1995; Genzen and Kenney 2009; Redmond et al. 2007).

Fungi producing distinctive clinical syndromes along with hydrocephalus are found in three major morphological forms:

1. *Small pseudomycetes (yeasts) causing leptomeningitis*: Because of their small size (*Cryptococci, Blastomycetes, Histoplasma, Coccidioidomycetes*), these fungi gain access to the cerebral microcirculation. From there they seed and infect the CSF and its containing leptomeninges. Fungi may reach the brain parenchyma along the Virchow-Robin spaces around the penetrating and perforating small cortical/cerebral vessels arising from the major vessels in the subarachnoid spaces. Therefore, these fungi may result in meningitis and/or meningoencephalitis which may lead to hydrocephalus due to alteration in CSF flow mechanism at the level of basal arachnoid and cisterns and hampered absorption due to scarring and coating of arachnoid granulation (Fig. 19.1).

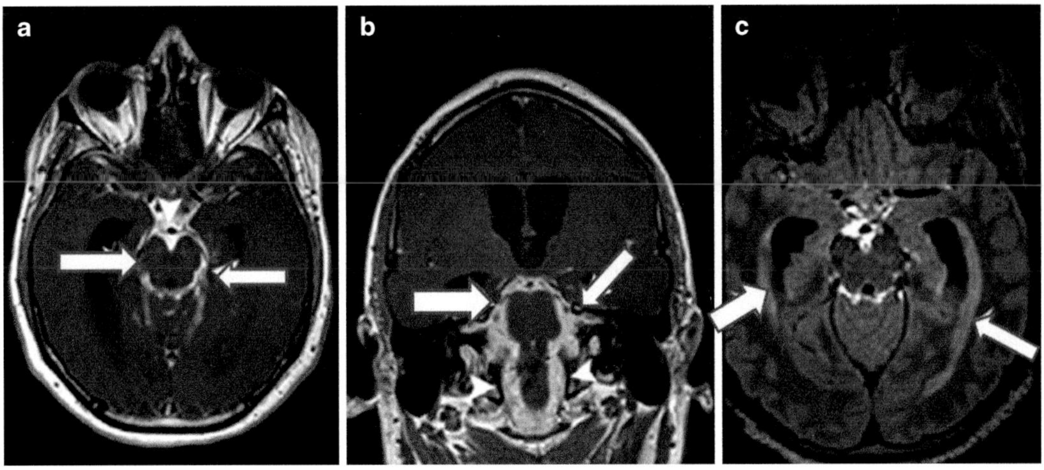

Fig. 19.1 Magnetic resonance imaging (MRI) T1-weighted contrast imaging of the brain of fungal meningitis patient in axial (**a**) and coronal (**b**) view showing marked leptomeningeal thickening with diffuse enhancement specially the basal cisterns (arrows). (**c**) FLAIR image axial view showing marked enlargement of lateral ventricles periventricular ooze of cerebrospinal fluid (CSF) (arrows)

2. *Large pseudomycetes (Candida) producing cerebral abscesses and granulomas*: These fungi are larger than 20 microns and can occlude cerebral arterioles. Such occlusions lead to focal cerebral ischemia and infarctions. Depending upon the virulence of the fungi and host resistance, a variety of the cerebral fungal lesions appear such as ischemic areas, focal infarctions, cerebritis, abscesses, granulomas, and combinations of these lesions. The tissue necrosis and highly virulent fungal infection rapidly convert infected cerebral areas into micro-abscesses, whereas a good host resistance but persistence of infection causes granulomatous inflammatory reactions in adjacent leptomeninges, neural parenchyma, or in both sites. This may result in hydrocephalus which needs to be treated promptly (Fig. 19.2).
3. *Septate (Aspergillus) and non-septate (Zygomycetes)*: Mycetes are very large in size and normally grow with large branched hyphae. Usually they infect juxta-cranial sites (paranasal sinuses, orbits, oral cavity, etc.) for a considerable period of time and then are capable of invading contiguous cranial bones, meningeal tissues, basal cerebral venous sinuses, etc., as well as intermediate- and large-sized intracranial arteries, and result in arterial thrombosis and occlusions which in turn causes extensive cerebral infarctions. These patients clinically present with cerebral stroke. The evolving hemorrhagic cerebral infarct is then converted to septic infarct with associated cerebritis and abscesses, whereas a good host defense results in granuloma formation. This granuloma may block directly or most of the time direct the way of the CSF flow pathway leading to hydrocephalus in some cases.

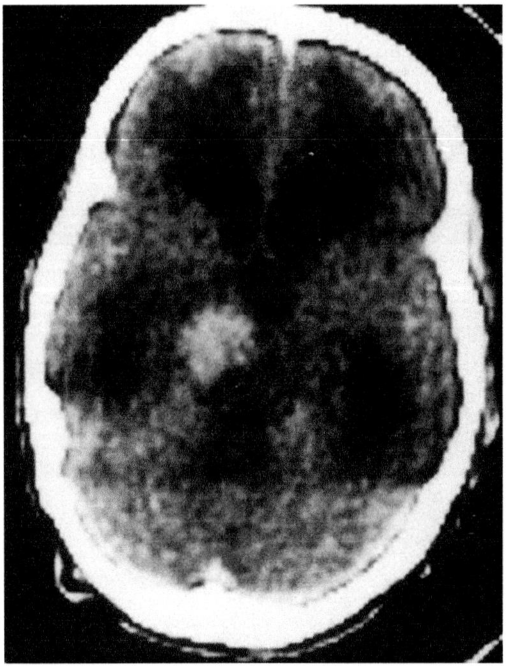

Fig. 19.2 Computed tomography (CT) scan head showing fungal granuloma causing compression and obstruction of CSF flow through third ventricle leading to hydrocephalus

19.3.2 Clinical Presentation of Fungal Hydrocephalus

Chronic fungal meningitis is common, whereas subacute meningitis is relatively less common, and acute fungal meningitis is distinctively rare except in intensive care unit (ICU) patients or in patients on ventilator for prolonged period or patients with severely immunocompromised states. Most of the pseudomycetes (yeasts) are capable of producing meningitis or meningoencephalitis. Clinical features of fungal meningitis and meningoencephalitis usually are headaches, nausea, vomiting, visual impairment, and papilloedema; later neck stiffness with fever, and personality changes may develop; and still later, seizures, deterioration in sensorium, cranial nerve palsies, and hydrocephalus may develop (Shankar et al. 2007; Zarei Mahmoudabadi 2002; Black and Baden 2007). In many patients, there are no focal or generalized physical signs. Fungal meningitis more frequently occurs with *Cryptococcus*, *Coccidioides*, *Blastomyces*, *Paracoccidioides*, *Sporotrichum*, *Histoplasma*, and *Candida* as compared to filamentous fungi such as *Aspergillus*, *Cladosporium* (phaeohyphomycosis), and *Zygomycetes*.

Candida also reaches CNS via colonization of the ventricular drains, shunt tubing, and central venous lines. Therefore, candidal meningitis can occur spontaneously as a complication of disseminated candidiasis or as a complication of an infected wound or ventriculostomy via direct inoculation of the organism into the CNS. Usually chronic but infrequently subacute, basal fungal meningitis causes obliteration of intracranial subarachnoid spaces and results in increased intracranial pressure with or without hydrocephalus (Zarei Mahmoudabadi et al. 2006; Zarrin and Najafi 2007; Hardesty et al. 2014; Pitisuttithum et al. 2005).

Various neurological manifestations, including headache, vomiting, visual impairment, mental change, gait ataxia, and deterioration of consciousness, may be associated with progressive hydrocephalus. These may be attributed to the infection itself, to hydrocephalus, or to both. These clinical findings are of little help in establishing the presence of hydrocephalus (Shankar et al. 2007; Zarei Mahmoudabadi 2002; Black and Baden 2007; Zarei Mahmoudabadi et al. 2006; Zarrin and Najafi 2007; Hardesty et al. 2014; Pitisuttithum et al. 2005). However, the presence of headache, visual impairment, mental change, gait ataxia, and deterioration of consciousness should raise the suspicion that hydrocephalus is present.

19.4 Management

19.4.1 Diagnostic Test

Fungal meningitis is defined as isolation of *fungal organism* from CSF culture, positive CSF fungal antigen titer, or positive results of CSF pathological fungal-specific staining studies and clinical features of meningitis with typical CSF features. Brain computed tomography (CT) and magnetic resonance imaging (MRI) are useful tools for rapid diagnosis of hydrocephalus (Baddley et al. 2002; Ito-Kuwa et al. 2008; Levitz 1991; Borha et al. 2009; Guarro and Gene 1995; Shankar et al. 2007). Hydrocephalus is usually diagnosed by the presence of a dilated temporal horn of the lateral ventricle, without obvious brain atrophy, and/or an Evans ratio of 10.3 on the initial and/or follow-up CT or MRI. Evans ratio is the ratio of the ventricular width of the bilateral frontal horn to the maximum biparietal diameter.

CSF opening pressure. The CSF opening pressure measured by lumbar puncture is recorded some time. There may be very high opening pressure (>350 mmH_2O) or a normal or moderately high pressure (<350 mmH_2O) (Hardesty et al. 2014).

CSF analysis. Samples of CSF obtained either by lumbar puncture or by the ventricular route are sent to the laboratory for cell analysis and determination of glucose, lactate, and protein levels and fungal antigen titer. In the analysis of the antigen titer, a titer of >1:1024 is considered to be high in *Cryptococcus* infection, whereas a titer of <1:1024 is considered to be low and a positive correlation between CSF features and outcome was observed by some researches (Zarei Mahmoudabadi 2002; Black and Baden 2007; Zarei Mahmoudabadi et al. 2006; Zarrin and Najafi 2007; Hardesty et al. 2014).

19.4.2 Treatment

19.4.2.1 Drug Treatment

Intravenous administration of antifungal drugs is the standard treatment for fungal meningitis. In Japan, miconazole and fluconazole have been used since 1989 to treat *Aspergillus* infection. CNS infections due to *Aspergillus* have a poor prognosis, because no drug has sufficiently effective activity against aspergillosis. Fluconazole is absorbed well from the gastrointestinal tract and also penetrates the blood-brain barrier well so is frequently used to treat fungal meningitis. No definitive method for the treatment of Aspergillus meningoencephalitis has yet been established, but fluconazole is sometime effective in some cases. The long-term use of antifungal agents is thought to be effective for the treatment of Aspergillus meningoencephalitis (Baddley et al. 2002; Zarrin et al. 2010; Speed and Dunt 1995; Kovoor et al. 2002; Pagano et al. 1997; Middleton et al. 1976; Shankar et al. 2007). Therefore, antifungal drugs should always be administered for the recommended duration.

Reliance only on Amphotericin B is not effective. Fortunately, during the same period, many useful antifungal drugs are discovered and introduced initially, the lipid-based formulations of the Amphotericin B, then the new triazoles, and, most recently, echinocandins. These medications are used, more and more in combinations, in seriously ill patients with invasive mycoses. Now evidence-based data are gathering together in favour of their important roles in the management of invasive fungal infections (Dubey et al. 2005; Black and Baden 2007; Zarrin and Najafi 2007; Hardesty et al. 2014).

But still there are many unanswered questions and controversies relating to their use. Unquestionably, CNS fungal infections pose serious challenges in their management with controversies surrounding their medical and surgical therapies. Surgical options are less controversial in cases of focal or localized superficial cortico-subcortical lesions (such as abscesses and granulomas) in the non-eloquent areas of the brain.

Currently the following classes of natural and synthetic antifungal drugs are commonly used:

1. Polyenes: Amphotericin B deoxycholate complex (Fungizone registered, Bristol-Myers Squibb), nystatin lipid formulations of Amphotericin B.
   (a) AmBisome.
   (b) Amphocil (Amphotericin B colloidal dispersion {cholesteryl sulphate}, ABCD).
   (c) Abelcet (Amphotericin B lipid complex, ABLC).
2. Pyrimidines: 5-Fluorocytosine (flucytosine).
3. Triazole drugs: Fluconazole, itraconazole, posaconazole, voriconazole.
4. Echinocandins: Caspofungin, anidulafungin, micafungin.
5. Miscellaneous: Imidazoles (clotrimazole, ketoconazole, etc.), oral polyenes (amphotericin, nystatin), griseofulvin, etc. For dermal, oropharyngeal, esophageal, intestinal, and vaginal infections, terbinafine is effective for nail and ring worm infections.

19.4.2.2 Surgical Treatment

The treatment of patients with fungal meningitis with hydrocephalus is essentially a diversion of ventricular CSF through a ventriculoperitoneal (VP) shunt or external ventricular drainage. The indications and timing for placement of a shunt in patients with fungal meningitis complicating hydrocephalus are not well understood or universally accepted (Black and Baden 2007; Zarei Mahmoudabadi et al. 2006; Zarrin and Najafi 2007; Hardesty et al. 2014; Pitisuttithum et al. 2005). Most authors suggest early shunt placement for hydrocephalus to avoid irreversible neurological complications. However, in some patients with fungal meningitis and hydrocephalus, diversion of CSF through a VP shunt does not result in any significant improvement. Thus, selecting patients who would benefit from a VP shunt becomes important. Some of the patients who were successfully treated with temporary external CSF drainage and medical therapy did not undergo permanent shunting. Similarly, some patients have been treated successfully with endoscopic third ventriculostomy; however, our personal experience is that third ventriculostomy is rarely successful in the setting of coccidioidomycosis (presumably due to basilar cisternal arachnoid scarring) (Hardesty et al. 2014; Pitisuttithum et al. 2005; Diamond and Bennett 1974; Tang 1990; Park et al. 1999).

19.4.2.3 Shunt Failure and Complication

The risk of shunt failure is high, and half of all patients in few series required one or more shunt revisions during the follow-up period, and 9% mortality rate during follow-up demonstrates the severity of this often-fatal disease process despite the best medical therapies (Black and Baden 2007; Zarei Mahmoudabadi et al. 2006; Zarrin and Najafi 2007; Hardesty et al. 2014; Pitisuttithum et al. 2005; Diamond and Bennett 1974; Tang 1990; Park et al. 1999; Lu et al. 1999). The most common (50–81%) cause of shunt failure is due to mechanical clogging of the drainage system. Coccidioidomycosis can lead to significant proteinaceous debris; considerable biofilms or focal abscesses have been observed on catheters or within valve tapping chambers at the time of shunt revision. Unfortunately, no data suggest a solution to improve shunt longevity, as they did not observe any differences among shunt valve brands.

Appropriate medical therapy with systemic anti-fungals is necessary in patients with hardware placed in a chronically infected space, and all these patients must be maintained on systemic antifungal medication. The role of intrathecal antifungals should be the focus of future study, and any benefit of intrathecal therapy on shunt failure rate should be evaluated. Despite low drainage pressures and adequate CSF diversion, many patients with fungal hydrocephalus experience persistent ventriculomegaly after shunt surgery. The mechanism for this is not well elucidated, but it may include an alteration in the compliance of the ventricular wall or entire brain parenchyma due to infectious scarring or altered extraventricular CSF circulation (Zarei Mahmoudabadi 2002; Black and Baden 2007; Zarei Mahmoudabadi et al. 2006; Zarrin and Najafi 2007; Hardesty et al. 2014; Pitisuttithum et al. 2005; Diamond and Bennett 1974; Tang 1990; Park et al. 1999). The clinical importance of this with regard to patient chronic headache or subtle cognitive function changes is unclear. However, it behoves the clinician treating patients with fungal hydrocephalus to assume that ventricular size does not necessarily indicate shunt failure or a functional shunt system.

19.5 Prognostic Factors and Outcome

Poor prognostic factors that influence the outcome of fungal meningitis are low CSF glucose level, high CSF lactate level, high CSF cryptococcal antigen titer (>1:1024), level of consciousness, hydrocephalus, and increased intracranial pressure. Factors that influence the outcome of VP shunt placement surgery to treat fungal meningitis with hydrocephalus have not been discussed in few studies. Poor Glasgow Coma Scale (GCS) score (<8) at the time of surgical intervention and prolonged duration (>48 hours) of deteriorated consciousness before surgery are associated with poor improvement and outcome after surgery (Hardesty et al. 2014). Extreme elevation of the intracranial pressure (>350 mmH_2O) is common in patients with fungal meningitis. In one series, 30% of patients were found to have extremely high intracranial pressure. Extremely high intracranial pressure is associated with increased early mortality. In one series, however, hydrocephalus and extremely elevated intracranial pressure did not correlate with poor outcome. It is likely that VP shunts remove a large amount of CSF and lower the intracranial pressure, thereby significantly improving the outcome.

In fact, extremely high intracranial pressure without hydrocephalus associated with fungal meningitis can also be resolved using a VP shunt. Patients with hydrocephalus who have poor consciousness (GCS score, 8 or <8) at the time of surgical intervention have poor outcome. Performing shunting procedures for these patients still does not result in a good outcome. Perhaps patients with poor consciousness and hydrocephalus already have irreversible brain tissue damage before hydrocephalus is corrected by use of a VP shunt (Chiou et al. 1994; Cruciani et al. 1992; Sanchez-Portocarrero et al. 1994). The duration of altered consciousness is also an important predictive factor of clinical outcome. A > 48 hours duration of deteriorated consciousness is associated with a poor response to VP shunting (Hardesty et al. 2014).

19.6 Conclusion

- Hydrocephalus is a serious cause of morbidity and mortality in patients with CNS fungal infection.
- Patients with immunocompromised status are at higher risk for the disease process.
- Shunt failure rates are high, usually due to obstruction.
- Not all patients' ventriculomegaly resolves, even with low-normal draining pressures.
- The use of VP shunts does not result in a good response or outcome if it is associated with a GCS score of 8 and below and duration of altered consciousness of more than 48 hours.
- Multidisciplinary teams of neurosurgeons and infectious disease specialists are required to treat these challenging patients.

References

Baddley JW, Salzman D, Pappas PG. Fungal brain abscess in transplant recipients: epidemiologic, microbiologic, and clinical features. Clin Trans. 2002;16(6):419–24.

Black KE, Baden LR. Fungal infections of the CNS: treatment strategies for the immunocompromised patient. CNS Drugs. 2007;21(4):293–318.

Borha A, Parienti JJ, Emery E, Coskun O, Khouri S, Derlon JM. Candida albicans cerebral granuloma in an immunocompetent patient. A case report. Neurochirurgie. 2009;55(1):57–62.

Casadevall A, Rosas AL, Nosanchuk JD. Melanin and virulence in Cryptococcus neoformans. Curr Opin Microbiol. 2000;3(4):354–8.

Chakrabarti A, Sharma SC. Paranasal sinus mycoses. Indian J Chest Dis Allied Sci. 2000;42:293–304.

Chakrabarti A, Das A, Mandal J. The rising trend of invasive zygomycosis in patients with uncontrolled diabetes mellitus. Med Mycol. 2006;44(4):335–42.

Chimelli L, Mahler-Araujo MB. Fungal infections. Brain Pathol. 1997;7(1):613–27.

Chiou CC, Wong TT, Lin HH. Fungal infection of ventriculoperitoneal shunts in children. Clin Infect Dis. 1994;19:1049–53.

Cruciani M, Di Perri G, Molesini M, Vento S, Concia E, Bassetti D. Use of fluconazole in the treatment of Candida albicans hydrocephalus shunt infection. Eur J Clin Microbiol Infect Dis. 1992;11:957.

Diamond RD, Bennett JE. Prognostic factors in cryptococcal meningitis. Ann Intern Med. 1974;80:176–81.

Dotis J, Iosifidis E, Roilides E. Central nervous system aspergillosis in children: a systematic review of reported cases. Int J Infect Dis. 2007;11(5):381–93.

Dubey A, Patwardhan RV, Sampth S, Santosh V, Kolluri S, Nanda A. Intracranial fungal granuloma: analysis of 40 patients and review of the literature. Surg Neurol. 2005;63(3):254–60.

Dupont B. Fungal infections of the central nervous system. In: Anaissie EJ, McGinnis MR, Pfaller MA, editors. Clinical mycology. 1st ed. New York: Churchill Livinstone; 2003. p. 539–53.

Feng B, Wang X, Hauser M. Molecular cloning and characterization of WdPKS1, a gene involved in dihydroxynaphthalene melanin biosynthesis and virulence in Wangiella (Exophiala) dermatitidis. Infect Immun. 2001;69(3):1781–94.

Fessler RD, Sobel J, Guyot L. Management of elevated intracranial pressure in patients with cryptococcal meningitis. J Acquir Immune Defic Syndr Hum Retrovirol. 1998;17:137–42.

Genzen JR, Kenney B. Central nervous system Aspergillus infection after epidural analgesia: diagnosis, therapeutic challenges, and literature review. Diagn Microbiol Infect Dis. 2009;65(3):312–8.

Guarro J, Gene J. Opportunistic fusarial infections in humans. Eur J Clin Microbiol Infect Dis. 1995;14:74–54.

Hardesty DA, Ramey W, Afrasiabi M a, Beck B, Gonzalez O, Moran A, Nakaji P. Patient outcomes and surgical complications in coccidioidomycosis-related hydrocephalus: an institutional review. J Neurosurg. 2014;121:785–9.

Ito-Kuwa S, Nakamura K, Valderrama B, Aoki S, Vidotto V, Osafune T. Diversity of laccase among Cryptococcus neoformans serotypes. Microbiol Immunol. 2008;52(10):492–8.

Jellinger KA, Setinek U, Drlicek M, Böhm G, Steurer A, Lintner F. Neuropathology and general autopsy findings in AIDS during the last 15 years. Acta Neuropathol. 2000;100(2):213 20.

Kantarcioglu AS, de Hoog GS. Infections of the central nervous system by melanised fungi: a review of cases presented between 1999 and 2004. Mycoses. 2004;47(1-2):4–13.

Kedziora K, Słomiński JM, Gil K, Porzezińska M, Gorzewska A. Invasive aspergillosis of the paranasal sinuses, lung and brain. Pneumonol Alergol Pol. 2008;76(5):400–6.

Kovoor JM, Mahadevan A, Narayan JP. Cryptococcal choroid plexitis as a mass lesion: MR imaging and histopathologic correlation. AJNR Am J Neuroradiol. 2002;23(2):273–6.

Levitz SM. The ecology of Cryptococcus neoformans and the epidemiology of cryptococcosis. Rev Infect Dis. 1991;13:1164–9.

Lu CH, Chang WN, Chang HW. The prognostic factors of cryptococcal meningitis in HIV-negative patients. J Hosp Infect. 1999;42:313–20.

Middleton FG, Jurgenson PF, Utz JP, Shadomy S, Shadomy J. Brain abscess caused by Cladosporium trichoides. Ann Int Med. 1976;136:444–8.

Moore CB, Sayers N, Mosquera J, Slaven J, Denning DW. Antifungal drug resistance in Aspergillus. J Infect. 2000;41(3):203–20.

Nakouzi A, Zhang T, Oscarson S, Casadevall A. The common Cryptococcus neoformans glucuronoxylomannan M2 motif elicits non-protective antibodies. Vaccine. 2009;27(27):3513–8.

Nguyen MH, Yu VL. Meningitis caused by Candida species: an emerging problem in neurosurgical patients. Clin Infect Dis. 1995;21(2):323–7.

Pagano L, Ricci P, Tonso A. Mucormycosis in patients with haematological malignancies: a retrospective clinical study of 37 cases. Br J Haematol. 1997;99(2):331–6.

Pappas PG, Pottage JC, Powderly WG. Blastomycosis in patients with acquired immunodeficiency syndrome. Ann Intern Med. 1992;116:847–53.

Park MK, Hospenthal DR, Bennett JE. Treatment of hydrocephalus secondary to cryptococcal meningitis by use of shunting. Clin Infect Dis. 1999;28:629–33.

Pitisuttithum P, Negroni R, Graybill JR. Activity of posaconazole in the treatment of central nervous system fungal infections. J Antimicrob Chemother. 2005;56(4):745–55.

Redmond A, Dancer C, Woods ML. Fungal infections of the central nervous system: a review of fungal pathogens and treatment. Neurol India. 2007;55:251–9.

Revankar SG, Sutton DA, Rinaldi MG. Primary central nervous system phaeohyphomycosis: a review of 101 cases. Clin Infect Dis. 2004;38(2):206–16.

Ribaud P, Chastang C, Latgé JP. Survival and prognostic factors of invasive aspergillosis after allogeneic bone marrow transplantation. Clin Infect Dis. 1999;28(2):322–30.

Sanchez-Portocarrero JP, Saldan CJ, Perzececilia E. Candida cerebrospinal fluid shunt infections: report of two cases and review of literature. Diag Microbiol Infect Dis. 1994;20:33–40.

Shankar SK, Mahadevan A, Sundaram C. Pathobiology of fungal infections of the central nervous system with special reference to the Indian scenario. Neurol India. 2007;55:198–215.

Singh N, Husain S. Infections of the central nervous system in transplant recipients. Transpl Infect Dis. 2001;2:101–11.

Speed B, Dunt D. Clinical and host differences between infections with the two varieties of Cryptococcus neoformans. Clin Infect Dis. 1995;21(1):28–36.

Tang LM. Ventriculoperitoneal shunt in cryptococcal meningitis with hydrocephalus. Surg Neurol. 1990;33:314–9.

Treseler CB, Sugar AM. Fungal meningitis. Infect Dis Clin N Am. 1990;4(4):789–808.

Venger BH, Landon G, Rose JE. Solitary Histoplasmoma of the thalamus: case report and literature review. Neurosurgery. 1987;20(5):784–7.

Verma A, Brozman B, Petito CK. Isolated cerebral mucormycosis: report of a case and review of literature. J Neurol Sci. 2006;240:65–9.

Wheat LJ, Batteiger BE, Sathapatayavongs B. Histoplasma capsulatum infections of the central nervous system, a clinical review. Medicine. 1990;69:244–60.

Wright D, Schneider A, Berger JR. Central nervous system opportunistic infections. Neuroimaging Clin N Am. 1997;7(3):513–25.

Zarei Mahmoudabadi A. Antifungal drugs. Iran: Vasef; 2002. p. 102–6.

Zarei Mahmoudabadi A, Farrahei F, Zarrin M. In vitro synergism between miconazole and griseofulvin against Candida species. Pak J Med Sci. 2006;22(4):454–6.

Zarrin M, Najafi M. In vitro activities of amphotericin B in combination with rifampin against Aspergillus species. Pak J Med Sci. 2007;23(3):323–5.

Zarrin M, Zarei Mahmoudabadi A. Invasive candidiasis; a review article. Jundishapur J Microbiol. 2009;2(1):1–6.

Zarrin M, Jamshidian M, Jafari M. In vitro interactions of miconazole with sulfametoxazole against Candida species. Pak J Med Sci. 2009;25:243–6.

Zarrin M, Jorfi M, Aamirrajab N, Rostami M. Isolation of Cryptococcus neoformans from pigeon droppings in Ahwaz, Iran. Turk J Med Sci. 2010;40(1):313–6.

Intracranial Space-Occupying Lesions

20

Erdal Kalkan, Fatih Erdi, Yasar Karatas, and Bülent Kaya

Abbreviations

CNS	Central nervous system
CSF	Cerebrospinal fluid
CT	Computed tomography
MRI	Magnetic resonance imaging
SOLs	Space-occupying lesions

20.1 Introduction

Fungal infections of the central nervous system (CNS) represent a diagnostic and therapeutic challenge with a generally poor outcome despite surgical and medical treatment attempts. Invasive systemic fungal pathogens including *Cryptococcus neoformans*, *Candida* spp., and *Aspergillus* spp. have been commonly associated with CNS involvement. While the species of *Candida* and *Aspergillus* remain the most common causes of invasive fungal infections, other yeasts, filamentous fungi, and opportunistic yeast-like fungi and molds are increasingly being recognized (Richardson and Lass-Flörl 2008). Immunocompetent individuals usually do not get infected by the fungal pathogens due to opportunistic nature of fungi including *Cryptococcus*, *Aspergillus*, *Zygomycetes*, and *Candida* (McKeever 2012). *Aspergillus* is the most common pathogen which causes intracranial granulomas (Naik et al. 2015). Fungal space-occupying lesions (SOLs) include intracranial fungal granulomas, abscesses, and cysts, particularly in the primary parenchymal location. These nonneoplastic fungal SOLs of the CNS can grow expansively and easily mimic their neoplastic counterparts in both clinical and radiological evaluations. Fungal granulomas are the most frequently encountered form of the disease in clinical practice, but fungal abscesses or a compound of these lesions can be seen in decreasing frequency. Intraparenchymal cysts which locate in basal ganglia typically occur in cryptococcal infection. *Candida*, *Aspergillus*, *Cladosporium*, and *Mucorales* commonly produce primary parenchymal fungal abscesses. Hematogenous dissemination of fungi from an extracranial site causes multiple foci of infection within the brain. Initial meningoencephalitis leads to vasculitis thrombosis and late hemorrhagic cerebral infarction. When an abscess develops, it may rapidly expand. Aspergillosis, histoplasmosis, blastomycosis, paracoccidioidomycosis, cladosporiasis, mucormycosis, and cryptococcosis may produce CNS fungal granulomas which mimic tuberculomas but differ by the presence of more

E. Kalkan (✉) · Y. Karatas · B. Kaya
Department of Neurosurgery, Medova Private Hospital, Konya, Turkey

F. Erdi
Department of Neurosurgery, Meram Faculty of Medicine, Necmettin Erbakan University, Konya, Turkey

M. Turgut et al. (eds.), *Fungal Infections of the Central Nervous System*,
https://doi.org/10.1007/978-3-030-06088-6_20

fibrosis. Frontal and temporal granulomas generally occur due to spread from paranasal sinuses as in aspergillosis and mucormycosis, whereas parietal granulomas occur due to hematogenous spread of other fungi (Raman Sharma 2010).

20.2 Epidemiology

The incidence of CNS fungal infections is similar to that of systemic fungal infections and has been rising due to increased life expectancy, large ageing population, malignancy, extensive use of immunosuppressive drugs, longer survival of patients, increased frequency of acquired immunodeficiency syndrome (AIDS), and poor nutritional status (Naik et al. 2015). The estimated annual incidences of invasive fungal infections caused by opportunistic pathogens per million of the population vary between 12 and 228 infections according to causative agent (Raman Sharma 2010). The Indian subcontinent has the highest reported frequency of histologically verified intracranial fungal mass lesions in geographic distribution with one to two cases per year. Hot and dry climate with high content of fungal spores in agrarian dust was blamed for endemic form of the disease in India, Africa, and California (Naik et al. 2015). Predisposing factors include diabetes, tuberculosis, HIV, steroids, immunosuppression, and chemotherapy (Naik et al. 2015). Intracranial fungal mass lesions had a 0.5–1% cumulative prevalence in transplant recipients (Rajshekhar 2007).

20.3 Pathogenesis

Infection usually spreads to the CNS via the bloodstream from a primary pulmonary infection, or it can extend directly from a close focus such as wound infection, otitis, osteomyelitis, or an infected cranial sinus (McKeever 2012). In the presence of an infected paranasal sinus, infection could spread gradually from the sinus to bone, extradural space, meninges, orbit, anterior and middle skull base, and parasellar region. Extension to the intracranial space can be via anatomical apertures such as orbital apex, and communicating perivascular spaces act as a bridge for spreading to subarachnoid space. Retrograde thrombophlebitis was also blamed for the development of cerebellopontine angle and cerebellar masses. Although fungal pathogens can cause meningitis, encephalitis, abscess formation, vasculitis, or granulomas, they tend to cause granulomatous meningitis following an acute phase of infection and can affect the meninges, calvarium, brain, and intracranial vessels in distinct forms, severity, and compositions (Naik et al. 2015).

20.4 Diagnosis

A high index of suspicion is critical for early diagnosis and avoidance from associated significant morbidity and mortality. Past medical history of the patient or the patient's close relatives should be taken into consideration. Like other intracranial space-occupying lesions, headache, nausea, vomiting, altered vision, and mental status, focal neurological deficits are commonly encountered presentations. Invasion of the cavernous sinus and orbital apex could cause visual symptoms, proptosis, ophthalmoplegia, superior orbital fissure syndrome, and cranial nerve palsies. Other uncommon manifestations include seizures, stroke, subarachnoid hemorrhage, and mycotic aneurysm formation (Naik et al. 2015).

20.5 Imaging Findings

Computed tomography (CT) scan is a common first-line investigation tool with a few characteristic findings. Irregular iso-/hyperdense lesion with perilesional edema and thin heterogeneous contrast enhancement are well-known features. In the case of primary sinus disease (Fig. 20.1), proximity of lesions, evidence of bone destruction, and infarcts due to arteritis may promote a fungal etiology (Naik et al. 2015). Primary parenchymal lesions showed heterogeneous attenuation with predominantly low-density areas, while dural-based lesions showed isodense to hyperdense attenuation (Saini et al. 2010).

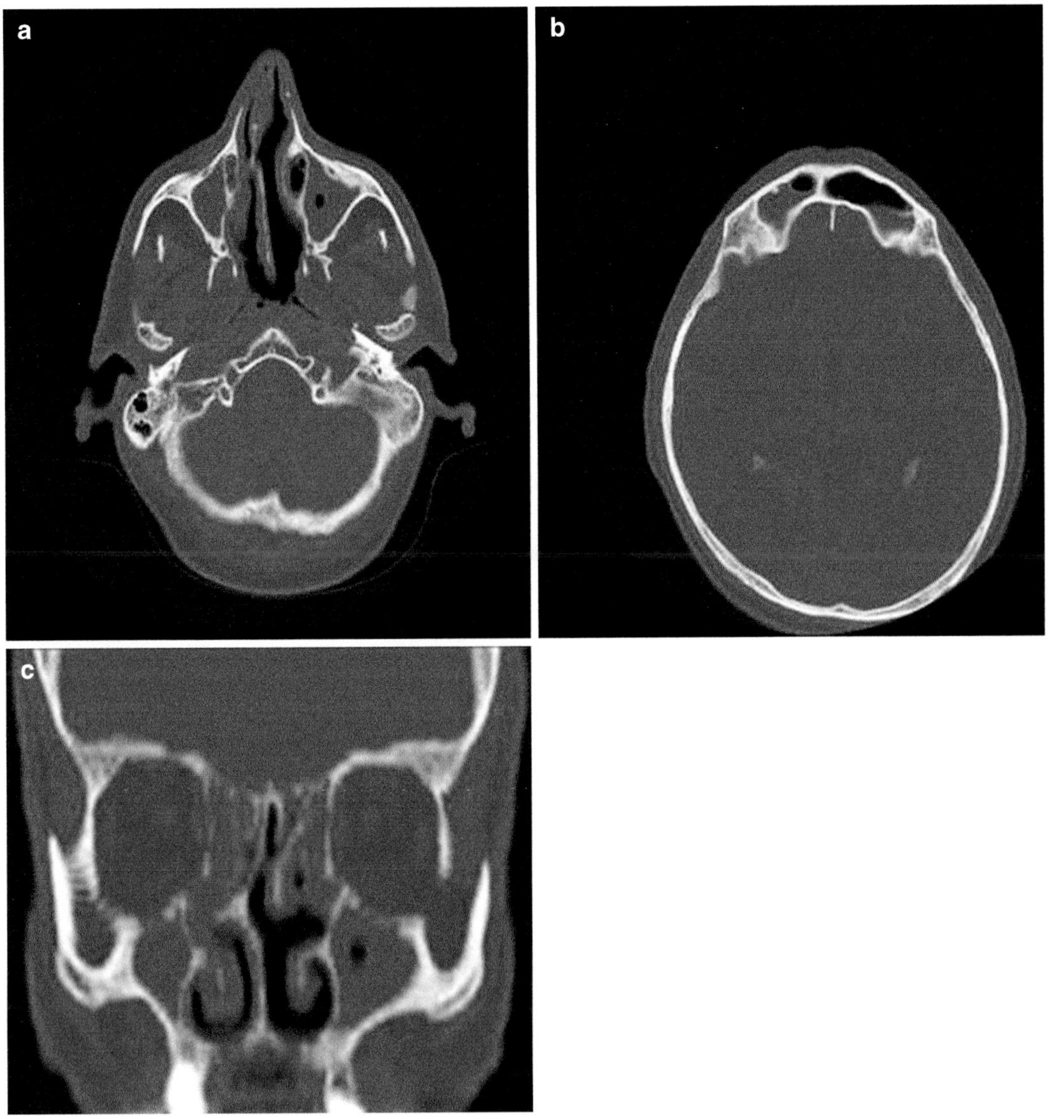

Fig. 20.1 Paranasal sinus computed tomography (CT) of a 45-year-old male patient with common variable immunodeficiency. Complete filling of maxillary (**a**) and frontal sinus with pus and pansinusitis appearance (**c**)

Multiple lesions in an immunocompromised patient should prompt further investigation with magnetic resonance imaging (MRI).

MRI findings have been reported to vary depending on the immunological status of the patients and on the age of the lesions. Again primary sinus disease gains importance for establishing correct diagnosis with thickened mucosa or complete filling appearance. Isointense to hypointense signals of the lesion on both T(1)-weighted (T1W) and T(2)-weighted (T2W) images are primary findings. Primary parenchymal lesions show heterogeneous signal intensity pattern with predominantly hypointense signal on T1W and hyperintense signal intensity on T2W images. The lesions could enhance contrast in a homogenous or peripheral ring pattern. There is commonly a lack of contrast enhancement or surrounding edema in immunocompromised patients, reflecting reduced immune response. The wall of the fungal abscess is usually regular and thin. Irregularity of the rim can vary depending on the aggressiveness of the fungus and the host's ability to exert an immune response (Hadley et al. 2017). Infiltration of the orbit, extraocular muscles, or cranial nerve compression can be detected with MRI. Restricted diffusion on diffusion-weighted imaging similar with pyogenic abscess, decreased perfusion on perfusion-weighted imaging, and presence of hemorrhage on gradient echo sequence gave worthy supporting data (Fig. 20.2) (Naik et al. 2015; Saini et al. 2010). The infarcts distribute commonly at the gray-white matter junction as well as basal ganglia, thalamus, corpus callosum, and perforating small artery territories in disseminated fungal infection (DeLone et al. 1999). The involvement of perforating arteries without involvement of the distal major arterial territories stresses the pathophysiologic difference between

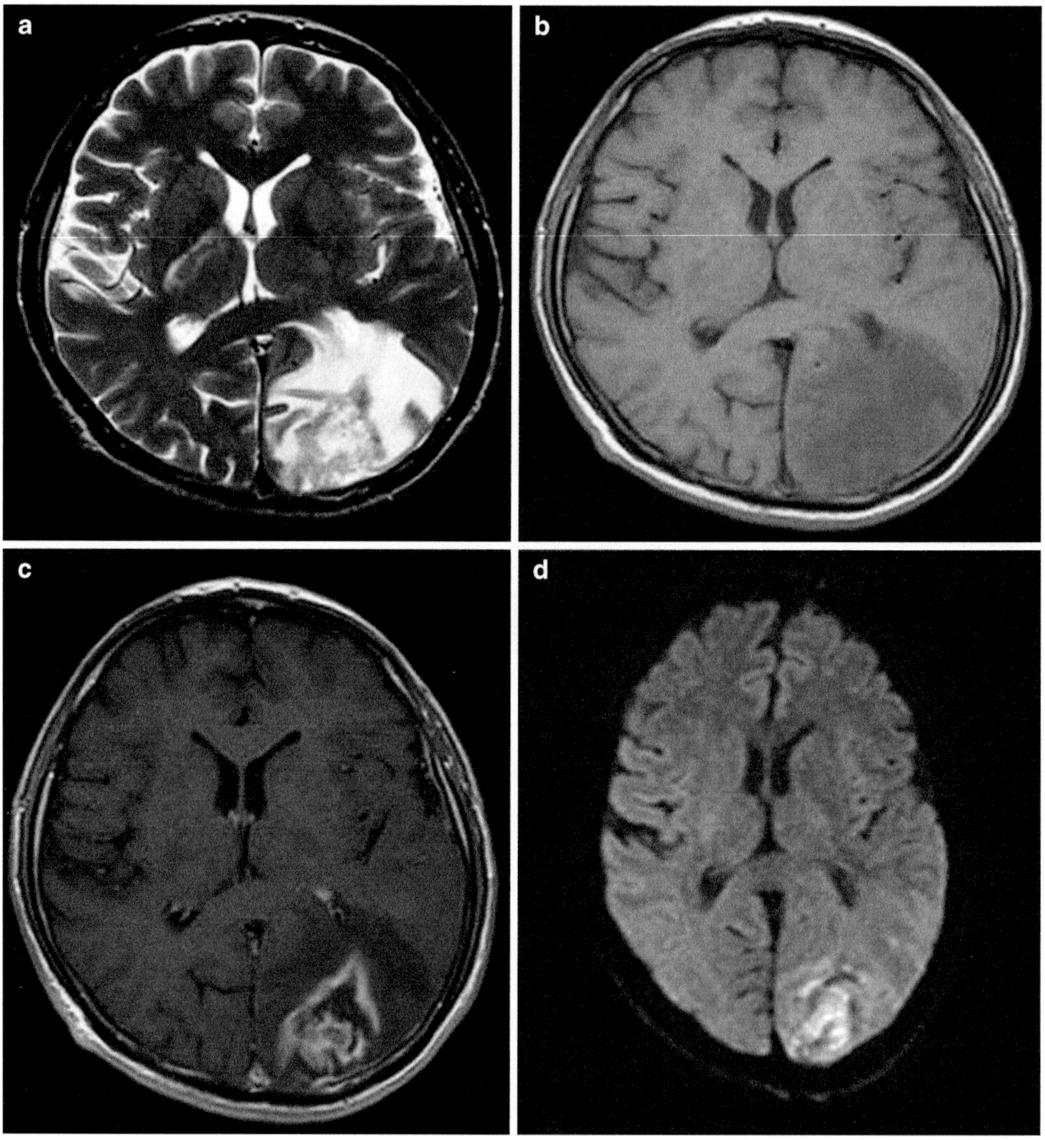

Fig. 20.2 T2-weighted pre-gadolinium (**a**), T1-weighted pre-gadolinium (**b**), and post-gadolinium (**c**) axial magnetic resonance imaging (MRI) sections showed a fungal space-occupying lesion (SOL) at the left occipital lobe of the same patient. Note the irregular rim pattern (**c**) and restricted diffusion on diffusion MRI (**d**)

septic fungal and thromboembolic infarction (Yamada et al. 2002). Corpus callosum involvement can be used for distinguishing fungal infection from pyogenic infection and thromboembolic infarction as the latter do not commonly involve the corpus callosum. But other processes such as glioblastoma, lymphoma, and multiple sclerosis should keep in mind for differential diagnosis (DeLone et al. 1999).

20.6 Management

Antifungal medications and surgery are the mainstay treatment options. Treatment modality preference depends on the primary location, size, and number of the lesions. General medical status of the patient carries high importance. Small fungal SOLs can be managed with aggressive antifungal medications and supportive care, whereas significantly large lesions that compress adjacent brain structures need radical surgical excision. Urgent decompression can be lifesaving in emergency situations. Surgical options include stereotactic procedures, craniotomy, shunt surgery, and mycotic aneurysm surgery. Indications of the stereotactic procedures include deep-seated lesions and lesions in the eloquent brain regions for the establishment of tissue diagnosis (Murthy and Sundaram 2014). Surgical excision reduces infection load, reduces mass effect, and improves efficacy of following medical treatment. Radical excision of lesions without excessive contamination of cerebrospinal fluid (CSF) spaces was advocated (Naik et al. 2015). Survival rates are much better in patients treated with combined medical and surgical treatment in patients treated with medical treatment only (Gonzalez et al. 2002). Adherence/invasion of the lesion to basal vessels and cranial nerves leads to specific challenges and complicates the postoperative course by leading to arteritis and infarcts, cavernous sinus thrombosis, meningoencephalitis, ventriculitis, etc. Shunt surgery could be imperative due to hydrocephalus with elevated intracranial pressure (Gonzalez et al. 2002). Ommaya reservoir insertion for intralesional administration of amphotericin B was reported in patients with sinocranial aspergillus granulomas with dense fibrous tissue (Murthy and Sundaram 2014). Surgical clipping or endovascular treatments with aggressive antifungal treatment are indicated for the patients with mycotic aneurysms (Rajshekhar 2007). Prognosis after treatment depends on the prompt recognition and management of the disease as well as preoperative neurologic status of patient, immunocompromised state, contamination of ventricular CSF during surgery, and renal failure (due to amphotericin B) (Naik et al. 2015). Previously reported gloomy surgical results (Dubey et al. 2005; Sharma et al. 1997; Yanai et al. 1985) were improving slowly (Naik et al. 2015). Naik et al. recommended preoperative antifungal treatment for 1–2 weeks, followed by radical surgery and antifungal treatment for the following 6 weeks (Naik et al. 2015).

20.7 Conclusion

It is concluded that:

- CNS fungal infections have been diagnosed increasingly over the last few decades, due to the increase of immunocompromised patients under risk.
- Although some improvements have been achieved, CNS fungal infections constitute a diagnostic and therapeutic challenge.
- Antifungal medications and surgery are the mainstay treatment options.
- Radical excision of SOLs without excessive contamination of CSF spaces improves outcome.

References

DeLone DR, Goldstein RA, Petermann G, et al. Disseminated aspergillosis involving the brain: distribution and imaging characteristics. AJNR Am J Neuroradiol. 1999;20:1597–604.

Dubey A, Patwardhan RV, Sampth S, et al. Intracranial fungal granuloma: analysis of 40 patients and review of the literature. Surg Neurol. 2005;63:254–60. https://doi.org/10.1016/J.SURNEU.2004.04.020.

Gonzalez CE, Rinaldi MG, Sugar AM. Zygomycosis. Infect Dis Clin North Am. 2002;16:895–914. https://doi.org/10.1016/S0891-5520(02)00037-5.

Hadley C, Haneef Mohamed AW, Singhal A. Central nervous system fungal infection in a young male with a history of intravenous drug abuse and hepatitis C. Radiol Case Rep. 2017;12:590–6. https://doi.org/10.1016/j.radcr.2017.03.016.

McKeever PE. Pathologic basis of central nervous system infections. Neuroimaging Clin N Am. 2012;22:773–90. https://doi.org/10.1016/j.nic.2012.06.001.

Murthy JMK, Sundaram C. Fungal infections of the central nervous system. Handb Clin Neurol. 2014;121:1383–401. https://doi.org/10.1016/B978-0-7020-4088-7.00095-X.

Naik V, Ahmed FU, Gupta A, et al. Intracranial fungal granulomas: a single institutional clinicopathologic study of 66 patients and review of the literature. World Neurosurg. 2015;83:1166–72. https://doi.org/10.1016/j.wneu.2015.01.053.

Rajshekhar V. Surgical management of intracranial fungal masses. Neurol India. 2007;55:267–73. https://doi.org/10.4103/0028-3886.35688.

Raman Sharma R. Fungal infections of the nervous system: current perspective and controversies in management. Int J Surg. 2010;8:591–601. https://doi.org/10.1016/j.ijsu.2010.07.293.

Richardson M, Lass-Flörl C. Changing epidemiology of systemic fungal infections. Clin Microbiol Infect. 2008;14(Suppl 4):5–24. https://doi.org/10.1111/j.1469-0691.2008.01978.x.

Saini J, Gupta AK, Jolapara MB, et al. Imaging findings in intracranial aspergillus infection in immunocompetent patients. World Neurosurg. 2010;74:661–70. https://doi.org/10.1016/j.wneu.2010.06.017.

Sharma BS, Khosla VK, Kak VK, et al. Intracranial fungal granuloma. Surg Neurol. 1997;47:489–97. https://doi.org/10.1016/S0090-3019(96)00209-1.

Yamada K, Shrier DA, Rubio A, et al. Imaging findings in intracranial aspergillosis. Acad Radiol. 2002;9:163–71.

Yanai Y, Wakao T, Fukamachi A, Kunimine H. Intracranial granuloma caused by Aspergillus fumigatus. Surg Neurol. 1985;23:597–604.

Invasive Fungal Diseases of the Skull Base

21

Manogaran Ravi Sankar, Mathialagan Arulalan, Amit K. Keshri, Arun K. Srivastava, Awadhesh K. Jaiswal, and Sanjay Behari

Abbreviations

AFRS	Allergic fungal rhinosinusitis
AISBFD	Acute invasive skull base fungal disease
CIGFD	Chronic invasive granulomatous fungal disease
CISBFD	Chronic invasive skull base fungal disease
CSF	Cerebrospinal fluid
CT scan	Computed tomographic scan
FDA	Food and Drug Administration
Ig E	Immunoglobulin E
MRI	Magnetic resonance imaging
PCR	Polymerase chain reaction
WI	Weighted images

21.1 Introduction

Fungal infection of the skull base is not uncommon in clinical practice. In the recent times, the incidence of this entity has been increasing due to increase in the prevalence of immunocompromised conditions like diabetes mellitus and haematological malignancies (Dubey et al. 2005). Rarely, it can be present in immunocompetent individuals also (Shah et al. 2017). Fungal infection of the central nervous system can manifest as meningitis, meningoencephalitis, vasculitis, abscess formation and granuloma formation (Mohindra et al. 2008). Skull base fungal pathologies present with headache, nasal symptoms, orbital symptoms, cranial nerve palsy and paresis. Isolated skull base involvement is rare; commonly, skull base is involved by the lesion spreading from the adjacent paranasal sinuses. The paranasal sinuses are closely related to the anterior and middle cranial base and also to vital structures like the orbit, optic nerve, internal carotid artery, pituitary gland, cavernous sinus and cranial nerves. Fungal diseases have a wide spectrum of acute-to-chronic clinical presentation. There are various fungal organisms involved in causing lesions of the skull base, like *Aspergillus*, *Scedosporium*, *Alternaria*, *Curvularia* and *Mucor*, and these are more abundant in the air and soil (Süslü et al. 2009; Tarkan et al. 2012; Zuniga and Turner 2014).

de Shazo et al. (1997) classified fungal diseases into two major categories, *non-invasive* and *invasive*, based on the histopathology. The non-invasive fungal diseases are further classified as *allergic fungal rhinosinusitis* (AFRS) and *chronic non-invasive diseases* (fungal ball).

M. Ravi Sankar · M. Arulalan · A. K. Keshri
Division of Neuro-otology, Department of Neurosurgery, Sanjay Gandhi Postgraduate Institute of Medical Sciences, Lucknow, Uttar Pradesh, India

A. K. Srivastava · A. K. Jaiswal · S. Behari (✉)
Department of Neurosurgery, Sanjay Gandhi Postgraduate Institute of Medical Sciences, Lucknow, Uttar Pradesh, India

M. Turgut et al. (eds.), *Fungal Infections of the Central Nervous System*,
https://doi.org/10.1007/978-3-030-06088-6_21

The *invasive fungal disease* has a spectrum that is classified as *acute fulminant invasive*, *chronic invasive* and *granulomatous invasive*.

The prognosis depends more on the type of infection and the host immunity and to a lesser extent on the type of the fungal species, but identification of the fungal species by culture does aid in the antifungal medication selection and the therapy administered.

21.2 Invasive Fungal Disease

Invasive fungal disease involving the skull base is classified based on the onset, duration and progression of the disease as chronic invasive and acute invasive.

21.2.1 Chronic Invasive Skull Base Fungal Disease (CISBFD)

Chronic or indolent fungal pathologies involving the skull base occur in both immunocompetent and immunocompromised individuals. The usual clinical course of these lesions is slowly progressive in nature, developing over weeks to months, in contrast to their acute counterparts. Any immunocompromised patient presenting with fever of unknown origin, headache, facial swelling, facial pain, nasal obstruction, nasal discharge, nasal bleed, nasal crusting, proptosis, diplopia and cranial nerve deficits should be suspected of having an invasive fungal pathology. In immunocompetent individuals, however, diplopia, painless proptosis and orbital complaints are the commonest presentations (Shah et al. 2017). All the suspected patients should undergo a complete cranial nerve examination followed by nasal endoscopy and oral cavity examination to look for a change in the colour of the mucosa or the presence of any mucosal ulceration or necrosis. A biopsy from the suspected site should be taken for histopathologic confirmation. Skull base involvement is usually secondary to the sinonasal involvement (Figs. 21.1, 21.2, and 21.3). Moreover, an isolated sphenoidal sinus (Fig. 21.4) involvement is more aggressive

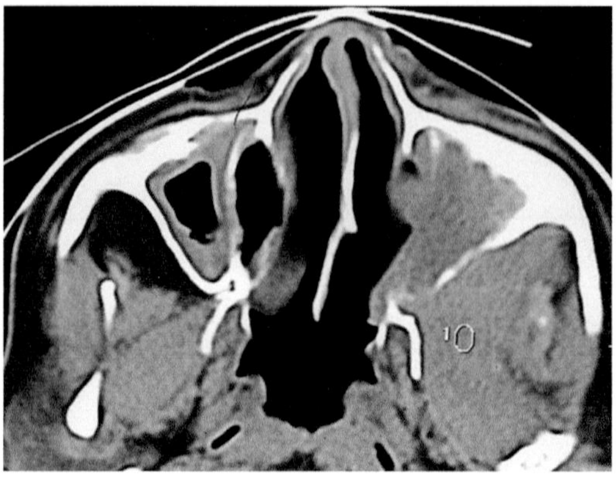

Fig. 21.1 CT scan shows a left maxillary sinus pathology with destruction of its posterior wall and an infra-temporal bone involvement

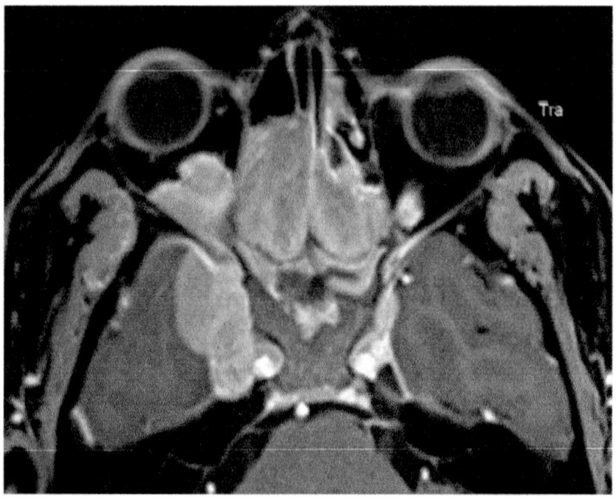

Fig. 21.2 T1W MRI showing a sphenoethmoidal lesion extending into the orbit and involving the skull base

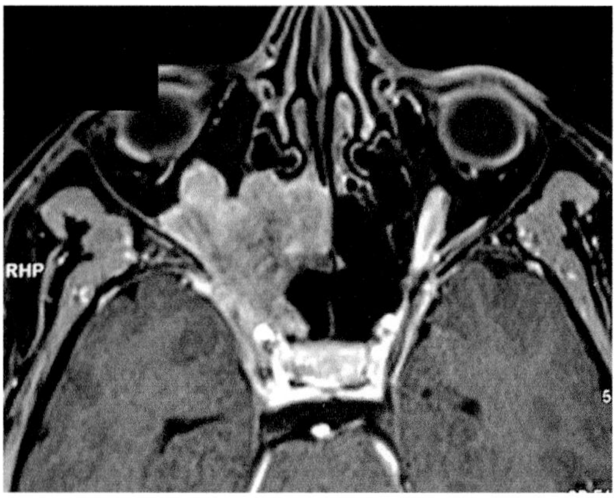

Fig. 21.3 An ethmoidal lesion spreading into the orbital apex and the superior orbital fissure

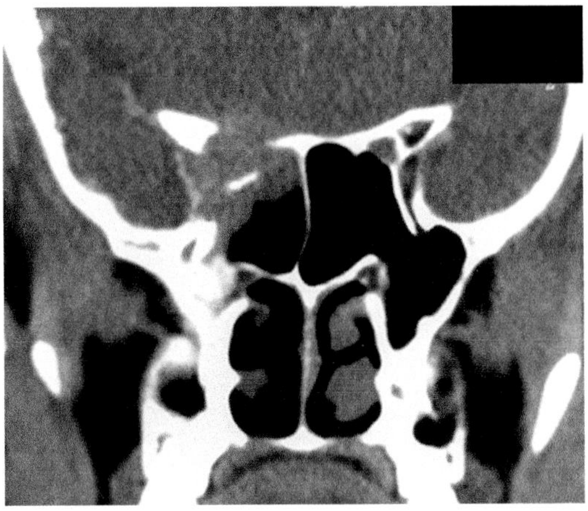

Fig. 21.4 An isolated sphenoidal pathology eroding the skull base

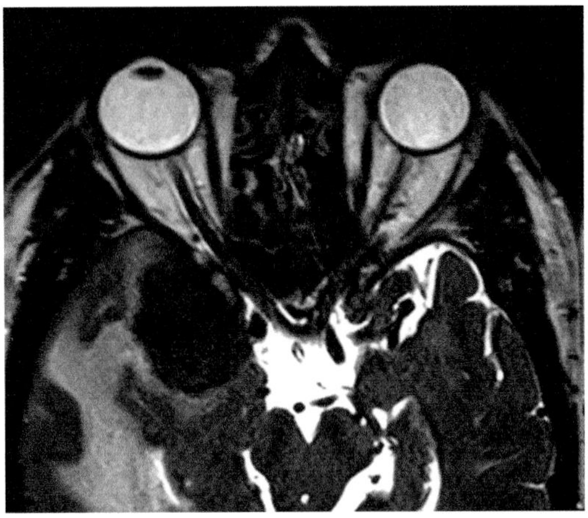

Fig. 21.6 MR T2 W image showing an isolated skull base aspergilloma

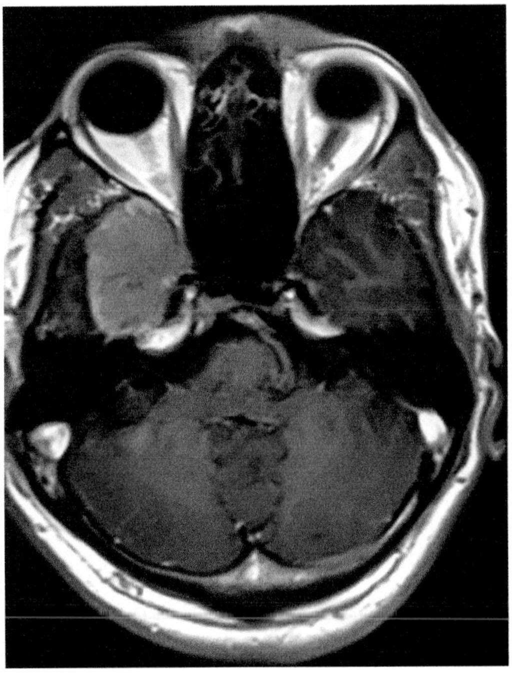

Fig. 21.5 MR T1W contrast-enhanced image showing an isolated skull base aspergilloma without sinus involvement

in nature because of its anatomical proximity to the orbital apex, optic nerve, carotid artery, cavernous sinus, pituitary gland and cranial nerves (Dhiwakar et al. 2003b). Rarely do we encounter isolated skull base involvement without sinonasal pathology (Figs. 21.5 and 21.6). In isolated skull base fungal pathology, it is difficult to differentiate the lesion from other pathologies like a meningioma and a tuberculoma (Mohindra et al. 2008).

Biopsy from the suspected lesion should be subjected to microscopy, fungal culture and histopathology. For fungal microscopy, the commonest strain used is potassium hydroxide (Fig. 21.7) and the calcofluor white (a special fluorescent stain that binds strongly to structures containing cellulose and chitin) method using fluorescence microscopy. For histopathology, the commonest stain used for fungal identification is Gomori methenamine silver staining (Schell 2000) (Fig. 21.8). The histopathological examination of the tissue establishes the presence and nature of the fungal hyphae (Fig. 21.9). In mucormycosis, the fungal elements are broad, ribbon-like, irregular and rarely septate, whereas aspergillosis shows narrow, regular septae with 45° branching patterns (Ferguson 2000; Gillespie and O'Malley 2000). Fungal elements should also be looked for in the submucosa. The presence of angio-invasion, tissue necrosis and recruitment of inflammatory cells should also be assessed (de Shazo 1998). One of the most striking differences between aspergillosis and mucormycosis is that the former causes angio-invasion but does not lead to vaso-occlusion, whereas mucormycosis is almost always associated with vaso-obliteration (Epstein and Kern 2008). Fungal culture is also important to initiate species-specific antifungal

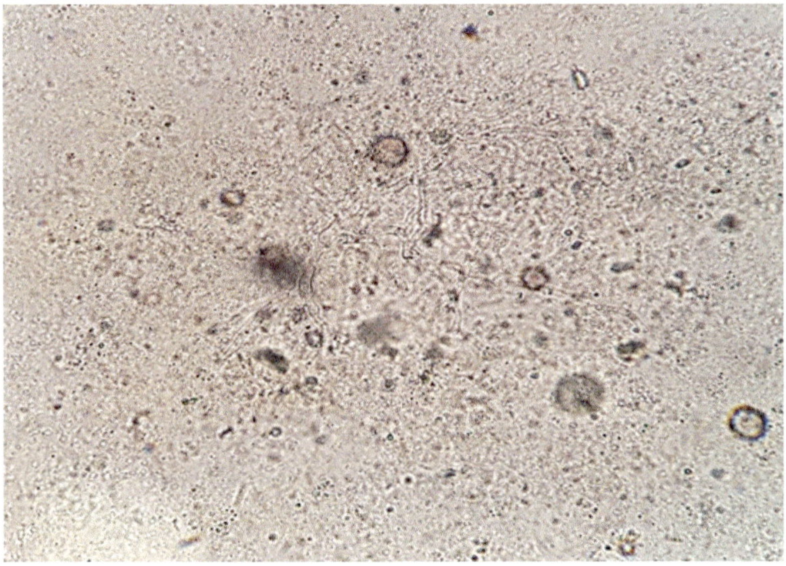

Fig. 21.7 10% KOH wet mount of the nasal tissue showing the hyaline septate with acute angle branching fungal hyphae suggestive of the *Aspergillus* species

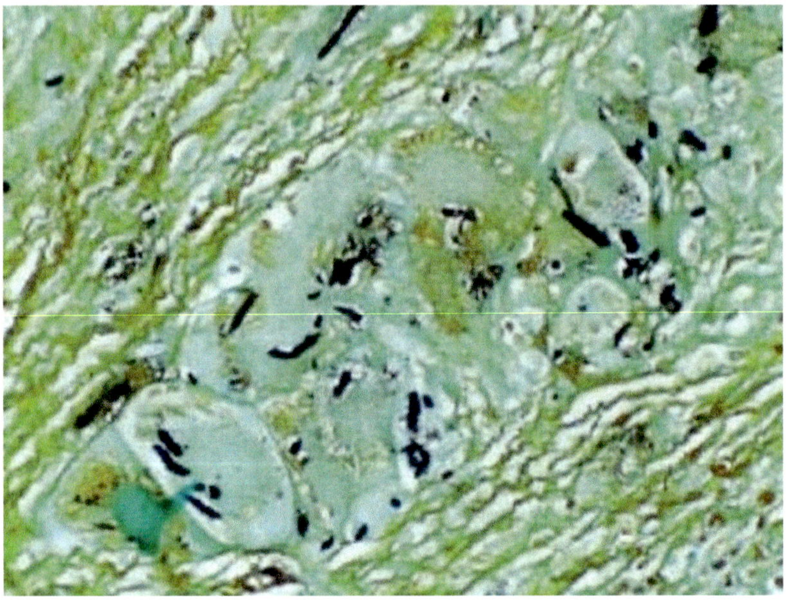

Fig. 21.8 *Aspergillus* seen on Gomori methenamine silver stain

therapy and to identify the additional rare fungal species causing skull base pathologies like the *Fusarium*, *Alternaria* and *Pseudallescheria* species (Kalkanci et al. 2006) (Figs. 21.10 and 21.11). Sometimes, the routine evaluation does not show any fungal infection; in these conditions, the newer modalities like identification of fungal cell wall markers in the serum like galactomannan (Chen et al. 2011; Schwartz et al. 2005), beta-D-glucan and mannan enzyme immunoassay may be done. These tests are more specific for detection of aspergillosis infection. Molecular testing method that uses the oligonucleotide probe and gene sequencing can be used for rapid identification of the fungal species. In case of frank intracranial involvement by invasive aspergillosis, the sensitivity of cerebrospinal fluid (CSF) polymerase chain reaction (PCR) is 100% as compared to the sensitivity of galactomannan, which is 80% (Chen et al. 2011).

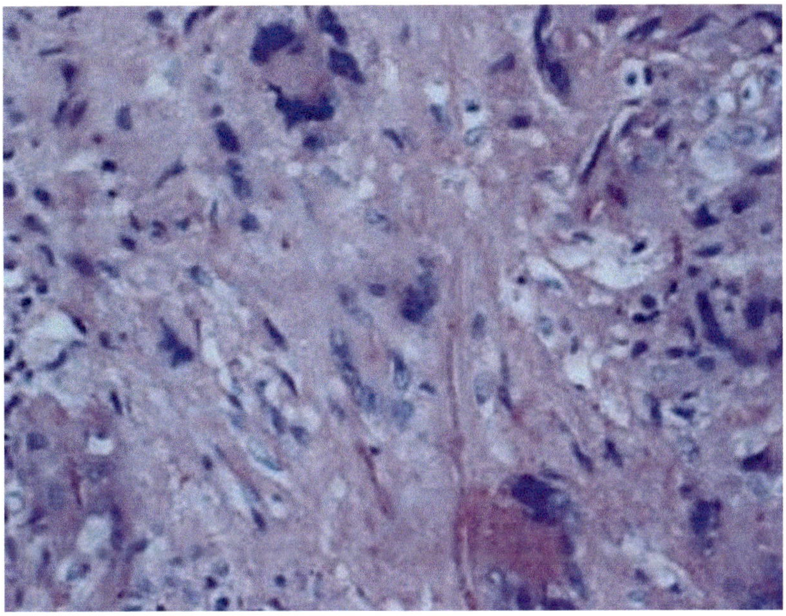

Fig. 21.9 Histopathological examination showing *Aspergillus* and its branching pattern

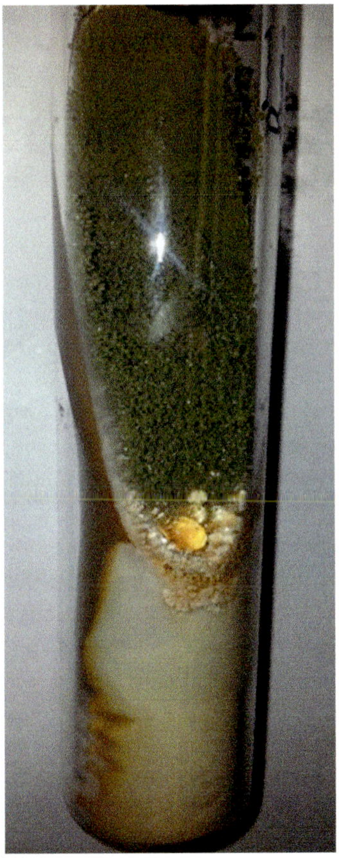

Fig. 21.10 Culture on Sabouraud's dextrose agar shows the velvety powdery greenish yellow colonies suggestive of *Aspergillus flavus*

To evaluate the extent of the lesion is as important as the clinical and laboratory confirmation of the fungal infection. The computed tomographic (CT) scan is the primary imaging modality in all the suspected cases harbouring a fungal pathology to assess for abnormalities in the paranasal sinuses and the skull base. The common findings are partial or complete sinus opacification with or without destruction of the bony wall and the sclerotic thickening of the sinus wall (Hoon et al. 2014). On contrast-enhanced CT scan images of the skull base, aspergilloma (Fig. 21.12) is present as an enhancing mass with irregular border with surrounding cerebral oedema (Jain et al. 2007). Contrast-enhanced magnetic resonance imaging (MRI) may be a better tool for establishing the diagnosis and to determine the extent of disease (Dubey et al. 2005; Yamada et al. 2002). On MRI, fungal lesions are isointense on T1-weighted images (WI) with a hypo-to-isointense signal intensity on T2WI. There is a uniform enhancement on contrast T1W1 (Hoon et al. 2014; Jain et al. 2007) (Fig. 21.13).

After confirming the diagnosis and the extent of pathology, the basic principles of management include correcting the immunocompromised condition, the surgical debridement (Selvam et al. 2010) (Figs. 21.14 and 21.15) and the start-

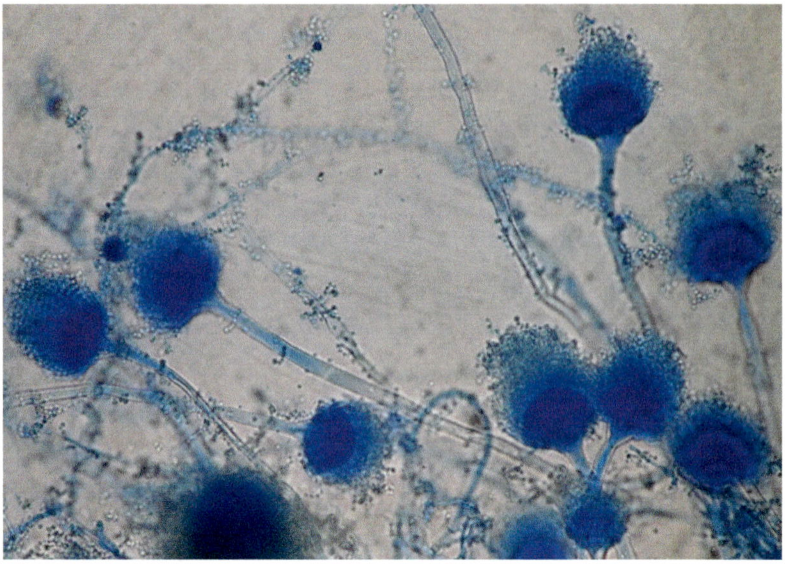

Fig. 21.11 Lactophenol cotton blue mount shows the septate fungal hyphae bearing conidiophores with radiating conidial heads; vesicles with biseriate phialides with chains of conidia are also seen

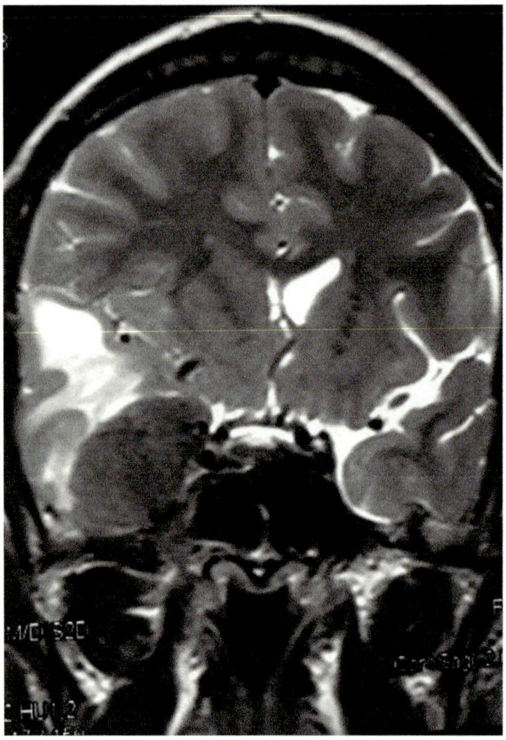

Fig. 21.12 T2 W MR scans showing evidence of skull aspergilloma with surrounding oedema

ing of the appropriate antifungal therapy. Among these, the most important issue is to take steps to cause reversal of the underlying co-morbid condition. In some cases, even an infusion of granulocytes is used to reverse the immune status of the patients (Martinez et al. 2013).

An aggressive surgical debridement is essential to reduce the disease load and for gaining a better outcome; however, due to the presence of vital structures in and around the skull base, like the optic nerve, carotid artery, cranial base dura, cavernous sinus and cranial nerves, radical debridement is often not possible. Lesions involving the orbital apex (Fig. 21.16) and the retrobulbar region warrant an orbital exenteration, but this is not required during the anterior and inferomedial involvement of the orbit (Dhiwakar et al. 2003a). Some studies have shown that the extent of debridement was not a significant factor in influencing the patient survival (Hoon et al. 2014). To tackle the residual disease, initiation of antifungal therapy is mandatory.

Antifungals like triazoles (fluconazole, itraconazole, voriconazole and posaconazole), echinocandidins (caspofungin, micafungin,

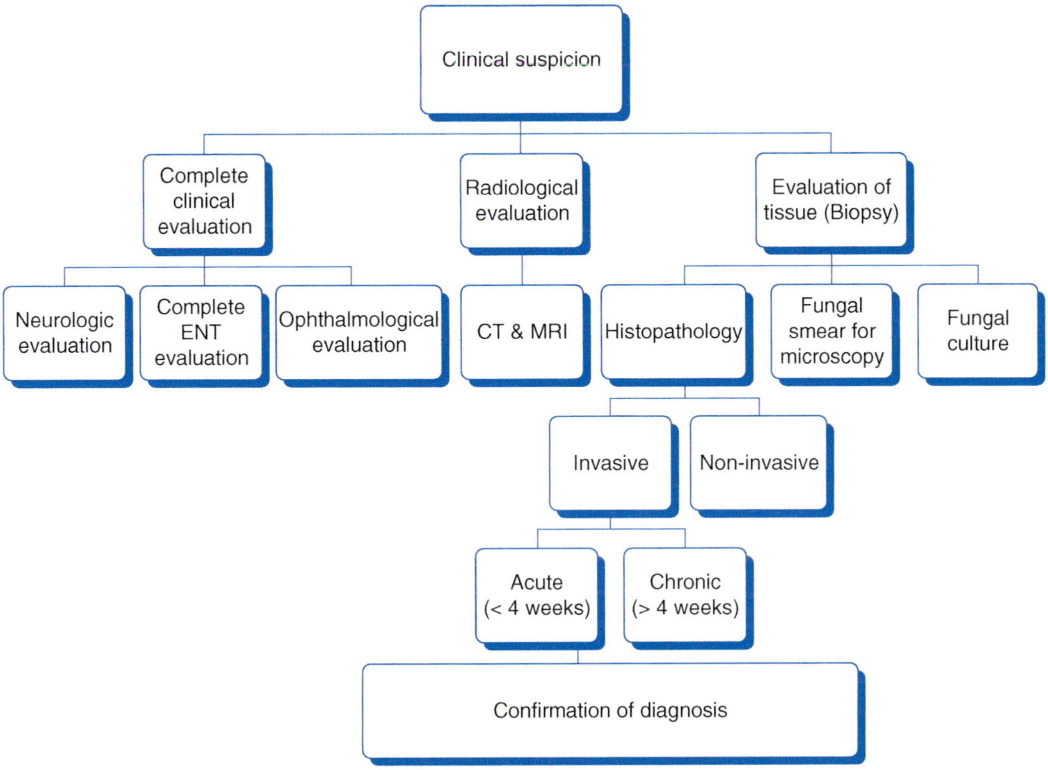

Fig. 21.13 Evaluation of clinically suspicious skull base fungal disease

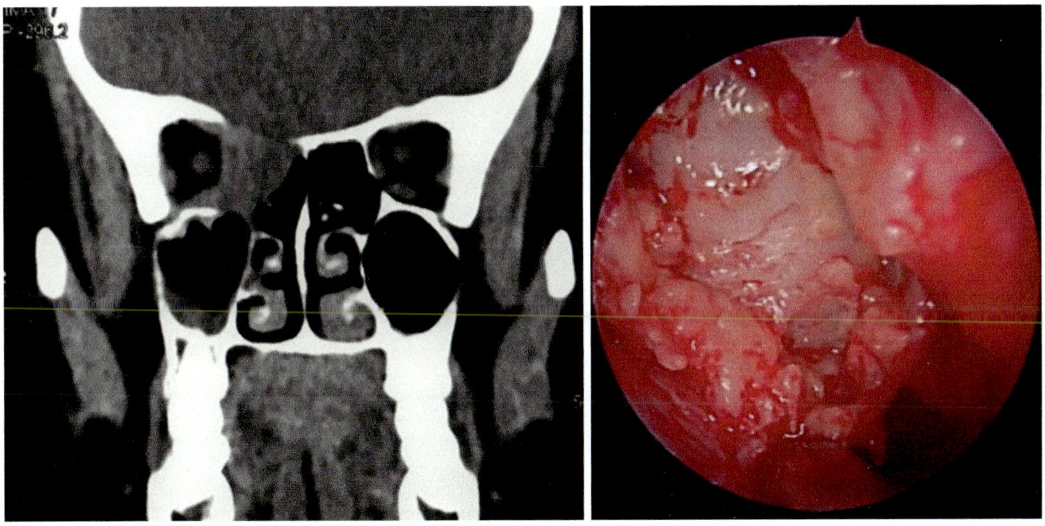

Fig. 21.14 Extradural clearance of the disease from anterior skull base with CT correlation

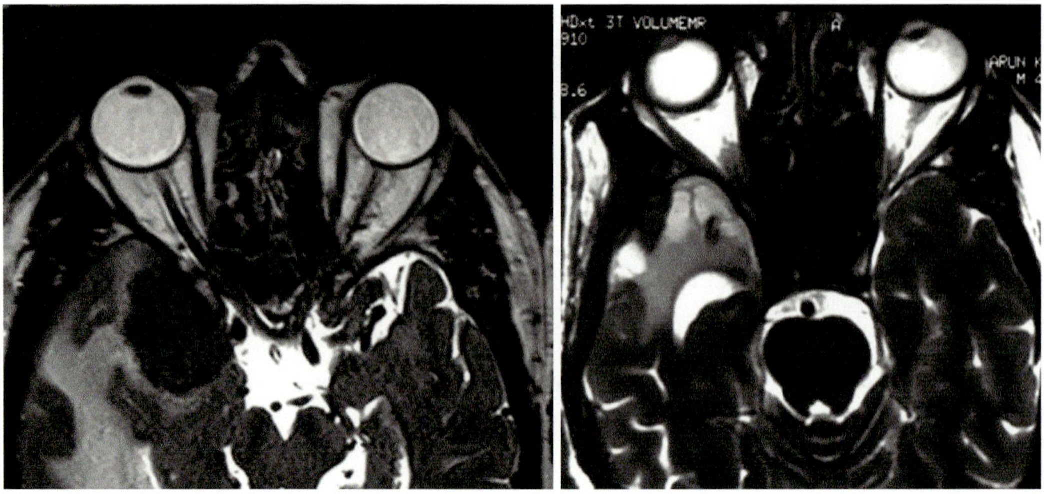

Fig. 21.15 Pre- and post-operative (6 months follow-up with voriconazole) images of the skull base aspergilloma

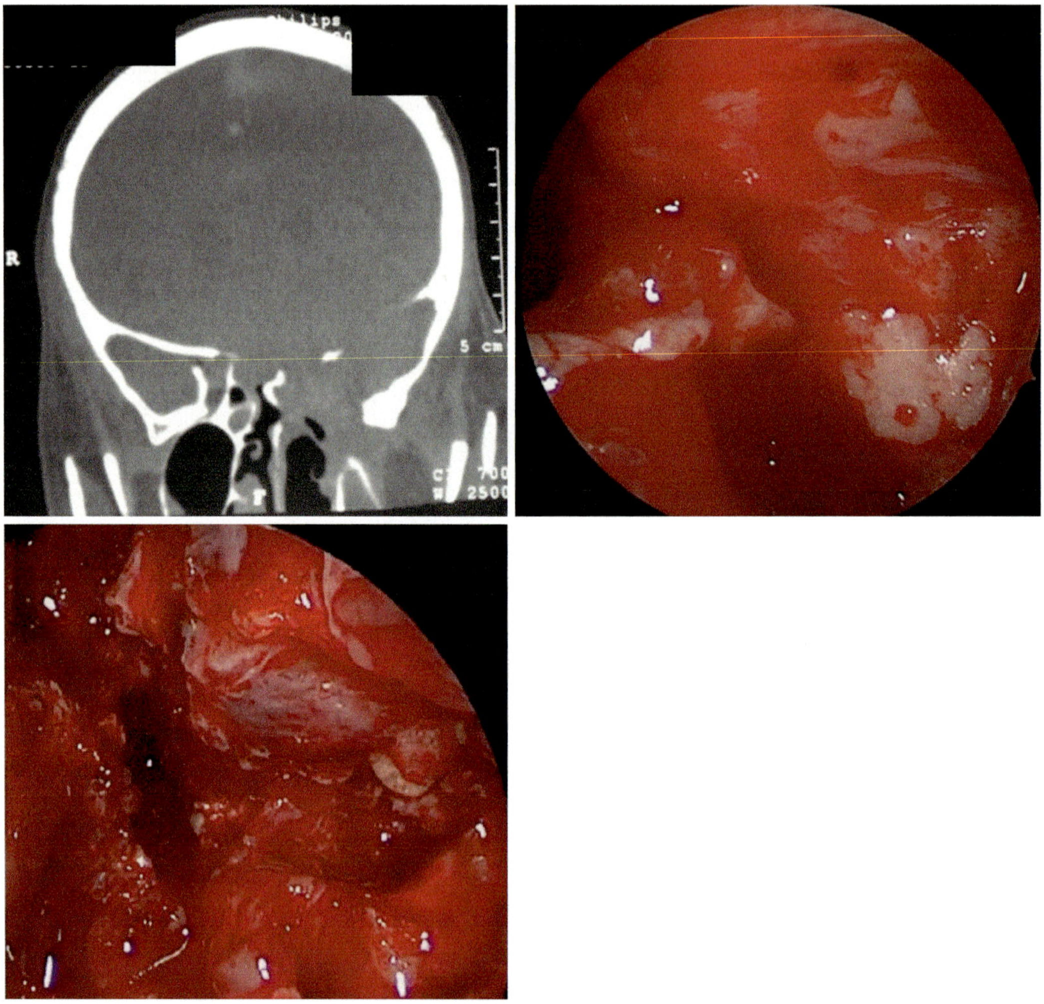

Fig. 21.16 The pterygopalatine fossa exposure and debulking of disease

anidulafungin), polyenes (amphotericin B) and flucytosine are available for the medical treatment of invasive fungal disease (Herbrecht et al. 2002; Kontoyiannis 2012; Redmond et al. 2007). Amphotericin B is the broad-spectrum fungicidal agent, but its toxicity limits its widespread and prolonged usage. The newer liposomal formulations are comparatively less toxic and can be used in higher dosages. Voriconazole, approved by the US Food and Drug Administration (FDA) in 2002, is more effective than amphotericin in invasive aspergillosis (Gillespie and O'Malley 2000). The duration of therapy is based on clinical and radiological response and varies from 3 to 6 months. Posaconazole has shown its efficacy as a salvage therapy in patients with end-stage renal disease caused due to diabetes (Mehta and Langston 2009).

Shah et al. (2017) and Mohindra et al. (2008) have described the protocol for the management of skull base invasive aspergillosis. Patient with skull base involvement with minimal invasion of the basal frontal lobe, cavernous sinus and the infratemporal fossa should be treated with extradural debridement followed by systemic antifungal therapy. Stable patients with massive intracranial invasion of the frontal or temporal lobes with cerebral oedema should be preloaded with liposomal amphotericin B of 2 g followed by debridement; and after debridement, they should be given a cumulative dose of up to 6 g. Patients who are not hemodynamically stable because of reasons like uncal herniation need immediate debridement without the requirement for preloading of antifungal medications. The debridement may followed by administration of 6–8 g of amphotericin B. After completion of the desired dose of amphotericin B, the patients should be started on azole group of drugs. The medicines are continued for 3–6 months (Fig. 21.17).

21.2.2 Acute Invasive Skull Base Fungal Disease (AISBFD)

Acute invasive fungal disease is also called as fulminant fungal disease. AISBFD results from rapid progression of the fungus into the paranasal sinus, orbit, vessels and nerves, the musculoskeletal system surrounding the skull base and the brain parenchyma. The time course of less than 4 weeks' duration differentiates this entity from the CISBFD. AISBFD is almost always common in individuals suffering from an immunocompromised condition like a haematological malignancy, uncontrolled diabetes mellitus, prolonged steroid use, organ transplantation or autoimmune deficiency syndrome (Abu El-Naaj et al. 2013; Kasapoglu et al. 2010). Although rare, this condition is also reported in immunocompetent individuals (Chopra et al. 2006; Gillespie and O'Malley 2000; Marple 2001; Saravanan et al. 2006). AISBFD is a condition that requires immediate management; otherwise the mortality can be as high as 50–80% (Gillespie et al. 1998; Kennedy et al. 1997). The most common organisms responsible are the *Aspergillus* species and the *Zygomycetes* species (Süslü et al. 2009; Tarkan et al. 2012). Patients with uncontrolled diabetes mellitus are more prone to developing mucormycosis infection because of their altered transferrin binding capacity (Spellberg et al. 2012). Any patient in an immunocompromised status with facial swelling, facial pain, headache, prolonged fever, orbital symptoms and cranial nerve palsies should be evaluated clinically, radiologically and pathologically to confirm the diagnosis. These patients require steps to revert the immunocompromised status, the surgical debridement and the administration of appropriate systemic antifungal therapy (Fig. 21.18).

21.2.3 Chronic Invasive Granulomatous Fungal Disease (CIGFD)

CIGFD is seen in immunocompetent individuals, and it is most commonly caused by *Aspergillus flavus* (Stringer and Ryan 2000). The most common presentation is unilateral proptosis. Other symptoms include nasal congestion, nasal obstruction, facial pain, headache and facial numbness (Stringer and Ryan 2000).

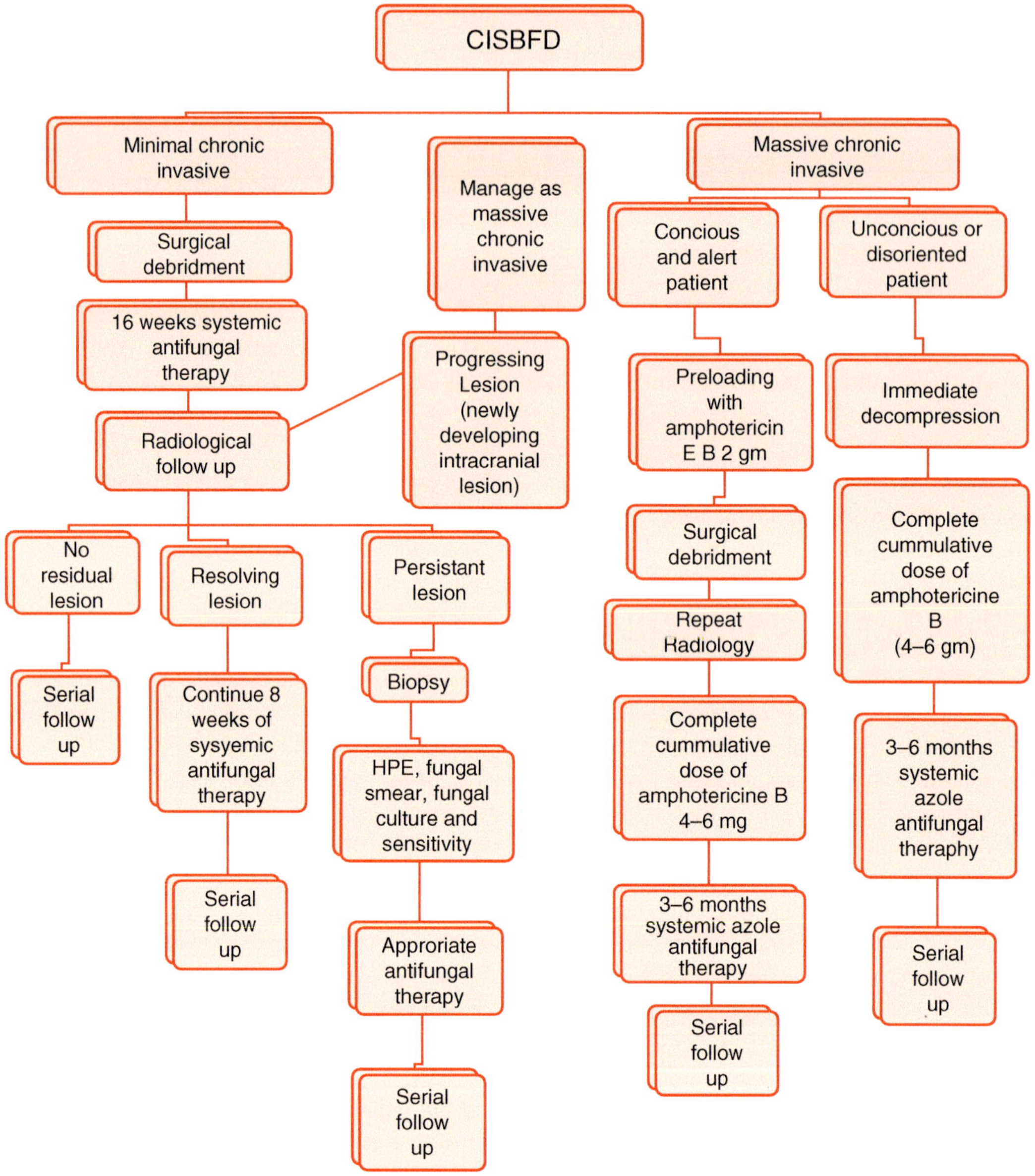

Fig. 21.17 Management protocol for chronic invasive skull base fungal disease

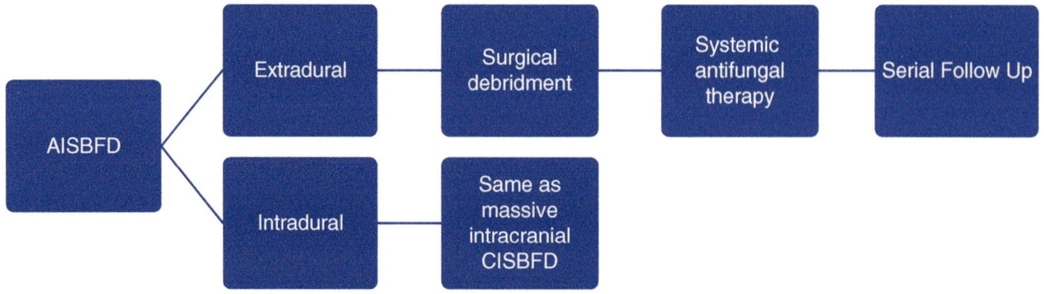

Fig. 21.18 Management protocol for acute invasive skull base fungal disease

On a CT scan, it presents as a unilateral isodense or hypodense lesion, whereas on MRI, it is isointense on T1WI and hypointense on T2WI (Reddy et al. 2010). On histopathology, CIGFD may be differentiated from chronic invasive fungal disease (CIFD) by the presence of non-caseating granulomas with fungal hyphae within the giant cells of the granuloma, with occasional invasion of blood vessels and adjoining tissues (Stringer and Ryan 2000). The treatment for CIGFD is still under debate, with the most accepted treatment being surgical debridement followed by oral antifungal agents (Halderman et al. 2014; Kim et al. 2012). Voriconazole is a very effective oral agent when there is involvement of skull base as there is good penetration of the CSF (Black and Baden 2007). There is no consensus on the duration for which oral antifungal treatment needs to be continued, but to prevent a relapse, most authors recommend treatment until complete remission is achieved (Black and Baden 2007; Halderman et al. 2014; Stringer and Ryan 2000).

21.3 The Non-invasive Fungal Diseases

Non-invasive fungal disease of the paranasal sinuses can involve the skull base, but these are usually extradural lesions that can cause symptoms based on the type and its location. Allergic fungal rhinosinusitis and fungal ball are the two types of non-invasive fungal diseases. AFRS is considered to be the sinonasal form of allergic bronchopulmonary aspergillosis (ABPA) (Marple 2001). Type I hypersensitivity to the fungal antigen is the proposed pathophysiology. The commonest fungi that are attributed to this disease are the *Alternaria*, *Bipolaris*, *Curvularia* and *Aspergillus* species (Kim et al. 2012). Manning and Holman analysed the serum from patients with AFRS and found 82% IgE antibodies (Halderman et al. 2014). In extensive disease with orbital involvement, patients present with proptosis, telecanthus as well as visual disturbance and cranial nerve palsy. When the anterior skull base and cavernous sinus are involved,

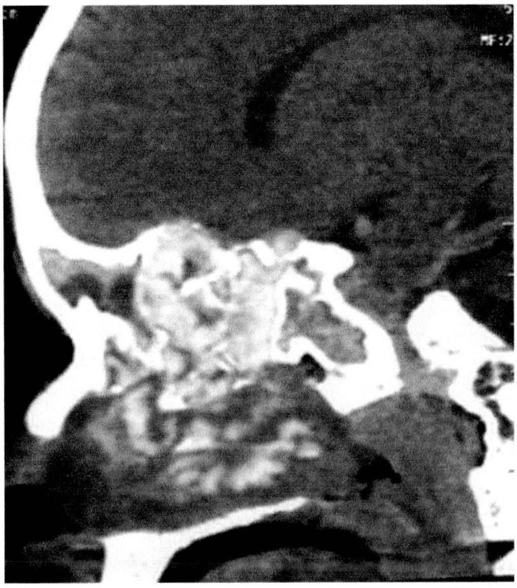

Fig. 21.19 AFRS eroding the skull base

these manifestations are mainly caused by the pressure effect of the expanding fungal tissue (Fig. 21.19). Studies by Saravan and colleagues and Diwakar and colleagues found considerably increased incidence of bony erosion and sinus expansion on the CT scan (Black and Baden 2007; Kennedy et al. 1997; Marple 2001; Saravanan et al. 2006; Stringer and Ryan 2000). Ghegan and colleagues showed that 56% of AFRS had skull base erosion (Ryan 2011; Süslü et al. 2009). Though this is not an invasive condition, surgery followed by intranasal steroid is the treatment modality of choice (Manning and Holman 1998). The role of systemic antifungal therapy (itraconazole) is controversial (Khalil et al. 2011; Seiberling and Wormald 2009). Fungal ball is a non-invasive lesion most commonly involving the maxillary sinus. It occurs in both immunocompetent and immunocompromised hosts. Sphenoid sinus fungal ball comprises of 13–25% of all fungal balls, and of that, about 50% of patients have visual complaints. The visual symptoms are caused because of neuritis, ischemic infiltrates or compression due to the fungal ball (Fig. 21.20). Surgical removal of the fungal ball is the definitive management. There is no role of antifungal therapy (Kim et al. 2016).

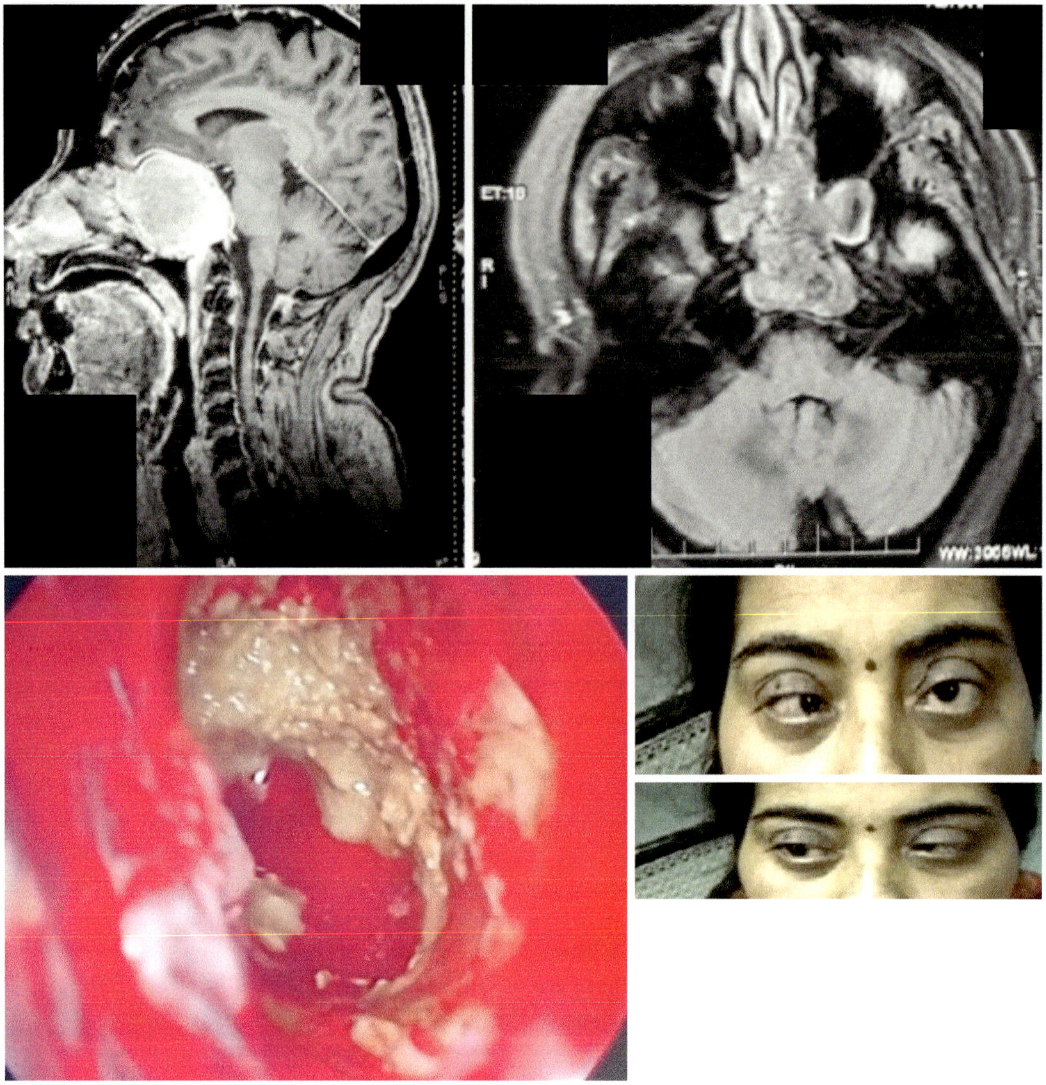

Fig. 21.20 A case of sphenoid fungal ball presenting with bilateral 6th nerve palsy and left-sided loss of vision

21.4 Conclusion

Fungal disease of the skull base covers the entire spectrum of diseases ranging from diseases with a lower morbidity status to extremely fatal conditions. In many cases, clinical suspicion and an adequate workup can make a huge impact on the outcome of the disease. Though surgery plays a very important role in the initial management, antifungal therapy and a serial follow-up are more important for a better long-term morbidity control.

References

Abu El-Naaj I, Leiser Y, Wolff A, Peled M. The surgical management of rhinocerebral mucormycosis. J Craniomaxillofac Surg. 2013;41(4):291–5.

Black KE, Baden LR. Fungal infections of the CNS: treatment strategies for the immunocompromised patient. CNS Drugs. 2007;21(4):293–318.

Chen S, Pu J-L, Yu J, Zhang J-M. Multiple Aspergillus cerebellar abscesses in a middle-aged female: case report and literature review. Int J Med Sci. 2011;8(7):635–9.

Chopra H, Dua K, Malhotra V, Gupta RP, Puri H. Invasive fungal sinusitis of isolated sphenoid sinus in immunocompetent subjects. Mycoses. 2006;49(1):30–6.

de Shazo RD. Fungal sinusitis. Am J Med Sci. 1998;316(1):39–45.
de Shazo RD, O'Brien M, Chapin K, Soto-Aguilar M, Gardner L, Swain R. A new classification and diagnostic criteria for invasive fungal sinusitis. Arch Otolaryngol Head Neck Surg. 1997;123(11):1181–8.
Dhiwakar M, Thakar A, Bahadur S. Invasive sino-orbital aspergillosis: surgical decisions and dilemmas. J Laryngol Otol. 2003a;117(4):280–5.
Dhiwakar M, Thakar A, Bahadur S, Sarkar C, Banerji U, Handa KK, et al. Preoperative diagnosis of allergic fungal sinusitis. Laryngoscope. 2003b;113(4):688–94.
Dubey A, Patwardhan RV, Sampath S, Santosh V, Kolluri S, Nanda A. Intracranial fungal granuloma: analysis of 40 patients and review of the literature. Surg Neurol. 2005;63(3):254–60.
Epstein VA, Kern RC. Invasive fungal sinusitis and complications of rhinosinusitis. Otolaryngol Clin North Am. 2008;41(3):497–524.
Ferguson BJ. Definitions of fungal rhinosinusitis. Otolaryngol Clin North Am. 2000;33(2):227–35.
Gillespie MB, O'Malley BW. An algorithmic approach to the diagnosis and management of invasive fungal rhinosinusitis in the immunocompromised patient. Otolaryngol Clin North Am. 2000;33(2):323–34.
Gillespie MB, O'Malley BW, Francis HW. An approach to fulminant invasive fungal rhinosinusitis in the immunocompromised host. Arch Otolaryngol Head Neck Surg. 1998;124(5):520–6.
Halderman A, Shrestha R, Sindwani R. Chronic granulomatous invasive fungal sinusitis: an evolving approach to management. Int Forum Allergy Rhinol. 2014;4(4):280–3.
Herbrecht R, Denning DW, Patterson TF, Bennett JE, Greene RE, Oestmann J-W, et al. Voriconazole versus amphotericin B for primary therapy of invasive aspergillosis. N Engl J Med. 2002;347(6):408–15.
Hoon D, Tae L, Yoon M, Kyoo J, Young L, Joo E, et al. Invasive fungal sinusitis of the sphenoid sinus. Clin Exp Otorhinolaryngol. 2014;7(3):181–7.
Jain KK, Mittal SK, Kumar S, Gupta RK. Imaging features of central nervous system fungal infections. Neurol India. 2007;55(3):241–50.
Kalkanci A, Kustimur S, Turkoz Sucak G, Senol E, Sugita T, Adams G, et al. Fulminating fungal sinusitis caused by Valsa sordida, a plant pathogen, in a patient immunocompromised by acute myeloid leukemia. Med Mycol. 2006;44(6):531–9.
Kasapoglu F, Coskun H, Ozmen OA, Akalin H, Ener B. Acute invasive fungal rhinosinusitis: evaluation of 26 patients treated with endonasal or open surgical procedures. Otolaryngol Head Neck Surg. 2010;143(5):614–20.
Kennedy CA, Adams GL, Neglia JP, Giebink GS. Impact of surgical treatment on paranasal fungal infections in bone marrow transplant patients. Otolaryngol Head Neck Surg. 1997;116(6 Pt 1):610–6.
Khalil Y, Tharwat A, Abdou AG, Essa E, Elsawy AH, Essawy AH, et al. The role of antifungal therapy in the prevention of recurrent allergic fungal rhinosinusitis after functional endoscopic sinus surgery: a randomized, controlled study. Ear Nose Throat J. 2011;90(8):E1–7.
Kim JS, Kim BK, Hong SD, Kim HJ, Kim HY. Clinical characteristics of sphenoid sinus fungal ball patients with visual disturbance. Clin Exp Otorhinolaryngol. 2016;9(4):326–31.
Kim TH, Jang HU, Jung YY, Kim JS. Granulomatous invasive fungal rhinosinusitis extending into the pterygopalatine fossa and orbital floor: a case report. Med Mycol Case Rep. 2012;1(1):107–11.
Kontoyiannis DP. Invasive mycoses: strategies for effective management. Am J Med. 2012;125:S25–38.
Manning SC, Holman M. Further evidence for allergic pathophysiology in allergic fungal sinusitis. Laryngoscope. 1998;108(10):1485–96.
Marple BF. Allergic fungal rhinosinusitis: current theories and management strategies. Laryngoscope. 2001;111(6):1006–19.
Martinez M, Chen V, Tong AJ, Hamilton K, Clemons KV, Stevens DA. Experimental evidence that granulocyte transfusions are efficacious in treatment of neutropenic hosts with pulmonary aspergillosis. Antimicrob Agents Chemother. 2013;57(4):1882–7.
Mehta AK, Langston AA. Use of posaconazole in the treatment of invasive fungal infections. Expert Rev Hematol. 2009;2(6):619–30.
Mohindra S, Mukherjee KK, Chhabra R, Gupta SK, Gupta R, Khosla VK. Invasive intracranial aspergillosis: the management dilemmas. Surg Neurol. 2008;69(5):496–505.
Reddy CEE, Gupta AK, Singh P, Mann SBS. Imaging of granulomatous and chronic invasive fungal sinusitis: comparison with allergic fungal sinusitis. Otolaryngol Neck Surg. 2010;143(2):294–300.
Redmond A, Dancer C, Woods ML. Fungal infections of the central nervous system: a review of fungal pathogens and treatment. Neurol India. 2007;55(3):251–9.
Ryan MW. Allergic fungal rhinosinusitis. Otolaryngol Clin North Am. 2011;44(3):697–710.
Saravanan K, Panda NK, Chakrabarti A, Das A, Bapuraj RJ. Allergic fungal rhinosinusitis: an attempt to resolve the diagnostic dilemma. Arch Otolaryngol Head Neck Surg. 2006;132(2):173–8.
Schell WA. Histopathology of fungal rhinosinusitis. Otolaryngol Clin North Am. 2000;33(2):251–76.
Schwartz S, Ruhnke M, Ribaud P, Corey L, Driscoll T, Cornely OA, et al. Improved outcome in central nervous system aspergillosis, using voriconazole treatment. Blood. 2005;106(8):2641–5.
Seiberling K, Wormald P-J. The role of itraconazole in recalcitrant fungal sinusitis. Am J Rhinol Allergy. 2009;23(3):303–6.
Selvam M, Pande A, Chakravarthy V, Ramamurthi R. Invasive rhino-cerebral fungal granuloma. Neurol India. 2010;58(2):270.
Shah SR, Keshri A, Patadia S, Marak RSK, Behari S. Invasive aspergillosis of anterior skull base in the immunocompetent host: outcomes with a combined

treatment modality—an institutional experience. Orig Artic. 2017;78:89–95.

Spellberg B, Kontoyiannis DP, Fredricks D, Morris MI, Perfect JR, Chin-Hong PV, et al. Risk factors for mortality in patients with mucormycosis. Med Mycol. 2012;50(6):611–8.

Stringer SP, Ryan MW. Chronic invasive fungal rhinosinusitis. Otolaryngol Clin North Am. 2000;33(2):375–87.

Süslü AE, Oğretmenoğlu O, Süslü N, Yücel OT, Onerci TM. Acute invasive fungal rhinosinusitis: our experience with 19 patients. Eur Arch Otorhinolaryngol. 2009;266(1):77–82.

Tarkan O, Karagün B, Ozdemir S, Tuncer U, Sürmelioğlu O, Cekiç E, et al. Endonasal treatment of acute invasive fungal rhinosinusitis in immunocompromised pediatric hematology-oncology patients. Int J Pediatr Otorhinolaryngol. 2012;76(10):1458–64.

Yamada K, Shrier DA, Rubio A, Shan Y, Zoarski GH, Yoshiura T, et al. Imaging findings in intracranial aspergillosis. Acad Radiol. 2002;9(2):163–71.

Zuniga MG, Turner JH. Treatment outcomes in acute invasive fungal rhinosinusitis. Curr Opin Otolaryngol Head Neck Surg. 2014;22(3):242–8.

Skull Base Clinical Syndromes

22

Jagarlapudi M. K. Murthy and Subhendu Parida

Abbreviations

CNS Central nervous system
CT Computed tomography
MRI Magnetic resonance imaging
SBO Skull base osteomyelitis

22.1 Introduction

Epidemiology of invasive fungal infections is rapidly increasing over the last few decades mostly due to the expansion of immunocompromised population at risk. Most of the systemic fungal pathogens have been associated with central nervous system (CNS) involvement, and involvement of CNS is associated with significant morbidity and mortality. To achieve good outcomes, early diagnosis and early institution of appropriate therapies are the key issues. Sometimes the presenting clinical syndrome can give a clue to the possible fungal pathogen (Murthy and Sundaram 2014).

The presenting clinical syndromes in patients with CNS fungal infections are protean and depend on the type of CNS pathology. Morphology and size of the fungus determine the pathology. Small-sized (diameter ~20 μm) yeast fungi (*Cryptococci, Coccidioides, Paracoccidioides, Blastomycetes, Histoplasma*) access the microcirculation from which they seed the subarachnoid space and produce meningitis/meningoencephalitis and subpial ischemic lesions. Intermediate (larger than 20 μm) sized fungi (*Candida*) can occlude the small vessels and produce local tissue necrosis and subsequent microabscess formation. Larger-sized fungi, septate (*Aspergillus*) *and non-septate* (*Mucorales*), usually infect juxta-cranial sites (paranasal sinuses, orbit, ear, oral cavity, etc.) (Murthy and Sundaram 2014; Shankar et al. 2007).

22.2 CNS Fungal Infections: Skull Base Syndromes

The pathological process in patients with skull base syndromes due to fungal infections can be chronic meningitis as in yeast infections, contiguous invasion of the cranial cavity as in infections with *Aspergillus* spp., and *Mucorales* spp., and spread of infection to cranial bones [skull base osteomyelitis (SBO)] as with *Aspergillus* spp., from the juxta-cranial sites (paranasal sinuses, nose, ear, etc.) (LeClerc et al. 2014; Murthy and Sundaram 2014; Spielmann et al. 2012). Various skull base syndromes of CNS fungal infections are given in Table 22.1 (Murthy 2007).

J. M. K. Murthy (✉)
CARE Institute of Neurosciences, CARE Hospitals, Hyderabad, India

S. Parida
Neuroradiology, CARE Institute of Neurosciences, CARE Hospitals, Hyderabad, India

M. Turgut et al. (eds.), *Fungal Infections of the Central Nervous System*,
https://doi.org/10.1007/978-3-030-06088-6_22

Table 22.1 Fungal infections of central nervous system: skull base syndromes (Murthy 2007)

• Optic neuropathy
• Cavernous sinus syndromes: unilateral or bilateral
• Orbital apex syndromes
• Proptosis with or without ocular palsies
• Polyneuritis cranialis
• Orbito-cranial syndromes

22.3 Chronic Fungal Meningitis

Small-sized (diameter up to 20 μm) yeast fungi (*Cryptococci, Coccidioides, Paracoccidioides, Blastomycetes, Histoplasma*), access the microcirculation from which they seed the subarachnoid space and produce meningitis/meningoencephalitis. Chronic meningitis and pachymeningitis can present with cranial neuropathies, including optic neuropathy. Of the 92 cases of *Aspergillus* meningitis reviewed, chronic meningitis or pachymeningitis accounted for 15 (16%) cases. Optic neuropathy, external ophthalmoplegia, lower cranial neuropathy, and deafness were the clinical syndromes (Antinori et al. 2013).

22.4 Sino-cranial Aspergillosis

Sino-cranial aspergillosis is most commonly described from countries with temperate climates like Saudi Arabia, Sudan, Pakistan, India, and some African countries and often in otherwise immunocompetent individuals (Murthy et al. 2000, 2001; Shamim et al. 2007; Sundaram et al. 2006).

Aspergillus spp. are ubiquitous in the environment and have a worldwide distribution and infect juxta-cranial sites: the paranasal sinuses, nose, and ear (Murthy and Sundaram 2014; Shankar et al. 2007). The conidia of *Aspergillus* are inhaled into the sinuses and lungs. The small size of the conidia of *A. fumigatus* facilitates its entry into pulmonary alveoli, whereas the larger conidial size of *A. flavus* gets it trapped in the sinuses. Similar may be the involvement of the nose and ears. The risks of exposure vary both temporally and geographically and are dependent on precipitation patterns, humidity, temperature, and wind conditions (Panackal et al. 2010).

Intracranial and orbital invasion from the juxta-cranial spaces, paranasal sinuses, nose, and ear can be by direct extension. This mode of spread is most commonly described in patients with sino-cranial aspergillosis (Murthy et al. 2001; Murthy and Sundaram 2014; Shankar et al. 2007; Sundaram et al. 2006). The pathology of sino-cranial aspergillosis is well-formed granulomas (Sundaram et al. 2006). Patients with sino-cranial aspergillosis may present with features of intracranial focal mass lesions, skull base syndromes as follows: orbital apex syndrome, cavernous sinus syndrome, proptosis with or without ocular nerve palsies, polyneuritis cranialis, and orbito-cranial syndromes (Table 22.1) (Murthy 2007) (Fig. 22.1).

Other large-sized fungi, *Mucorales* spp., also infect juxta-cranial sites and invade the cranial cavity by contiguous spread. Skull base syndromes are unusual presenting features of

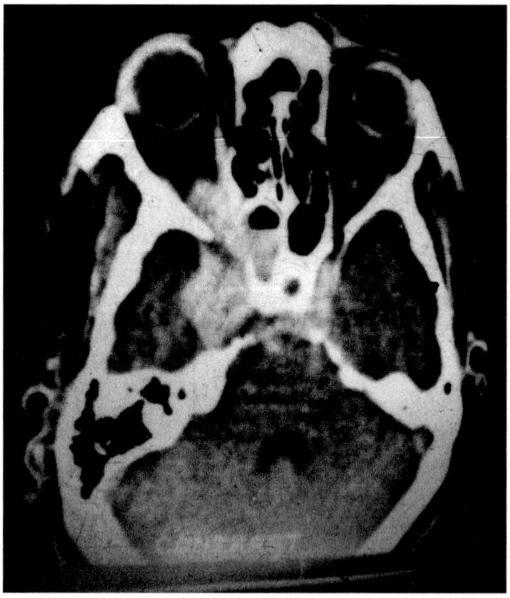

Fig. 22.1 Non-contrast computed tomography (CT) scan image showing hyperdense lesion in the region of right cavernous sinus and anterior extension of the cavernous sinus lesion into the right orbit. Hyperdensity with possible fluid level noted within the sphenoid sinus. There is less severe involvement of left cavernous sinus on CT. The histopathology in this patient showed aspergillus granuloma

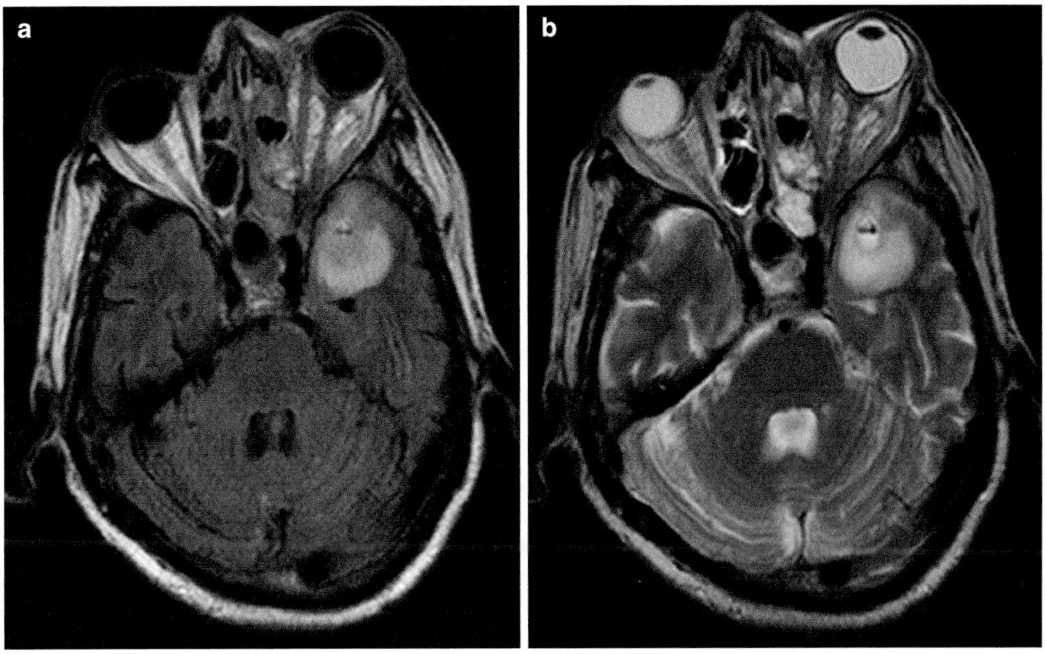

Fig. 22.2 FLAIR axial (**a**) and T2 axial (**b**) magnetic resonance imaging (MRI) sections show mucosal thickening and hyperintensity within the left sided ethmoidal air cells, fat stranding is noted within the left orbit, probably due to extension of inflammation through the lamina papyracea, there is intracranial extension into the left middle cranial fossa with signs of cerebritis and focal abscess formation in the anterior aspect of left temporal lobe. There is proptosis of left globe. The causative fungal pathogen in this patient was *Mucorale* spp.

mucormycosis. The common presenting clinical forms are cerebral and rhinocerebral (Roden et al. 2005) (Fig. 22.2). Manifestations of the disease may reflect the sequential involvement of the nose, sinuses, eye, and brain. Manifestations of cavernous sinus thrombosis include loss of vision and internal and external ophthalmoplegia. Thrombosis of the internal carotid artery also can occur and causes contralateral hemiplegia (Murthy and Sundaram 2014; Roden et al. 2005).

22.5 Fungal Skull Base Osteomyelitis

Central SBO or atypical SBO refers to osteomyelitis that affects the sphenoid and occipital bone, often centered on the clivus and can be sinugenic or otogenic. Central SBO typically affects middle-aged males, with underlying diabetes mellitus and immunocompromised being predisposing factors (Johnson and Batra 2014). About half of the central SBO cases are caused by microorganisms other than *Pseudomonas aeruginosa* including fungi (Ridder et al. 2015). Of the SBO cases, fungal SBO account for 10% (LeClerc et al. 2014; Spielmann et al. 2012). The true incidence of fungal SBO may be higher than what has been reported. Of the histologically confirmed invasive aspergillosis, 80% were culture negative (Stoduslski et al. 2006). The reported fungal pathogens associated with SBO include most commonly *Aspergillus* spp. and, less commonly, *Mucor* spp. and *Scedosporium* spp. (Blyth et al. 2011).

The most common symptoms at initial presentation in patients with central SBO are headaches and/or facial pain. Cranial nerve involvement most commonly include VI, IX, X, and VII (Blyth et al. 2011) (Fig. 22.3). Only one-fourth of the patients complain classic sinonasal symptoms, such as congestion and discharge. Fever is relatively uncommon on presentation (Johnson and Batra 2014). There are some distinct differences between bacterial SBO and fungal SBO. Fungal SBO is

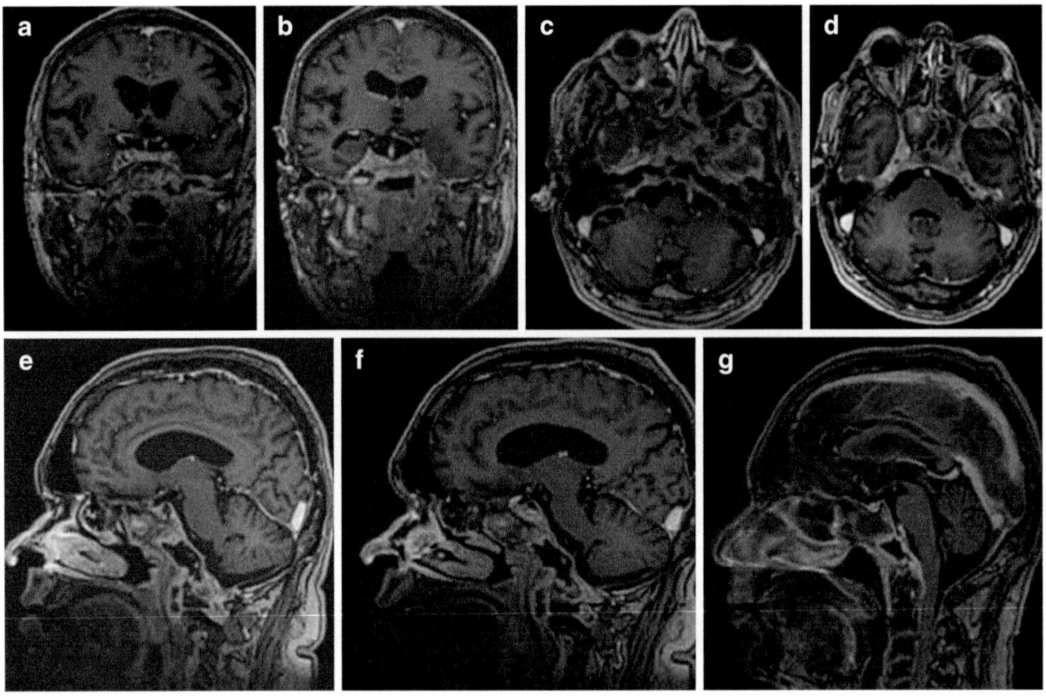

Fig. 22.3 (**a**–**g**) Post contrast T1 coronal and axial MRI showing heterogenously enhancing lesion filling the sphenoid sinus spreading laterally to cavernous sinus and eroding floor of left middle cranial fossa (**a**–**d**); Post contrast T1 MRI showing destruction of most anterior portion of clivus with sclerotic changes in the rest of the clivus, enhancing craniovertebral junction with abscess in prevertebral space (**e**, **f**); Post contrast T1 MRI showing partial resolution following treatment. The causative fungal pathogen in this patient was *Aspergillus fumigatus*

frequently associated with underlying chronic sinusitis, sinonasal pain, facial/periorbital swelling and nasal stuffiness or discharge, and the absence of purulent ear discharge (Blyth et al. 2011).

22.6 Conclusion

In countries with temperate climates, fungal pathology should be considered in patients presenting with skull base syndromes, more so with juxta-cranial infections in the paranasal sinuses, nose, and ears. The most common pathogen is *Aspergillus* spp.

References

Antinori S, Corbellino M, Meroni L, Resta F, Sollima S, Tonollni M, Tortorano AM, Millazzo L, Bello L, Furfaro E, Galli M, Viscoli C. Aspergillus meningitis: a rare clinical manifestation of central nervous systemic aspergillosis. Case report and review of 92 cases. J Infect. 2013;66:218–38.

Blyth CC, Games L, Sorrell TC, da Cruz M, Sud A, Chen SCA. Skull-base osteomyelitis: fungal vs. bacterial infection. Clin Microbiol Infect. 2011;17:306–11.

Johnson AK, Batra PS. Central skull base osteomyelitis: an emerging clinical entity. Laryngoscope. 2014;124:1084–8.

LeClerc N, Verilaud B, Duet M, Gulchard JP, Herman P, Kania R. Skull base osteomyelitis incidence of resistance, morbidity, and treatment strategy. Laryngoscope. 2014;124:2013–6.

Murthy JMK, Sundaram C, Prasad VS, Purohit AK, Rammurti S, Laxmi V. Aspergillosis of central nervous system: a study of 21 patients seen in a university hospital in south India. J Assoc Physicians India. 2000;48:677–81.

Murthy JMK, Sundaram C, Prasad VS, Purohit AK, Rammurti S, Laxmi V. Sinocranial aspergillosis: a form of central nervous system aspergillosis in south India. Mycoses. 2001;44:141–5.

Murthy JMK. Fungal infections of the central nervous system: the clinical syndromes. Neurol India. 2007;55:221–5.

Murthy JMK, Sundaram C. Fungal infections of the central nervous system. In: Biller J, Ferro JM, editors. Handbook clinical neurology. Vol 121 (3rd series);

Neurological aspects of systemic disease part III, vol. 121. Amsterdam: Elsevier BV; 2014. p. 1383–401.
Panackal AA, Li H, Kontoyiannis DP, Mori M, Pergo CA, Boeckh M, Marr KA. Geoclimatic influences on invasive Aspergillosis after hematopoietic stem cell transplantation. Clin Infect Dis. 2010;50:1588–97.
Ridder GJ, Breunig C, Kaminsky J, Pfeiffer J. Central skull base osteomyelitis: new insights and implications for diagnosis and treatment. Eur Arch Otorhinolaryngol. 2015;272:1269–76.
Roden MM, Zaoutis TE, Buchanan WL, Knudsen TA, Schaufele RL, Sein M, Sein T, Chu JH, Kontoviannis DP, Walsh TJ. Epidemiology and outcome of zygomycosis: a review of 929 reported case. Clin Infect Dis. 2005;41:634–53.
Shamim MS, Siddiqui AA, Enam SA, Shah AA, Jooma R, Anwar S. Craniocerebral aspergillosis in immunocompetent hosts: surgical perspective. Neurol India. 2007;55:274–81.
Shankar SK, Mahadevan A, Sundaram C, Sarkar C, Chacko G, Lanjewar DN, Santosh V, Yasha TC, Radhakrishnan VV. Pathobiology of fungal infections of the central nervous system with special reference to the Indian scenario. Neurol India. 2007;55: 198–215.
Spielmann PM, Yu R, Neeff M. Skull base osteomyelitis current microbiology and management. J Laryngol Otol. 2012;127:S8–S12.
Stoduslski D, Kawalska B, Stankiewicz C. Otogenic skull base osteomyelitis caused by invasive fungal infection. Eur Arch Otorhinolaryngol. 2006;263: 1070–6.
Sundaram C, Umabala P, Laxmi V, Purohit AK, Prasad VS, Panigrahi M, Sahu BP, Sarathi MV, Kaul S, Borghain R, Meena AK, Jayalakshimi SS, Suvarna S, Mohandas S, Murthy JMK. Pathology of fungal infections of the central nervous system: 17 years' experience from Southern India. Histopathology. 2006;49:396–405.

23 Orbito-Rhinocerebral Syndrome

Gauri S. Mankekar, Rahul Mehta, and Daniel W. Nuss

Abbreviations

AIDS	Acquired immunodeficiency syndrome
AFRS	Allergic fungal rhinosinusitis
AIFRS	Acute invasive fungal rhinosinusitis
CGFRS	Chronic granulomatous fungal rhinosinusitis
CIFRS	Chronic invasive fungal rhinosinusitis
CT	Computed tomography
H&E	Hematoxylin and eosin
IFRS	Invasive fungal rhinosinusitis
KOH	Potassium hydroxide
MRI	Magnetic resonance imaging
ROCS	Rhino-orbito-cerebral syndrome

23.1 Introduction

Fungi are ubiquitous in the environment and are deposited in the nose and paranasal sinuses during routine respiration (Green et al. 2005). In most people, the fungi do not cause disease. However, sometimes, they can cause mild to even fulminant paranasal sinusitis progressing to orbital complications, intracranial invasion, and even death. The immune status of the individual appears to be a key factor involved in the progression of paranasal fungal infection (Soler and Schlosser 2012). Fungi are apparently unable to invade the mucosal or epithelial lining in immunocompetent individuals (Cheng et al. 2012; Hontelez et al. 2012) although cases of invasive fungal rhinosinusitis (IFRS) have also been reported in immunocompetent individuals (Bhattacharyya et al. 1992; Gillespie and O'malley 2000; Chopra et al. 2006; Sridhara et al. 2005).

The highest incidence of rhino-orbito-cerebral syndrome (ROCS) is amongst immunocompromised patients with diabetes mellitus, especially in those presenting with ketoacidosis (Prabhu and Patel 2004; Ingram et al. 1989; Morduchowicz et al. 1986; Jiménez et al. 2002), followed by hematologic malignancies (Kontoyiannis et al. 2000; Spellberg et al. 2005), solid organ transplants (Jiménez et al. 2002) and those on immunosuppressive therapy (steroids or chemotherapy) (Kontoyiannis et al. 2000). In these patients, the fungal infection progresses rapidly from the nose to the paranasal sinuses and then to the orbits or intracranially either by direct extension or due to angioinvasion. Skip lesions can also occur. Early diagnosis and aggressive multidisciplinary team approach involving otolaryngologists, ophthalmologists, neurosurgeons, medical intensiv-

G. S. Mankekar (✉)
Neurotology and Skull Base Surgery,
Our Lady of the Lake, Baton Rouge, LA, USA

Louisiana State University Health Sciences Center,
New Orleans, LA, USA

R. Mehta • D. W. Nuss
Department of Otolaryngology,
Louisiana State University Health Sciences Center,
New Orleans, LA, USA
e-mail: rmeht1@lsuhsc.edu; DNuss@lsuhsc.edu

M. Turgut et al. (eds.), *Fungal Infections of the Central Nervous System*,
https://doi.org/10.1007/978-3-030-06088-6_23

ists, and infectious disease specialists have been shown to decrease mortality (Mankekar 2014; Palejwala et al. 2016). The role of the microbiologist and pathologist in the early identification of the type of fungus causing ROCS cannot be underestimated.

23.2 Classification of Paranasal Sinus Fungal Infections

Paranasal sinus fungal infections have been classified by de Shazo et al. (deShazo et al. 1997; deShazo and Swain 1995) as invasive and noninvasive. They further classified IFRS into three distinct entities based on clinical presentations, acute invasive (fulminant) fungal rhinosinusitis (AIFRS), chronic invasive fungal rhinosinusitis (CIFRS), and chronic granulomatous fungal rhinosinusitis (CGFRS), while noninvasive fungal rhinosinusitis was classified as allergic fungal rhinosinusitis (AFRS) and sinus mycetoma or fungal ball.

IFRS, by definition, means demonstrable fungal hyphae within the mucosa, submucosa, bone, and blood vessels on histopathology (deShazo et al. 1997). ROCS which follows the spread of paranasal sinus fungal infection to the orbit and intracranial structures is associated with ophthalmic and neurological manifestations. It is typically seen with the AIFRS.

23.2.1 Pathogenesis

In immunocompromised individuals, the fungi from the nose and paranasal sinuses cause inflammation. Qualitative and quantitative neutrophil, macrophage, and monocyte abnormalities along with altered iron metabolism are postulated to contribute to the pathogenesis of ROCS (Gamaletsou et al. 2012). From the ethmoid sinus, the infection can extend via the lamina papyracea into the extraocular muscles, orbital apex (Anders et al. 2015), and optic nerve (Gamaletsou et al. 2012). Vascular invasion causes spread of infection through the ethmoidal and ophthalmic arteries to the cavernous sinus (Gamaletsou et al. 2012), internal carotid artery (Bae et al. 2012), and brain (Bae et al. 2012; Koc et al. 2007).

23.2.2 Causative Agents

The fungi involved in causing AIFRS and, therefore, ROCS are often similar in particular forms of fungal disease, although there is a geographic variation (Montone et al. 2012). AIFRS is uniformly associated with *A. fumigatus*, *A. flavus*, and *Rhizopus* sp. worldwide (Epstein and Kern 2008; Panda et al. 1998; Das et al. 2009). In 80% of patients with diabetes, *Rhizopus* spp., *Rhizomucor* spp., *Absidia* spp., and *Mucor* spp. are responsible for AIFRS (Gillespie et al. 1998). *Aspergillus spp* is responsible for 80% of AIFRS cases in patients with neutropenia, e.g., post-chemotherapy or steroids, hematologic malignancies, and organ transplantation, or in patients with acquired immunodeficiency syndrome (AIDS) (Gillespie et al. 1998). A few cases due to *Cunninghamella bertholletiae*, *Apophysomyces elegans*, and *L. corymbifera* have also been reported (Diwakar et al. 2007; Chakrabarti et al. 2006). *Apophysomyces elegans* has been reported to cause AIFRS in immunocompetent patients (Sridhara et al. 2005; Garcia-Covarrubias et al. 2001).

23.3 Clinical Presentation

The symptoms of ROCS in AIFRS are initially restricted to the nose and paranasal sinuses with persistent nasal blockage accompanied by bloody, serosanguineous rhinorrhea and cough (Mankekar 2014). Subsequent symptoms include periorbital cellulitis (Dhiwakar et al. 2003a), orbital pain, facial numbness and headache. Spread of disease to the orbit is associated with conjunctival chemosis, blurring of vision, proptosis, ptosis, visual loss, and ophthalmoplegia. Fever not responding to antibiotics in a neutropenic patient is a presenting feature of AIFRS (Talbot et al. 1991).

Once the orbital and ophthalmic arteries are involved, infection can reach the cavernous sinus and internal carotid artery. Clinically this manifests as cranial nerve palsies, especially involving cranial nerves II, III, IV, V, and VI with cavernous sinus thrombosis. In advanced cases, hemiparesis, hemiplegia, convulsions, delirium, and finally death can occur (Bae et al. 2012; Epstein and Kern 2008; Yohai et al. 1994; Maheshwari et al. 2013).

23.4 Diagnosis

ROCS diagnosis is based on a high index of suspicion and clinical examination, corroborated by microbiological and histopathological studies. Imaging studies are not diagnostic but provide information about the anatomy, extent of the disease, and complications.

An immunocompromised individual presenting with unexplained fever, cough, acute sinusitis, nasal congestion, or orbital apex syndrome or ophthalmoplegia should raise the suspicion of potential IFRS (Deshazo 2009) (Fig. 23.1).

A cursory nasal and oral examination may not reveal any pathology. It is therefore essential for an otolaryngologist to decongest the nose and perform a rigid nasal endoscopy. Whitish discoloration (due to tissue ischemia) of the nasal mucosa with serosanguineous discharge may be present. Often black eschar due to ischemic tissue necrosis is a distinct warning sign for AIFRS (Idris and Lim 2012) (Fig.23.2). These mucosal changes are commonly seen on the middle turbinate, followed by the septum, hard palate, and inferior turbinate (Gillespie and O'malley 2000). It is important to watch for skip lesions which occur due to the spread of infection along the intima of blood vessels (Mankekar 2014). Invasive mucormycosis of the maxillary sinus presents with features which are often different from ethmoid sinus mucormycosis (Gamaletsou et al. 2012). While maxillary sinus infection extends into the oral cavity which is seen as a black necrotic ulcer on the hard palate, ethmoid sinus infection extends into the orbit or intracranially. An oral examination may reveal gingival or palatal or lingual eschar which is clinically distinctive for AIFRS. In some cases, facial hyperesthesia or anesthesia may present even prior to the appearance of other symptoms.

An ophthalmological examination is mandatory at the beginning and throughout the treatment course in all patients suspected to have AIFRS. It is important to test not only the visual acuity but also document the field of vision to exclude ophthalmoplegia and examine the retina for chorioretinitis. Blurring of vision, diplopia, and ophthalmoplegia may be earliest manifestations of cavernous sinus thrombosis, even before the appearance of changes on imaging studies (Gamaletsou et al. 2012).

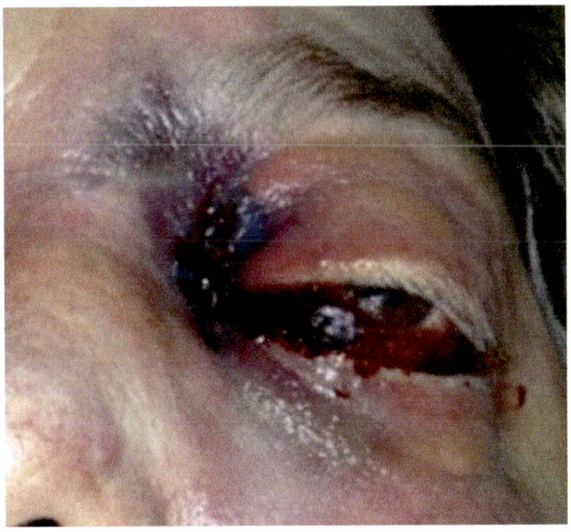

Fig. 23.1 Clinical appearance of patient with rhino-orbito-cerebral syndrome (ROCS) (Courtesy Dr. DW Nuss)

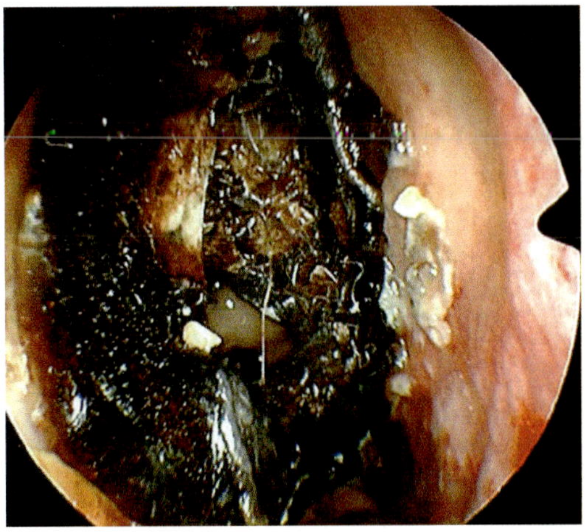

Fig. 23.2 Endoscopic appearance of black, devascularized nasal mucosa in a patient with ROCS (Courtesy Dr. DW Nuss)

Neurological examination for cranial nerve palsies, facial asymmetry, facial paresthesia or anesthesia, motor and sensory weakness, and signs of meningitis is essential during initial evaluation as well as during the entire treatment course.

Rapid diagnosis can be obtained with a potassium hydroxide (KOH), calcofluor wet mount (Figs. 23.3 and 23.4). Fungal culture and in situ hybridization aid not only in the diagnosis but are also the only methods to definitively identify the fungal species (Schwartz 2011).

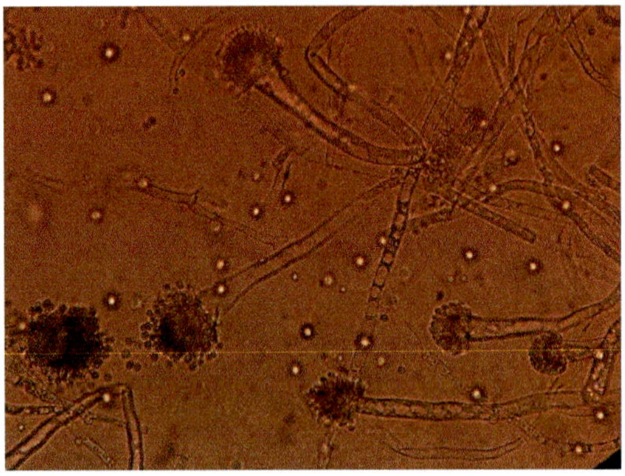

Fig. 23.3 Potassium hydroxide (KOH) mount of *Aspergillus* showing septate hyphae (Reproduced from Invasive Fungal Rhinosinusitis, ed. Mankekar, Springer, India, 2014)

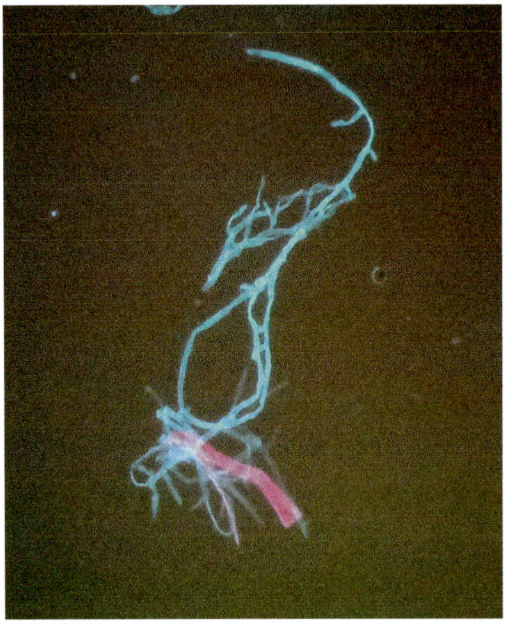

Fig. 23.4 Calcofluor preparation showing aseptate fungal filaments (Reproduced from Invasive Fungal Rhinosinusitis, ed. Mankekar, Springer, India, 2014)

Thin axial and coronal computed tomography (CT) scans of the paranasal sinuses must be obtained in all patients with suspected AIFRS and ROCS to determine the extent of disease (Spellberg et al. 2005; Mankekar 2014; Epstein and Kern 2008; Kim et al. 2015). Intravenous contrast may be required to detect intra-orbital and intracranial involvement. However, magnetic resonance imaging (MRI) is preferred to CT in evaluating patients with altered sensorium, ophthalmoplegia, stroke, or cranial nerve palsies with possible intra-orbital and intracranial involvement. It can evaluate the spread of disease to the retro-antral, intra-orbital (Fig. 23.5), and intracranial regions (Fig. 23.6) but can be time-consuming and could therefore delay definitive diagnosis (Soler and Schlosser 2012). Ischemic tissue necrosis is seen as non-enhancing lesions on gadolinium-enhanced MRI scans (Mankekar 2014) and is recommended for early diagnosis, determining the extent of surgical debridement required and for follow-up (Kim et al. 2015).

The earliest imaging finding in rhinocerebral mucormycosis is the infiltration of the periantral fat planes. This may be accompanied by soft tissue attenuation along the sinus walls. There is

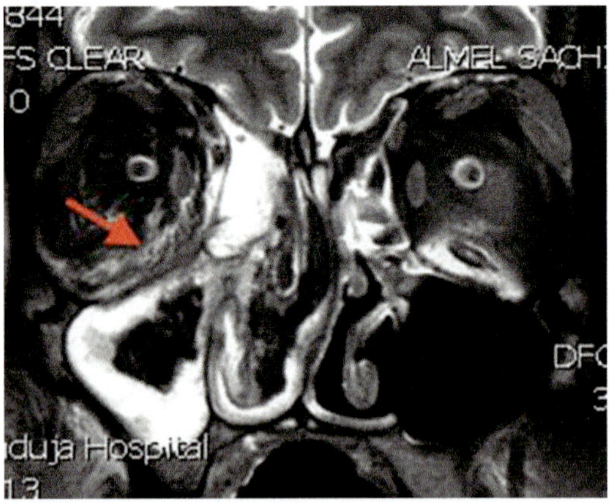

Fig. 23.5 Magnetic resonance imaging (MRI) T2W coronal image showing right ethmoid and maxillary mucormycosis, with infiltration into the right orbit (arrow) (Reproduced from Invasive Fungal Rhinosinusitis, ed. Mankekar, Springer, India, 2014)

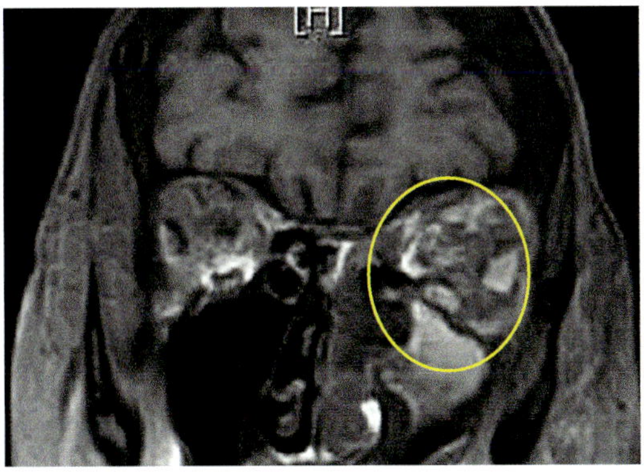

Fig. 23.6 T2W coronal MRI showing intracranial extension of rhino-orbito-cerebral mucormycosis through the cribriform plate (Courtesy Dr. DW Nuss)

obliteration of the normal fat planes in the pterygopalatine fossa, pterygomaxillary fissure, and infratemporal fossa due to soft tissue infiltration. Features of orbital invasion include lateral displacement and thickening of the medial rectus (Fig. 23.5), cellulitis, subperiosteal abscess, orbital abscess, and even cavernous sinus thrombosis. Intracranial imaging findings are secondary to vascular thrombosis, abscesses, or mycotic emboli. This can present as epidural or subdural abscesses and cavernous or sagittal sinus thrombosis.

The standard method for diagnosing AFIRS is histologic examination of tissue samples (Schwartz 2011). Early examination with rigid nasal endoscopy along with frozen section biopsy of suspicious (Gillespie and O'malley 2000) discolored, ischemic areas of the middle and inferior turbinate or septum should be performed. Blind samples obtained from the nasal vestibule delay the diagnosis and should be avoided. Hematoxylin and eosin (H &E) stain can identify the fungal elements. However, special stains like periodic acid Schiff and Gomori's silver methenamine preparation identify the causative fungi easily. In fact, it is recommended that a silver stain should be performed before releasing a negative diagnosis for invasive fungal infection (Schell 2000). *Mucor* spp can be identified with silver stains with its broad, ribbonlike aseptate hyphae, while *Aspergillus* spp has narrow, regularly septate hyphae which branch at 45°.

23.5 Management

The treatment of ROCS requires a multidisciplinary approach. The principles of treatment include early identification, reversal and adequate control of predisposing risk factors, surgical debridement, and appropriate antifungal therapy. Patients with hematological diseases require a complex sequence of decisions and extremely individualized care (Kontoyiannis et al. 2011). Tiny lesions, when diagnosed early, can be surgically debrided. This will prevent progression of the disease to the orbit or brain. In the absence of rapid diagnostic tests, a high index of suspicion is required to diagnose these cases early. The outcome relies on the severity of the immunosuppression, early diagnosis, location and extent of the infection, optimal therapy, and follow-up.

23.6 Medical Management

Systemic antifungal therapy is often prescribed in high-risk patients suspected to have AIFRS to prevent progression to ROCS. This is done concomitantly with histopathology, microbiology, and imaging studies. Correction of diabetic ketoacidosis or neutropenia is also initiated concurrently with the antifungal therapy. Deferoxamine or immunosuppressive agents like steroids or chemotherapy may have to be discontinued if ROCS is diagnosed (Spellberg et al. 2005; Skiada et al. 2013).

Intravenous amphotericin B at doses of 0.25–1 mg/kg/day is initiated in patients with ROCS due to *Mucor* species, after recording baseline blood urea nitrogen and creatinine levels. In patients with poor renal function, the dose of amphotericin may have to be decreased or replaced with liposomal amphotericin B. Despite its high cost, liposomal amphotericin B is preferred in patients with elevated levels of serum creatinine. Intravenous voriconazole is more effective compared to amphotericin B in AIFRS caused by *Aspergillus spp* (Herbrecht et al. 2002).

Patients responding to parenteral amphotericin B can be transitioned over several days to oral posaconazole for maintenance or secondary prophylaxis (Kontoyiannis et al. 2011).

Posaconazole has also been reported to be useful as salvage therapy in patients of invasive aspergillosis refractory to or intolerant to previous antifungal treatment (Walsh et al. 2014). However, it is important to monitor serum concentrations of the drug to reduce incidence of breakthrough or relapsing mucormycosis due to inadequate serum concentration.

The duration of systemic antifungal therapy has not yet been defined and is determined by the resolution of all associated clinical symptoms and findings (Skiada et al. 2013). Maintenance therapy or secondary prophylaxis has been recommended in persistently immunocompromised patients (Skiada et al. 2013).

Anticoagulant therapy has been considered a standard part of cavernous sinus thrombosis which can occur in rhinocerebral mucormycosis. Advocates of anticoagulation believe that it can prevent propagation of thrombus and help improve blood flow. However, use of anticoagulants is controversial as it could potentially be associated with the risk of cerebral and systemic hemorrhage.

Granulocyte colony-stimulating factor is useful in reversing neutropenia in patients with hematologic malignancies (Gillespie and O'malley 2000; Spellberg et al. 2005; Skiada et al. 2013). Adjuvant treatment with hyperbaric oxygen has been reported to improve survival in cases of ROCS as the higher concentration of tissue oxygen increases neutrophil antifungal activity and the oxidative killing mechanism caused by polyenes (Walsh et al. 2014; Garcia-Covarrubias et al. 2002; Price and Stevens 1980), although it has not been recommended for routine use due to insufficient data (Skiada et al. 2013).

23.7 Surgery

Concurrent to antifungal therapy, aggressive surgical debridement is essential to treat and prevent the progression of AIFRS to ROCS. To adequately treat the disease, radical debulking is necessary (Soler and Schlosser 2012; Epstein and Kern 2008; Walsh et al. 2008). The goal is to remove all necrotic tissue until healthy-appearing and bleeding tissue is visualized. So far, no specific criteria for the extent or range of debulking have been established. Reports of surgical debulking range from endoscopic debridement of affected sinus, nasal, and orbital tissues (Fig. 23.7) to radical surgery such as enucleation of the eyeball and maxillectomy (Dhiwakar et al. 2003a, b; Epstein and Kern 2008; Songu et al. 2008) (Fig. 23.8).

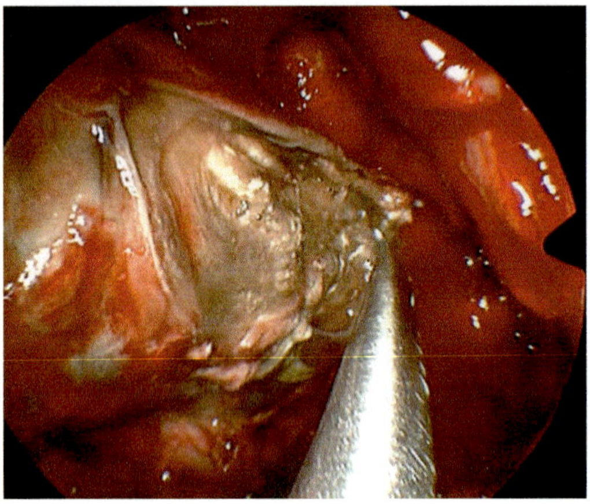

Fig. 23.7 Nasal endoscopic debridement of devitalized orbital periosteum and tissues in a patient with ROCS (Courtesy Dr. DW Nuss)

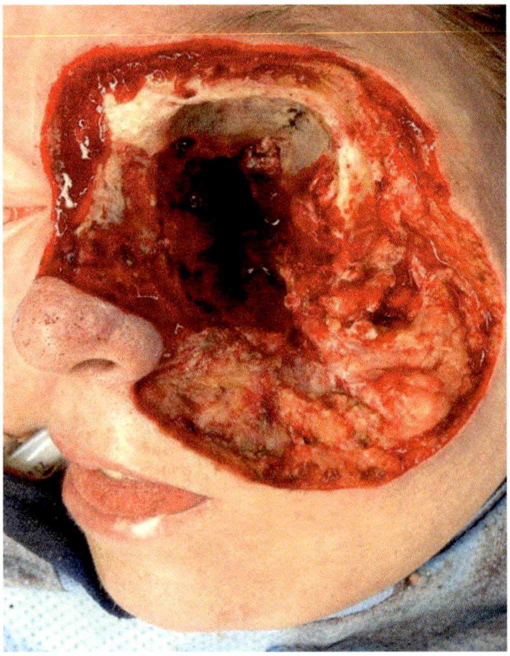

Fig. 23.8 Naso-orbital resection in a patient with rhino-orbito-cerebral mucormycosis (Courtesy Dr. DW Nuss)

The dilemma of whether orbital exenteration is indicated in ROCS continues (Songu et al. 2008; Hargrove et al. 2006; Nishimura et al. 2017) with several authors recommending removal in patients with orbital apex syndrome (Hargrove et al. 2006; Plowes Hernandez et al. 2015), while others report successful treatment without it (Nishimura et al. 2017; Kohn and Hepler 1985). As outcomes of intracranial extension of disease are poor, it is rarely treated with surgical resection (Peterson et al. 1997).

Endoscopic debridement of the nose and paranasal sinuses, besides providing tissue for microbiology and histopathological diagnosis, decreases the fungal load, slows disease progression (Gillespie and O'malley 2000), and controls local disease (Vironneau et al. 2014). The pterygopalatine fissure and sphenopalatine foramen are considered reservoirs of invasive mucormycosis, and exposure of this fissure with removal of the posterior wall of the maxilla is recommended by several authors (Songu et al. 2008; Plowes Hernandez et al. 2015) for adequate disease control. Nishimura et al. (Nishimura et al. 2017) have reported a novel combined endoscopic-sinus approach to the nose and orbit for surgical management of ROCS due to invasive aspergillosis.

Repeated endoscopic debridement in the operating room and bedside examination of the nose and sinuses daily has been recommended until macroscopic resolution of disease and crusting with remucosalization of the sinuses (Otto and DelGaudio 2006).

23.8 Prognosis

Data regarding outcomes is derived mainly from retrospective, institutional studies or case reports. The prognosis of ROCS is reported to be better in patients with diabetic ketoacidosis compared to those with neutropenia (Parikh et al. 2004), and intracranial extension of disease with failure to reverse immunosuppression is associated with higher incidence of mortality (Thompson and Patterson 2012). Parikh et al. (2004) reported that patients with ROCS due to *Mucor* spp had a higher incidence of mortality compared to those with invasive aspergillosis. Overall, the mortality rate is less than 20% (Parikh et al. 2004) in AIFRS and almost 100% in patients with intracranial extension and symptoms of the disease (Gillespie and O'malley 2000).

23.9 Conclusion

ROCS is associated with invasive fungal sinus disease caused by *A. fumigatus*, *A. flavus*, and *Rhizopus* spp. although a few other fungi have also been implicated. Its incidence is higher among immunocompromised individuals with diabetic ketoacidosis or neutropenia secondary to hematologic malignancies, human immune deficiency virus, solid organ, and stem cell transplantation. A high index of clinical suspicion and early diagnosis are essential to prevent the rapid spread of the disease from the nose and paranasal sinuses to the orbit and brain. A multidisciplinary approach with aggressive surgical debridement and systemic antifungal therapy is required to achieve favorable outcomes.

References

Anders UM, Taylor EJ, Martel JR, Martel JB. Acute orbital apex syndrome and rhino-orbito-cerebral mucormycosis. Int Med Case Rep J. 2015;8:93–6.

Bhattacharyya AK, Deshpande AR, Nayak SR, Kirtane MV, Ingle MV, Vora IM. Rhinocerebral mucormycosis: an unusual case presentation. J Laryngol Otol. 1992;106(1):48–9.

Chakrabarti A, Das A, Mandal J, Shivaprakash MR, George VK, Tarai B, et al. The rising trend of invasive zygomycosis in patients with uncontrolled diabetes mellitus. Med Mycol. 2006;44:335–42.

Cheng SC, Joosten LAB, Kullberg BJ, Netea MG. Interplay between Candida albicans and the mammalian innate host defense. Infect Immun. 2012;80:1304–13.

Chopra H, Dua K, Malhotra V, Gupta RP, Puri H. Invasive fungal sinusitis of isolated sphenoid sinus in immunocompetent subjects. Mycoses. 2006;49(1):30–6.

Das A, Bal A, Chakrabarti A, Panda N, Joshi K. Spectrum of fungal rhinosinusitis; histopathologist's perspective. Histopathology. 2009;54(7):854–9.

Deshazo RD. Syndromes of invasive fungal sinusitis. Med Mycol. 2009;47(Suppl 1):S309–14.

deShazo RD, Swain RE. Diagnostic criteria for allergic fungal sinusitis. J Allergy Clin Immunol. 1995;96(1):24–35. Available from: http://www.ncbi.nlm.nih.gov/pubmed/7622760

deShazo RD, O'Brien M, Chapin K, Soto-Aguilar M, Gardner L, Swain R. A new classification and diagnostic criteria for invasive fungal sinusitis. Arch Otolaryngol Head Neck Surg. 1997;123(11):1181–8. Available from: http://www.ncbi.nlm.nih.gov/entrez/query.fcgi?cmd=Retrieve&db=PubMed&dopt=Citation&list_uids=9366697

Dhiwakar M, Thakar A, Bahadur S. Invasive sino-orbital aspergillosis: surgical decisions and dilemmas. J Laryngol Otol. 2003a;117(4):280–5.

Dhiwakar M, Thakar A, Bahadur S. Improving outcomes in rhinocerebral mucormycosis—early diagnostic pointers and prognostic factors. J Laryngol Otol. 2003b;117(11):861–5.

Diwakar A, Dewan RK, Chowdhary A, Randhawa HS, Khanna G, Gaur SN. Zygomycosis—a case report and overview of the disease in India. Mycoses. 2007;50(4):247–54. Available from: http://www.ncbi.nlm.nih.gov/pubmed/17576314

Epstein VA, Kern RC. Invasive fungal sinusitis and complications of rhinosinusitis. Otolaryngol Clin N Am. 2008;41(3):497–524.

Gamaletsou MN, Sipsas NV, Roilides E, Walsh TJ. Rhino-orbital-cerebral mucormycosis. Curr Infect Dis Rep. 2012;14(4):423–34.

Garcia-Covarrubias L, Bartlett R, Barratt DM, Wassermann RJ. Rhino-orbitocerebral mucormycosis attributable to apophysomyces elegans in an immunocompetent individual: case report and review of the literature. J Trauma. 2001;50(2):353–7.

Garcia-Covarrubias L, Barratt DM, Bartlett R, Metzinger S, Van Meter K. Invasive aspergillosis treated with adjunctive hyperbaric oxygenation: a retrospective clinical series at a single institution. South Med J. 2002;95(4):450–6. Available from: http://www.ncbi.nlm.nih.gov/entrez/query.fcgi?cmd=Retrieve&db=PubMed&dopt=Citation&list_uids=11958246

Gillespie MB, O'malley BW. An algorithmic approach to the diagnosis and management of invasive fungal rhinosinusitis in the immunocompromised patient. Otolaryngol Clin N Am. 2000;33:323–34.

Gillespie MB, O'Malley BW, Francis HW. An approach to fulminant invasive fungal rhinosinusitis in the immunocompromised host. Arch Otolaryngol Head Neck Surg. 1998;124(5):520–6.

Green BJ, Sercombe JK, Tovey ER. Fungal fragments and undocumented conidia function as new aeroallergen sources. J Allergy Clin Immunol. 2005;115(5):1043–8.

Hargrove RN, Wesley RE, Klippenstein KA, Fleming JC, Haik BG. Indications for orbital exenteration in mucormycosis. Ophthal Plast Reconstr Surg. 2006;22(4):286–91.

Herbrecht R, Denning DW, Patterson TF, Bennett JE, Greene RE, Oestmann J-W, et al. Voriconazole versus amphotericin B for primary therapy of invasive aspergillosis. N Engl J Med. 2002;347(6):408–15. Available from: http://www.nejm.org/doi/abs/10.1056/NEJMoa020191

Hontelez S, Sanecka A, Netea MG, van Spriel AB, Adema GJ. Molecular view on PRR cross-talk in antifungal immunity. Cell Microbiol. 2012;14:467–74.

Idris N, Lim LHY. Nasal eschar: a warning sign of potentially fatal invasive fungal sinusitis in immunocompromised children. J Pediatr Hematol Oncol. 2012;34(4):e134–6.

Ingram CW, Sennesh J, Cooper JN, Perfect JR. Disseminated zygomycosis: report of four cases and review. Rev Infect Dis. 1989;11(5):741–54.

Jiménez C, Lumbreras C, Paseiro G, Loinaz C, Romano DR, Andrés A, et al. Treatment of mucor infection after liver or pancreas-kidney transplantation. Transplant Proc. 2002;34(1):82–3.

Kim JH, Kang BC, Lee J-H, Jang YJ, Lee B-J, Chung Y-S. The prognostic value of gadolinium-enhanced magnetic resonance imaging in acute invasive fungal rhinosinusitis. J Infect. 2015;70(1):88–95.

Koc Z, Koc F, Yerdelen D, Ozdogu H. Rhino-orbital-cerebral mucormycosis with different cerebral involvements: infarct, hemorrhage, and ophthalmoplegia. Int J Neurosci. 2007;117(12):1677–90.

Kohn R, Hepler R. Management of limited rhino-orbital mucormycosis without exenteration. Ophthalmology. 1985;92(10):1440–4.

Kontoyiannis DP, Wessel VC, Bodey GP, Rolston KV. Zygomycosis in the 1990s in a tertiary-care cancer center. Clin Infect Dis. 2000;30(6):851–6.

Kontoyiannis DP, Lewis RE, Spellberg B, Edwards J, Ibrahim A, Roden M, et al. How I treat mucormycosis. Blood. 2011;118(5):1216–24. Available from: https://www.ncbi.nlm.nih.gov/pubmed/21622653

Bae MS, Kim EJ, Lee KM, Choi WS. Rapidly progressive rhino-orbito-cerebral mucormycosis complicated with unilateral internal carotid artery occlusion: a case report. Neurointervention. 2012;7:45–9.

Maheshwari M, Richa D, Kaur R. Invasive Aspergillus sinusitis in a young immunocompetent host: call for early diagnosis and treatment. Ann Trop Med Public Heal. 2013;6(1):120. Available from: http://www.atmph.org/article.asp?issn=1755-6783

Mankekar G. Invasive fungal rhinosinusitis; 2014. p. 1–93. https://www.springer.com/us/book/9788132215295

Montone KT, Livolsi VA, Feldman MD, Palmer J, Chiu AG, Lanza DC, et al. Fungal rhinosinusitis: a retrospective microbiologic and pathologic review of 400 patients at a Single University Medical Center. Int J Otolaryngol. 2012;2012:1–9.

Morduchowicz G, Shmueli D, Shapira Z, Cohen SL, Yussim A, Block CS, et al. Rhinocerebral mucormycosis in renal transplant recipients: report of three cases and review of the literature. Rev Infect Dis. 1986;8(3):441–6.

Nishimura K, Takahashi Y, Yamagishi Y, Banno S, Uchida Y, Tanigawa T, et al. Advanced surgical technique for invasive fungal sinusitis: endoscopic orbit-sinus combined approach. Minim Invasive Ther Allied Technol. 2017;26(5):307–13.

Otto K, DelGaudio J. Invasive fungal rhinosinusitis: what is the appropriate follow-up? Am J Rhinol. 2006;20(6):582–5. Available from: http://www.ingentaconnect.com/content/ocean/ajr/2006/00000020/00000006/art00007

Palejwala S, Zangeneh T, Goldstein S, Lemole GM. An aggressive multidisciplinary approach reduces mortality in rhinocerebral mucormycosis. Surg Neurol Int. 2016;7(1):61. Available from: http://surgicalneurologyint.com/surgicalint_articles/an-aggressive-multidisciplinary-approach-reduces-mortality-in-rhinocerebral-mucormycosis/

Panda NK, Sharma SC, Chakrabarti A, Mann SB. Paranasal sinus mycoses in north India. Mycoses. 1998;41:281–6. Available from: http://ovidsp.ovid.com/ovidweb.cgi?T=JS&PAGE=reference&D=emed4&NEWS=N&AN=1998412993

Parikh SL, Venkatraman G, DelGaudio JM. Invasive fungal sinusitis: a 15-year review from a single institution. Am J Rhinol. 2004;18(2):75–81.

Peterson KL, Wang M, Canalis RF, Abemayor E. Rhinocerebral mucormycosis: evolution of the disease and treatment options. Laryngoscope. 1997;107(7):855–62. Available from: http://ovidsp.ovid.com/ovidweb.cgi?T=JS&PAGE=reference&D=med4&NEWS=N&AN=9217119

Plowes Hernandez O, Prado Calleros HM, Soberon Marmissolle Daguerre GS, Sadek Gonzalez A. Rhino-orbito-cerebral mucormycosis. Management strategies to avoid or limit intracraneal affection and improve survival. Acta Otorrinolaringol Esp. 2015;66(6):348–52.

Prabhu RM, Patel R. Mucormycosis and entomophthoramycosis: a review of the clinical manifestations, diagnosis and treatment. Clin Microbiol Infect. 2004;10(Suppl 1):31–47.

Price JC, Stevens DL. Hyperbaric oxygen in the treatment of rhinocerebral mucormycosis. Laryngoscope. 1980;90:737–47. Available from: http://ovidsp.ovid.com/ovidweb.cgi?T=JS&PAGE=reference&D=emed1ab&NEWS=N&AN=1980129271

Schell WA. Histopathology of fungal rhinosinusitis. Otolaryngol Clin N Am. 2000;33:251–76.

Schwartz LE. Acute invasive fungal rhinosinusitis. Pathol Case Rev. 2011;16(6):230–3.

Skiada A, Lanternier F, Groll AH, Pagano L, Zimmerli S, Herbrecht R, et al. Diagnosis and treatment of mucormycosis in patients with hematological malignancies: guidelines from the 3rd European Conference on Infections in Leukemia (ECIL 3). Haematologica. 2013;98(4):492–504.

Soler ZM, Schlosser RJ. The role of fungi in diseases of the nose and sinuses. Am J Rhinol Allergy. 2012;26(5):351–8.

Songu M, Unlu HH, Gunhan K, Ilker SS, Nese N. Orbital exenteration: a dilemma in mucormycosis presented with orbital apex syndrome. Am J Rhinol. 2008;22(1):98–103. Available from: http://wustl.library.ingentaconnect.com.beckerproxy.wustl.edu/content/ocean/ajr/2008/00000022/00000001/art00021?token=0054182ad32ed8a1437a63736a6f3547354c486667776a23796f644a467b4d616d3f4e4b348505c0506e

Spellberg B, Edwards J, Ibrahim A. Novel perspectives on Mucormycosis: pathophysiology, presentation, and management. Clin Microbiol Rev. 2005;18(3):556–69.

Sridhara SR, Paragache G, Panda NK, Chakrabarti A. Mucormycosis in immunocompetent individuals: an increasing trend. J Otolaryngol. 2005;34(6):402–6. Available from: http://www.ncbi.nlm.nih.gov/pubmed/16343400

Talbot GH, Huang A, Provencher M. Invasive aspergillus rhinosinusitis in patients with acute-leukemia. Rev Infect Dis. 1991;13(2):219–32.

Thompson GR, Patterson TF. Fungal disease of the nose and paranasal sinuses. J Allergy Clin Immunol. 2012;129:321–6.

Vironneau P, Kania R, Morizot G, Elie C, Garcia-Hermoso D, Herman P, et al. Local control of rhino-orbito-cerebral mucormycosis dramatically impacts survival. Clin Microbiol Infect. 2014;20(5):O336–9.

Walsh TJ, Anaissie EJ, Denning DW, Herbrecht R, Kontoyiannis DP, KA M, et al. Treatment of aspergillosis: clinical practice guidelines of the Infectious Diseases Society of America. Clin Infect Dis. 2008;46(3):327–60.

Walsh TJ, Skiada A, Cornely OA, Roillides E, Ibrahim A, Zaoutis T, et al. Development of new strategies for early diagnosis of mucormycosis from bench to bedside. Mycoses. 2014;57(03):2–7.

Yohai RA, Bullock JD, Aziz AA, Markert RJ. Survival factors in rhino-orbital-cerebral mucormycosis. Surv Ophthalmol. 1994;39:3–22.

24 Cavernous Sinus Syndrome

Forhad Hossian Chowdhury,
Mohammod Raziul Haque,
Mohammod Zahed Hossain,
and Mainul Haque Sarker

Abbreviations

CNS	Central nervous system
CS	Cavernous sinus
CST	Cavernous sinus thrombosis
CT	Computed tomography
CTA	Computed tomographic angiogram
DSA	Digital subtraction angiography
EC-IC	Extracranial-intracranial
FLAIR	Fluid attenuated inversion recovery
ICA	Internal carotid artery
MCA	Middle cerebral artery
MRA	Magnetic resonance angiogram
MRI	Magnetic resonance imaging
PNS	Paranasal sinuses

24.1 Introduction

The cavernous sinus (CS) is a small but complex structure consisting of a venous plexus, the carotid artery, cranial nerves, and sympathetic fibers. Broad categories of diseases involving the cavernous sinus can cause the so-called cavernous sinus syndrome; these diseases include bacterial or fungal infections, non-infectious inflammation, vascular lesions, and neoplasms (Lee et al. 2003).

Intracranial fungal infection of the CS is a condition that usually affects immunocompromised individuals and is rarely seen in immunocompetent individuals. It is a potentially life-threatening condition which requires prompt treatment (Ng et al. 2017).

24.2 Anatomy of Cavernous Sinus

The CS is a complex and loculated venous space, which lies between periosteal and meningeal layers of dura adjacent to the sphenoid bone. It is a paired structure lying on either side of the sella turcica. The two halves communicate freely via the two intercavernous sinuses, which pass anterior and posterior to the pituitary gland. The CS extends anteriorly from the superior orbital fissure to the apices of the petrous temporal bones. Superiorly is the diaphragma sellae, and inferiorly is the greater wing of sphenoid. The sinus is bounded laterally by dura. As there are no lateral bony boundaries, all diseases of the CS cause volume expansion and thus lateral bulging of its walls, which is best seen on coronal examinations (Fig. 24.1). The symptoms of CS syndrome correlate with the involved structures of the venous space. Medially within the CS is the internal carotid artery (ICA) with its periarterial sympathetic plexus, involvement of which may cause

F. H. Chowdhury (✉) · M. Z. Hossain
Department of Neurosurgery, National Institute of Neurosciences and Hospital, Dhaka, Bangladesh

M. R. Haque · M. H. Sarker
Neurosurgery, Dhaka Medical College and Hospital, Dhaka, Bangladesh

M. Turgut et al. (eds.), *Fungal Infections of the Central Nervous System*,
https://doi.org/10.1007/978-3-030-06088-6_24

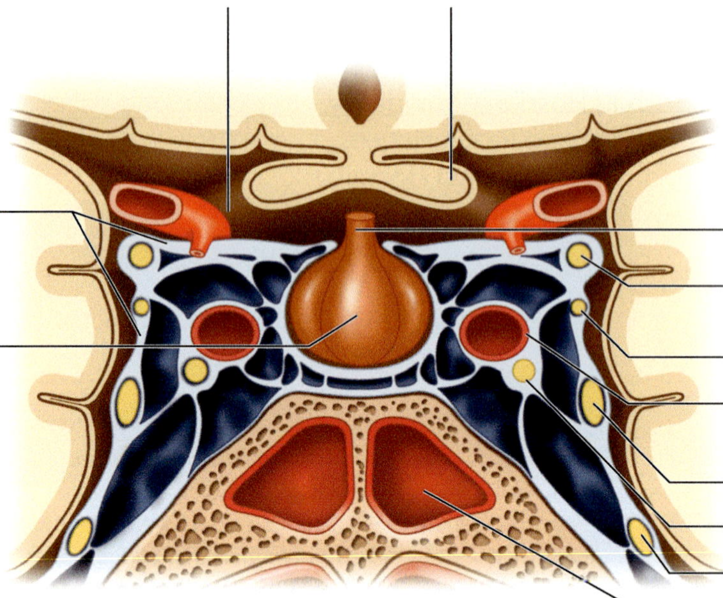

Fig. 24.1 Schematic drawing of cross-sectional (coronal) anatomy of both cavernous sinuses (CS) at midsellar region showing boundary-related structures and contents

Horner's syndrome. Inferolateral to the ICA is the abducens nerve. Within the lateral dural border of the CS lie the ophthalmic and maxillary divisions of the trigeminal nerve, oculomotor nerve, and trochlear nerve (Figs. 24.1, 24.2, 24.3, and 24.4). Involvement of these cranial nerves can cause ophthalmoplegia or facial sensory loss. Compromise of venous drainage may give rise to chemosis and proptosis. The CS has complex, valveless, venous communications. It communicates directly or indirectly with almost every important venous structure in the head and neck. Draining into the CS are the superior and inferior ophthalmic veins, sphenoparietal sinuses, and middle meningeal vein. The CS communicates with the facial vein and pterygoid venous plexus via the superior and inferior ophthalmic veins. This communication explains how CS thrombosis may result from facial infections. Draining from the CS are the superior and inferior petrosal sinuses, which eventually drain into the sigmoid sinus and internal jugular vein. The CSs are connected via two intercavernous sinuses (Chowdhury et al. 2012; Tang et al. 2010).

24.3 Etiopathogenesis

24.3.1 Causative Fungus

Of the more than 400,000 known fungal species, approximately 400 are human pathogens, only 50 of which cause systemic or central nervous system (CNS) infection. Many of these fungi are ubiquitous in our environment. Although many people are colonized by fungi, an intact immune system prevents subsequent infection. Although several fungi have been implicated to cause sinus infection, *Aspergillus*, *Bipolaris*, and *Rhizopus* species are more commonly implicated organisms causing fungal sinusitis (Thompson and Patterson 2011).

Apart from the species of *Aspergillus* which is isolated from a majority of such cases, dematiaceous hyphomycetes, *Pseudallescheria boydii*, *Candida*, *Fusarium*, *Hyphomycetes*, and *Zygomycetes* are also reported. The changing terminology for mucormycosis and of its causative agents has complicated data retrieval and created

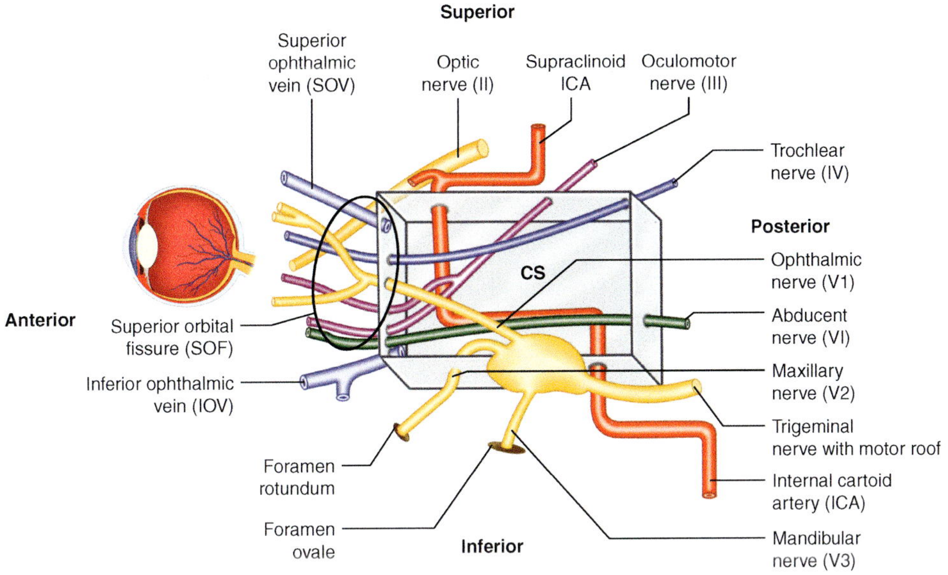

Fig. 24.2 Schematic drawing of left CS lateral view structures and boundaries with their relation and contents of CS

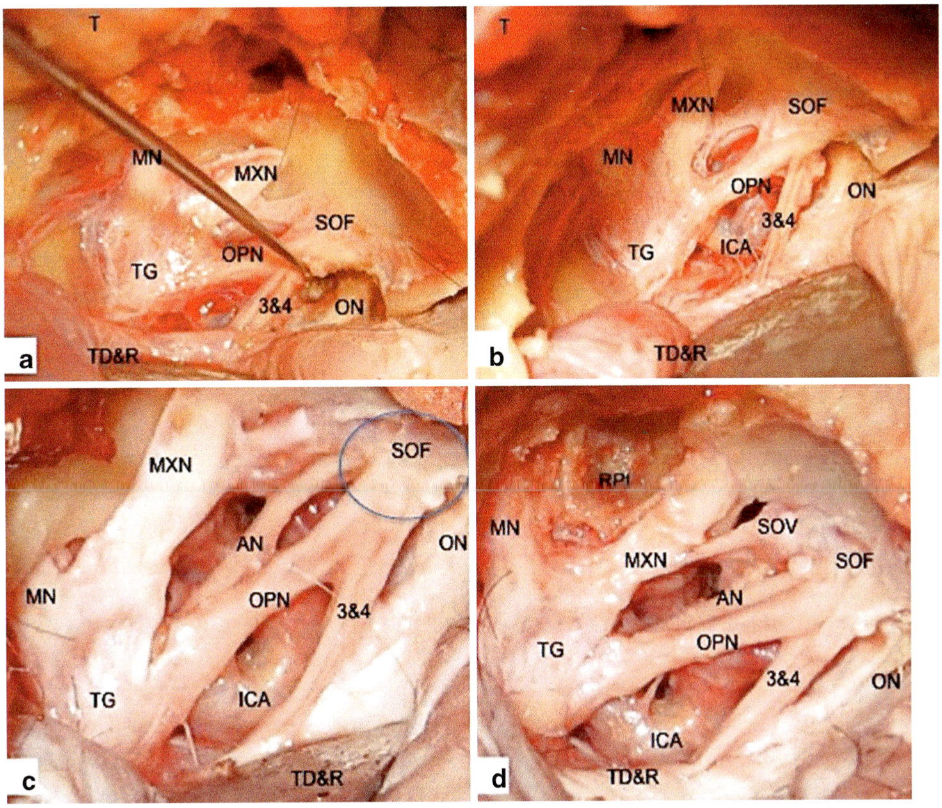

Fig. 24.3 (**a–d**) Sequential cadaveric temporal extradural dissection of left CS with drilling out of anterior clinoid process. *T* temporalis muscle, *TD&R* temporal dura and retractor, *TG* trigeminal ganglion, *MN* mandibular nerve, *MXN* maxillary nerve, *OPN* ophthalmic nerve, *ON* optic nerve, *AN* abducens nerve, *3 and 4* oculomotor and trochlear nerve, *ICA* internal carotid artery (cavernous segment), *SOF* superior orbital fissure, *SOV* superior ophthalmic vein, and *RPt* root of pterygoid

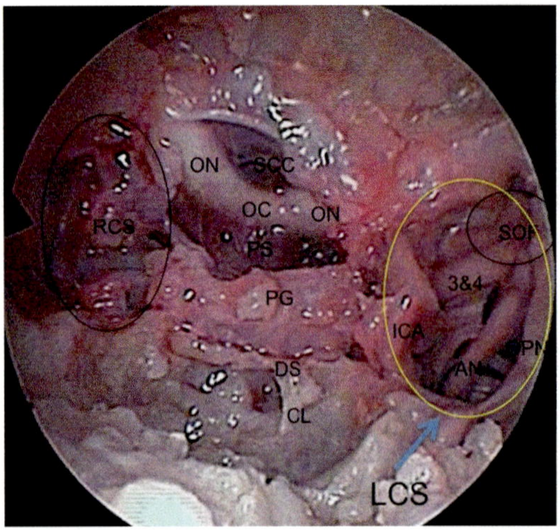

Fig. 24.4 Endoscopic endonasal extended transsphenoidal exposure of CS, sella, and suprasellar region with dissection of left CS in cadaver. *RCS* right cavernous sinus, *LCS* left CS, *ON* optic nerve, *OC* optic chiasma, *SCC* suprachiasmatic cistern, *PS* pituitary stalk, *PG* pituitary gland, *DS* dorsum sella, *CL* clivus, *ICA* medially mobi lized internal carotid artery, *AN* abducens nerve, *OPN* ophthalmic nerve, *3 and 4* oculomotor and trochlear nerve, and *SOF* superior orbital fissure

confusion amongst the clinicians. All the agents of mucormycosis belong to the order *Mucorales*. The classification of the genera that contain the agents of mucormycosis in man is *Zygomycetes* (class) and *Mucorales* (order). *Mucorales* order has six families.

Family Genus:

1. *Cunninghamallaceae Cunninghamella.*
2. *Mortierellaceae Mortierella.*
3. *Mucoraceae Rhizopus*, *Absidia*, *Rhizomucor*, *Mucor*, *Apophysomyces.*
4. *Saksenaceae Saksenaea.*
5. *Syncephalastraceae Syncephalastrum.*
6. *Thamnidiaceae Cokeromyces* (Rao et al. 2006).

24.3.2 Risk Factors

The risk factors are solid organ transplantation, leukemia, lymphoma, myeloma, diabetes mellitus, extensive burns, renal insufficiency, hepatic cirrhosis, antineoplastic chemotherapy, chronic use of corticosteroids or immunosuppressive therapy, radiotherapy, malnutrition, primary immunodeficiency syndromes, etc. The development of mucormycosis is rare in other immunosuppressive states such as in acquired immunodeficiency syndrome (AIDS) or in immunocompetent patients (Haber et al. 2008).

24.3.3 Mode of Spread

The extension in CS is one of the most dreaded complications of fungal sinusitis with high mortality rates. The fungus generally spreads into CS through direct extension, hematogenous route, perineural invasion of cranial nerve, penetrating injury, and rarely surgery or blood transfusion.

Direct extension: This is the most common mode of extension. Due to the location of the sphenoid sinus, the infection can easily spread to the cavernous sinus. The fungus causes osteitis and osteomyelitis of the sinus wall/pressure necrosis and subsequent erosion leading to the extension in the CS.

As the fungus is known to be angioinvasive, it digests the elastic tissue and penetrates the vessel wall, causing arteritis and intramural spread. In direct arterial involvement, the endothelial cells engulf the organism, and subsequently the internal elastic lamina is infiltrated and destroyed.

Hematogenous spread: It is more insidious and asymptomatic. There is also formation of mycotic emboli and thrombus due to extension of fungal hyphae. The fungus usually involves more proximal portions of the cavernous internal carotid artery causing vascular damage in large areas. These are more common in immunocompromised patients. The thrombus or the emboli lead to cerebral infarction. The primary could be in the lungs, as in the case of *Aspergillus* spp. It is also likely in patients with artificial valves in the heart. This spread could lead to vasculitis and cavernous sinus thrombosis (CST).

Perineural spread: It occurs along the nerves and their foramina resulting in cranial nerve palsies and skull base spread.

The infection can also spread through the cribriform plate into the anterior skull base. Rarely, a blood transfusion can cause such infection. It has also been reported to spread by surgery, especially transsphenoidal surgery (Shah and Rathore 2009).

24.3.4 Pathology (Shah and Rathore 2009)

Fungal sinusitis is the inflammation of the sinus mucosa, caused by a wide variety of fungi. *Aspergillus spp* is the most common, and *Rhizopus*, *Mucor*, *Cladosporium*, *Candida*, and *Cryptococcus species* are among the others. The noninvasive ones are, generally, dematiaceous molds including *Curvularia*, *Bipolaris*, *Alternaria*, *Fusarium*, *Aspergillus*, etc. These cause intracranial complications in about 20% of the patients.

There are broadly two types of fungal infection of the sinuses:

- Noninvasive (extramucosal).
  - Allergic fungal sinusitis.
  - Mycetoma.
- Invasive.
  - Acute.
  - Chronic indolent.
  - Chronic granulomatous.

Noninvasive: These generally do not invade the bone or tissues and, more often, are a result of hypersensitivity skin reactions. But a long-term disease can eventually erode the bone by pressure necrosis and hence cause an intracranial or intraorbital complication. It occurs in an immunocompetent host and is characterized by the presence of allergic mucin, Charcot-Leyden crystals and eosinophils, etc.

Invasive: The more fatal variety is known to penetrate the mucosa and cause tissue destruction and lead to intracranial extension. These are known to occur in immunocompromised hosts in about 50% of the cases. The most common is *Aspergillus spp* followed by *Mucor*, *Rhizopus*, *Cryptococcus*, etc. The mortality rates are high in such infections (85–100%).

The acute variety rapidly progresses in few hours to days and progresses to fulminant intracranial infections. Mostly, these are caused by *Mucor*, *Absidia*, *Fusarium*, etc. Some authors prefer to call such infections as rhinocerebral mucormycosis. These often occur in patients with diabetes having ketoacidosis. The chronic one has an indolent course and could be granulomatous also. The species implicated are *Alternaria*, *Curvularia*, *Mucor*, *Bipolaris*, etc. These are slow growing and cause slow tissue destruction and subsequent invasion (Shah and Rathore 2009).

24.4 Clinical Presentation

Cavernous sinus syndrome is characterized by multiple cranial neuropathies. The clinical presentation includes impairment of ocular motor nerves leading to ophthalmoplegia, Horner's syndrome, and sensory loss of the first or second divisions of the trigeminal nerve in various combinations. The pupil may be involved or spared or may appear spared with concomitant oculosympathetic and parasympathetic involvement. Various degrees of pain may be involved (Lee et al. 2003).

A good history along with symptoms of any systemic ailments should be elicited. A sinusitis patient not responding to conventional antibiotics should arouse the suspicion of fungal sinusitis. Diagnostic nasal endoscopy should be performed, and one should look for allergic mucin, blackish/brownish discharge, erosion of palate, pale/dark nasal mucosa, etc.

The most common symptoms are nasal obstruction, nasal discharge, headache, vomiting, nausea, epistaxis, periorbital pain, facial pain, facial swelling, anosmia, altered sensorium, seizures, and weakness of limbs, diplopia, visual disturbance, and fever. The signs depend upon the areas involved like ophthalmoplegia, chemosis, proptosis, lateral/medial rectus palsy, and hemiparesis (Shah and Rathore 2009).

24.5 Investigations

24.5.1 Radiology

Since fungal infections are rapidly on the rise resulting in disastrous outcomes, one has to diagnose them early with the aid of radiology. The computed tomography (CT) scan and magnetic resonance imaging (MRI) of the paranasal sinus (PNS) and brain are the mainstay in diagnosing these infections.

There is generally a homogenous mass with areas of lesser density, linear interlacing pattern, or dense in center with low attenuation at periphery. There could be expansion, thinning, erosion, or remodeling of the bone with intracranial/intraorbital extension. On contrast adminstration, enhancement is seen. For intracranial extension, an axial cut is also needed (Shah and Rathore 2009) (Figs. 24.5, 24.6, 24.7a–c, and 24.8).

24.5.1.1 CT Findings of Sinus Lesions

The early stages resemble chronic rhinosinusitis showing mucosal thickening which is hypoattenuated. Since the fungus may spread by blood vessels, bone erosion or mucosal thickening might be absent. In chronic cases, a hyperattenuating soft tissue collection can be seen in one or more sinuses. It often gives a masslike appearance, resembling a malignancy with destruction and erosion of the bony walls of the sinuses and extension to the surrounding tissues. In case of allergic fungal sinusitis, there is opacification of multiple sinuses with expansion. There are areas of hyperattenuation in the sinuses due to the presence of allergic mucin. It is essential to have both bone window and soft tissue windows to appreciate the "double density." When a fungal ball is present, it appears as hyperattenuation due to dense matted fungal hyphae and may show punctate calcification. There is mottling seen in some cases with sclerotic walls of the sinus, along with thinning due to pressure necrosis (Shah and Rathore 2009).

24.5.1.2 CT Findings of CS Lesions

The CT scan findings of PNS and orbit show bone destruction, and variable contrast-enhancing mass can be seen in cavernous sinus. On CT angiogram, cavernous ICA may be stenosed or blocked, or there may be mycotic aneurysm. There may be ischemia, infarcts, or multiple small embolic infarcts on the same-sided cerebral hemisphere due to involvement of cavernous ICA. Distal mycotic aneurysm can also be seen (Shah and Rathore 2009).

24.5.1.3 MRI Findings of Sinus Lesions

Since a CT scan only reveals a bony destruction, MRI is needed for assessing the CS and intracranial and intraorbital spread. In acute cases, one should look for obliteration of periantral fat planes. Sometimes, leptomeningeal enhancement is seen with intracranial spread. The granulomas may appear as hypointense masses on T1-T2-weighted images with very little enhancement on contrast. In diagnosing chronic invasive cases, infiltration of periantral soft tissue around the maxillary sinus should be looked for. The T2-weighted images have markedly low intensity. In case of acute fungal sinusitis, there are hyperintensity on T1 and hypointensity on T2 of the sinus contents. The inflamed mucosa shows hyperintensity on T2 and enhancement on contrast. The center is devoid of the enhancement, unlike a malignancy (Figs. 24.5, 24.6, and 24.7a–c).

A fungal ball is hypointense on both T1 and T2 and shows signal void on T2 due to calcification and paramagnetic metals like iron, magnesium, and manganese (Shah and Rathore 2009).

24.5.1.4 MRI Findings of CS Lesions

Invasive aspergillosis may affect the sphenoid sinus in immunocompromised patients and may extend intracranially with invasion of the CS. This infection shows low signal intensity on both T1- and T2-weighted images, which is attributed to the presence of ferromagnetic elements and calcium in the fungal and mucous concretions. It exhibits intense inhomogeneous contrast enhancement (Aribandi et al. 2007; Parikh et al. 2004; Stringer and Ryan 2000).

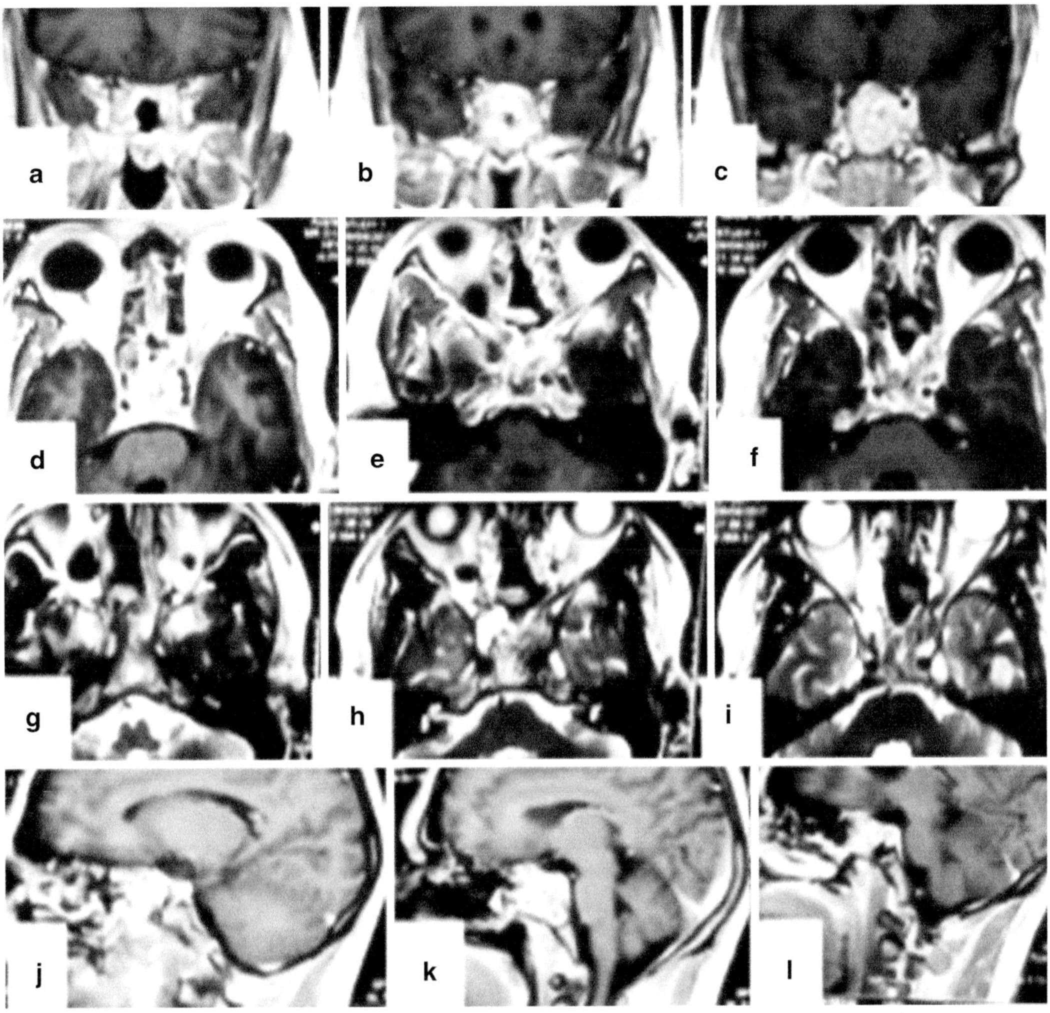

Fig. 24.5 Magnetic resonance imaging (MRI) of the head. (**a–c**) contrast coronal images; (**d–f**) axial contrast images; (**g–i**) axial T2W images; (**j–l**) sagittal contrast images showing bilateral CS aspergillosis (left > right) with bilateral involvement of paranasal sinuses and orbits in a diabetic patient of 35 years (confirmed by histopathology and fungal culture)

Rhinocerebral mucormycosis is often an acute fulminant opportunistic infection, which may affect the orbits and paranasal sinuses. The MRI findings include enhancing soft tissue masses in the orbital apex and CS, with thickening and lateral displacement of the medial rectus muscle and involvement of the neighboring ethmoid sinus (Chan et al. 2000; Goldberg et al. 1983; Mandava et al. 2001). Extension into the CS may result in thrombosis and thickening of the ICA walls, with narrowing of its lumen. Its MRI features are nonspecific (Ohta et al. 2002; Pagliani et al. 2006). These infections should always be considered in immunosuppressed patients who present with any type of paranasal sinus disease that

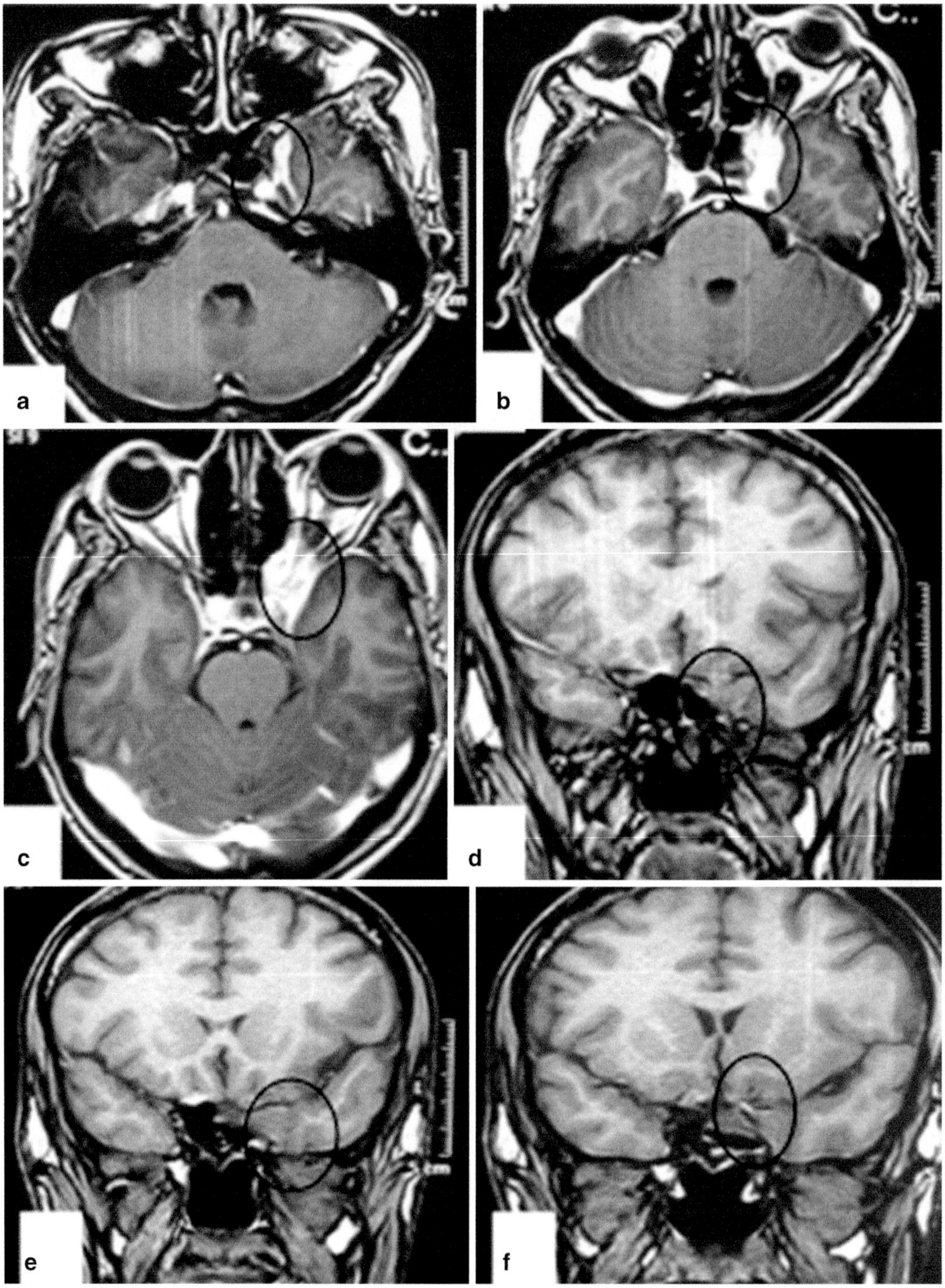

Fig. 24.6 MRI of the head of a 35-year-old apparently immunocompetent patient; (**a**–**c**) contrast axial images; (**d**–**f**) T1W coronal images; (**g**–**i**) contrast sagittal images showing aspergillosis of the left cavernous sinus, left orbital apex, and left sphenoidal sinus (confirmed by histopathology and culture)

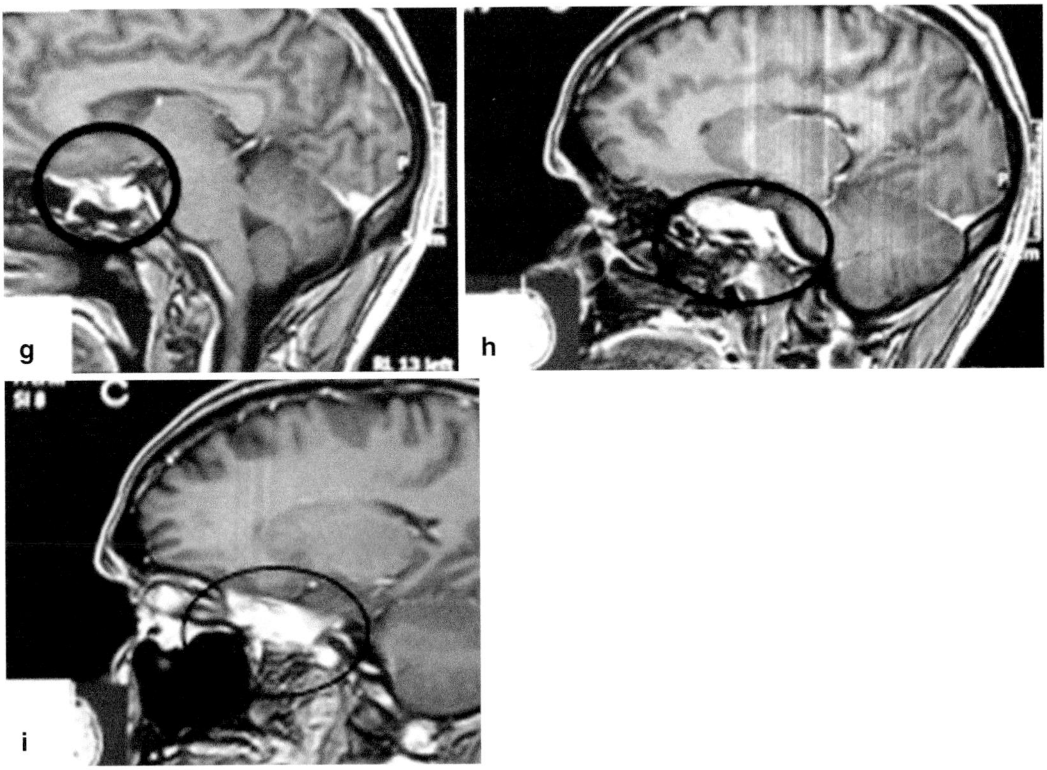

Fig. 24.6 (continued)

extends beyond the bony walls of that sinus (Figs. 24.5, 24.6, and 24.7a–c) (Razek and Castillo 2009).

24.5.1.5 Radiological Differential Diagnosis of Fungal CS Lesion

Differential diagnoses of CS fungal infection are tuberculosis, pyogenic chronic abscess (Fig. 24.9), sarcoidosis, lymphoma, myeloma, metastasis, meningioma, pseudotumor, inflammatory lesion, Tolosa-Hunt syndrome, etc.

24.5.2 Fungal Culture and Biopsy

There are special stains required for detecting the fungus. These include Gomori methenamine silver for *Mucor*, *Rhizopus*, and *Absidia*. The *Aspergillus* has uniform septate hyphae branching at 45°. The *Mucor* shows nonseptate, nonuniform branching at 90°. The allergic mucin is characteristic of allergic fungal sinusitis, and one has to stain deeply to look for fungal hyphae. The culture used is Sabouraud media. The biopsy can be taken using endoscopic endonasal approach from PNS especially from sphenoid sinuses (when sinuses are involved) and from CS. Where endonasal endoscopic biopsy is not available or suitable, then transcranial open biopsy may be needed. All the material including soft tissue and bones should be sent for histopathological examination (Shah and Rathore 2009). *Aspergillus* cultured optimally on Sabouraud agar demonstrates characteristic conidiophores. However, blood and cerebrospinal fluid cultures, even in disseminated disease, are frequently negative (Nadkarni and Goel 2005).

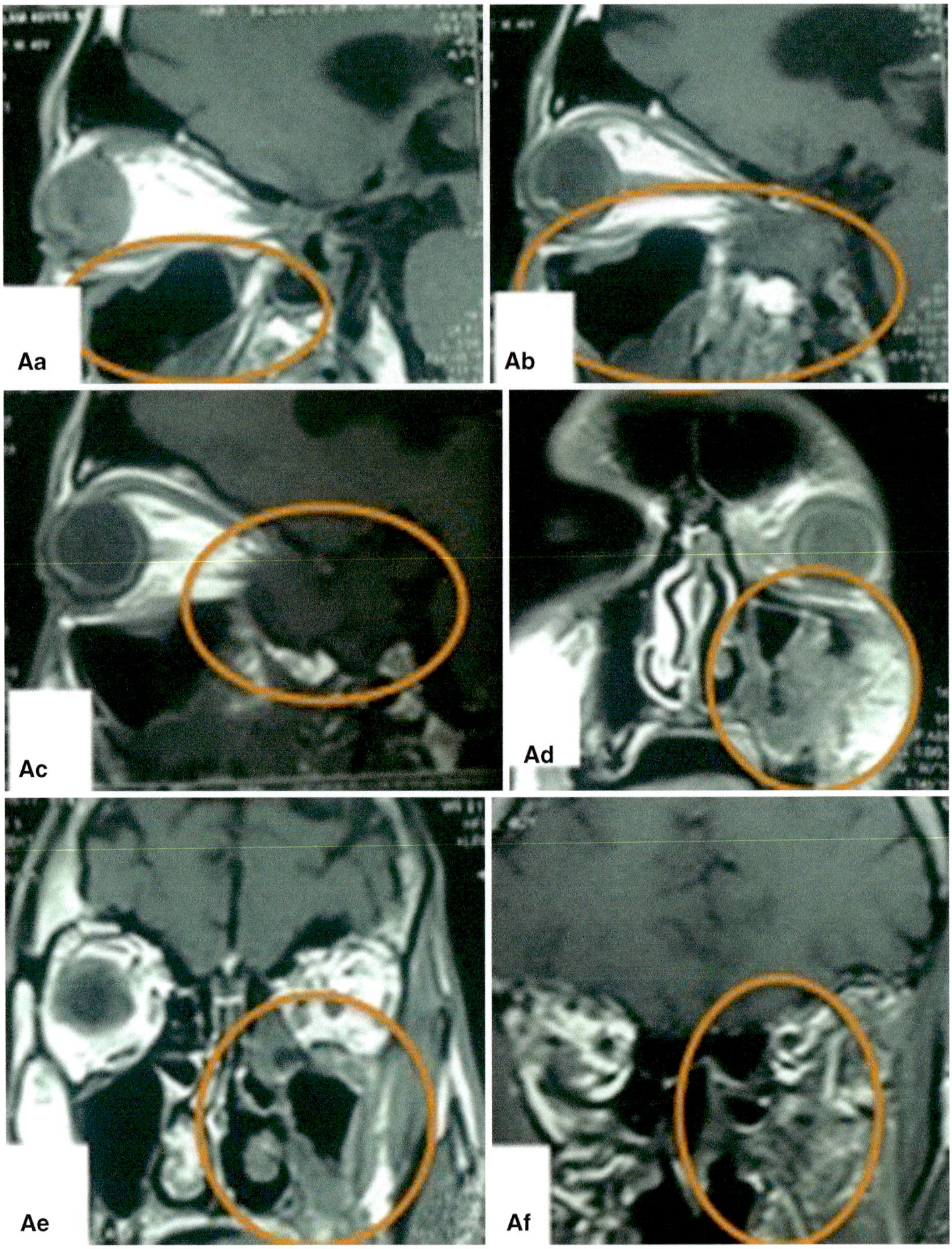

Fig. 24.7 (**a**) MRI of the head of a young diabetic patient. (**a**–**c**) T1W sagittal images; (**d**–**f**) contrast coronal images; and (**g**–**i**) contrast axial images showing mucormycosis involving right-sided maxillary sinus, ethmoid sinuses, sphenoidal sinus, orbital apex, and CS with proptosis (confirmed by histopathology and culture). (**b**) MRI of the head of patient of (**a**). (**a**–**d**) Axial FLAIR images showing mucormycosis involving right-sided maxillary sinus, ethmoid sinuses, sphenoidal sinus, orbital apex, and CS with proptosis. (**c**) MRI of the head of patient of (**a**). (**a**–**d**) Axial DW images showing multiple embolic infarcts in the left cerebral hemisphere from left cavernous ICA stenosis by invasion of mucormycosis. (**f**–**i**) MR angiogram showing left ICA stenosis form invasion of mucormycosis on arterial wall

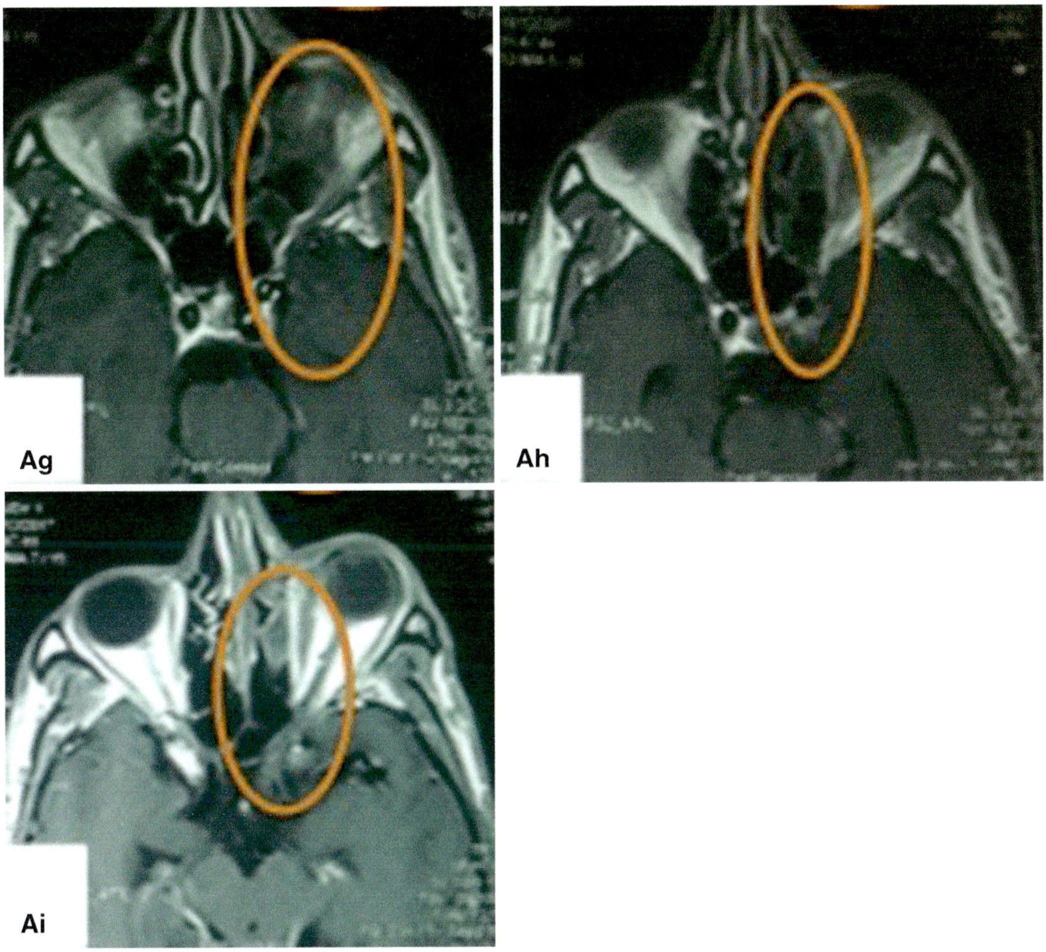

Fig. 24.7 (continued)

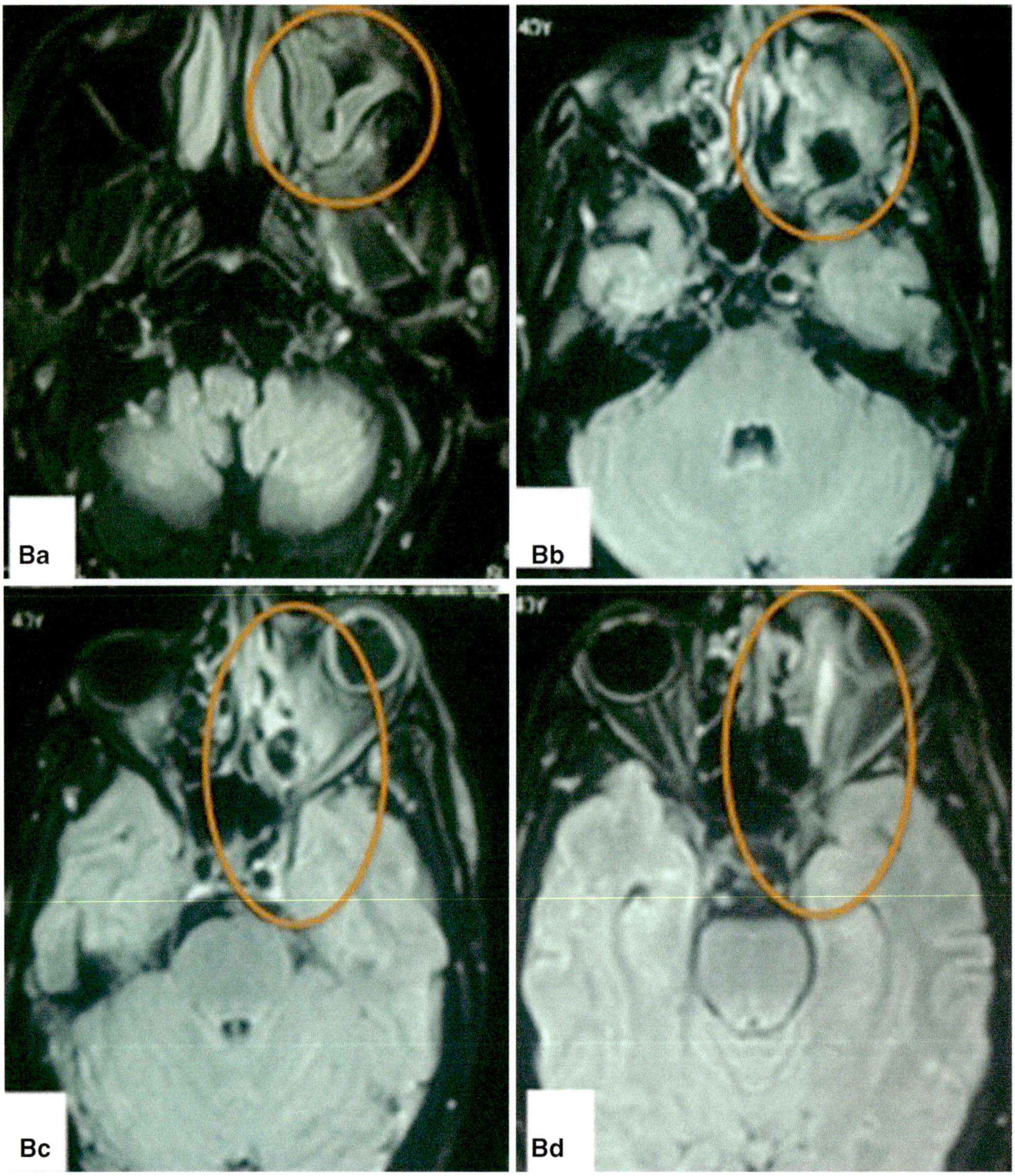

Fig. 24.7 (continued)

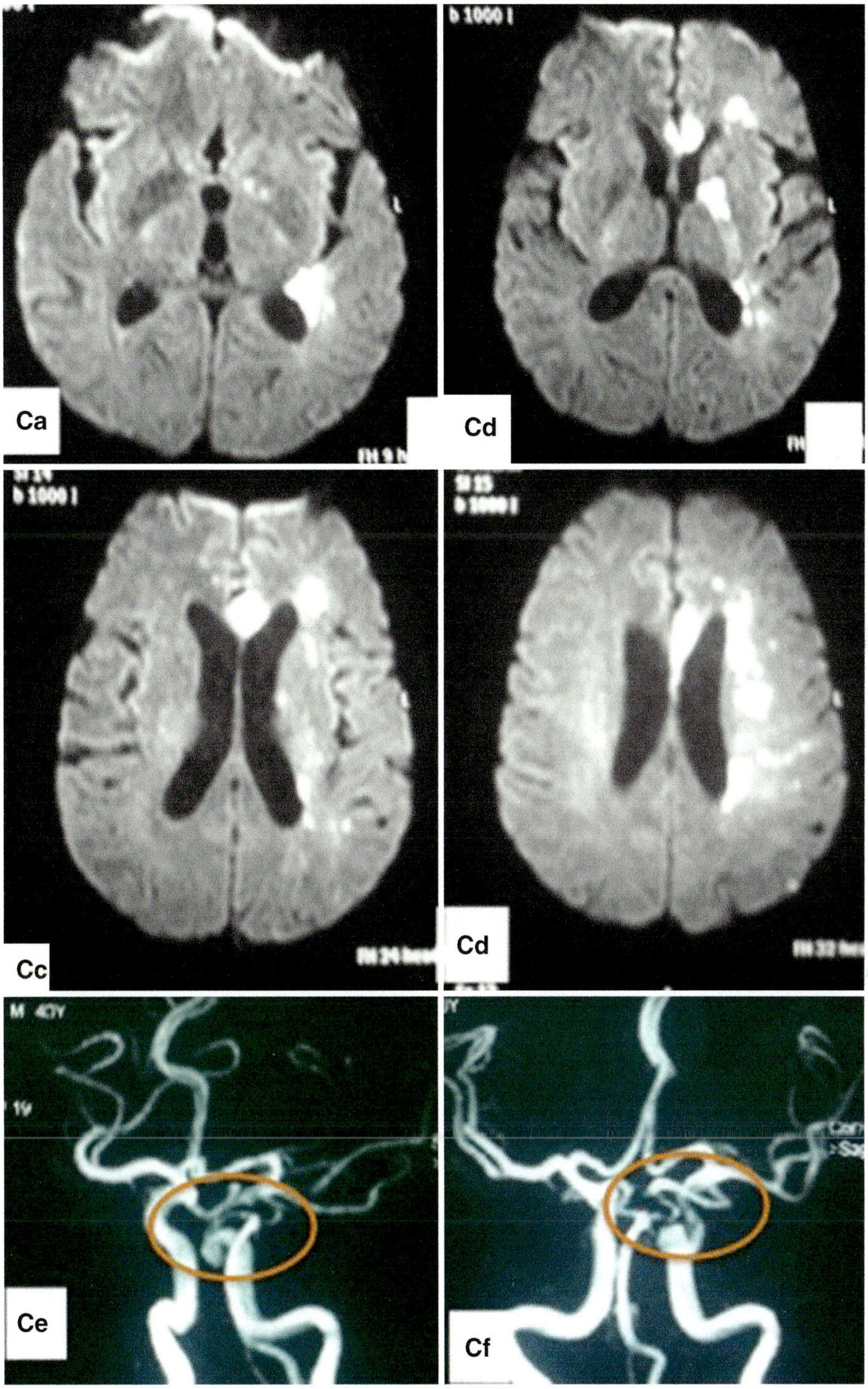

Fig. 24.7 (continued)

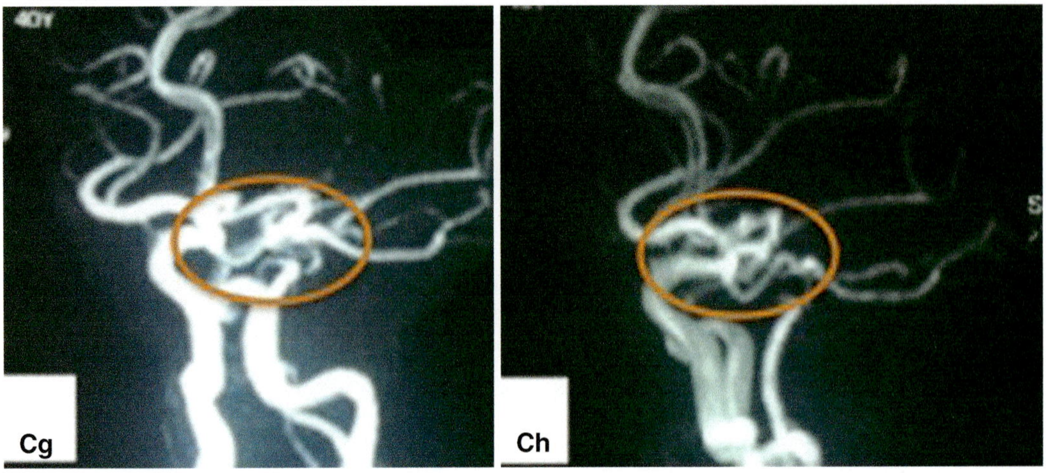

Fig. 24.7 (continued)

24.5.3 Serologic Tests

Serial serologic tests (i.e., double diffusion counterimmunoelectrophoresis, immunofluorescence, or enzyme-linked immunosorbent assay) significantly help in arriving at a diagnosis. Immunoassay may detect the disease early but these tests are rarely done. Serologic testing has been unreliable for *A. fumigatus*, except in leukemia patients followed prospectively (Nadkarni and Goel 2005).

24.6 Treatment

An initial biopsy and culture (endoscopic directed) is taken to confirm the presence and type of fungal involvement (from PNS and/or CS). If sinus tissue is absent, open biopsy can be taken from cavernous sinus. In cases of obvious clinical fungal sinusitis, endoscopic sinus surgery with removal of all fungal debris should be performed even at the initial stage when sending material for histopathology and microbiologic studies.

24.6.1 Medical Treatment

The mainstay of treatment is antifungal therapy with amphotericin B or other antifungal drugs (e.g., itraconazole, voriconazole, posaconazole) usually with surgery. Amphotericin B combines with the ergosterol in fungal cell membrane and manifests its antifungal properties. The maximum dose is 2–4 g/day. Due to its toxic effects, the liposomal amphotericin B is preferable, as it is less toxic. Due to its high cost, it is generally used in patients having creatinine > 2.5 mg. The required dosage is 4 mg/kg/day and could be increased up to 10–15 mg/kg/day (Shah and Rathore 2009).

24.6.2 Surgical Treatment

Once the infection is identified, aggressive management is necessary. Unfortunately, the response rate to medical therapy is only 40–60% (Choi et al. 2008; Mauriello Jr et al. 1995). The mortality rate of invasive sino-orbital aspergillosis is also 40–75% despite maximal management including surgical debridement and antifungal therapy (Choi et al. 2008; Mauriello Jr et al. 1995; Sivak-Callcott et al. 2004). Initially patient can be treated with antifungals including amphotericin, itraconazole, voriconazole, and posaconazole, but if the infection does not respond or progressed despite the therapies, surgical treatment is needed. Surgery includes debridement in the form of resection of the cavernous sinus and a portion of the petrous apex with or without extracranial-intracranial (EC-IC) bypass. Cavernous sinus resection carries significant morbidity and a mortality rate that can approach 25% (Couldwell et al. 2014). Indications for cavernous sinus resection are rare and poorly defined; progressive fungal infection despite treatment may represent one of them. The decision to proceed with CS resection should be approached with marked caution and deliberation. This deliberation should include planning to address the cranial

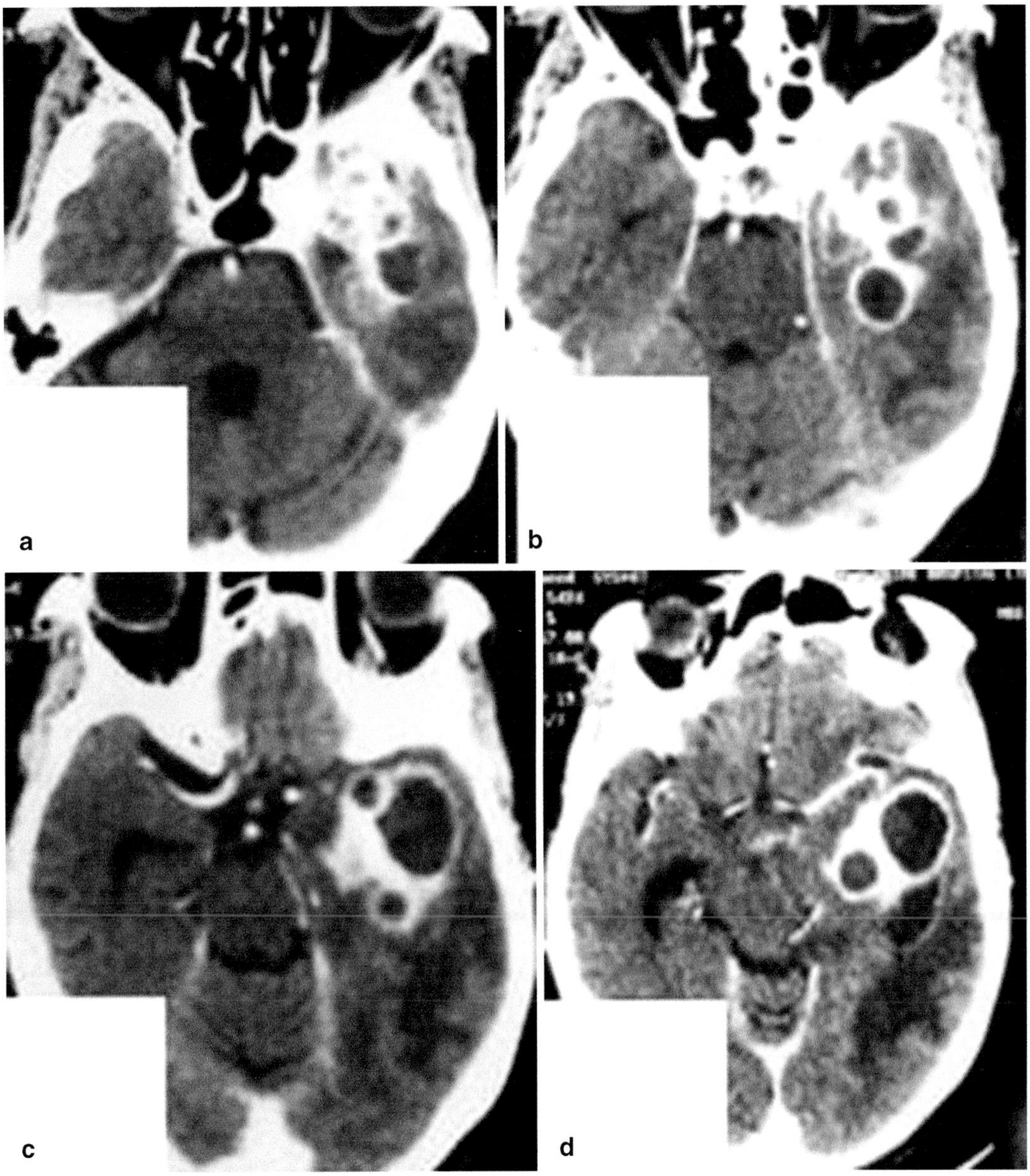

Fig. 24.8 (**a**–**d**) Preoperative contrast axial computed tomography (CT) scan of the head in a 55-year-old female showing left CS and temporal lobe fungal (aspergillus) lesion (confirmed by histopathology and culture). (**e**–**h**) Postoperative (2.5 months after operation and after antifungal therapy). CT scan of the head of the same patient showing resolution of the lesion

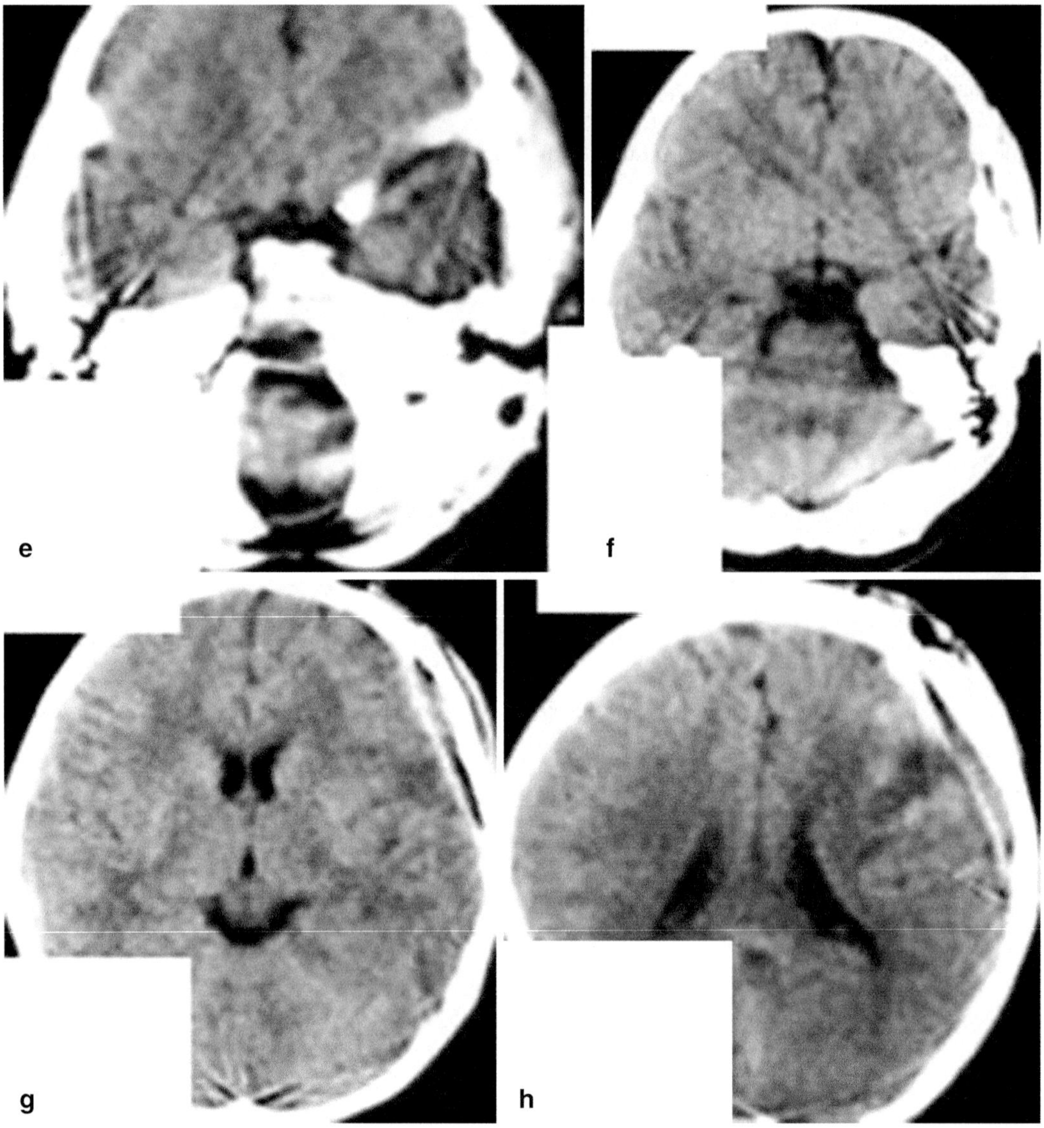

Fig. 24.8 (continued)

nerves and the carotid artery and reconstruction of the skull base defect. For complete unilateral cavernous sinus resection, cranial nerves II–VI will be resected. In such cases, a new cranial nerve deficit is not a major consideration; for example, in the present case, the patient had preoperative blindness and ophthalmoplegia in the affected eye. In cases of infection, care should be employed to ensure that all infected tissue is removed, especially if the infection involves proximal or distal cranial nerve tissue (e.g., the root entry zone or beyond the foramen rotundum or ovale with resection of cranial nerve V). Similarly, management of the carotid artery should be planned in detail prior to resection. In general, carotid artery sacrifice will be necessary for cavernous sinus resection based on the pathology. Proceeding with revascularization is controversial. A selective approach including balloon occlusion testing can be used (Taussky and Couldwell 2010). There is limited literature regarding the risk of bypass specific to carotid sacrifice for skull base lesions, but

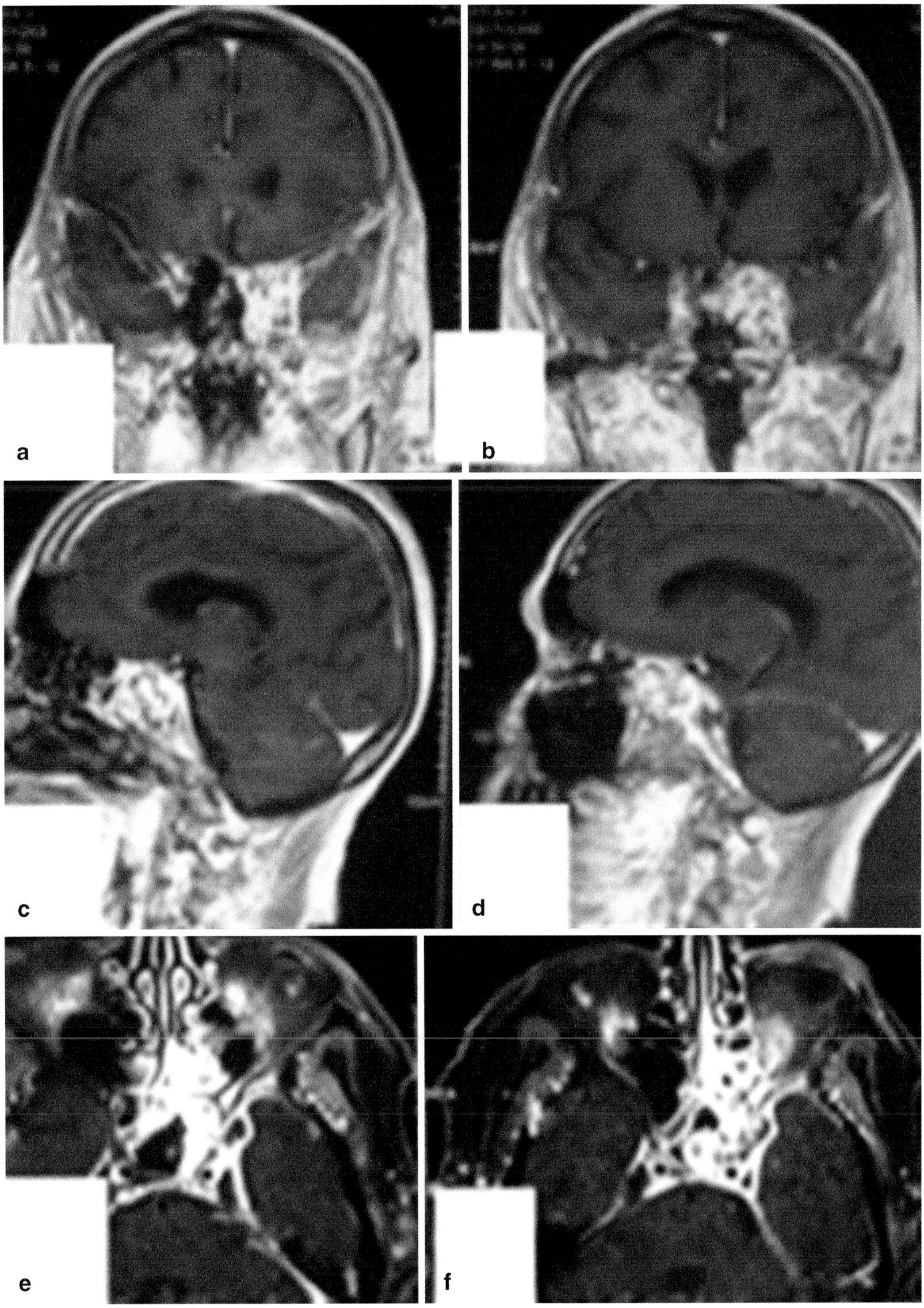

Fig. 24.9 Contrast MRI of the head in an 80-year-old lady. (**a**, **b**) Contrast coronal images; (**c**, **d**) contrast sagittal images; and (**e–h**) contrast axial images showing infection involving left-sided ethmoid, sphenoid sinus, orbit, and CS with proptosis. It was thought to be due to fungal infection. But histopathology reported inflammatory lesion and culture confirmed Methicillin-resistant *Staphylococcus aureus* (MRSA) infection

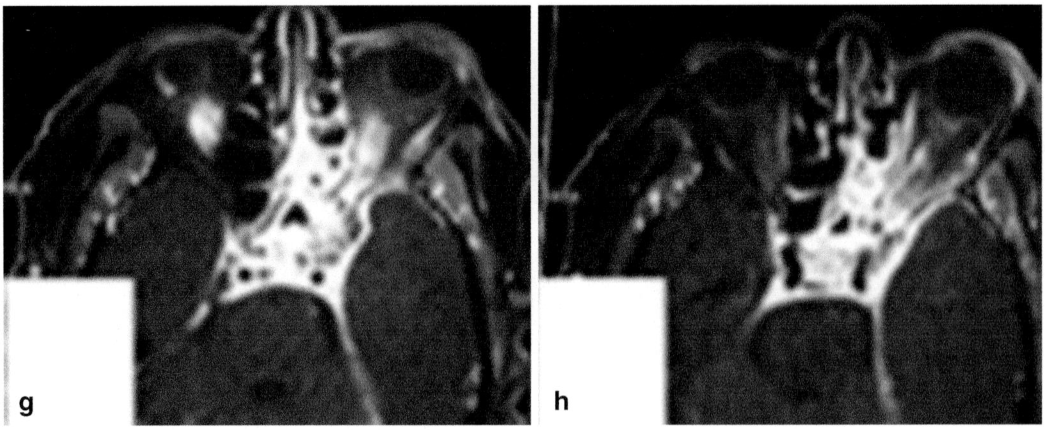

Fig. 24.9 (continued)

the published rates of morbidity are 3–20%, and mortality rates of less than 6% have been reported (Abdulrauf 2005; Kalani et al. 2013; Lawton and Spetzler 1996; Mendelowitsch et al. 2004). These risks should be weighed against the risk of carotid sacrifice in skull base lesions without bypass, for which there are neurological morbidity of 17% and mortality of 7% (Mendelowitsch et al. 2004). The middle cerebral artery (MCA) distal site ensures an anastomosis remote from the infection. Previous experience with bypass grafts in patients with fungal infections with arterial involvement has indicated that anastomosis sites even a short distance from the infection may result in higher thrombosis (Neil et al. 2016). A regular follow-up (clinical and neuroimaging) and endoscopic examination are essential. For sinusitis, the patient is asked to do nasal wash. Postoperative neurologic follow-up and assessment are critical. Often serial scans are required to confirm the presence or spread of disease postoperatively (Shah and Rathore 2009).

24.7 Special Situations in CS Fungal Infection

24.7.1 Cavernous Sinus Thrombosis (CST) Syndrome

It is a rare and serious complication secondary to invasive fungal sinusitis but rarer still in cases of allergic fungal sinusitis (McGinn et al. 2009) or non-invasive fungal infection in sphenoid sinus (Devèze et al. 2005). Current recommendations for CST are controversial, especially regarding anticoagulation, secondary to the rarity of the diagnosis. Early surgical debridement and intravenous antibiotics are crucial to prevent mortality and decrease morbidity. Because thrombosis is thought to be caused by a bacterial superinfection, which follows a response to *Aspergillus*, antifungals may not be necessary. Despite the controversy, most physicians opt to treat with anticoagulation (McGinn et al. 2009).

The most common clinical features are purulent or bloody rhinorrhea, mostly unilateral, with fever, headache, general discomfort, blepharitis, diplopia, decrease in visual acuity, unilateral or bilateral rhinorrhea, proptosis, chemosis, periorbital cellulitis, alteration of the intrinsic and extrinsic ocular motoricity, and amaurosis. Features of cerebral ischemia or infarction may be present when ICA is involved (Haber et al. 2008).

The CST diagnosis is made both with clinical signs and radiologic evaluation by CT and/or MRI, and the latter is more sensitive to the diagnosis. This exam may reveal direct signs of CST such as changes in the signal intensity, size and contour of the CS and indirect signs like the thickening and enhancement of the contrast on the lateral wall of the CS (Haber et al. 2008). CTA or MRA may show ICA narrowing or occlusion.

Treatment is surgery and aggressive antifungal therapy.

24.7.2 Mucormycosis and CST

The first description of mucormycosis was made by Paultauf in 1885 (Paulltauf 1885). This is a necrotizing disease caused by fungi of the *Zygomycetes* class and *Mucorales* order. From these, the most common genders found are *Rhizopus* (about 70% of the cases), *Absidia*, *Mucor*, *Rhizomucor*, *Apophysomyces*, *Saksenaea*, *Cunninghamella*, *Cokeromyces*, and *Syncephalastrum* (Yohai et al. 1994). The main route of infection is inhalatory. The mucormycosis is a rare and opportunist disease in immunocompromised person, specially in poorly controlled diabetes mellitus. Before the 1960s the mucormycosis was almost always fatal, and with the discovery of amphotericin B and its wide use associated with surgical debridement, the mortality rate was reduced to approximately 40% (Yohai et al. 1994). This potentially fatal evolution is due to a certain specific characteristic of these fungi, which is vascular tropism, that initially invades the arteries and causes thrombosis and ischemic injuries (Fig. 24.7a–c). Then there occurs vein and lymphatic node invasion (Van Johnson et al. 1988). The mucormycosis may present as rhino-orbito-cerebral form which is the most common presentation (Prabhu and Patel 2004). The infection may be disseminated to the CNS through the orbital apex and the cribriform plate or cause thrombosis in arteries that supply the CNS. The CNS manifeatations characterized by a change in the conscience level, convulsion, and/or hemiplegia are associated with a worse prognosis (Ferry 1961). A potential intracranial complication of mucormycosis is the CST. In the mucormycosis and CST, the diagnosis must be early with aggressive therapy. The mucormycosis is a more fatal acute fungal infection for mankind, with mortality rate from 15 to 34% (Fairley et al. 2000). The mucormycosis rhino-orbito-cerebral form, when present in the nasal cavity or in the PNS, may spread to the orbit through the nasolacrimal duct, through natural dehiscences in the papyraceous blade, or through arteries and veins in the orbital wall (Ferry 1961). The fungal invasion may commit the ocular globe and the retina artery and produce amaurosis (Yohai et al. 1994). The initial complaints of the CST are retro-orbital pain, periorbital edema, chemosis, proptosis, palpebral ptosis, and diplopia. Such symptoms are not specific and may be present in other affections as in the orbital cellulitis. However, the presence of sepsis, paralysis of cranial nerves, and bilateral ocular involvement are important signs for the CST. The early visual loss favors the suspicion of the retina artery involvement by mucormycosis, but the amaurosis caused by the CST occurs more lately (Bray et al. 1987; Van Johnson et al. 1988). The patient is treated clinically with systemic antifungal agents (amphotericin B), with intravenous antibiotics (initially ceftriaxone and after with vancomycin), with heparinization, and with intranasal and paranasal sinus surgery with debridement of the nasal mucosa necrosis areas. In the suspicion of acute invasive fungal rhinosinusitis (mucormycosis), the treatment must be carried out quickly and aggressively, by surgery for removal of the necrotic areas of the nasal mucosa and the use of intravenous systemic antifungal agents. Even so, there is a high rate of mortality and morbidity (Haber et al. 2008).

24.7.3 Internal Carotid Artery Involvement with Fungal Infection

Sphenoid sinus fungal infection results in invasion to ICA and worsens the patient's prognosis by cerebral infarction (Hase et al. 2013), especially mucormycosis which has vascular tropism that initially invades the arteries and causes thrombosis and ischemic injuries (Haber et al. 2008). So early diagnosis and treatment are important. For diagnosis CTA, MRA or DSA is needed (Fig. 24.7a–c). Systemic antifungal with anticoagulant with EC-IC bypass and trapping/excision of ICA may be needed with or without CS excision specially in ICA occlusion with malignant cavernous sinus fungal infection (Neil et al. 2016).

24.8 Prevention of Fungal Infection in CS (with PNS)

Invasive fungal infections (IFIs) represent significant complications in patients with hematological malignancies and other immunodeficiencies. Chemoprevention of IFIs may be important in this setting, but most antifungal drugs have demonstrated poor efficacy, particularly in the prevention of invasive aspergillosis. Antifungal prophylaxis in hematological patients is currently regarded as the gold standard in situations with a high risk of infection, such as acute leukemia, myelodysplastic syndromes, and autologous or allogeneic hematopoietic stem cell transplantation. Over the years, a series of recommendations for antifungal prophylaxis based on prospective studies performed with different drugs were tried to establish protocols. However, the prescription of each agent must be personalized, adapting its administration to the characteristics of individual patients and taking into account possible interactions with concomitant medication. The availability of new triazoles (e.g., voriconazole, posaconazole), characterized by a wider spectrum, may have modified the role of antifungal prophylaxis in recent times (Vazquez 2016).

24.9 Conclusion

Fungal infection of CS is a lethal infective condition especially in immunocompromised or uncontrolled diabetic patient. Any lesion in the CS in immunodeficient patient especially with PNS infection should be investigated aggressively by keeping in mind that it can be of fungal origin and if proved of fungal etiology, should be treated (surgical and medical) aggressively without delay to avoid high mortality and morbidity.

References

Abdulrauf SI. Extracranial-to-intracranial bypass using radial artery grafting for complex skull base tumors: technical note. Skull Base. 2005;15:207–13.

Aribandi M, McCoy V, Bazan C. Imaging features of invasive and noninvasive fungal sinusitis: a review. Radiographics. 2007;27:1283–96.

Bray WH, Giangiacomo J, Ide CH. Orbital apex syndrome. Surv Ophthalmol. 1987;32(2):136–40.

Chan LL, Singh S, Jones D, et al. Imaging of mucormycosis skull base osteo-myelitis. AJNR Am J Neuroradiol. 2000;21:828–31.

Choi HS, Choi JY, Yoon JS, Kim SJ, Lee SY. Clinical characteristics and prognosis of orbital invasive aspergillosis. Ophthal Plast Reconstr Surg. 2008;24:454–9.

Chowdhury F, Haque M, Kawsar K, Ara S, Mohammod Q, Sarker MH, Goel A. Transcranial microsurgical and endoscopic endonasal cavernous sinus (CS) anatomy: a cadaveric study. J Neurol Surg A. 2012;73:296–306.

Couldwell WT, Macdonald JD, Taussky P. Complete resection of the cavernous sinus-indications and technique. World Neurosurg. 2014;82:1264–70.

Devèze A, Facon F, Latil G, Moulin G, Payan-Cassin H, Dessi P. Cavernous sinus thrombosis secondary to non-invasive sphenoid aspergillosis. Rhinology. 2005;43(2):152–5.

Fairley C, Sullivan TJ, Bartley P, et al. Survival after rhino-orbital cerebral mucormycosis in an immunocompetent patient. Ophthalmology. 2000;107:555.

Ferry AP. Cerebral mucormycosis (phycomycosis). Ocular findings and review of the literature. Surv Ophthalmol. 1961;6:1.

Goldberg AL, Tievsky AL, Jamshidi S. Wegener's granulomatosis invading the cavernous sinus: a CT demonstration. J Comput Assist Tomogr. 1983;7:701–3.

Haber DM, Fernandes AM, Neto DDS, Schiavetto RR. Rhino-orbitocerebral mucormycosis associated with cavernous sinus thrombosis: case report. Int Arch Otorhinolaryngol. 2008;12(4):574–8.

Hase T, Kurita H, Matsumoto E, Kuroda H, Hashimoto M, Shinoda S. A case of cavernous sinus aspergillosis. No Shinkei Geka. 2013;41(10):901–6.

Kalani MY, Kalb S, Martirosyan NL, Lettieri SC, Spetzler RF, Porter RW, et al. Cerebral revascularization and carotid artery resection at the skull base for treatment of advanced head and neck malignancies. J Neurosurg. 2013;118:637–42.

Lawton MT, Spetzler RF. Internal carotid artery sacrifice for radical resection of skull base tumors. Skull Base Surg. 1996;6:119–23.

Lee JH, Lee HK, Park JK, Choi CG, Suh DC. Cavernous sinus syndrome: clinical features and differential diagnosis with MR imaging. AJR Am J Roentgenol. 2003;181:583–90. https://doi.org/10.2214/ajr.181.2.1810583.

Mandava P, Chaljub G, Patterson K, et al. MR imaging of cavernous sinus invasion by mucormycosis: a case study. Clin Neurol Neurosurg. 2001;103:101–4.

Mauriello JA Jr, Yepez N, Mostafavi R, Barofsky J, Kapila R, Baredes S, et al. Invasive rhinosino-orbital aspergillosis with precipitous visual loss. Can J Ophthalmol. 1995;30:124–30.

McGinn JD, Isaacson JE, Scurry WC, Cheung EJ. Cavernous sinus thrombosis secondary to allergic fungal sinusitis. Rhinology. 2009;47-51:105–8.

Mendelowitsch A, Taussky P, Rem JA, Gratzl O. Clinical outcome of standard extracranial-intracranial bypass surgery in patients with symptomatic atherosclerotic occlusion of the internal carotid artery. Acta Neurochir (Wien). 2004;146:95–101.

Nadkarni T, Goel A. Aspergilloma of the brain: an overview. J Postgrad Med. 2005;51(Suppl S1):37–41.

Neil JA, Orlandi RR, Couldwell WT. Malignant fungal infection of the cavernous sinus: case report. J Neurosurg. 2016;124:861–5. https://doi.org/10.3171/2015.2.JNS142668.

Ng BHK, Kho GS, Sim SK, Liew DNS, Tang IP. Cavernous sinus fungal infection: a rare case. Br J Neurosurg. 2017:1–2. https://doi.org/10.1080/02688697.2017.1335857. Accessed 09 Jun 2017

Ohta S, Nishizawa S, Namba H, et al. Bilateral cavernous sinus actinomycosis resulting in painful ophthalmoplegia: case report. J Neurosurg. 2002;96:600–2.

Pagliani L, Campi L, Cavallini GM. Orbital actinomycosis associated with painful ophthalmoplegia: actinomycosis of the orbit. Ophthalmologica. 2006;220:201–5.

Parikh SL, Venkatraman G, DelGaudio JM. Invasive fungal sinusitis: a 15-year review from a single institution. Am J Rhinol. 2004;18:75–81.

Paulltauf A. Mycosis mucorina. Virchows Arch. 1885;102:543–9.

Prabhu RM, Patel R. Mucormycosis and entomophthoramycosis: a review of the clinical manifestations, diagnosis and treatment. Clin Microbiol Infect. 2004;10(suppl 1):31.

Rao SP, Kumar KR, Rokade VR, Khanna V, Pal C. Orbital apex syndrome due to mucormycosis caused by Rhizopus microsporum. Indian J Otolaryngol Head Neck Surg. 2006;58(1):83–8.

Razek AA, Castillo M. Imaging lesions of the cavernous sinus. AJNR Am J Neuroradiol. 2009;30(3):444–52. https://doi.org/10.3174/ajnr.A1398.

Shah NJ, Rathore A. Intracranial extension of fungal sinusitis. Otorhinolaryngol Clin. 2009;1(1):55–61.

Sivak-Callcott JA, Livesley N, Nugent RA, Rasmussen SL, Saeed P, Rootman J. Localised invasive sino-orbital aspergillosis: characteristic features. Br J Ophthalmol. 2004;88:681–7.

Stringer SP, Ryan MW. Chronic invasive fungal rhinosinusitis. Otolaryngol Clin N Am. 2000;33:375–87.

Tang Y, Booth T, Steward M, Solbach T, Wilhelm T. The imaging of conditions affecting the cavernous sinus. Clin Radiol. 2010;65:937–45.

Taussky P, Couldwell W. Decision-making strategies for EC-IC bypass in the treatment of skull base tumors. In: Abdelrauf SI, editor. Cerebral revascularization: techniques in extracranial-to-intracranial bypass surgery. Philadelphia: Saunders; 2010. p. 349–54.

Thompson GR, Patterson TF. Fungal disease of the nose and paranasal sinuses. J Allergy Clin Immunol. 2011;129:321–6.

Van Johnson E, Kline LB, Julian BA. Bilateral cavernous sinus thrombosis due to mucormycosis. Arch Ophthalmol. 1988;106(8):1089–92.

Vazquez L. Antifungal prophylaxis in immunocompromised patients. Mediterr J Hematol Infect Dis. 2016;8(1):e2016040. https://doi.org/10.4084/MJHID.2016.040.

Yohai RA, Bullock JD, Aziz AA, Markert RJ. Survival factors in rhino-orbital-cerebral mucormycosis. Surv Ophthalmol. 1994;39(1):3–22.

Intracranial Fungal Aneurysms

25

Ali Akhaddar and Sylma Diabira

Abbreviations

CNS	Central nervous system
CSF	Cerebrospinal fluid
CT	Computed tomography
ICA	Internal carotid artery
IFA	Intracranial fungal aneurysm
IIA	Intracranial infectious aneurysm
MR	Magnetic resonance

25.1 Introduction

Infectious intracranial aneurysms (IIA) or so-called mycotic aneurysms or microbial aneurysms are rare cerebrovascular lesions that occur through microbial infection of the brain arterial wall (Akhaddar 2017a). The term "mycotic" was first used by Osler in 1885 because of the resemblance of such lesion with "fungal vegetation" (Osler 1885). Although they can be secondary to fungal pathogen, most infectious intracranial aneurysms are bacterial (Choi et al. 2014; Ducruet et al. 2010).

It is well known that intracranial fungal aneurysm (IFA) is among the most serious complications of central nervous sytem (CNS) fungal infections with a high mortality rate (Azar et al. 2016; Kannoth et al. 2007; Kunimatsu et al. 2015). The first publication of a histologically verified IFA was reported in 1965, when Stehbens described a 35-year-old woman with a history of acute leukemia who was found to have an intracranial internal carotid artery (ICA) fusiform aneurysm due to proliferation of mucormycosis. This patient presented with an episode of meningitis (Stehbens 1965). Since Stehbens's description, reports of IFAs are very rare and largely confined to isolated case reports and small series.

For this chapter we will focus on IIA secondary to fungal infections. Although there is a paucity of data in the current literature regarding IFA, we will provide in this report a practical review regarding these potentially fatal cerebrovascular lesions and their management strategies.

25.2 Epidemiology

Among IIA, fungal forms are known to be rare representing about 1% of all infectious aneurysms (Brown et al. 1984). But, in the past few years, the literature in this field has increased in

A. Akhaddar (✉)
Department of Neurosurgery, Avicenne Military Hospital of Marrakech, Mohammed V University of Rabat, Rabat, Morocco

S. Diabira
Department of Neurosurgery, Avicenne Military Hospital of Marrakech, Mohammed V University of Rabat, Rabat, Morocco

Spine Surgery Unit, Private Hospital of Saint-Grégoire, Rennes, France

M. Turgut et al. (eds.), *Fungal Infections of the Central Nervous System*,
https://doi.org/10.1007/978-3-030-06088-6_25

complexity and quantity owing to the recent increase in the number of immunocompromised patients and those with fungal paranasal sinusitis (Azar et al. 2016; Muraoka et al. 2016; Ogawa et al. 2015; Radotra et al. 2015; Shinya et al. 2015; Yamaguchi et al. 2016). In Kannoth's series published in 2007, IFA represented 16 % (4 cases) of all 25 cases of IIA (Kannoth et al. 2007). More recently, a literature review performed by Choi et al. estimated that 4% of all IIA were fungal in origin (Choi et al. 2014). At least, half of these patients were immunocompromised. Knouse et al., reported that 14% of all carotid IIA were fungal in origin (Knouse et al. 2002). The difficulty in estimating the exact incidence of IFA is due to the undefined natural history of these vascular lesions.

IFA are less common in infants than in adults without apparent sex predominance (Ahmad et al. 2006; Choi et al. 2014; Goldman et al. 1979; Loeys et al. 1999; Marazzi et al. 2008). Unlike the bacterial ones, IFA arise mostly in the setting of an extravascular infection (paranasal sinusitis, orbital cellulitis, meningitis, and post-craniotomy infections) especially in an immunocompromised host (Azar et al. 2016; Corvisier et al. 1987; Hurst et al. 2001; Morriss and Spock 1970; Negoro et al. 2013; Okada et al. 1998; Piotrowski et al. 1990; Takeshita et al. 1992; Yip et al. 2012). Fungal infections are unusually encountered in the context of endocarditis (Ahmad et al. 2014; Takeda et al. 1998).

25.3 Pathogenesis and Pathology

As is the case for all other forms of IIA, three recognized sources of fungal intracranial aneurysmal formation were previously suggested (Akhaddar 2017a; Kannoth and Thomas 2009): (1) from a remote extracranial site (hematogenous dissemination), (2) through a contiguous cranial focus (direct invasion), or (3) from a contamination secondary to improper neurosurgical procedures, especially following pituitary surgery (Horten et al. 1976; Kasliwal et al. 2009; Okada et al. 1998; Radotra et al. 2015; Visudhiphan et al. 1973). However, some primary forms could be cryptogenic without obvious definite source of fungal infection (Abecassis et al. 2013). Direct invasion from adjacent skull base structures (such as paranasal sinuses, orbit, or the ear) is more likely encountered involving proximal segments of the intracranial arterial vasculature (Corvisier et al. 1987; Gulshan et al. 1978; Morriss and Spock 1970; Takeda et al. 1998; Watson et al. 1999). In the opposite, hematogenous dissemination is likely associated with distal branching aneurysm (Choi et al. 2014).

Most invasive skull base fungal infections have a propensity to invade the ICA, cavernous sinus, and the adjacent brain vasculature (Akhaddar 2017b, 2008). This can result in thrombosis, stenosis or aneurysmal formations including their own cerebrovascular complications (Hurst et al. 2001; Muraoka et al. 2016). Also, IFA may be associated with a granulomatous inflammation of the brain and meninges, causing granuloma formation, meningitis, or meningoencephalitis (Kannoth et al. 2007; Negoro et al. 2013). In a study of 11 patients with fungal ICA aneurysms, 7 were confirmed to be secondary to direct invasion from a paranasal sinus, and the sphenoid sinus was the most frequently involved sinus (4 cases among 7) (Hot et al. 2007).

Unlike the non- infectious aneurysm, size seems not a reliable predictor of potential rupture for IFA. It was observed that even small IIA can rupture and bleed fatally, while many IIA may enlarge and produce progressive symptoms (Choi et al. 2014).

Aspergillus species, *Candida albicans*, and *Mucor* species are the three most common pathogens causing IFA (Abecassis et al. 2013; Azar et al. 2016; Hot et al. 2007). Aspergillosis may be involved in more than 2/3 of all fungal forms. Other reported fungi include *Pseudallescheria boydii*, *Coccidioides*, and *Scedosporium* species (Kannoth and Thomas 2009; Ong et al. 2011). Aspergillosis has a special vasocentric tropism in deep fungi. Elastase produced by this fungus can induce aneurysm formation. Elastase decomposes elastin, a major component of the vascular wall, and induces inflammation and fragility in all layers of the vascular wall (Kothary et al. 1984; Paris et al. 1997). Furthermore, the intraluminal vascular extension of fungal hyphae may cause in situ thrombosis and occlusion with resulting infarction of the affected larger vascular distribution (Ho and Deruytter 2004; Kikuchi et al. 1985; Muraoka et al. 2016). A combination of fungal and bacterial components in the same IIA was previously described by Abecassis et al. (2013).

25.4 Clinical Features

Clinical presentations cannot be categorized as being typical and may vary widely. However, the most common signs and symptoms of IFA are those related to aneurysm bleeding (subarachnoid and/or intraparenchymal hemorrhage) and their causative origin (Ducruet et al. 2010; Yamaguchi et al. 2016). IFA can present with headache, seizures, meningitis, focal neurological signs, or altered mental status. However, fever occurs unusually (Ahmad et al. 2006).

It is often difficult to diagnose a patient with an IFA before it ruptures because its clinical manifestations are insidious. Among 18 patients with fungal aneurysms reported by Yamagushi et al., just five patients were diagnosed before its rupture (Yamaguchi et al. 2016). Patients with IFA occurring from an extravascular origin tend to have symptoms and signs of more local or regional infections with no aneurysmal rupture. In these patients clinical features are those related to skull base, paranasal, orbital, or orbito-cerebral invasion. Some cases with extracranial hemorrhage have been reported, especially severe epistaxis (Hot et al. 2007; Hurst et al. 2001; Kim et al. 2012).

It's important to have a high index of suspicion of an IFA in patients with other fungal infections in the body, particularly those with fungal paranasal sinusitis, cavernous sinus, and orbital apex syndromes. Screening of the whole body should be done to look for concomitant systemic and/or local infectious sources (Ahmad et al. 2014; Marazzi et al. 2008).

25.5 Diagnosis

Digital subtraction angiography continues to be the gold standard for the diagnosis of IFA (Yamaguchi et al. 2016), although computed tomography (CT) scan angiography and magnetic resonance (MR) angiography can be used. On the other hand, parenchymal changes (cerebral infarction and/or hemorrhage) associated with the aneurysmal lesion are better assessed on MR imaging (Muraoka et al. 2016).

All IIA are typically thin-walled and friable, often with a wide or absent neck and a high tendency to rupture and bleed (Akhaddar 2017a; Ducruet et al. 2010). Classically, fungal mycotic aneurysms tend to be solitary, larger, and longer than bacterial ones and located in major cerebral artery trunks (like internal carotid and basilar arteries) as opposed to bacterial intracranial aneurysms that are small and located in the distal branches of the middle cerebral artery consistent with their pathogenesis in which septic emboli lodge within the blood vessel (Fig. 25.1) (Kasliwal et al. 2009; Negoro et al. 2013; Ogawa et al. 2015; Piotrowski et al. 1990; Zanaty et al. 2013). Multiple IFAs are infrequent (Kasliwal et al. 2009; Kim et al. 2012; Kikuchi et al. 1985; Yip et al. 2012). Change in the size of the aneurysm or appearance of new aneurysmal lesion on follow-up angiogram may also predict an IFA (Kojima et al. 1989).

Definitive diagnosis is often difficult and should be made by direct examination and culture of the vascular lesion although it is not always an easy option. Determining species is critical to choose the most appropriate antifungal drug (Akhaddar 2017b). Despite serial blood and cerebrospinal fluid (CSF) cultures, pathogenic agents are rarely identified (Kojima et al. 1989; Negoro et al. 2013; Yip et al. 2012). Leukocytosis, elevated erythrocyte sedimentation rates (ESR), and elevated C-reactive protein (CRP) levels are not specific in cases of fungal infection. In some cases, clinical evidence has been limited to surrogate markers like galactomannan in CSF for diagnosis of brain aspergillosis (Mennink-Kersten et al. 2004; Verweij et al. 1999). Biopsy of extracranial suspected lesions may be helpful but often requiring multiple interventions (Ahsan et al. 2009).

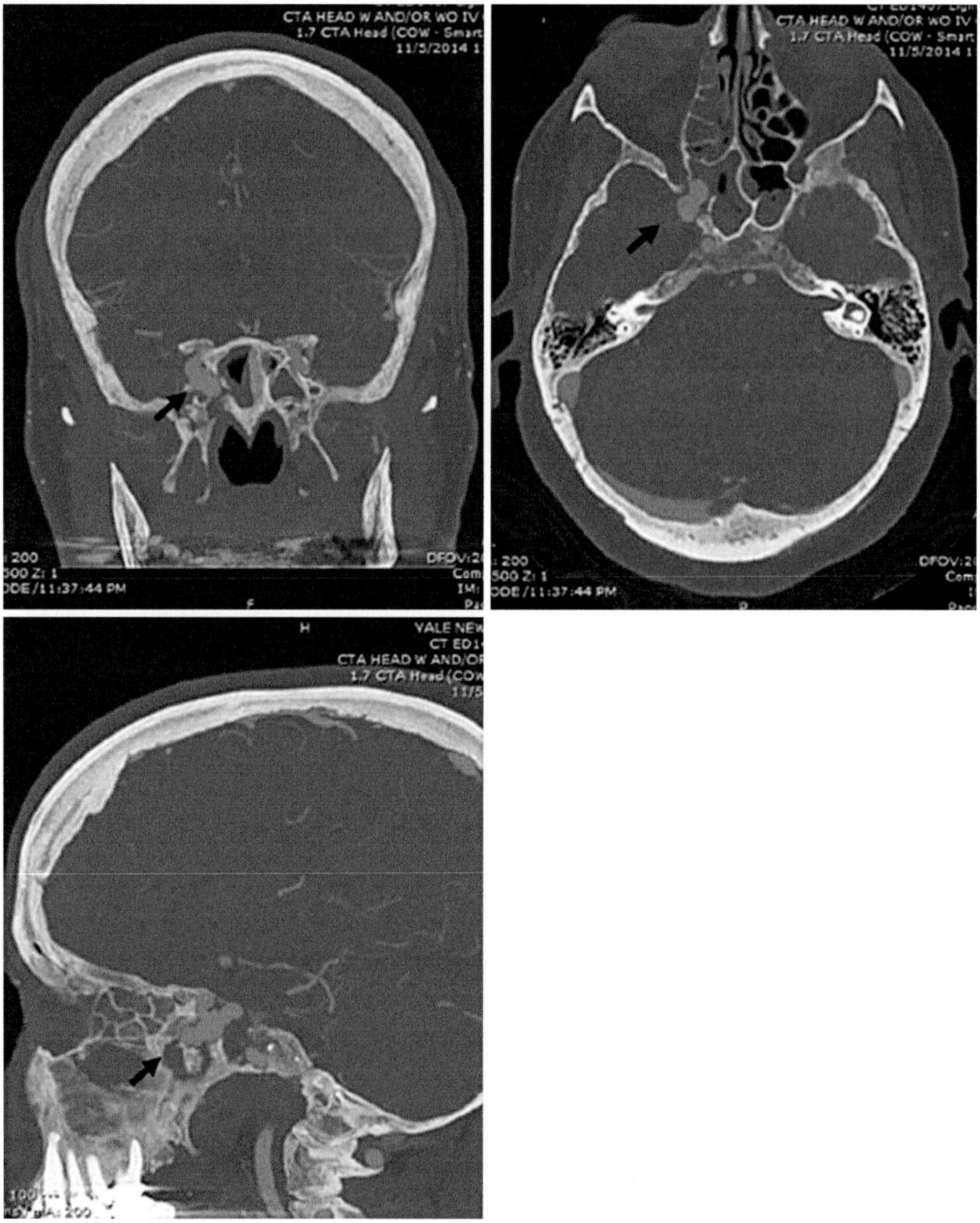

Fig. 25.1 Computed tomography (CT) scan of the brain shows a 1.2 × 0.8 cm bilobed aneurysm (arrows) arising from the cavernous part of the right internal carotid artery (ICA) and eroding into the sphenoid sinus [Reproduced from Azrar MM et al. Mycopathologia (2016)181:425-33; with permission]

25.6 Treatment Options

All the patients with IFA would require treatment with appropriate antifungal agents. There is no clear accepted procedure for management which may differ according to specific details of individual patients with IFA such as the character and position of the aneurysm itself as well as the clinical condition. In the past, the presence of fungal intracranial aneurysmal lesion was a relative indication for conservative nonsurgical management. However, since the last few decades, open surgical and/or endovascular procedures have been generally accepted (Ducruet et al. 2010; Hot et al. 2007).

The duration of antifungal therapy required for cure has not been well defined (between 6 weeks and up to 6 months). It seems that bacterial intracranial aneurysms respond more favorably to anti-infectious therapy than fungal ones (Ahsan et al. 2009). The net state of immunosuppression, the involved fungal pathogen (mucormycosis being more difficult to cure than aspergillosis), and the adequacy of source control are key factors to consider in determining treatment discontinuation (Azar et al. 2016).

Concerning open surgery, because of the very friable nature of the IFA, clip ligation may not always be feasible (not easy and/or hazardous). In this case, wrapping the aneurysm dome is a surgical treatment option, as is trapping the parent artery (Choi et al. 2014). For proximal aneurysms, such as ICA lesions, carotid ligation with distal revascularization may be an option (Yamaguchi et al. 2016).

Treatment of the causal predisposing infection is an important part of therapy.

Recent publications recommend initiating antifungal therapy and serial angiography or MR angiography for all unruptured fungal aneurysms to monitor the progression of the aneurysmal lesion closely. If a non- ruptured fungal aneurysm fails to resolve, enlarges, or ruptures, then the patient should be evaluated for endovascular therapy or open microvascular surgery to prevent bleeding. Several case reports have shown that ruptured IFA treated with surgery and antifungal therapy fare better than those treated with antifungal drugs alone (Choi et al. 2014; Ho and Deruytter 2004; Kannoth et al. 2007). Over the last decade, advancements in coil and stent design, embolic agents, guide catheters, and microwires have facilitated the treatment of IFA and have provided a safe and effective first approach especially in critically ill patients at high surgical risk, and preliminary studies have shown encouraging results (Fig. 25.2) (Azar et al. 2016; Eddleman et al. 2008; Grandhi et al. 2014; Hot et al. 2007; Kim et al. 2012; Zanaty et al. 2013).

25.7 Outcomes

Compared to bacterial IIA, fungal ones lead to a poor outcome because of a mixture of difficulty in making a correct diagnosis, poor favorable response to antifungal drugs, proximal site of the aneurysms, adjacent artery thrombosis, immunocompromised status, serious medical comorbidities, and often a friable arterial wall. Generally, patients with no ruptured aneurysm had better outcomes than those with aneurysmal rupture (Choi et al. 2014; Shinya et al. 2015).

In the past, patients with IFA had a very poor outcome with a mortality rate greater than 90% despite medical or surgical treatment (Ahsan et al. 2009; Kojima et al. 1989; Negoro et al. 2013). But, in most recent case series, mortality was much lower (between 58 and 12%) especially for patients managed with modern endovascular therapy (Hot et al. 2007; Kannoth and Thomas 2009; Kim et al. 2012; Yamaguchi et al. 2016).

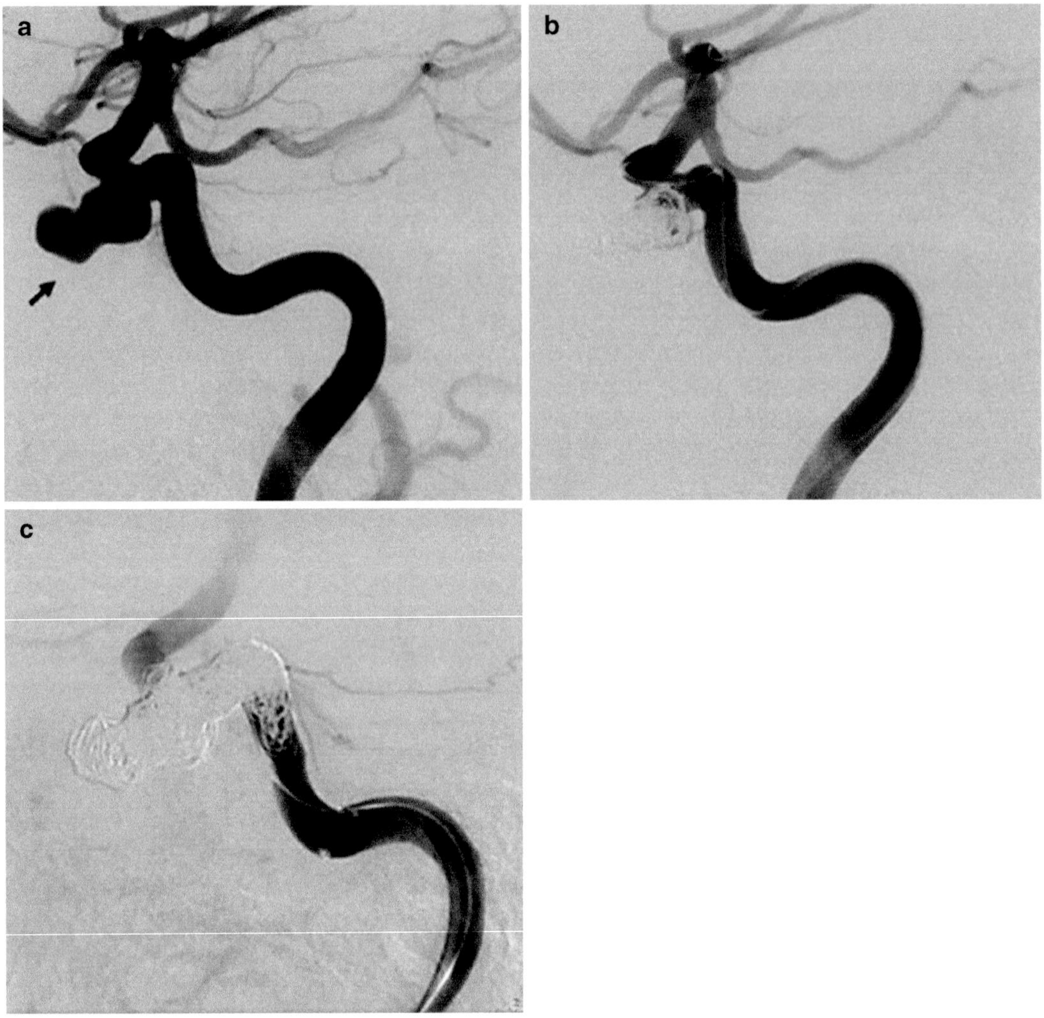

Fig. 25.2 Angiography of the right carotid artery and cerebral circulation. The aneurysm (arrow) is shown arising from the horizontal segment of the cavernous right ICA (**a**). Coil embolization of the aneurysm (**b**) and the parent vessel (**c**) is shown. Completion angiography shows successful exclusion of the aneurysm (**c**) [Reproduced from Azrar MM et al. Mycopathologia (2016)181:425-33; with permission]

25.8 Conclusion

Among the cerebrovascular lesions, fungal intracranial aneurysm has been reported as very rare with high mortality rate. Diagnosis and management of this complex form of infectious intracranial aneurysms is a true challenge because they are unpredictable and often occur in a clinical context that is neither specific nor alarming. IFAs require a high index of suspicion, multidisciplinary team approach for expeditious and accurate diagnosis, appropriate antifungal therapy, surgical/endovascular intervention if necessary, and treatment of any underlying disorder. The patient's initial clinical condition and the potential concomitant diseases are the strongest predictors of the outcome.

References

Abecassis IJ, Adel JG, Ayer A, Batjer HH. A ruptured infectious intracranial aneurysm with a combined fungal and bacterial etiology. Clin Neurol Neurosurg. 2013;115(11):2393–6. https://doi.org/10.1016/j.clineuro.2013.08.026.

Ahmad FU, Mahajan H, Mahapatra AK, Suri A. Mycotic aneurysm. An unusual cause of pyrexia of unknown origin in an immunodeficient infant. Pediatr Neurosurg. 2006;42(4):237–9.

Ahmad RA, Hussain ST, Tan CD, Pettersson GB, Clair D, Gordon SM. Successful surgical treatment of rare Aspergillus terreus prosthetic valve endocarditis complicated by intracranial and mesenteric artery mycotic aneurysms. J Thorac Cardiovasc Surg. 2014;148(5):e221–3. https://doi.org/10.1016/j.jtcvs.2014.06.084.

Ahsan H, Ajmal F, Saleem MF, Sonawala AB. Cerebral fungal infection with mycotic aneurysm of basilar artery and subarachnoid haemorrhage. Singapore Med J. 2009;50(1):e22–5.

Akhaddar A. Intracranial Infectious Aneurysms. In: Akhaddar A, editor. Atlas of infections in neurosurgery and spinal surgery. 1st ed. Cham: Springer International Publishing; 2017a. p. 143–8. https://doi.org/10.1007/978-3-319-60086-4_15.

Akhaddar A. Fungal infections of the Central Nervous System. In: Akhaddar A, editor. Atlas of infections in neurosurgery and spinal surgery. 1st ed. Cham: Springer International Publishing; 2017b. p. 317–23. https://doi.org/10.1007/978-3-319-60086-4_29.

Akhaddar A, Gazzaz M, Albouzidi A, Lmimouni B, Boucetta M. Invasive Aspergillus terreus sinusitis with orbitocranial extension: case report. Surg Neurol. 2008;69(5):490–5. discussion 495. https://doi.org/10.1016/j.surneu.2007.02.059.

Azar MM, Assi R, Patel N, Malinis MF. Fungal mycotic aneurysm of the internal carotid artery associated with sphenoid sinusitis in an immunocompromised patient: a case report and review of the literature. Mycopathologia. 2016;181:425–33. https://doi.org/10.1007/s11046-015-9975-1.

Brown SL, Busuttil RW, Baker JD, Machleder HI, Moore WS, Barker WF. Bacteriologic and surgical determinants of survival in patients with mycotic aneurysms. J Vasc Surg. 1984;1:541–7.

Choi H, Hall WA, Deshaies EM. Infectious intracranial aneurysms. In: Hall WA, KIM PD, editors. Neurosurgical infectious disease. Surgical and nonsurgical management. New York: Thieme; 2014. p. 133–46.

Corvisier N, Gray F, Gherardi R, Lebras F, Blanc CM, Nyugen JP, et al. Aspergillosis of ethmoid sinus and optic nerve, with arteritis, and rupture of the internal carotid artery. Surg Neurol. 1987;28:311–5.

Ducruet AF, Hickman ZL, Zacharia BE, Narula R, Grobelny BT, Gorski J, et al. Intracranial infectious aneurysms: a comprehensive review. Neurosurg Rev. 2010;33:37–46. https://doi.org/10.1007/s10143-009-0233-1.

Eddleman CS, Surdell D, DiPatri A Jr, Tomita T, Shaibani A. Infectious intracranial aneurysms in the pediatric population: endovascular treatment with Onyx. Childs Nerv Syst. 2008;24(8):909–15. https://doi.org/10.1007/s00381-008-0614-8.

Goldman JA, Fleischer AS, Leifer W, Parent A, Schwarzman SW, Raggio J. Candida albicans mycotic aneurysm associated with systemic lupus erythematosus. Neurosurgery. 1979;4:325–8.

Grandhi R, Zwagerman NT, Linares G, Monaco EA 3rd, Jovin T, Horowitz M, et al. Onyx embolization of infectious intracranial aneurysms. J Neurointerv Surg. 2014;6(5):353–6. https://doi.org/10.1136/neurintsurg-2013-010755.

Gulshan KA, Neeraj J, Malini V, Subimal R. Cerebral mycotic aneurysm of fungal origin. Case report. J Neurosurg. 1978;49:107–10.

Ho CL, Deruytter MJ. CNS aspergillosis with mycotic aneurysm, cerebral granuloma and infarction. Acta Neurochir (Wien). 2004;146:851–6.

Horten BC, Abbott GF, Porro RS. Fungal aneurysms of intracranial vessels. Arch Neurol. 1976;33:577–9.

Hot A, Mazighi M, Lecuit M, Poirée S, Viard JP, Loulergue P, et al. Fungal internal carotid artery aneurysms: successful embolization of an Aspergillus-associated case and review. Clin Infect Dis. 2007;45(12):e156–61. https://doi.org/10.1086/523005.

Hurst RW, Judkins A, Bolger W, Chu A, Loevner LA. Mycotic aneurysm and cerebral infarction resulting from fungal sinusitis: imaging and pathologic correlation. AJNR Am J Neuroradiol. 2001;22:858–63.

Kannoth S, Thomas SV. Intracranial microbial aneurysm (infectious aneurysm): current options for diagnosis and management. Neurocrit Care. 2009;11:120–9. https://doi.org/10.1007/s12028-009-9208-x.

Kannoth S, Iyer R, Thomas SV, Furtado SV, Rajesh BJ, Kesavadas C, et al. Intracranial infectious aneurysm: presentation, management and outcome. J Neurol Sci. 2007;256(1-2):3–9.

Kasliwal MK, Reddy VS, Sinha S, Sharma BS, Das P, Suri V. Bilateral anterior cerebral artery aneurysm due to mucormycosis. J Clin Neurosci. 2009;16(1):156–9. https://doi.org/10.1016/j.jocn.2008.04.019.

Kikuchi K, Watanabe K, Sugawara A, Kowada M. Multiple fungal aneurysms: report of a rare case implicating steroid as predisposing factor. Surg Neurol. 1985;24(3):253–9.

Kim YC, Lee H, Ryu HH, Beom SH, Yang Y, Kim S, et al. Aspergillus-associated cerebral aneurysm successfully treated by endovascular and surgical intervention with voriconazole in lupus nephritis patient. J Korean

Med Sci. 2012;27(3):317–20. https://doi.org/10.3346/jkms.2012.27.3.317.
Knouse MC, Madeira RG, Celani VJ. Pseudomonas aeruginosa causing a right carotid artery mycotic aneurysm after a dental extraction procedure. Mayo Clin Proc. 2002;77:1125–30.
Kojima Y, Saito A, Kim I. The role of serial angiography in the management of bacterial and fungal intracranial aneurysms—report of two cases and review of the literature. Neurol Med Chir (Tokyo). 1989;29(3):202–16.
Kothary MH, Chase T Jr, Macmillan JD. Correlation of elastase production by some strains of Aspergillus fumigatus with ability to cause pulmonary invasive aspergillosis in mice. Infect Immun. 1984;43(1):320–5.
Kunimatsu A, Tsuji S, Saito N. Recurrent cerebral aneurysm formation and rupture within a short period due to invasive aspergillosis of the nasal sinus; pathological analysis of the catastrophic clinical course. Int J Clin Exp Pathol. 2015;8(10):13510–22.
Loeys BL, Van Coster RN, Defreyne LR, Leroy JG. Fungal intracranial aneurysm in a child with familial chronic mucocutaneous candidiasis. Eur J Pediatr. 1999;158(8):650–2.
Marazzi MG, Bondi E, Giannattasio A, Strozzi M, Savioli C. Intracranial aneurysm associated with chronic mucocutaneous candidiasis. Eur J Pediatr. 2008;167:461–3.
Mennink-Kersten MA, Donnelly JP, Verweij PE. Detection of circulating galactomannan for the diagnosis and management of invasive Aspergillosis. Lancet Infect Dis. 2004;4:349–57.
Morriss FH Jr, Spock A. Intracranial aneurysm secondary to mycotic orbital and sinus infection: report of a case implicating penicillium as an opportunistic fungus. Am J Dis Child. 1970;119:357–62.
Muraoka S, Araki Y, Izumi T, Takeuchi K, Okamoto S, Wakabayashi T. Cerebral infarction and subarachnoid hemorrhage caused by central nervous system Aspergillus infection. World Neurosurg. 2016;90:705.e9–705.e13. https://doi.org/10.1016/j.wneu.2016.03.021.
Negoro E, Morinaga K, Taga M, Kaizaki Y, Kawai Y. Mycotic aneurysm due to Aspergillus sinusitis. Int J Hematol. 2013;98(1):4–5. https://doi.org/10.1007/s12185-013-1369-x.
Ogawa M, Sakurai K, Kawaguchi T, Naiki-Ito A, Nakagawa M, Okita K, et al. Internal carotid artery blister-like aneurysm caused by Aspergillus—case report. Pol J Radiol. 2015;80:159–63. https://doi.org/10.12659/PJR.893050.
Okada Y, Shima T, Nishida M, Yamane K, Yoshida A. Subarachnoid hemorrhage caused by Aspergillus aneurysm as a complication of transcranial biopsy of an orbital apex lesion—case report. Neurol Med Chir (Tokyo). 1998;38(7):432–7.
Ong A, Blyth CC, Bency R, Vicaretti M, Harun A, Meyer W, et al. Fatal mycotic aneurysms due to Scedosporium and Pseudallescheria infection. J Clin Microbiol. 2011;49(5):2067–71. https://doi.org/10.1128/JCM.02615-10.
Osler W. Goulstonian lectures on malignant endocarditis. Brit Med J. 1885;1:467–70.
Paris S, Boisvieux-Ulrich E, Crestani B, Houcine O, Taramelli D, Lombardi L, et al. Internalization of Aspergillus fumigatus conidia by epithelial and endothelial cells. Infect Immun. 1997;65(4):1510–4.
Piotrowski WP, Pilz P, Chuang IH. Subarachnoid hemorrhage caused by a fungal aneurysm of the vertebral artery as a complication of intracranial aneurysm clipping. Case report. J Neurosurg. 1990;73(6):962–4.
Radotra BD, Salunke P, Parthan G, Dutta P, Vyas S, Mukherjee KK. True mycotic aneurysm in a patient with gonadotropinoma after trans-sphenoidal surgery. Surg Neurol Int. 2015;6:193. https://doi.org/10.4103/2152-7806.172697.
Shinya Y, Miyawaki S, Nakatomi H, Okano A, Imai H, Shin M, et al. Recurrent cerebral aneurysm formation and rupture within a short period due to invasive aspergillosis of the nasal sinus; pathological analysis of the catastrophic clinical course. Int J Clin Exp Pathol. 2015;8(10):13510–22.
Stehbens WE. Atypical cerebral aneurysms. Med J Aust. 1965;1(21):765–6.
Takeda S, Wakabayashi K, Yamazaki K, Miyakawa T, Arai H. Intracranial fungal aneurysm caused by Candida endocarditis. Clin Neuropathol. 1998;17:199–203.
Takeshita M, Izawa M, Kubo O, Tanikawa T, Onda H, Wanifuchi H, Tamura Y, Kagawa M. Aspergillotic aneurysm formation of cerebral artery following neurosurgical operation. Surg Neurol. 1992;38:146–51.
Verweij PE, Brinkman K, Kremer HP, Kullberg BJ, Meis JF. Aspergillus meningitis: diagnosis by non-culture-based microbiological methods and management. J Clin Microbiol. 1999;37:1186–9.
Visudhiphan P, Bunyaratavej S, Khantanaphar S. Cerebral aspergillosis. Report of three cases. J Neurosurg. 1973;38:472–6.
Watson JC, Myseros JS, Bullock MS. True fungal mycotic aneurysm of the basilar artery: a clinical and surgical dilemma. Cerebrovasc Dis. 1999;9:50–3.
Yamaguchi J, Kawabata T, Motomura A, Hatano N, Seki Y. Fungal internal carotid artery aneurysm treated by trapping and high-flow bypass: a case report and literature review. Neurol Med Chir (Tokyo). 2016;56(2):89–94. https://doi.org/10.2176/nmc.cr.2015-0206.
Yip CM, Hsu SS, Liao WC, Chen JY, Liu SH, Chen CH. Orbital apex syndrome due to aspergillosis with subsequent fatal subarachnoid hemorrhage. Surg Neurol Int. 2012;3:124. https://doi.org/10.4103/2152-7806.102349.
Zanaty M, Chalouhi N, Starke RM, Tjoumakaris S, Gonzalez LF, Hasan D, et al. Endovascular treatment of cerebral mycotic aneurysm: a review of the literature and single center experience. Biomed Res Int. 2013;2013:151643. https://doi.org/10.1155/2013/151643.

Acute Ischemic or Hemorrhagic Stroke Syndromes

26

Arsovska Anita and Arsovski Zoran

Abbreviations

AIDS	Acquired immunodeficiency syndrome
CNS	Central nervous system
CSF	Cerebrospinal fluid
CT	Computed tomography
GI	Gastrointestinal
HIV	Human immunodeficiency virus
i.v	Intravenous
MCA	Middle cerebral artery
MR	Magnetic resonance
rtPA	Recombinant tissue plasminogen activator
WHO	World Health Organization

26.1 Introduction

Acute stroke is a medical emergency; it is the leading cause of adult physical disability and second most common cause of death worldwide (Murray et al. 2012). According to the World Health Organization (WHO), there are 15 million people in the world who suffer from stroke every year. The two main types of stroke are ischemic stroke that occurs in 80–85% of the cases and hemorrhagic stroke that occurs in 15–20%. The risk factors for stroke (modifiable and nonmodifiable) have already been established and are well known; however, in certain cases, the epidemiology of stroke cannot be sufficiently explained only by their presence (Grau et al. 2010). Presence of certain infections may add a higher risk for stroke occurrence (Wolf et al. 1991). Actually, the relationship between stroke and infection is bidirectional, infections can cause stroke, and on the other hand, the rate of infection is increased after stroke.

26.2 Epidemiology

The exact incidence and prevalence of acute ischemic and hemorrhagic stroke syndromes related to fungal infections are unknown (Fugate et al. 2014). They occur rarely. Case reports and case series have been reported (Kalita et al. 1999; Calli et al. 1999; Goel et al. 1999; Murthy et al. 2000). Ischemic strokes related to fungal infections are more common compared to hemorrhagic strokes.

A. Anita (✉)
University Clinic of Neurology, Medical Faculty, University of Ss. Cyril and Methodius, Skopje, Republic of North Macedonia

A. Zoran
University Clinic of Pulmonology and Allergy, Medical Faculty, University of Ss. Cyril and Methodius, Skopje, Republic of North Macedonia

M. Turgut et al. (eds.), *Fungal Infections of the Central Nervous System*,
https://doi.org/10.1007/978-3-030-06088-6_26

26.3 Etiology and Pathogenesis

Fungal infection is a possible trigger for stroke, and it can act independently or in association with traditional vascular risk factors. Invasion and occlusion of arteries, large vessel vasculitis, embolization, and intracerebral/subarachnoid hemorrhage after rupture of mycotic aneurysms are cerebrovascular complications of central nervous system (CNS) fungal infections.

Ischemic stroke in CNS fungal infections can occur as a result of arterial narrowing (cerebral vasculitis, vasospasm, intra-arterial thrombosis) or infective endocarditis causing embolism. Fungal infections of the intracranial arteries may cause continuous vascular inflammation, necrosis of the vessel wall, occlusion, and ischemia. Severe infections may also activate the coagulation pathway and cause cytokine-mediated and immune deposition.

Intracerebral and/or subarachnoid hemorrhage occurs when mycotic aneurysms rupture, which are located in distal branches of intracranial arteries.

Gradual contiguous involvement of the skull base structures in cases of prolonged paranasal fungal sinusitis (commonly aspergillosis, zygomycosis, cladosporiosis, etc.) leads to angioinvasion which in turn results in fungal vasculitis, and thereafter the thrombotic occlusions occur in the major branches of the cerebral blood vessels of the anterior and posterior circulation. The hyphae invade the vessel walls causing cerebral arterial thrombosis, cerebral infarction, and cerebritis. The hemorrhagic infarcts may convert into septic infarcts. In the study by Sharma et al. of 170 patients, there were 45 cases of major cerebral artery thrombosis, either in the territory of internal carotid artery or in the basilar artery (Sharma et al. 2006).

On the other hand, ischemic (cardioembolic stroke) can be caused by fungal endocarditis, which accounts for 1.3–6% of infective endocarditis (Bayer and Scheld 2000; Karchmer 2000). Fungal endocarditis can occur at any age, but it generally affects individuals older than 50 years of age. The treatment of fungal endocarditis is based on the specific fungal type causing the infection. The mainstay of treatment is through antifungal medication; surgery may be required in some cases. Untreated fungal endocarditis can lead to an extremely poor prognosis and can almost always be fatal. With appropriate early diagnosis and treatment, the outcomes are better. However, the prognosis also depends upon a set of factors including the type of fungi causing infection, the health status of the individual, and the presence of any heart illness, among other factors. Other risk factors include medical procedures, such as oral surgery, tooth extraction, abdominal surgery, and genitourinary surgery; prostate resection; diagnostic procedures such as upper gastrointestinal (GI) endoscopy, colonoscopy, and barium enema; transesophageal echocardiography; placement of intravascular catheters; poor oral hygiene and aggressive brushing of teeth; heart valve related, placement of an artificial (prosthetic) valve, heart valve repaired with a prosthetic material, age-related degeneration of the heart valves, valvulopathy, or heart valve disease, arising in a transplanted heart; and heart related, previous history of endocarditis, certain congenital heart diseases, human immunodeficiency virus (HIV), and acquired immunodeficiency syndrome (AIDS) patients, because of suppressed immune system, poorly controlled diabetes, and long-standing corticosteroid therapy. Several types of fungi may cause endocarditis: *Candida albicans* (usually seen in intravenous (i.v) drug users or those with compromised immune system such as AIDS-affected individuals), *Histoplasma capsulatum*, and *Aspergillus* spp. (Pierrotti and Baddour 2002; Challa et al. 2004).

Rarely, disseminated fungal cardiac emboli lodging in the peripheral cerebral vasculature leads to intracranial fungal mycotic aneurysms, solitary or multiple, which may present with extremely rare and usually fatal complications of subarachnoid hemorrhage/intracerebral hemorrhage with and without cerebral infarctions (McKee 1950; Corvisier et al. 1987; Lau et al. 1991).

Intracranial aneurysms of fungal etiology are extremely rare, and often the diagnosis is established at autopsy. Fungal mycotic intracranial aneurysms are usually found in the setting of disseminated hematogenous infection and fungal endocarditis (Horten et al. 1976; Iihara et al. 1990; Piotrowski et al. 1990; Chou et al. 1993; Radhakrishnana et al. 1994; Kurino et al. 1994; Suzuki et al. 1995; Takeda et al. 1998; Watson et al. 1999; Ho and Deruytter 2004). Rarely, they can occur following surgery and rarely from contiguous spread from the paranasal sinuses (Takeshita et al. 1992; Hurst et al. 2001). In the first two settings, the host is immunocompromised, and in the latter settings, the host is otherwise immunocompetent. The majority of intracranial fungal mycotic aneurysms are in the proximal portion of the major arteries at the base of the brain and have been described with *Aspergillus* spp., *Candida* spp., and *Zygomycetes* spp. infections (Horten et al. 1976; Iihara et al. 1990).

Histoplasma capsulatum, *Rhizopus* spp., *Cryptococcus neoformans*, and *Exserohilum rostratum* have been related to the occurrence of ischemic stroke, while *Mucormycetes* and *Rhizopus* spp. have been related to hemorrhagic stroke. *Aspergillus* spp. and *Coccidioides immitis* have been associated with the occurrence of both types of stroke (Murthy 2007).

Sometimes ischemic and hemorrhagic stroke can present simultaneously in the same patient. Endo et al. described a case of fatal subarachnoid hemorrhage, with brain stem and cerebellar infarction, caused by *Aspergillus* infection after cerebral aneurysm surgery (Endo et al. 2002). Extremely rarely intracerebral hemorrhage can be the complication of fungal infections of the CNS.

There are three types of fungi that are implicated in stroke: single-celled yeasts, hyphae-forming molds, and dimorphic fungi that take the form of molds at ambient temperature and yeasts at human body temperature. Yeasts usually cause fungal meningitis and may cause large vessel vasculopathy, obstruction of the venous outflow, and endarteritis leading to stroke (Rosario et al. 2012; Ludmerer et al. 1993; Saul et al. 1986). They can also form focal brain parenchymal abscesses associated with hemorrhage. Molds carry enzymes that invade the wall of the cerebral blood vessels and tend to cause strokes hematogenously. Molds directly invade the cerebral vasculature, causing mycotic arteritis or aneurysms. Systemic fungal infection can also lead to septic embolic showers to the brain.

Molds: *Aspergillus* spp. are the most important human pathogenic molds associated with stroke. Aspergillosis is the most common form of angioinvasive mycosis. Most of the published cases describe aspergillosis in patients with AIDS, neutropenia, tuberculosis, cancer, or alcoholism, causing cerebral thrombosis, intracranial mycotic aneurysms, and subarachnoid hemorrhage. *Aspergillus* enzyme elastase digests the internal elastic lamina of cerebral arteries leading to focal micro-hemorrhages. Mycotic aneurysm formation may occur in the weakened walls of the cerebral arteries causing their rupture and consecutive intracerebral and/or subarachnoid hemorrhage. *Aspergillus spp* has a predilection for the small perforating arteries, causing their occlusion, with consecutive brain infarction with hemorrhagic transformation and embolism. Commonly involved brain structures are the thalamus, basal ganglia, and corpus callosum (Ashdown et al. 1994; Dayal et al. 1974; Seton et al. 2008).

Rhinocerebral mucormycosis, caused by *Mucor* spp. or *Rhizopus* spp., is a craniofacial infection that can cause ischemic stroke or hemorrhage. The highly destructive organisms can invade the walls of major intracranial arteries, including the basilar artery, predisposing to stroke and aneurysmal rupture (Rangel-Guerra et al. 1996). Fu et al. published a case report of a 38-year-old man with a basilar artery stroke due to invasive fungal sphenoid sinusitis caused by rhinocerebral form of mucormycosis (Fu et al. 2015). The rhinocerebral form can be rapidly progressive and invasive with a high mortality rate. The lumbar puncture revealed eosinophilic pleocytosis with a mildly elevated total protein and borderline low glucose level. Computed tomography (CT) scan revealed a left medullary and cerebellar infarct confirmed by magnetic resonance (MR) imaging. MR imaging also displayed a diffuse marrow signal abnormality in the clivus with contiguous sinus disease. Endoscopic sinus surgery confirmed that the fungal sinusitis was mucormycosis of the *Rhizopus* genus, which had affected the left sphenoid sinus, invaded through the skull base, and involved the basilar artery. He was given liposomal amphotericin (500 mg i.v.) with posaconazole (400 mg i.v. twice daily). Due to the severity of the invasion and poor prognosis, the patient was discharged with comfort care measures.

Exserohilum rostratum (*Setosphaeria rostrata*), a ubiquitous pigmented mold, is a rare cause of human disease but was implicated in hundreds of cases of iatrogenic nervous system infections from contaminated epidural steroid injections. Twelve percent of meningitis cases presented with posterior circulation strokes (Bell et al. 2013; Smith et al. 2013). Stroke types were ischemic or hemorrhagic and caused by mycotic arteritis.

Yeasts: *Cryptococcus* spp. and *Candida* spp. are the most important yeast infections in the CNS. Stroke, either ischemic or hemorrhagic, might arise as a rare complication of candida infection (Grouhi et al. 1998; Wasserman et al. 2009). Disseminated candidiasis can also provoke arteritis, subarachnoid hemorrhage, and multiple brain microabscesses.

Cryptococcus is the most common yeast infection in the CNS and usually happens in immunocompromised conditions, although immunocompetent hosts exist (Browne et al. 2012). *Cryptococcus* spp. invade the meninges and parenchyma to result in meningitis and, subsequently, abscesses. Strokes can occur by irritation of subarachnoid blood vessels, resulting in vasospasm and ischemic damage (Rosario et al. 2012). Alternatively, endarteritis from inflammation can result in small vessel ischemic strokes, usually in the basal ganglia, internal capsule, and thalamus (Lan et al. 2001).

Dimorphic Fungi: Major dimorphic fungi are *Histoplasma capsulatum* (*Ajellomyces capsulatus*), *Blastomyces dermatitidis* (*Ajellomyces dermatitidis*), *Coccidioides immitis*, *Paracoccidioides brasiliensis*, *Sporothrix schenckii*, and *Penicillium marneffei* (*Talaromyces marneffei*). CNS involvement by these infections is unusual; stroke is reported in only a few cases. The only reported cases of stroke were caused by blastomycosis (Elias et al. 2005; Bariola et al. 2010; Bush et al. 2013). Histoplasmosis of the nervous system usually manifests as meningitis, but pontine stroke secondary to small vessel vasculitis has been reported as a result of septic emboli in immunocompetent patients (Saccente 2008). Coccidioidomycosis can cause cerebral ischemia from septic emboli and meningeal inflammation, particularly around the basal meninges, and can be complicated by vasculitis and stroke (Williams et al. 1992). In a retrospective study of 62 patients with CNS coccidioidomycosis, nearly 40% had ischemic infarction; however only 1 case had concomitant basilar meningitis (Arsura et al. 2005).

26.4 Diagnosis

Diagnosis is established with the detailed history, clinical examination, neuroimaging methods (CT and MR imaging of the brain, CT angiography, MR angiography, conventional pancerebral angiography) and laboratory testing (specific antibodies in blood), lumbar puncture (cerebrospinal fluid (CSF) culture and microscopy), and if possible brain biopsy. Diagnostic criteria to distinguish infectious vasculitis from other causes of stroke have not been well established in the literature and need further review and standard guidelines.

26.4.1 When to Investigate for Infectious Causes

Patients who have had strokes caused by infection might be misdiagnosed if lumbar puncture is not performed. However, lumbar puncture is not indicated when evaluating a typical stroke patient, except in the setting of a subarachnoid hemorrhage. The clinical symptoms that might indicate infectious causes include a history of fever, rash, and known prior infections. For immunocompromised patients, the suspicion should be higher, and lumbar puncture should be performed. Cerebrospinal fluid (CSF) analysis is indicated when focal neurological symptoms and signs appear gradually, rather than hyperacutely, and if other classic features of CNS infection are present, such as fever, neck stiffness, and impaired consciousness. In patients with focal neurologic deficits, brain imaging should be obtained if possible before a lumbar puncture is done. Brain imaging findings might assist in the decision to do a lumbar puncture. We should also take into account possible contraindications to perform lumbar puncture. Meningeal enhancement or multifocal infarctions, particularly ones that do not respect traditional arterial or venous territories, could raise the suspicion for infectious or inflammatory pathologies.

Besides the clinical picture of stroke, the occurrence of headache, seizures, and encephalopathy in a patient who has multiple cerebral ischemic involvement, hemorrhages, or multiple white matter lesions on a brain scan should lead to the suspicion of cerebral vasculitis. An infectious origin should be considered in those patients with progressive headache, seizures, recurrent strokes, fever, infectious risk factors and findings of increased cells and proteins in CSF, and the detection of multiple cerebral artery stenoses or mycotic aneurysms on neuroimaging.

The clinical presentation varies, depending on the severity, location, and extension of stroke. Usual symptoms and signs include consciousness impairment, focal motor neurological deficit (hemiparesis, hemiplegia, quadriparesis, quadriplegia), visual field impairment (hemianopia), cerebellar symptoms, brain stem signs, and epileptic seizures. Primary infections of the CNS may be further complicated with cerebritis, cerebral edema, and hydrocephalus. Infectious vasculitis may be complicated with recurrent ischemic strokes and multiple brain hemorrhagic lesions.

Initial brain CT scan helps to rule out intracerebral hemorrhage, but it has a lower sensitivity for visualization of subarachnoid hemorrhage. MR imaging is a preferred diagnostic method; it can detect the size and distribution of deep ischemic lesions and signs of mural inflammation. Unenhanced axial T1-weighted images may depict luminal narrowing and wall thickening compared to contralateral arteries. Contrast-enhanced T1-weighted MR imaging is a sensitive test to detect large vessel vasculitis. Gadolinium enhancement is a classical sign of inflammation of vessel wall, and wall enhancement can be seen in the intracranial vessels of circle of Willis in various forms or arteritis. Gadolinium-enhanced MR imaging may also help during the follow-up of patients, since decrease of contrast enhancement is expected to be seen during convalescence. MR images can show enhancing intraparenchymal lesions with perilesional edema, enhancing or nonenhancing lesions of the meninges, choroid plexus or ependyma, hydrocephalus, white matter edema, and cerebral infarcts with or without hemorrhage. Invasive *Zygomycetes/Phycomycetes* and *Aspergillus* may cause characteristic lesions at the inferior area of frontal lobes adjacent to posterior sinuses (Arsura et al. 2005). Fungal microabscesses may appear hypointense on T2-weighted images and may show ring enhancement after contrast administration.

Enhancement of contrast, wall thickening, and lumen narrowing may be seen on CT angiography, MR angiography, and cerebral angiography, in patients with meningitis complicated with stroke. Different vascular abnormalities have been reported, such as narrowing of supraclinoid internal carotid artery, middle cerebral artery (MCA), anterior cerebral arteries, etc. Nowadays, cerebral angiography, as the invasive technique, is only used in selected cases; CT angiography and MR angiography are preferred methods. Also, it is important to know that these vascular abnormalities seen in infectious vasculitis are not specific. Unfortunately, these neuroimaging techniques cannot provide a diagnosis of vasculitis, but only vasculopathy. Vascular abnormalities can also be observed in noninfectious vasculitis and in other conditions, including intracranial atherosclerosis, cerebral reversible vasoconstriction syndrome, hypercoagulable states, and intravascular lymphoma. For this reason, the analysis of inflammatory markers, blood cultures, and CSF analysis, in the appropriate clinical context, may be needed. Brain biopsy should also be considered in the diagnosis in those cases with severe, progressive, and even life-threatening presentation. In many cases, a brain biopsy may be the only way to make certain of a vasculitis diagnosis, and pathological examination of brain/meningeal tissue may be necessary to distinguish between infectious CNS vasculitis and other diseases and to begin appropriate treatment.

Transcranial Doppler ultrasound is a noninvasive tool that may be helpful to detect focal acceleration of cerebral blood flow in stenotic vessels and may detect changes in arteries velocity in the circle of Willis (Topcuoglu 2012). It can be used for long-term follow-up of the patients.

26.5 Treatment

Management of fungal-related strokes focuses on treatment of the underlying infection with appropriate antifungal drugs and prevention of medical complications. Treatment of systemic infections that precede or accompany stroke requires prompt initiation of effective antifungal therapy. The treatment of specific pathogens should generally follow established guidelines wherever they exist. Similarly, guidelines for stroke prevention, treatment, and rehabilitation are best followed as usual unless a specific contraindication exists. There are no reference guidelines for the management of CNS fungal infections concerning the best method for monitoring the response and the length of drug treatment. These patients need to be closely followed up and CT scan repeated if obstructive hydrocephalus is suspected.

26.5.1 Specific Treatment

Any CNS fungal infection should be treated with an effective and specific antifungal therapy. Early antifungal therapy should be initiated in immunocompromised patient when fungal infection is suspected or when mycotic aneurysm is detected in the context of fungal infection. Azoles, flucytosine, and amphotericin B deoxycholate are therapeutic options to treat fungal infections (Johnson and Perfect 2010).

26.5.2 Corticosteroids

We might consider adjunctive corticosteroid therapy for reducing the neuroinflammation and cerebral edema (Panackal and Williamson 2015). However, the role of oral or intravenous steroids alongside antimicrobial drugs with infections and new stroke is also unclear and needs further elucidation. Data are lacking regarding the best therapeutic approach to treat infectious cerebral vasculitides. There is a need for appropriate efficacy analysis regarding the use of steroids and other anti-inflammatory drugs in infectious cerebral vasculitis.

26.5.3 Antiaggregation, Thrombolytic, Anticoagulation, and Other Therapies for Acute Stroke

Acute stroke management should be done according to contemporary guidelines; however, data are lacking regarding the use of acute stroke therapy in the setting of infection-associated stroke (Powers et al. 2018). Neurologists and stroke physicians should be aware of the recognized risk of intracerebral hemorrhage associated with both antiaggregation and thrombolytic therapy in the setting of infectious cerebral vasculitis. Actually, the efficacy and safety of antiaggregation medication for secondary stroke prevention in patients with infectious vasculitis have not been validated, and the number of studies is really low. It is usually recommended for secondary prevention, along with all usual measures to improve stroke risk factors such as regulation of blood pressure and blood sugar management.

The efficacy and safety of endovascular vasodilator treatment as adjunctive intervention in patients with meningitis-associated vasculopathy need further investigations. Although commonly used in subarachnoid hemorrhage-related vasospasm, this therapy has been used only occasionally in some patients with parainfectious cerebral vasospasm (Taqui et al. 2014).

Recombinant tissue plasminogen activator (rtPA) is the only approved thrombolytic treatment for acute ischemic stroke. Infection is not an official contraindication; however, formal recommendations for treatment cannot be made because of insufficient clinical data. The clinical experience with rtPA in infectious vasculitis is very limited. When there is a high degree of suspicion of infective endocarditis, the use of rtPA should be avoided. There is a risk of bleeding from mycotic aneurysms when using thrombolytic treatment in the setting of endocarditis. Case series of infective endocarditis patients treated with rtPA reported that most patients developed multifocal intracranial hemorrhages (Ferro and Fonseca 2014; Mateen et al. 2013). However, at the time of acute presentation, the underlying cause of stroke (echocardiogram, cultures) may not be available at the moment, even in highly developed centers.

Anticoagulation has a role in stroke therapy in specific cases, such as in cardioembolic stroke. No convincing evidence proves that anticoagulation prevents embolization in either native or prosthetic valve-related infectious endocarditis; in fact, the risk of intracranial hemorrhage is probably increased with anticoagulation (Tornos et al. 1999). Because of unproven benefit and possibly increased risk, most patients with infectious endocarditis should not be given anticoagulation drugs, unless a separate indication exists. The study of Kang et al. suggested a benefit of early cardiac surgery in 76 patients with severe left-sided infectious endocarditis with large valvular vegetations, but the appropriate timing of surgery for most patients with infectious endocarditis is controversial (Kang et al. 2012).

Each patient is individually assessed according to own risk, whether antiaggregation, anticoagulation, or thrombolytic treatment should be applied or not.

26.5.4 Endovascular and Surgical Treatment

Some patients may need urgent neurosurgical intervention, especially those who have acute neurological deterioration due to hydrocephalus, cerebral hematoma, or significant mass effect. Ventriculoperitoneal shunt may be needed in some patients to decompress ventricles.

26.6 Prognosis

In general, fungal infections of the CNS are associated with poor outcome and high mortality, and therefore, early diagnosis and treatment are necessary.

26.7 Conclusion

The incidence of fungal infections causing ischemic and hemorrhagic strokes is underestimated. Use of contemporary neuroimaging techniques (diffusion-weighted MRI and time of flight MR angiography) could result in a higher proportion of confirmed cases of vasculitis and stroke in patients with CNS fungal infections. CSF analysis only offers moderate help in the diagnosis as negative CSF cultures can occur in 10–30% of these patients. Guidelines about optimal length of drug treatment and the method for monitoring the response for treatment are still lacking. There is a need for new epidemiological and clinical studies to fully understand the complexity of fungal infections and stroke syndromes, in order to recognize the exact incidence, triggers, associated risk factors, the optimal treatment, and prognosis.

References

Arsura EL, Johnson R, Penrose J, et al. Neuroimaging as a guide to predict outcomes for patients with coccidioidal meningitis. Clin Infect Dis. 2005;40(4):624–7.

Ashdown BC, Tien RD, Felsberg GJ. Aspergillosis of the brain and paranasal sinuses in immunocompromised patients: CT and MR imaging findings. Am J Roentgenol. 1994;162:155–9.

Bariola JR, Perry P, Pappas PG, et al. Blastomycosis of the central nervous system: a multicenter review of diagnosis and treatment in the modern era. Clin Infect Dis. 2010;50:797–804.

Bayer A, Scheld M. Endocarditis and intravascular infections. In: Mandell GL, Bennett JE, Dolin R, editors. Mandell Douglas and Bennett's principles and practice of infectious diseases. Philadelphia, PA: Churchill Livingstone; 2000. p. 857–902.

Bell WR, Dalton JB, McCall CM, et al. Iatrogenic exserohilum infection of the central nervous system: mycological identification and histopathological findings. Mod Pathol. 2013;26:166–70.

Browne SK, Burbelo PD, Chetchotisakd P, et al. Adult-onset immunodeficiency in Thailand and Taiwan. N Engl J Med. 2012;367:725–34.

Bush JW, Wuerz T, Embil JM, et al. Outcomes of persons with blastomycosis involving the central nervous system. Diagn Microbiol Infect Dis. 2013;76:175–81.

Calli C, Savas R, Parildar M, Pekindil G, Alper H, Yunten N. Isolated pontine infarction due to rhinocerebral mucormycosis. Neuroradiology. 1999;41:179–81.

Challa S, Prayaga AK, Vemu L, Sadasivan J, Jagarlapudi MK, Digumarti R, et al. Fungal endocarditis: an autopsy study. Asian Cardiovasc Thorac Ann. 2004;12:95–8.
Chou SM, Chong YY, Kinkel R. A proposed pathogenetic process in the formation of Aspergillus mycotic aneurysm in the central nervous system. Ann Acad Med Singapore. 1993;22:518–25.
Corvisier N, Gray F, Gherardi R, Lebras F, Blanc CM, Nguyen JP, et al. Aspergillosis of ethmoid sinus and optic nerve, with arteritis and rupture of the internal carotid artery. Surg Neurol. 1987;28:311–5.
Dayal Y, Weindling HK, Price DL. Cerebral infarction due to fungal embolus. A complication of Aspergillus infection on an aortic valve prosthesis. Neurology. 1974;24:76–9.
Elias J Jr, dos Santos AC, Carlotti CG Jr, et al. Central nervous system paracoccidioidomycosis: diagnosis and treatment. Surg Neurol. 2005;63:S13–2.
Endo T, Tominaga T, Konno H, Yoshimato T. Fatal subarachnoid hemorrhage, with brainstem and cerebellar infarction, caused by Aspergillus infection after cerebral aneurysm surgery: case report. Neurosurgery. 2002;50:1147–51.
Ferro JM, Fonseca AC. Infective endocarditis. Handb Clin Neurol. 2014;119:75–91.
Fu K, Nguyena P, Sanossiana N. Basilar artery territory stroke secondary to invasive fungal sphenoid sinusitis: a case report and review of the literature. Case Rep Neurol. 2015;7:51–8.
Fugate JE, Lyons JL, Thakur KT, et al. Infectious causes of stroke. Lancet Infect Dis. 2014;14:869–80.
Goel D, Kalita J, Misra UK. Basilar artery occlusion in Cryptococcal meningitis. Neurol India. 1999;47:245–6.
Grau AJ, Urbanek C, Palm F. Common infections and the risk of stroke. Nat Rev Neurol. 2010;6:681–94.
Grouhi M, Dalal I, Nisbet-Brown E, Roifman CM. Cerebral vasculitis associated with chronic mucocutaneous candidiasis. J Pediatr. 1998;133:571–4.
Ho CL, Deruytter MJ. CNS aspergillosis with mycotic aneurysm, cerebral granuloma and infarction. Acta Neurochir (Wien). 2004;146:851–6.
Horten BC, Abbort GF, Porro RS. Fungal aneurysms of intracranial vessels. Arch Neurol. 1976;33:577–9.
Hurst RW, Judkins A, Bolger W, Chu A, Loevner LA. Mycotic aneurysm and cerebral infarction resulting from fungal sinusitis: imaging and pathologic correlation. AJNR Am J Neuroradiol. 2001;22:858–63.
Iihara K, Makita Y, Nabeshima S, Tei T, Keyaki A, Nioka H. Aspergillosis of the central nervous system causing subarachnoid hemorrhage from mycotic aneurysm of the basilar artery—case report. Neurol Med Chir. 1990;30:618–23.
Johnson MD, Perfect JR. Use of antifungal combination therapy: agents, order, and timing. Curr Fungal Infect Rep. 2010;4:87–95.
Kalita J, Bansal R, Ayagiri A, Misra UK. Midbrain infarction: a rare presentation of cryptococcal meningitis. Clin Neurol Neurosurg. 1999;101:23–5.
Kang D, Kim Y, Kim S, et al. Early surgery versus conventional treatment for infective endocarditis. N Eng J Med. 2012;366:2466–73.
Karchmer AM. Infection on prosthetic valves and intravascular devices. In: Mandell GL, Bennett JE, Dolin R, editors. Mandell Douglas and Bennett's principles and practice of infectious diseases. Philadelphia, PA: Churchill Livingstone; 2000. p. 903–17.
Kurino M, Kuratsu J, Yamaguchi T, Ushio Y. Mycotic aneurysm accompanied by aspergillotic granuloma: a case report. Surg Neurol. 1994;42:160–4.
Lan SH, Chang WN, Lu CH, Lui CC, Chang HW. Cerebral infarction in chronic meningitis: a comparison of tuberculous meningitis and cryptococcal meningitis. QJM. 2001;94:247–53.
Lau AH, Takeshita M, Ishii N. Mycotic (Aspergillus) arteritis resulting in fatal subarachnoid hemorrhage: a case report. Angiology. 1991;42:251–5.
Ludmerer SW, Wright DJ, Schimmel P. Purifi cation of glutamine tRNA synthetase from Saccharomyces cerevisiae. A monomeric aminoacyl-tRNA synthetase with a large and dispensable NH2-terminal domain. J Biol Chem. 1993;268:5519–23.
Mateen FJ, Sweeney EM, Thakur KT, et al. IV-tissue plasminogen activator (IV-TPA) for acute ischemic stroke (AIS) in HIV+ adults (abstract S414). Ann Neurol. 2013;74(suppl):S17.
McKee EE. Mycotic infection of the brain with arteritis and subarachnoid hemorrhage: report of case. Am J Clin Pathol. 1950;20:381–4.
Murray CJ, Vos T, Lozano R, et al. Disability-adjusted life years (DALYs) for 291 diseases and injuries in 21 regions, 1990-2010: a systematic analysis for the Global Burden of Disease Study 2010. Lancet. 2012;380:2197–223.
Murthy J. Fungal infections of the central nervous system: the clinical syndromes. Neurol India. 2007;55: 221–5.
Murthy JM, Sundaram C, Prasad VS, Purohit AK, Rammurti S, Laxmi V. Aspergillosis of central nervous system: a study of 21 patients seen in a university hospital in south India. J Assoc Physicians India. 2000;48:677–81.
Panackal AA, Williamson PR. Fungal infections of the Central Nervous System. Continuum (Minneap Minn). 2015;21(6 Neuroinfectious Disease): 1662–78.
Pierrotti LC, Baddour L. Fungal endocarditis, 1995-2000. Chest. 2002;122:302–10.
Piotrowski WP, Pilz P, Chuang IH. Subarachnoid hemorrhage caused by a fungal aneurysm of the vertebral artery as a complication of intracranial aneurysm clipping: case report. J Neurosurg. 1990;73: 962–4.

Powers WJ, Rabinstein AA, Ackerson T, et al., on behalf of the American Heart Association Stroke Council. 2018 Guidelines for the early management of patients with acute ischemic stroke: a guideline for Healthcare Professionals from the American Heart Association/American Stroke Association. Stroke. 2018;49(3):e46–e110.

Radhakrishnana VV, Saraswathy A, Rout D, Mohan PK. Mycotic aneurysms of the intracranial vessels. Indian J Med Res. 1994;100:228–31.

Rangel-Guerra RA, Martinez HR, Saenz C, Bosques-Padilla F, Estrada-Bellmann I. Rhinocerebral and systemic mucormycosis. Clinical experience with 36 cases. J Neurol Sci. 1996;143:19–30.

Rosario M, Song SX, McCullough LD. An unusual case of stroke. Neurologist. 2012;18:229–32.

Saccente M. Central nervous system histoplasmosis. Curr Treat Options Neurol. 2008;10:161–7.

Saul RF, Gallagher JG, Mateer JE. Sudden hemiparesis as the presenting sign in cryptococcal meningoencephalitis. Stroke. 1986;17:753–4.

Seton M, Pless M, Fishman JA, Caruso PA, Hedley-Whyte ET. Case records of the Massachusetts General Hospital. Case 18-2008. A 68-year-old man with headache and visual changes after liver transplantation. N Engl J Med. 2008;358:2619–28.

Sharma RR, Lad SD, Pawar SJ, Gurusinghe NT, Bhagwati SN, Mahapatra AK. Surgical management of fungal infections of the central nervous system. In: Schmidek HH, Roberts DW, editors. Schmidek Sweet's operative neurosurgical techniques, indications, methods and results. 5th ed. Philadelphia, PA: Saunders Elsevier; 2006. p. 1633–71.

Smith RM, Schaefer MK, Kainer MA, et al. Fungal infections associated with contaminated methylprednisolone injections. N Engl J Med. 2013;369: 1598–609.

Suzuki K, Iwabuchi N, Kuramochi S, Nakanoma J, Suzuki Y, Serizawa H, et al. Aspergillus aneurysm of the middle cerebral artery causing a fatal subarachnoid hemorrhage. Intern Med. 1995;34:550–3.

Takeda S, Wakabayashi K, Yamazaki K, Miyakawa T, Arai H. Intracranial fungal aneurysm caused by Candida endocarditis. Clin Neuropathol. 1998;17:199–203.

Takeshita M, Izawa M, Kubo O, Tanikawa T, Onda H, Wanifuchi H, et al. Aspergillotic aneurysm formation of cerebral artery following neurosurgical operation. Surg Neurol. 1992;38:146–51.

Taqui A, Koffman L, Hui F, et al. Intra-arterial vasodilator therapy for parainfectious cerebral vasospasm. J Neurol Sci. 2014;340:225–9.

Topcuoglu MA. Transcranial Doppler ultrasound in neurovascular diseases: diagnostic and therapeutic aspects. J Neurochem. 2012;123(suppl 2):39–51.

Tornos P, Almirante B, Mirabet S, et al. Infective endocarditis due to Staphylococcus aureus: deleterious effect of anticoagulant therapy. Arch Intern Med. 1999;159:473–5.

Wasserman AM, Sarantopoulos GP, Khanna D. Fungal leukocytoclastic vasculitis as a presentation of systemic vasculitis in a patient with systemic lupus erythematosus. J Clin Rheumatol. 2009;15: 383–6.

Watson JC, Myseros JS, Bullock MR. True fungal mycotic aneurysm of the basilar artery: a clinical and surgical dilemma. Cerebrovasc Dis. 1999;9:50–3.

Williams PL, Johnson R, Pappagianis D, et al. Vasculitic and encephalitic complications associated with Coccidioides immitis infection of the central nervous system in humans: report of 10 cases and review. Clin Infect Dis. 1992;14:673–82.

Wolf PA, D'Agostino RB, Belanger AJ, Kannel WB. Probability of stroke: a risk profile from the Framingham study. Stroke. 1991;22:312–8.

Spinal Syndromes 27

Álynson Larocca Kulcheski, Xavier Soler I. Graells, and André Luís Sebben

27.1 Abbreviations

CT Computed tomography
HIV Human immonodeficiency virus
MRI Magnetic resonance imaging
ODI Oswestry disability index
VAS Visual analog scale

27.2 Introduction

Spinal infection is an ancient entity with some descriptions dating from the Iron Age (Tayles and Buckley 2004). Historically, they were devastating diseases with exceedingly high morbidity and mortality rates. With the advent of new diagnostic techniques, multidrug antimicrobial chemotherapy, and improvements in surgical techniques, the prognosis has improved dramatically in recent years.

Spinal infections are rare and comprise approximately 1% of bone infectious involvement (Ghanayem and Zdeblick 1996). Most of these infections are of pyogenic or tuberculous origin.

Staphylococcus aureus is the most common cause of spinal infections in general (Sapico and Montgomerie 1979).

Á. L. Kulcheski (✉) · X. S. I. Graells · A. L. Sebben
Orthopedics and Traumatology Service, Hospital de Clínicas, Universidade Federal do Paraná (UFPR), Curitiba, Paraná, Brazil

Non-pyogenic infections are even rarer. The main non-pyogenic infections are due to *Mycobacteria*, fungi, *Brucella*, and syphilis, and they induce granulomatous reactions.

In this chapter, we review about the fungal spinal infections and discuss the clinical presentation, diagnosis, complications, and treatment.

27.3 Epidemiology

In 1928, the first case of a fungal osteomyelitis was described by Conor. He reported a patient with *Monilia psilosis* osteomyelitis (Conner 1928). Since then, the incidence of fungal infections in general has increased substantially over the past several decades but is still extremely rare (Broner et al. 1996; Van den Bergh et al. 1999). Consequently, the number of the spinal infections also rose. Fungal spinal infections can range from a relatively simple discitis to more complicated and destructive osteomyelitis with large abscesses and sometimes marked deformity. Numerous risk factors for their development have been described, generally related to immunosuppressive states (Frazier et al. 2001). The main risk factors are diabetes mellitus, corticosteroid usage, chemotherapy, human immunodeficiency virus (HIV), organ transplantation, malnourished people, intravenous drug users, alcohol abuse, long-term catheters, sepsis, oncological therapies, extensive use of antibiotics, and oth-

M. Turgut et al. (eds.), *Fungal Infections of the Central Nervous System*,
https://doi.org/10.1007/978-3-030-06088-6_27

ers (Frazier et al. 2001; Salvalaggio et al. 2003; Salloum et al. 2004).

The most common fungal organisms causing spondylodiscitis include *Aspergillus* spp., *Candida* spp., and *Cryptococcus. neoformans*. These species are ubiquitous. *Coccidioides immitis* and *Blastomyces dermatitidis* are less frequent and are restricted to some specific geographical areas. *Blastomyces* mainly lives in areas of the United States and Canada surrounding the Ohio and Mississippi River valleys and the Great Lakes, but cases have also been reported in Central and South America, Africa, and the Middle East. The first is most commonly seen in the desert regions of the Southwestern United States and in Central and South America (Kim et al. 2006).

27.4 Pathogenesis

Fungi profoundly grow in the environment with abundance of organic matter and water. The fungus exists in its mycelia l phase in the soil. Humans become infected most commonly by inhalation of the spores (conidia) or less commonly through abrasions of the skin. Person-to-person transmission is rare (Crum et al. 2004).

Spinal infections can occur mainly in two ways. The first is the hematogenous spread due to fungemia, and the second is the contiguous dissemination from a soft tissue infection or by direct inoculation of the organism at the time of a surgical intervention (Frazier et al. 2001; Kim et al. 2006).

27.5 Clinical Manifestations

In general, the symptoms are nonspecific. The insidious onset of back pain, with or without the presence of other systemic symptoms, is the hallmark.

Fungal infections of the spine may present as intradural, extradural, and/or vertebral lesions. Extradural and vertebral lesions are relatively more frequent (Sharma 2010).

Spinal meningitis, spinal arachnoiditis, radiculopathy, and fungal myelitis may occur. Progressive myelopathic syndromes may be due to mass effect producing compressive spinal lesions such as granulomas or intramedullary abscess (Sharma 2010).

In fungal spondylodiscitis, back pain is the most frequent complaint, while neurological impairment appears to be relatively infrequent. Kyphosis is also uncommon due to the indolent nature of the infection. Involvement of the vertebral bodies can lead to vertebral compression fractures and deformity of the spine. In addition, spread of infection along the anterior longitudinal ligament can lead to psoas muscle or paravertebral abscesses (Skaf et al. 2010).

Hematogenous dissemination of fungal infections causes constitutional symptoms like fever, headache, malaise, anorexia, night sweats, lethargy, musculoskeletal pains, etc. (Sharma 2010).

Kulcheski et al. reported an atypical case of *Candida albicans* spondylodiscitis. That occurred after blunt chest contusion and progressed with necrotizing fasciitis of the anterior region of the chest and osteomyelitis of the sternum. Through contiguity, it also affected the upper thoracic spine. The patient evolved with neurological alterations and recovered satisfactorily after appropriate treatment with surgical decompression of the spinal cord and specific antibiotic therapy (Kulcheski et al. 2015).

27.6 Differential Diagnosis

Despite the increasing numbers of immunocompromised patients, the majority of osteomyelitis/discitis cases are caused by bacterial gram-positive organisms, mainly *Staphylococcus aureus*.

Fungal spondylodiscitis closely mimics mycobacterial infections and should be considered in the differential diagnoses of the osteolytic, granulomatous, or abscess-producing lesions of the spine (Broner et al. 1996).

27.7 Diagnosis

Often there is a long delay in diagnosis, mainly because other medical conditions may mask the diagnosis and because fungal spondylodiscitis characteristically runs an indolent course and is nonspecific. So, mycotic spinal infections can be difficult to recognize in the early stages (Frazier et al. 2001).

Literature reports a delay of 2–6 months between first symptoms and diagnosis (Frangen et al. 2006; Butler et al. 2006; Tsiodras and Falagas 2006).

The inflammatory markers such as white cell count, erythrocyte sedimentation rates, and C-reactive protein levels can be elevated. These are not specific for fungal infections, but they are used for monitoring the response to the treatment (Frazier et al. 2001). Antibody tests are seldom helpful in the diagnosis of spinal infections due to ubiquitous fungi such as *Candida* and *Aspergillus* (Yeo and Wong 2002).

All patients need to be investigated with imaging exams. Plain X-rays of the spine show osteolytic lesions, spinal deformities and instability as well as soft tissue shadow of the paraspinal abscesses and granulomas. The spinal computed tomography (CT) scan demonstrates the findings seen on the plain X-rays more clearly as well as shows the surrounding soft tissue involvement more precisely (Figs. 27.1 and 27.2). Magnetic resonance imaging (MRI) scans of the fungal spondylitis show discal hypointensity with relative preservation of the intranuclear cleft on T2-weighted images, as compared to hyperintensity of the intervertebral discs with loss of intranuclear cleft in pyogenic spondylitis in these images. In general, fungal and tubercular granulomatous lesions cause more pronounced destructive vertebral lesions with relative sparing of the intervertebral discs in the initial stages of infection, whereas the pyogenic infection destroys both the vertebral bodies and the discs (Sharma 2010).

Definitive diagnosis rests on the evaluation of a tissue specimen. Biopsies must be evaluated with fungal stains, as well as cultures, because the latter may be negative or take several weeks or months before identification is possible. Closed biopsy was reported to be positive in only 50% of cases, whereas open biopsy was positive in all cases in the series of Campbell and colleagues (Frazier et al. 2001).

27.8 Therapy

Nonsurgical treatment has been met with varied success in the treatment of fungal spinal infections. Successfully treated patients experience

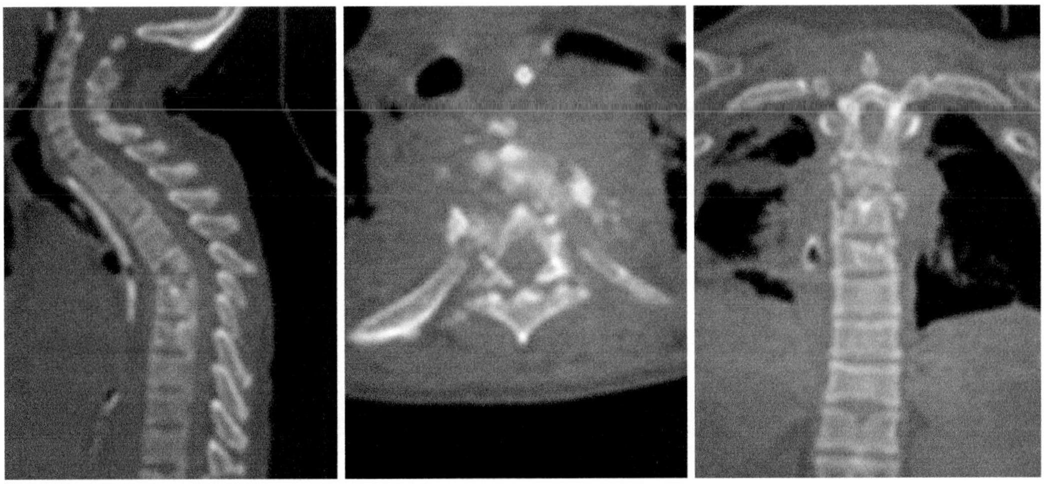

Fig. 27.1 *Candida albicans* spondylodiscitis. Computed tomography (CT) scan images in sagittal, axial, and coronal

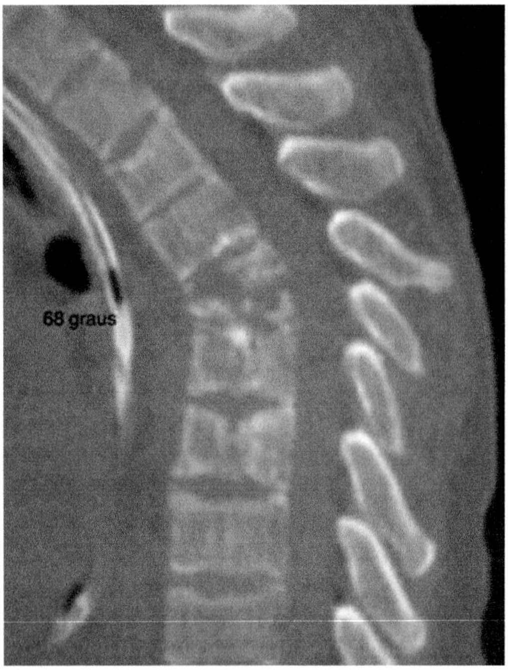

Fig. 27.2 *Candida albicans* spondylodiscitis. Destruction of the vertebral bodies in the upper thoracic spine showing kyphosis of 68°

resolution of spine pain and often fuse spontaneously. Nonoperative treatment includes the institution of antifungal agents, spinal immobilization, and early ambulation. Kim et al. suggested a protocol of treatment for the main fungal spinal infections (Table 27.1) (Kim et al. 2006).

Despite the fact that the antifungal agents may be toxic and the majority of the patients have other comorbidities and are immunosuppressed (Kim et al. 2006), evaluation by an infectious disease specialist should always be considered, because the treatment is prolonged and sometimes the drugs should be changed because of side effects.

Surgical intervention is indicated in the presence of neurological deficits, spinal cord compression, instability, deformity, abscess formation, and/or failure of conservative management. These patients will benefit from debridement and stabilization. We currently use and recommend hardware in cases of instability preoperative or due to an aggressive debridement (Fig. 27.3) (Ganesh et al. 2015). When there is a

Table 27.1 Preferred pharmacotherapeutic options for fungal infections of the spine (Kim et al. 2006)

Disease	Treatment regimen
Coccidioidomycosis	Preferred treatment
	(1) Fluconazole 400–1000 mg/day postoperatively
	(2) Itraconazole 400–600 mg/day postoperatively for up to 6 months
	Alternative
	Amphotericin B 1–2.5 g/day intravenously
Blastomycosis	Preferred treatment
	Amphotericin B in a 1.5–2.5 g/day for lite threatening diseases
	Intraconazole 200–400 mg/day for 6–12 months
	Alternative treatment
	(1) Ketoconazole or fluconazole 400–800 mg/day postoperatively for 6–12 months
Cryptococcosis	Preferred treatment
	(1) Amphotericin B 0.7–1 mg/kg/day and flucytosine 100 mg/kg/day for 2 weeks: then fluconazole 400 mg/day for minimum 10 weeks
	(2) Amphotericin B 0.7–1 mg/kg/day; and flucytosine 100 mg/kg/day for 10 weeks
	(3) Amphotericin B 0.7–1 mg/kg/day tor 6–10 weeks
	(4) Lipid formulation of amphotericin B 3–6 mg/kg/day for 6–10 weeks
Candidiasis	Preferred treatment
	(1) Fluconazole 6 mg/kg/day for 6–12 months: or
	(2) Amphotericin B 0.5–1 mg/kg/day for 6–10 weeks
	Alternative
	(1) Amphotericin B 0.5–1.0 mg/kg/day for 2–3 weeks: then fluconazole 6 mg/kg/day for 6–12 months
Aspergillosis	Preferred treatment
	(1) Amphotericin B deoxycholate 1–1.5 mg/kg/day for 2–3 years
	(2) Lipid formulation of amphotericin B 3–6 mg/kg/day
	(3) Itraconazole 200–400 mg/day

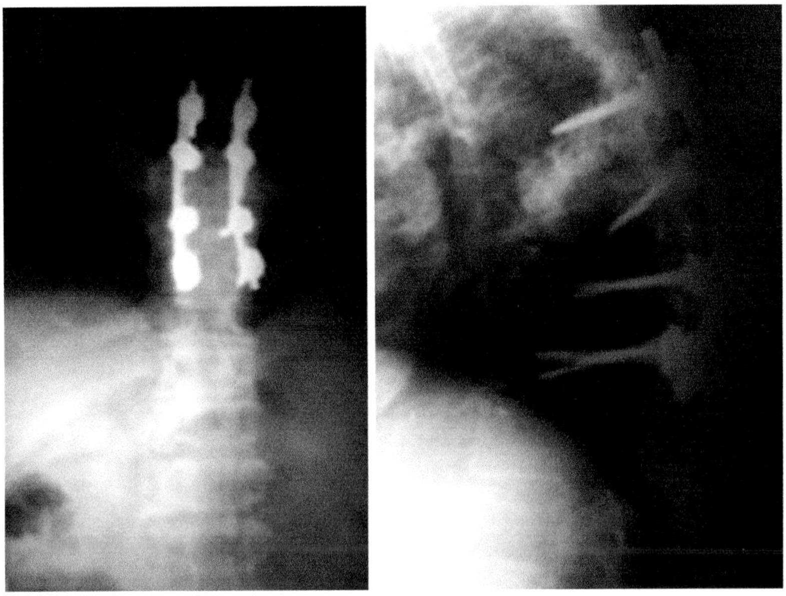

Fig. 27.3 Postoperative image of a patient with *Candida albicans* spondylodiscitis that had instability due to destruction of vertebral bodies and kyphosis

high degree of destruction of the vertebral body, an anterior decompression, bone graft, and fusion with posterior stabilization are the preferred treatment methods. In selected cases, it is possible to perform the debridement of the anterior vertebral elements through either an extracavitary or costotransversectomy approach and posterior fusion. An important advantage of these approaches is that they avoid entering the thoracic cavity (Kim et al. 2006).

27.9 Conclusion

Patients treated clinically and surgically after spinal infections should be evaluated for their clinical outcome. There are scales that allow this continuous evaluation. The most commonly used are the visual analog scale (VAS) for pain and the Oswestry Disability Index (ODI) (Mc Cormack et al. 1988; Fairbank et al. 1980). The first evaluates the patient's pain, ranging from 0 to 10. The last measures permanent functional disability. With these tools including VAS and ODI, in addition to a more detailed follow-up, in addition to a more detailed follow-up, the literature database will be increased and, in this way, fungal infections of the spine can be increasingly managed better.

References

Broner FA, Garland DE, Zigler JE. Spinal infections in the immunocompromised host. Orthop Clin North Am. 1996;27(1):37–46.3.

Butler JS, et al. Nontuberculous pyogenic spinal infection in adults: a 12-year experience from a tertiary referral center. Spine (Phila Pa 1976). 2006;31(23):2695–700.

Conner CL. Monilia from osteomyelitis. J Infect Dis. 1928;43:108–16.

Crum NF, Lederman ER, Stafford CM, Parrish JS, Wallace MR. Coccidioidomycosis: a descriptive survey of a reemerging disease. Clinical characteristics and current controversies. Medicine (Baltimore). 2004;83:149–75.

Fairbank JC, Couper J, Davies JB. The Oswestry low back pain questionnaire. Physiotherapy. 1980;66:271–3.

Frangen TM, et al. Surgical management of spondylodiscitis. An analysis of 78 cases. Unfallchirurg. 2006;109(9):743–53.

Frazier DD, Campbell DR, Garvey TA, et al. Fungal infections of the spine. Report of eleven patients with long-term follow-up. J Bone Joint Surg Am. 2001;83:560–5.

Ganesh D, Gottlieb J, Chan S, Martinez O, Eismont F. Fungal infections of the spine. Spine. 2015;40(12):E719–28.

Ghanayem AJ, Zdeblick TA. Cervical spine infections. Orthop Clin North Am. 1996;27(1):53–67.2.

Kim CW, Perry A, Currier B, Yaszemski M, Garfin SR. Fungal infections of the spine. Clin Orthop Relat Res. 2006;444:92–9.

Kulcheski AL, Graells XS, Benato ML, Santoro PG, Sebben AL. Espondilodiscite fúngica por *Candida albicans*: um caso atípico e revisão da literatura. Rev Bras Ortop. 2015;50(6):739–42.

Mc Cormack HM, Horne DJ, Sheather S. Clinical applications of visual analogue scales: a critical review. Psychol Med. 1988;18:1007–19.

Salloum A, Rao S, Havasi A. Aspergillus rib and vertebral osteomyelitis in a former intravenous drug user. Am J Med. 2004;116:208–9.

Salvalaggio PR, Bassetti M, Lorber MI. Aspergillus vertebral osteomyelitis after simultaneous kidney-pancreas transplantation. Transpl Infect Dis. 2003;5:187–90.

Sapico FL, Montgomerie JZ. Pyogenic vertebral osteomyelitis: report of nine cases and review of the literature. Rev Infect Dis. 1979;1:754–76.

Sharma RR. Fungal infections of the nervous system: current perspective and controversies in management. Int J Surg. 2010;8:591–601.

Skaf GS, Kanafani ZA, Araj GF, Kanj SS. Non-pyogenic infections of the spine. Int J Antimicrob Agents. 2010;36:99–105.

Tayles N, Buckley HR. Leprosy and tuberculosis in iron age southeast Asia? Am J Phys Anthropol. 2004;125(3):239–56.

Tsiodras S, Falagas ME. Clinical assessment and medical treatment of spine infections. Clin Orthop Relat Res. 2006;444:38–50.

Van den Bergh MF, Verweij PE, Voss A. Epidemiology of nosocomial fungal infections: invasive aspergillosis and the environment. Diagn Microbiol Infec Dis. 1999;34:221–7.

Yeo SF, Wong B. Current status of nonculture methods for diagnosis of invasive fungal infections. Clin Microbiol Rev. 2002;15:465–84.

Part IV

Radiological Findings of Fungal Infections Involving Central Nervous System and Its Coverings

Imaging of Fungal Infections of the Brain

28

Subhendu Parida

Abbreviations

CNS	Central nervous system
CSF	Cerebrospinal fluid
CT	Computed tomography
DSA	Digital subtraction angiography
DTI	Diffusion tensor imaging
DWI	Diffusion-weighted imaging
FDG	Fluorodeoxyglucose
FLAIR	Fluid-attenuated inversion recovery
HIV-AIDS	Human immunodeficiency virus-acquired immunodeficiency syndrome
MRI	Magnetic resonance imaging
MRS	Magnetic resonance spectroscopy
MT	Magnetization transfer
PET-CT	Positron emission tomography-computed tomography
ppm	Parts per million
SWI	Susceptibility-weighted imaging
VR	Virchow-Robin

28.1 Introduction

Fungal pathogens are ubiquitous organisms and are found worldwide. Most of the systemic fungal infections are associated with involvement of the central nervous system (CNS). Increasing recognition of fungal infections over the last two decades is due to expansion of the immunosuppressed population at risk and due to improved diagnostic facilities. This chapter reviews the radiological and imaging features of various fungal infections of the CNS. Certain fungal infections have very characteristic image morphology, thus helping the clinicians in early diagnosis. The imaging features may also help in predicting the outcomes (Kourbeti and Mylonakis 2014; Scully et al. 2008; Schwartz et al. 2018).

The radiological features partly depend on the type of fungal pathogen and the route of spread. The relevant CNS fungal pathogens are of three categories: yeasts, molds or filamentous fungi (septate, aseptate, or minimally septate), dematiaceous or pigmented fungi, and dimorphic fungi. Small-sized yeast fungi (*Blastomyces*, *Coccidioides*, *Paracoccidioides*, *Histoplasma*, *Cryptococcus*, *Candida*) access the microcirculation from which they seed the subarachnoid space and produce meningitis and subpial ischemic lesions. Intermediate-sized yeast fungi (*Candida*) occlude the small vessels and produce local tissue necrosis and subsequent abscess formation. Larger-sized fungi septate and aseptate, *Aspergillus*, *Cladosporium*, and *Mucorales*, obstruct large- and intermediate-sized arteries

S. Parida (✉)
Department of Radiology, CARE Hospitals, Hyderabad, India

Department of Neurology, CARE Hospitals, Hyderabad, India
e-mail: subhendu@neuroimaging.in

M. Turgut et al. (eds.), *Fungal Infections of the Central Nervous System*,
https://doi.org/10.1007/978-3-030-06088-6_28

and on occasions veins, resulting in large infarcts (Chimelli and Mahler-Araújo 1997; Shankar et al. 2007). CNS fungal infections are usually secondary to infections elsewhere in the body by hematogenous spread, most commonly from the lung. CNS invasion can be by direct extension from the adjacent structures; sinuses, nose, and ear canal. This mode of spread is most commonly described in patients with sino-cranial aspergillus granulomas (Chimelli and Mahler-Araújo 1997; Shankar et al. 2007; Murthy et al. 2001). Rhinocerebral infection of *Mucorales* spp. is from the nasal infection. Spread can also be via penetrating wounds and neurosurgical procedures. Often the CNS infections occur in the immunocompromised individuals. Rarely infection may occur in immunocompetent individuals (Sundaram et al. 2006; Mathur et al. 2012; Starkey et al. 2014; Lee et al. 1996).

28.2 Techniques and General Features in Imaging

The presenting clinical syndromes in patients with CNS fungal infections include meningitis, meningoencephalitis, sino-cranial syndrome, sino-orbital syndrome, rhinocerebral syndromes, parenchymal mass lesions, and vascular syndromes. Depending upon the presentation, the imaging protocol can be tailored to demonstrate the pathology optimally. Meningeal and parenchymal pathologies can be demonstrated using various magnetic resonance imaging (MRI) sequences including contrast studies.

28.2.1 Meningitis

Leptomeningeal enhancement refers to the superficial enhancement that closely follows the surface of the cerebral and cerebellar hemispheres and brain stem. Such enhancement may be uniform, predominantly basal, or more prominent along the cerebral convexities. Enhancement of the basal cisternal meninges, sometimes referred as leptomeningeal thickening, is seen in patients with basal meningitis, typically cryptococcal meningitis. An etiological diagnosis may not be possible from the demonstration of leptomeningeal enhancement, but in a population at risk, fungal meningitis should be considered (Lee et al. 2016; Smirniotopoulos et al. 2007; Kamran et al. 2004). Magnetization transfer (MT) imaging has demonstrated differing MT ratios within the leptomeningeal thickening both in tubercular and fungal meningitis but has been inconsistent as to which has higher values; furthermore it is difficult to reliably calculate MT ratios within the regions of interest (Kamran et al. 2004; Gupta et al. 1999). The sensitivity to detect leptomeningeal enhancement increases with the use of

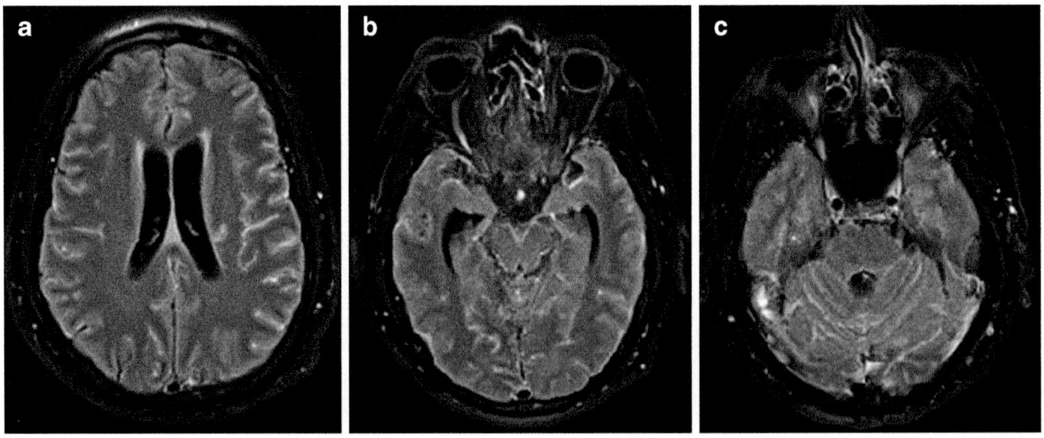

Fig. 28.1 Contrast enhanced fluid-attenuated inversion recovery (FLAIR) images in a patient of Candidial leptomeningitis, leptomeningeal enhancement is not seen in most patients, however some may show enhancement better identified on contrast enhanced FLAIR images. Enhancement is seen along the cerebral sulci upto their depths (**a**), on the surface of brainstem (**b**) and along the cerebellar foliae (**c**)

contrast-enhanced fluid-attenuated inversion recovery (FLAIR). FLAIR is very sensitive to minor changes in composition in cerebrospinal fluid (CSF); it does not show enhancement in normal vascular structures and hence may be superior to routinely used postcontrast T1 images (Fig. 28.1) (Lee et al. 2016; Smirniotopoulos et al. 2007). Parenchymal spread occurs through the Virchow-Robin (VR) (perivascular) spaces from the basal cisterns in *Cryptococcus*. Production of excess amounts of mucoid material leads to cystic enlargement of the perivascular spaces. Intensity remains similar to CSF and hence is very well demonstrated on T2 sequences (Starkey et al. 2014; Lee et al. 1996).

28.2.2 Parenchymal Lesions

Parenchymal lesions include acute infarcts, cerebritis, focal abscesses, and fungal granulomas (Sundaram et al. 2006; Mathur et al. 2012).

Cerebritis refers to an area of focal cerebral inflammation due to fungal invasion either by hematogenous dissemination or by direct invasion from an extra-axial source. It is often seen as an ill-defined area of focal T2/FLAIR hyperintense parenchymal swelling with varying amounts of surrounding edema. Lesions may demonstrate heterogeneous diffusion restriction. Only minimal or no postcontrast enhancement has been reported (Starkey et al. 2014; Tung and Rogg 2003; Marzolf et al. 2016). Host immune system restricts the infection, further evolving to fungal abscess. On imaging fungal abscesses are seen as defined lesions with T2 hypointense rim and hyperintense center with surrounding vasogenic edema.

Diffusion restriction may be seen in these lesions; the foci of restriction can be central and heterogenous, peripheral, or diffusely punctate; in contrast pyogenic abscesses generally have uniform high degree of diffusion restriction at the center of the lesion (Starkey et al. 2014; Tung and Rogg 2003; Marzolf et al. 2016).

Poor contrast enhancement is noted; contrast enhancement depends on the host immune status. In the immunocompetent patients, the contrast enhancement may be homogenous and dense. Fungal abscesses have been reported to have lobulated or crenated margins as compared to smooth-walled pyogenic and tubercular abscesses. They may also have non-enhancing projections along their inner walls unlike pyogenic or tubercular abscesses; these projections have been demonstrated to show diffusion restriction (Luthra et al. 2007). On susceptibility-weighted imaging (SWI) images fungal abscesses may show complete smooth or irregular rim and occasionally low signal at the center (Antulov et al. 2014). Parenchymal fungal granulomas have been commonly reported with *Aspergillus* spp. and *Mucor* spp. Frontal lobe is the most common location of intra-axial granulomas (Mathur et al. 2012; Starkey et al. 2014). The lesions mostly show nonspecific imaging features; clues to fungal ethology include isointense to hypointense signal on T2-weighted images. A thin rim of contrast enhancement may be seen (Michael et al. 1985).

There are few reports of magnetic resonance spectroscopy (MRS) findings in fungal parenchymal lesions; abscesses have been reported to show peaks of cytosolic amino acids such as valine, leucine, and isoleucine and lactate at 0.9 ppm and multiple peaks of trehalose between 3.6 and 4 parts per million (ppm) (Fig. 28.2) (Oner et al. 2006; Gupta et al. 2013). Diffusion tensor imaging (DTI) metrics have been evaluated for usefulness in pyogenic abscesses; however such evidence for fungal lesions is lacking (Nath et al. 2007).

28.2.2.1 Extra-axial: Sino-nasal and Skull Base Syndromes

MRI with a dedicated "skull base" protocol should be the imaging modality in patients with sino-nasal and skull base syndromes. The protocol should include thin section fat-saturated T1 and T2 sequences in coronal, axial, and sagittal planes and postcontrast fat-saturated T1 images in all planes (Herrera et al. 2009; Hudgins and Baugnon 2017). These sequences can optimally demonstrate sinus disease, bone infiltration in skull base, and perineural spread.

Thin section skull base computed tomography (CT) offers better resolution and demonstration of signs of focal bone destruction. Maxillary and ethmoidal sinuses are the sinuses most commonly affected. Sinus lesions appear as center hyperdense surrounded by hypodense thickened

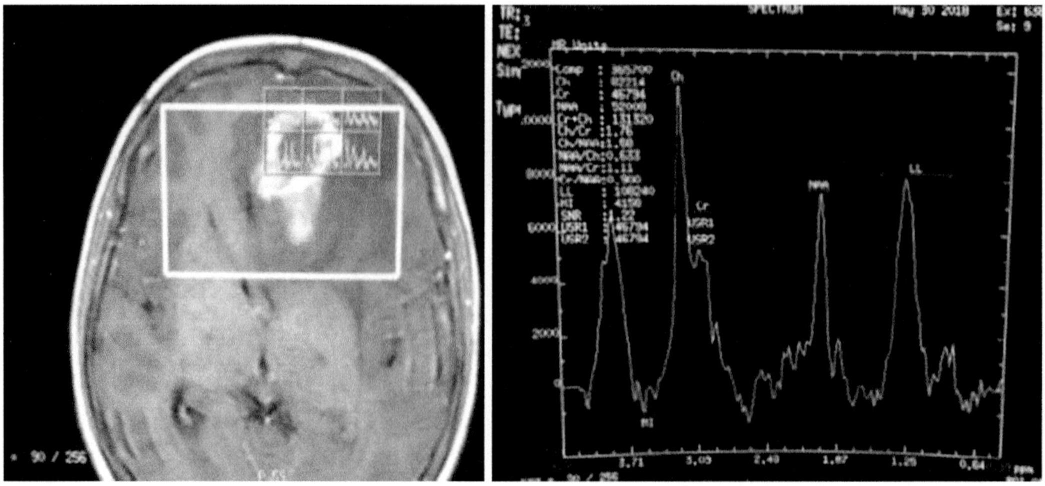

Fig. 28.2 Magnetic resonance spectroscopy (MRS) (TE 135 ms) in a case of left frontal aspergilloma, shows a prominent lipid peak at 1.3 parts per million (ppm) and characteristic Trehalose peak at 3.6–3.8 ppm

mucosa. Extra-sinus spread may be fat stranding or mass-like lesion even without frank destruction of the sinus walls; this is due to spread through blood vessels (Mathur et al. 2012; Starkey et al. 2014; Laine et al. 1990). Skull base foramina such as foramen ovale, foramen rotundum, Vidian canal, etc. may appear enlarged in case of perineural spread along the branches of fifth cranial nerve passing through them (Kandpal et al. 2008).

MRIs show mucosal thickening in the affected sinuses, with central signal loss which is due to the high mineral content of the fungal concretions. In case of extra-sinus extension, soft tissue intensity is noted in the surroundings such as masticator space in case of maxillary sinus disease. Postcontrast may show heterogeneous mucosal enhancement (Mathur et al. 2012; Starkey et al. 2014). Normal bright enhancement of the mucosa may not be seen due to angioinvasion, "black turbinate" sign described in nasal cavity disease (Safder et al. 2010).

28.2.2.2 Vascular Manifestations

Filamentous fungi such as *Aspergillus* and *Mucor* have a propensity for angioinvasion. Angioinvasion involves larger vessels at the skull base through direct invasion from paranasal sinuses and cavernous sinus (Marzolf et al. 2016). Smaller lenticulostriate and distal cerebral vessel involvement occurs with hematogenous spread of the infection. *Aspergillus* spp. produce the enzyme elastase that lyses elastin in the arterial walls resulting in loss in integrity. The consequences of angioinvasion include stenosis, thrombosis, or aneurysm formation (Mathur et al. 2012). Stenosis and thrombosis may result in ischemia and infarction in the area of the arterial territory. T2/FLAIR imaging show infarct as hyperintense lesion with diffusion restriction in the acute stage. Hemorrhagic transformation is common with CNS aspergillosis (Marzolf et al. 2016; Oner et al. 2006).

Fungal mycotic aneurysm is a rare complication; the possible pathogenetic mechanisms include compromise of vasa vasorum, direct invasion of vessel wall, immune complex deposition in the vessel wall, and subsequent damage (Ahuja et al. 1978; Hurst et al. 2001). Bacterial mycotic aneurysms may be single or multiple, are usually small, and located in the distal segments of the vessels, whereas fungal mycotic aneurysms are proximal, fusiform, and larger (Ahuja et al. 1978).

28.3 Specific Central Nervous System Fungal Infections: Radiology

28.3.1 Candidiasis

Increasing incidence of invasive CNS candida infections is due to the expansion of immunocompromised population at risk (Neves et al.

2014; Fennelly et al. 2013). Candida cerebral abscess is common in infants and young individuals (Ahuja et al. 1978). Brain involvement in candida infection is hematogenous; blood cultures isolate the organism in about half the cases (Fennelly et al. 2013). The clinical presenting features of CNS candida infection include microabscesses; macroabscesses; leptomeningitis with or without complications such as hydrocephalus, arteritis, and related infarcts; and mycotic aneurysms (Figueiredo et al. 2014). Microabscesses are innumerable, most often less than 3 mm in size, and indistinctly demarcated from the rest of the cerebral parenchyma. They may show mild perilesional edema and diffusion restriction. Nodular or discoid postcontrast enhancement is the feature (Fig. 28.3) (Mathur et al. 2012; Starkey et al. 2014; Hurst et al. 2001). Macroabscesses can be single or multiple of different sizes and peripheral in location. These can be variably hypointense on T1 images and hyperintense on T2 images. Some of the lesion may show intralesional bleeding. Most often the lesions show peripheral ring enhancement. Contrast study may be useful in delineation of smaller lesions. MRS findings may be nonspecific. Diagnosis is by biopsy and/or CSF analysis (Gupta et al. 2013; Fennelly et al. 2013; Figueiredo et al. 2014).

Diagnosis of leptomeningitis diagnosis is difficult on imaging; FLAIR hyperintensity on sulcal spaces and leptomeningeal pattern of enhancement on postcontrast are suggestive of leptomeningitis, though it is not specific for any etiology (Fig. 28.1) (Lee et al. 2016; Smirniotopoulos et al. 2007; Kamran et al. 2004). Vascular involvement due to arteritis causes luminal compromise or focal weakening of the vessel wall resulting in the formation of mycotic aneurysms. Luminal stenosis may cause ischemic stroke, predominantly localized to basal ganglia. In the acute stage, the lesions appear hyperintense on T2 or FLAIR with uniform diffusion restriction (Mathur et al. 2012; Starkey et al. 2014). Mycotic aneurysms have been rarely reported in cerebral candida infection. Subarachnoid hemorrhage and intraventricular

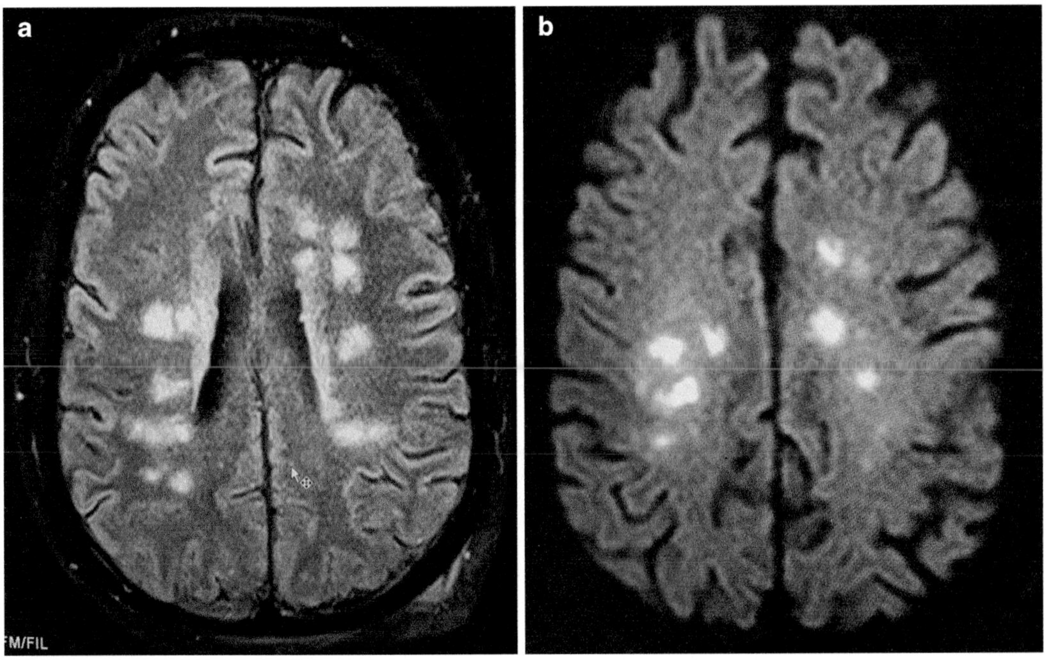

Fig. 28.3 A 65 years old diabetic patient presented with altered consciousness. Axial FLAIR image (**a**) reveals multiple rounded lesions in the periventricular and deep white matter, showing diffusion restriction on the diffusion-weighted imaging (DWI) (**b**), suggestive of abscesses. Contrast could not be administered to the patient due to poor renal function. Candida spp was isolated from cerebrospinal fluid (CSF), consistent with the diagnosis of candidial micro and macrobascesses

hemorrhage can be identified as hyperattenuation on unenhanced CT scan or as hyperintensity within the subarachnoid space on FLAIR. SWI images may show blooming (Ahuja et al. 1978; Hurst et al. 2001). Aneurysms are demonstrated often by CT angiography; digital subtraction angiography (DSA) is usually reserved for endovascular treatment planning.

28.3.2 Aspergillosis

Aspergillus spp. can affect both immunocompetent and immunocompromised individuals. Skull base and sino-orbital syndromes are mostly described from countries with temperate climates and in otherwise immunocompetent individuals. Hematogenous dissemination is more often in immunocompromised patients (Marzolf et al. 2016).

Angioinvasion is the primary pathology in cerebral involvement. Perforator arteries at the base of the brain are primarily involved. This results in infarcts in the corresponding arterial territories and subsequent fungal invasion. Findings on imaging depend on the stage of involvement and hence reflect the progression (Sundaram et al. 2006; Shaikh and Sundararajan 2015; Muraoka et al. 2016). The location of infarcts in aspergillosis include basal ganglia, thalami, brain stem as these regions are supplied by perforating arteries. *Aspergillus* abscesses are seen in deeper regions such as basal ganglia and thalami and also at the gray-white junction. In immunocompromised patients, the lesions are ill-defined with minimal perilesional edema. The lesions are usually T1 hypointense, and hyperintensity seen in some of the lesions is due to blood or minerals such as manganese and iron found abundantly in fungal hyphae. Central areas of necrosis seen are of nearly fluid intensity. T2 images show heterogenous intensity; the periphery can be T2 hypointense with central areas approaching fluid signal (Shaikh and Sundararajan 2015; Muraoka et al. 2016; Tempkin et al. 2006; Almutairi et al. 2009). Peripheral diffusion restriction may be noted (Fig. 28.4). SWI shows peripheral blooming due to blood or minerals. Postcontrast enhancement is marked in immunocompetent patients and may be absent or minimal in immunocompromised patients (Figs. 28.3 and 28.5) (Sundaram et al. 2006; Gupta et al. 2013; Shaikh and Sundararajan 2015; Tempkin et al. 2006; Almutairi et al. 2009).

Parenchymal lesions can however be mistaken for lymphoma or glioblastoma due to their varying appearances. It may be difficult to prospectively diagnose a fungal granuloma in such atypical lesions; imaging in such patients is useful in planning biopsy and for subsequent follow-up (Sidani et al. 2013; Kumar et al. 2018).

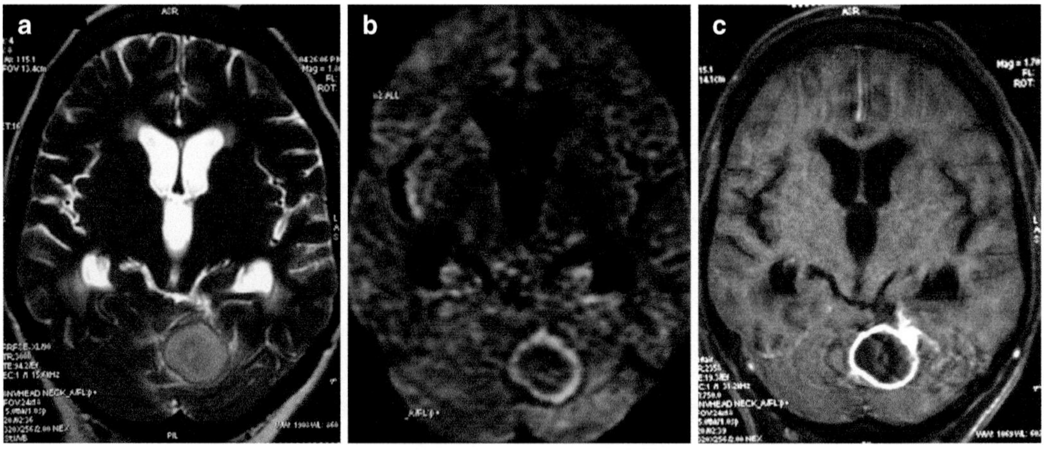

Fig. 28.4 A case of cerebellar aspergillus abscess. The axial T2 images (**a**) reveals a hyperintense left cerebellar lesion with thin hypointense wall and showing characteristic restricted diffusion along the wall of the abscess on DWI images (**b**). Mild perilesional edema is noted. Post contrast study shows uniform peripheral enhancement

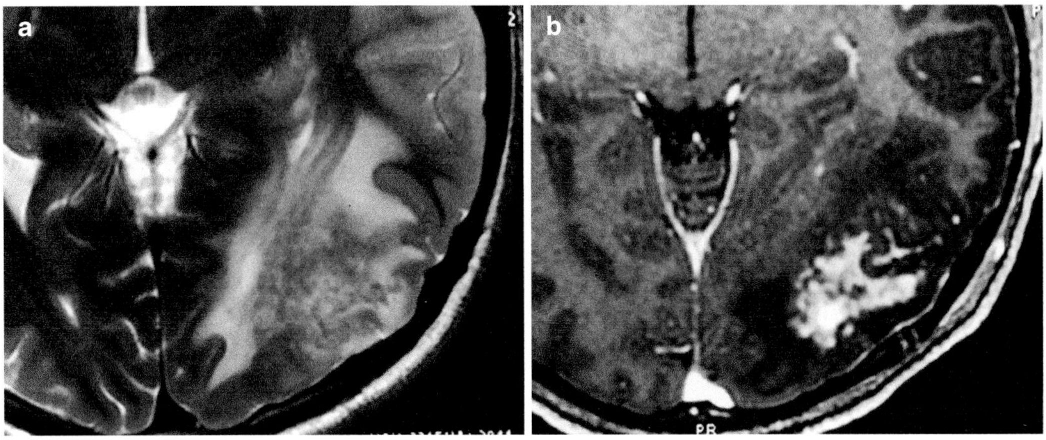

Fig. 28.5 A case of parenchymal aspergillus granuloma. Image (**a**) reveals a heterogenous ill defined lesion in the left temporal-occipital region, showing peripheral T2 isointense rim and central hyperintensity surrounded by edema. The post contrast scan (image **b**) reveals heterogeneous enhancement of the lesion

Infiltration of skull base leading to skull base osteomyelitis and focal granuloma formation may be seen as a direct extension from sino-nasal disease or from an infection in the ear. They present as focal lytic lesions or an area of permeative pattern of bone destruction on unenhanced CT scan. The lesion may be hypointense on T2 images, heterogeneous postcontrast is often seen, and there may be contiguous extension into the cavernous sinuses and orbits (Hudgins and Baugnon 2017; Laine et al. 1990).

28.3.3 Mucormycosis

Rhinocerebral-orbital mucormycosis is the most common localized form of invasive disease caused by *Mucorales* sp. and is more common in patients with poorly controlled diabetes. The infection usually starts in the sinuses (more commonly maxillary sinus) and ethmoidal air cells, and further spread occurs commonly through macroscopically intact sinus walls via angioinvasion of vessels, perineural invasion, small dehiscences, or foramina (Sundaram et al. 2006). Extension into orbits, cavernous sinus, and middle ear – petrous mastoid region – and intradural intraparenchymal extension can occur (Herrera et al. 2009; Moll et al. 1994). Similar to *Aspergillus* sp., angioinvasion is a pathologic feature, this leads to occlusion of the blood vessels and ischemia and infarction in the corresponding arterial tertiaries, and this includes sinuses and cerebral parenchyma (Moll et al. 1994; Mandava et al. 2001; Koc et al. 2007). Imaging is reflective of these changes. Sinusitis appears as mucosal thickening; the involved sinuses may have internal iso-attenuating or hypo-attenuating areas. Inspissated secretions may appear hyperdense on non-contrast scans. Spread beyond maxillary sinuses appears as fat stranding or soft tissue attenuation in the masticator space or subcutaneous region of face. Further spread into the pterygopalatine fossa appears as obliteration of the normal fat attenuation seen within it (Horger et al. 2006; Orguc et al. 2005; Raz et al. 2015). Focal bone erosions may be seen in mucormycosis; however, bone erosions are more common with suggestive of an *Aspergillus* infection (Nithyanandam and Correa 2010). MRI is more helpful to demonstrate the extent, especially in depicting soft tissue involvement, intracranial extension, and perineural spread. Involved sinuses show mucosal thickening. Sinus cavities often contain concretions that show signal loss and require examination on multiple sequences to differentiate from normal signal void of air. Extra-sinus extension appears as fat stranding or replacement of fat by soft tissue intensity (Fig. 28.6) (Raz et al. 2015).

Perineural spread has been documented in 70–90% of cases in pathological case series

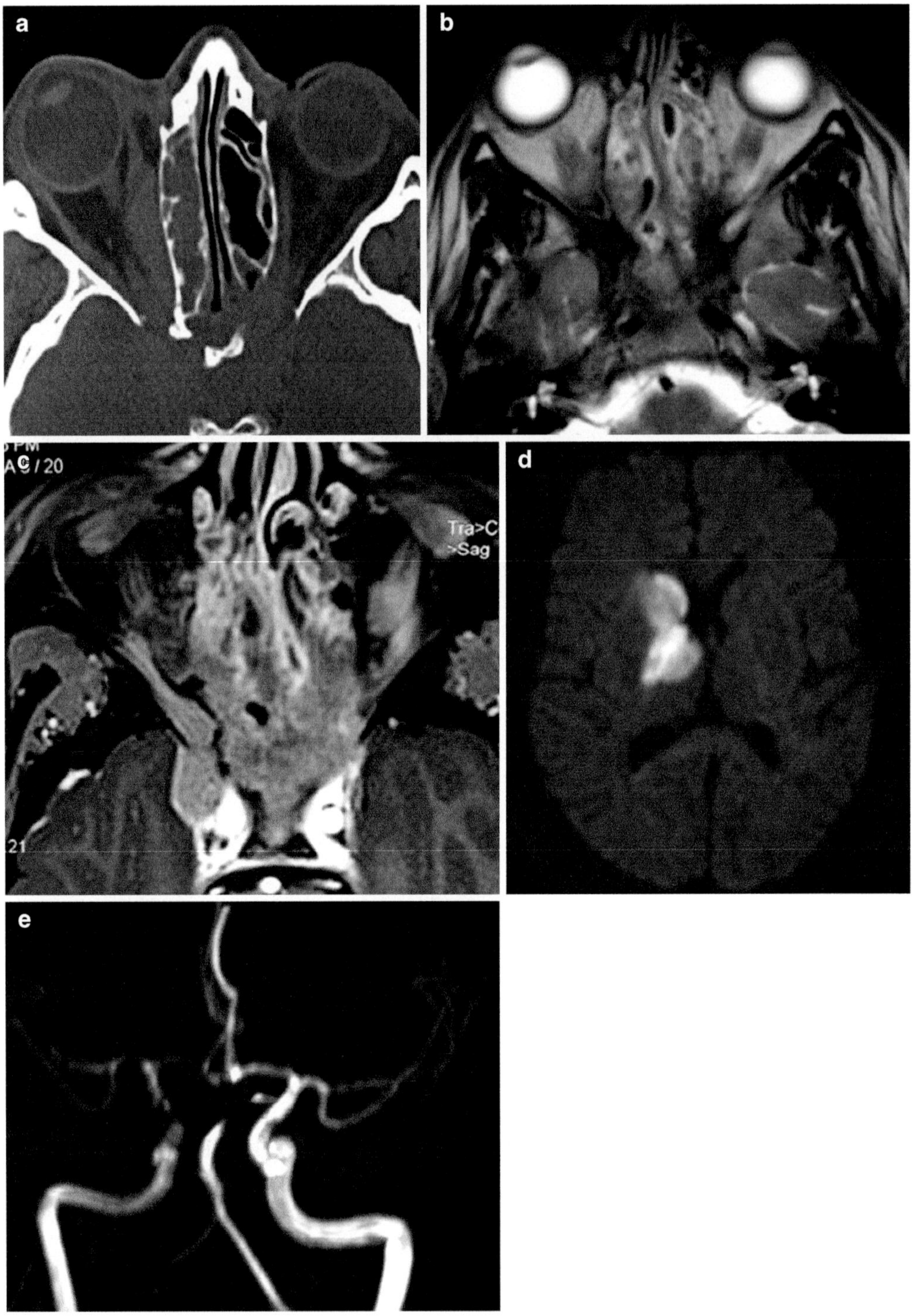

Fig. 28.6 A 55 years old diabetic female patient with rhinocerebral mucormycosis. The computed tomography images (**a**) revealed ill definded soft tissue attenuating lesion at right ethmoidal sinus and right medial extraconal orbital space. The T2 (**b**) & post contrast T1 (**c**) images reveals extension of lesion to bilateral ethmoidal, nasopharynx and right parasellar region with infiltration of the right cavernous sinus. The DWIs (**d**) reveal acute right basal ganglia and anterior thalamic infarct. The time-of-flight magnetic resonance angiography images reveal (**e**) irregularity of supraclinoid right internal carotid artery and the M1 segment of right middle cerebral artery. Basilar artery flow signal is normal, loss of signal at its apex is artifactual

(Sravani et al. 2014; Cornely et al. 2014). This mode of spread is uncommonly demonstrated on imaging. The imaging findings include thickness of the nerves, postcontrast enhancement, and atrophy of muscles supplied by the nerves. The foramina through which the nerves egress the skull are often enlarged. The nerve involved in the perineural spread depends on the lesion location: infraorbital nerve in maxillary sinus lesions; the nerves involved depend on the tissue extension of the lesion, for example, a lesion in the maxillary sinus may involve the infraorbital nerve, and for lesion in the masticator space or middle cranial fossa, floor 2nd division of trigeminal nerve may be involved. Cases have been reported where perineural spread of the nerve reached up to the lateral aspect of the pons in its lateral aspect (McLean et al. 1996).

28.3.4 Cryptococcosis

Cryptococcosis of the CNS mostly occurs in immunocompromised subjects, and the spread is by hematogenous route. Neurological manifestations include leptomeningitis and brain parenchyma lesions (Lee et al. 1996). Imaging of leptomeningitis is nonspecific, as the basal exudates either poorly enhance or do not enhance postcontrast. T2 sequence may show increased signal of the basal regions of the brain near the anterior perforated substance, the "hazy brain base sign." Communicating hydrocephalus may be seen (Katchanov et al. 2016). A small proportion of patients with cryptococcal meningitis may present with acute infarcts in the territory of the lenticulostriate arteries predominantly in the basal ganglia and thalami. It may be due to direct invasion of the lenticulostriate arteries; vasculitis has been demonstrated angiographically in previous studies. Other mechanisms include vessel spasm, vessel entrapment by exudate, and thrombus formation (Starkey et al. 2014; Katchanov et al. 2016; Offiah and Naseer 2016).

Parenchymal lesions include gelatinous pseudocysts, multiple small ill-defined T2 hyperintense lesions found predominantly in the vicinity of VR spaces, miliary lesions, and cryptococcomas. Gelatinous pseudocysts are a common manifestation of parenchymal lesions, as the organism enters the parenchyma through the VR spaces, and the expansion of the VR spaces is due to the abundant mucoid material of the capsule of *Cryptococcus*. These appear as multiple closely spaced cystic lesions in the basal ganglia, thalami, or midbrain with signal intensity similar to CSF with no perilesional edema. These lesions usually do not show contrast enhancement (Fig. 28.7). One should have a high index of suspicion while interpreting the images of patients with human immunodeficiency virus-acquired immunodeficiency syndrome (HIV-AIDS) infection since prominent VR spaces may be dismissed as an innocuous or age-related finding.

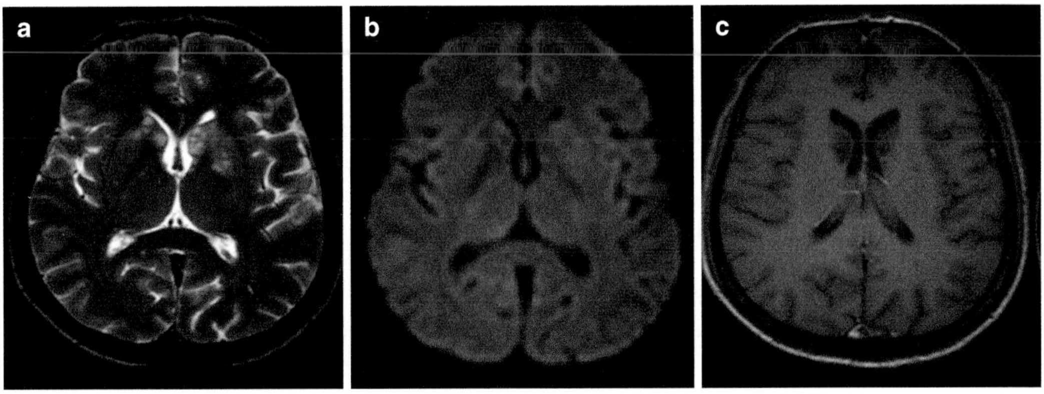

Fig. 28.7 A 34 years old immunocompromised patient presented with fever and headache. Axial T2 images (**a**) reveal multiple rounded hyperintense lesions at bilateral basal ganglia showing no diffusion restriction (**b**) or post contrast enhancement (**c**), suggestive of gelatinous pseudocysts. CSF study confirmed the presence of *Cryptococcus*

Smaller parenchymal lesions may be seen appearing hypointense on T1 images and hyperintense on T2 with variable amounts of perifocal edema and postcontrast enhancement. In situations of very poor immune response, e.g. those in patients with HIV-AIDS, these lesions may be numerous resembling a miliary pattern of disease (Lee et al. 1996; Katchanov et al. 2016; Offiah and Naseer 2016; Tore et al. 2010; Costa et al. 2013). Cryptococcomas are usually seen in immunocompetent subjects; it appears as a lobulated mass within the parenchyma, both in supra- and infratentorial spaces; and it may be multiloculated T1 hypointense and T2 hyperintense lesion. These lesions show central diffusion restriction and perifocal edema. Enhancement is peripheral and can be smooth and/or irregular nodular. It may mimic a cystic necrotic tumor (Liu et al. 2015).

28.3.5 Blastomycosis, Histoplasmosis, Coccidioidomycosis, and Phaeohyphomycosis

Blastomycosis is caused by *Blastomyces dermatitidis* and is endemic in certain parts of North America. CNS manifestations include meningitis, intracranial mass lesions, and epidural abscess. The mass lesions may be single or multiple (Bariola et al. 2010). MRI is the imaging modality for demonstration of leptomeningeal enhancement. Intracranial mass lesions have intense peripheral enhancement with internal foci of diffusion restriction. It is difficult to differentiate such lesions from other fungal lesions. Brain parenchymal lesions of *Histoplasma*, histoplasmomas present as peripheral contrast-enhancing multiple small rounded lesions. They may be widely scattered in the brain parenchyma. Appearance on T1 and T2 images is nonspecific. CNS manifestation of *Coccidioides immitis* infection (coccidioidomycosis) is basal meningitis and rarely parenchymal mass lesions (Stavrakis et al. 2015). Phaeohyphomycosis of the CNS is caused by phaeoid fungi such as *Bipolaris* sp. and *Cladophialophora* sp. Neurological manifestations include multiple cerebral abscesses or granulomatous encephalitis. The lesions may mimic high-grade glial tumors. Leptomeningitis and ischemic stroke probably due to arteritis have also been reported (Filizzola et al. 2003; Moja et al. 2000; Hauck et al. 2008; Buxi et al. 1996).

28.3.6 Current Role of Fluorodeoxyglucose-Positron Emission Tomography in Fungal Infections

Positron emission tomography-computed tomography (PET-CT) has been reported to be useful in the diagnosis and follow-up of invasive fungal infections including the assessment of treatment response; however owing to the high physiological uptake of fluorodeoxyglucose (FDG) by the brain parenchyma, the role of FDG-PET in the evaluation of fungal infections of brain is limited (Ankrah et al. 2016; Sharma et al. 2014). There is a report of PET-CT use in the diagnosis, biopsy planning, and follow-up in a case of rhino-orbital mucormycosis. The lesion could be correctly identified as an FDG avid area in the orbit, periorbital tissues, and ethmoidal air cells; treatment was adjusted according to response until follow-up PET-CT revealed resolution of lesions (Liu et al. 2013). The routine use of FDG-PET in the evaluation of CNS fungal infections is however rare and needs further evaluation.

28.4 Conclusion

Fungi cause meningeal and parenchymal diseases predominantly in immunocompromised individuals and occasionally in immunocompetent patients. The imaging findings are relatively nonspecific. Yeasts like *Cryptococcus* spp. and *Candida* spp. cause leptomeningitis predominantly; hyphal organisms cause paranasal sinus, skull base, and brain parenchymal disease. Angioinvasion may lead to infarcts in the basal ganglia, thalami, and areas supplied by lenticulostriate arteries. Parenchymal lesions of *Aspergillus* spp. include granulomas and abscesses; peripheral diffusion restriction is seen in fungal abscesses in contrast to pyogenic abscesses. Imaging is helpful in raising a suspicion of fungal infection, assessing the extent of involvement, planning biopsy, and monitoring response to therapy.

References

Ahuja GK, Jain N, Vijayaraghavan M, Roy S. Cerebral mycotic aneurysm of fungal origin: case report. J Neurosurg. 1978;49(1):0107–10.

Almutairi BM, Nguyen TB, Jansen GH, Asseri AH. Invasive aspergillosis of the brain: radiologic-pathologic correlation. Radiographics. 2009;29(2):375–9.

Ankrah AO, Sathekge MM, Dierckx RA, Glaudemans AW. Imaging fungal infections in children. Clin Transl Imaging. 2016;4(1):57–72.

Antulov R, Dolic K, Fruehwald-Pallamar J, Miletic D, Thurnher MM. Differentiation of pyogenic and fungal brain abscesses with susceptibility-weighted MR sequences. Neuroradiology. 2014;56(11):937–45.

Bariola JR, Perry P, Pappas PG, Proia L, Shealey W, Wright PW, Sizemore JM, Robinson M, Bradsher RW Jr. Blastomycosis of the central nervous system: a multicenter review of diagnosis and treatment in the modern era. Clin Infect Dis. 2010;50(6):797–804.

Buxi TB, Prakash K, Vohra R, Bhatia D. Imaging in phaeohyphomycosis of the brain: case report. Neuroradiology. 1996;38(2):139–41.

Chimelli L, Mahler-Araújo MB. Fungal infections. Brain Pathol. 1997;7(1):613–27.

Cornely OA, Arikan-Akdagli S, Dannaoui E, Groll AH, Lagrou K, Chakrabarti A, Lanternier F, Pagano LI, Skiada A, Akova M, Arendrup MC. ESCMID and ECMM joint clinical guidelines for the diagnosis and management of mucormycosis 2013. Clin Microbiol Infect. 2014;20:5–26.

Costa CH, Ribeiro JC, Nunes-Filho LP, Rabelo MG, Almeida-Neto WS. Soap bubble appearance in brain magnetic resonance imaging: cryptococcal meningoencephalitis. Rev Soc Bras Med Trop. 2013;46(5):658–9.

Fennelly AM, Slenker AK, Murphy LC, Moussouttas M, Desimone JA. Candida cerebral abscesses: a case report and review of the literature. Med Mycol. 2013;51(7):779–84.

Figueiredo SM, Campolina S, Rosa CA, Gontijo M, Tirone T, Assunção CB, Freire TF, Christo PP, Caligiorne RB. Cerebral macroabscess caused by Candida albicans in an immunocompetent patient: a diagnostic challenge. Med Mycol Case Rep. 2014;3:17–9.

Filizzola MJ, Martinez F, Rauf SJ. Phaeohyphomycosis of the central nervous system in immunocompetent hosts: report of a case and review of the literature. Int J Infect Dis. 2003;7(4):282–6.

Gupta RK, Kathuria MK, Pradhan S. Magnetization transfer MR imaging in CNS tuberculosis. Am J Neuroradiol. 1999;20(5):867–75.

Gupta RK, Jobanputra KJ, Yadav A. MR spectroscopy in brain infections. Neuroimaging Clin. 2013;23(3):475–98.

Hauck EF, McGinnis M, Nauta HJ. Cerebral phaeohyphomycosis mimics high-grade astrocytoma. J Clin Neurosci. 2008;15(9):1061–6.

Herrera DA, Dublin AB, Ormsby EL, Aminpour S, Howell LP. Imaging findings of rhinocerebral mucormycosis. Skull Base. 2009;19(2):117.

Horger M, Hebart H, Schimmel H, Vogel M, Brodoefel H, Oechsle K, Hahn U, Mittelbronn M, Bethge W, Claussen CD. Disseminated mucormycosis in haematological patients: CT and MRI findings with pathological correlation. Br J Radiol. 2006;79(945):e88–95.

Hudgins PA, Baugnon KL. Head and neck: skull base imaging. Neurosurgery. 2017;82(3):255–67.

Hurst RW, Judkins A, Bolger W, Chu A, Loevner LA. Mycotic aneurysm and cerebral infarction resulting from fungal sinusitis: imaging and pathologic correlation. Am J Neuroradiol. 2001;22(5):858–63.

Kamran S, Bener AB, Alper D, Bakshi R. Role of fluid-attenuated inversion recovery in the diagnosis of meningitis: comparison with contrast-enhanced magnetic resonance imaging. J Comput Assist Tomogr. 2004;28(1):68–72.

Kandpal H, Aneesh MK, Seith A, Sharma S. Symptomatic perineural extension of fungal sinusitis in an immunocompetent person: imaging features. Singap Med J. 2008;49(7):171–4.

Katchanov J, Branding G, Jefferys L, Arastéh K, Stocker H, Siebert E. Neuroimaging of HIV-associated cryptococcal meningitis: comparison of magnetic resonance imaging findings in patients with and without immune reconstitution. Int J STD AIDS. 2016;27(2):110–7.

Koc Z, Koc F, Yerdelen D, Ozdogu H. Rhino-orbital-cerebral mucormycosis with different cerebral involvements: infarct, hemorrhage, and ophthalmoplegia. Int J Neurosci. 2007;117(12):1677–90.

Kourbeti IS, Mylonakis E. Fungal central nervous system infections: prevalence and diagnosis. Expert Rev Anti-Infect Ther. 2014;12(2):26.

Kumar D, Nepal P, Singh S, Sheoran R, Bansal SK, Patil S. CNS aspergilloma mimicking tumors: review of CNS aspergillus infection imaging characteristics in the immunocompetent population. J Neuroradiol. 2018;45(3):169–76.

Laine FJ, Nadel L, Braun IF. CT and MR imaging of the central skull base. Part 2. Pathologic spectrum. Radiographics. 1990;10(5):797–821.

Lee EK, Lee EJ, Kim S, Lee YS. Importance of contrast-enhanced fluid-attenuated inversion recovery magnetic resonance imaging in various intracranial pathologic conditions. Korean J Radiol. 2016;17(1):127–41.

Lee SC, Dickson DW, Casadevall A. Pathology of cryptococcal meningoencephalitis: analysis of 27 patients with pathogenetic implications. Hum Pathol. 1996;27(8):839–47.

Liu BX, Dai XJ, Liu H, Gong HH, Wang YX, Zhang LL. Cerebellar cryptococcosis characterized by a space-occupying lesion in an immunocompetent non-HIV patient. Neuropsychiatr Dis Treat. 2015; 11:21.

Liu Y, Wu H, Huang F, Fan Z, Xu B. Utility of 18F-FDG PET/CT in diagnosis and management of mucormycosis. Clin Nucl Med. 2013;38(9):e370–1.

Luthra G, Parihar A, Nath K, Jaiswal S, Prasad KN, Husain N, Husain M, Singh S, Behari S, Gupta RK. Comparative evaluation of fungal, tubercular, and pyogenic brain abscesses with conventional and diffusion MR imaging and proton MR spectroscopy. Am J Neuroradiol. 2007;28(7):1332–8.

Mandava P, Chaljub G, Patterson K, Hollingsworth JW. MR imaging of cavernous sinus invasion by mucormycosis: a case study. Clin Neurol Neurosurg. 2001;103(2):101–4.

Marzolf G, Sabou M, Lannes B, Cotton F, Meyronet D, Galanaud D, Cottier JP, Grand S, Desal H, Kreutz J, Schenck M. Magnetic resonance imaging of cerebral aspergillosis: imaging and pathological correlations. PLoS One. 2016;11(4):e0152475.

Mathur M, Johnson CE, Sze G. Fungal infections of the central nervous system. Neuroimaging Clin N Am. 2012;22(4):609–32.

McLean FM, Ginsberg LE, Stanton CA. Perineural spread of rhinocerebral mucormycosis. Am J Neuroradiol. 1996;17(1):114–6.

Michael MA, Rushovich AM, Ciric I. Magnetic resonance imaging of cerebral aspergillosis. Comput Radiol. 1985;9(2):85–9.

Moja M, Muthuphei MN, van der Westhuizen LR, Gledhill RF. Multiple infarcts in a patient with cerebral phaeohyphomycosis: CT and MRI. Neuroradiology. 2000;42(4):261–6.

Moll GW, Raila FA, Liu GC, Conerly AW. Rhinocerebral mucormycosis in IDDM: sequential magnetic resonance imaging of long-term survival with intensive therapy. Diabetes Care. 1994;17(11):1348–53.

Muraoka S, Araki Y, Izumi T, Takeuchi K, Okamoto S, Wakabayashi T. Cerebral infarction and subarachnoid hemorrhage caused by central nervous system Aspergillus infection. World Neurosurg. 2016;90:705–e9.

Murthy JM, Sundaram C, Prasad VS, Purohit AK, Rammurti S, Laxmi V. Sinocranial aspergillosis: a form of central nervous system aspergillosis in south India. Mycoses. 2001;44(5):141–5.

Nath K, Husain M, Trivedi R, Kumar R, Prasad KN, Rathore RK, Gupta RK. Clinical implications of increased fractional anisotropy in meningitis associated with brain abscess. J Comput Assist Tomogr. 2007;31(6):888–93.

Neves N, Santos L, Reis C, Sarmento A. Candida albicans brain abscesses in an injection drug user patient: a case report. BMC Res Notes. 2014;7(1):837.

Nithyanandam S, Correa MA. Rhino-orbital mucormycosis and aspergillosis: differences in outcome, clinical and imaging characteristics. Eur Arch Otorhinolaryngol. 2010;267(1):161–2.

Offiah CE, Naseer A. Spectrum of imaging appearances of intracranial cryptococcal infection in HIV/AIDS patients in the anti-retroviral therapy era. Clin Radiol. 2016;71(1):9–17.

Oner AY, Celik H, Akpek S, Tokgoz N. Central nervous system aspergillosis: magnetic resonance imaging, diffusion-weighted imaging, and magnetic resonance spectroscopy features. Acta Radiol. 2006;47(4):408–12.

Orguc S, Yücetürk AV, Demir MA, Goktan C. Rhinocerebral mucormycosis: perineural spread via the trigeminal nerve. J Clin Neurosci. 2005;12(4):484–6.

Raz E, Win W, Hagiwara M, Lui YW, Cohen B, Fatterpekar GM. Fungal sinusitis. Neuroimaging Clin. 2015;25(4):569–76.

Safder S, Carpenter JS, Roberts TD, Bailey N. The "black turbinate" sign: an early MR imaging finding of nasal mucormycosis. Am J Neuroradiol. 2010;31(4):771–4.

Schwartz S, Kontoyiannis DP, Harrison T, Ruhnke M. Advances in the diagnosis and treatment of fungal infections of the CNS. Lancet Neurol. 2018;17(4):362–72.

Scully EP, Baden LR, Katz JT. Fungal brain infections. Curr Opin Neurol. 2008;21(3):347–52.

Shaikh AG, Sundararajan S. Angioinvasive aspergillosis of the central nervous system. Can J Neurol Sci. 2015;42(1):64–5.

Shankar SK, Mahadevan A, Sundaram C, Sarkar C, Chacko G, Lanjewar DN, Santosh V, Yasha TC, Radhakrishnan VV. Pathobiology of fungal infections of the central nervous system with special reference to the Indian scenario. Neurol India. 2007;55 (3):198.

Sharma P, Mukherjee A, Karunanithi S, Bal C, Kumar R. Potential role of 18F-FDG PET/CT in patients with fungal infections. Am J Roentgenol. 2014;203(1):180–9.

Sidani C, Freiser ME, Saigal G, Sklar E. Unusual case of cerebral aspergillosis with clinical and imaging findings mimicking lymphoma. Neuroradiol J. 2013;26(3):290–6.

Smirniotopoulos JG, Murphy FM, Rushing EJ, Rees JH, Schroeder JW. Patterns of contrast enhancement in the brain and meninges. Radiographics. 2007;27(2):525–51.

Sravani T, Uppin SG, Uppin MS, Sundaram C. Rhinocerebral mucormycosis: pathology revisited with emphasis on perineural spread. Neurol India. 2014;62(4):383.

Starkey J, Moritani T, Kirby P. MRI of CNS fungal infections: review of aspergillosis to histoplasmosis and everything in between. Clin Neuroradiol. 2014;24(3):217–30.

Stavrakis C, Narayan A, Voronel O. Cerebral blastomycosis: radiologic-pathologic correlation of solitary CNS blastomycosis mass-like infection. J Clin Imaging Sci. 2015;5:30.

Sundaram C, Umabala P, Laxmi V, Purohit AK, Prasad VS, Panigrahi M, Sahu BP, Sarathi MV, Kaul S, Borghain R, Meena AK. Pathology of fungal infections of the central nervous system: 17 years' experience from Southern India. Histopathology. 2006;49(4):396–405.

Tempkin AD, Sobonya RE, Seeger JF, Oh ES. Cerebral aspergillosis: radiologic and pathologic findings. Radiographics. 2006;26(4):1239–42.

Tore O, Akcaglar S, Kazak E, Heper Y, Akalin H, Hakyemez B, Ener B, Boekhout T, Hagen F. Multiple intracranial abscesses due to Cryptococcus neoformans: an unusual clinical feature in an immunocompetent patient and a short review of reported cases. Med Mycol. 2010;48(2):398–401.

Tung GA, Rogg JM. Diffusion-weighted imaging of cerebritis. Am J Neuroradiol. 2003;24(6):1110–3.

Imaging Findings of Fungal Infections of the Cranial and Peripheral Nerves

29

Ahmet T. Turgut, Elif Başbay Gündoğdu, Can Başaloğlu, and Mehmet Turgut

Abbreviations

AIDS	Acquired immunodeficiency syndrome
CNS	Central nervous system
CSF	Cerebrospinal fluid
DWI	Diffusion weighted imaging
HIV	Human immunodeficiency virus
MRI	Magnetic resonance imaging

29.1 Introduction

Fungal infections of the central nervous system (CNS) are rare, but their incidence has increased in recent years despite many advances in medical technology and public health measures because of increasing rate of immunocompromised populations. Neutropenia (especially hematological malignancies), acquired immunodeficiency syndrome (AIDS), organ transplantations, and widespread use of corticosteroids and cytotoxic drugs are possibly risk factors (Chakrabarti 2007; Scully et al. 2008). Fungal infections are more frequent in immunocompromised patients, but sinocranial aspergillosis may be seen in otherwise immunocompetent individuals (Chakrabarti 2007; Murthy 2007; Murthy and Sundaram 2014; Shih and Koeller 2015). Interestingly, some fungi have specific geographical distribution, although some of the fungi have worldwide distribution (Murthy and Sundaram 2014). Even today, despite new diagnostic tools and new therapies, morbidity and mortality rates of fungal infections of CNS still remain a significant problem in certain regions of the world, particularly in Africa, due to delay in the diagnosis (Murthy and Sundaram 2014; Shih and Koeller 2015). Therefore, early diagnosis and appropriate therapy and management are important (Scully et al. 2008).

Radiologically, there are nonspecific neuroimaging findings of fungal infections in the CNS because of the absence of typical inflammatory response, and hence making a definitive diagnosis is difficult and needs confirmatory laboratory tests, including cerebrospinal fluid (CSF) analysis (Shih and Koeller 2015). However, there are some specific findings for some agents and their knowledge helps in differential diagnosis. A high degree of suspicion concerning the possibility

A. T. Turgut (✉)
Department of Radiology, Istinye University Faculty of Medicine, İstanbul, Turkey

E. B. Gündoğdu
Department of Radiology, Osmangazi University, Eskişehir, Turkey

C. Başaloğlu
Department of Radiology, İzmir Dr. Suat Eren Chest Diseases and Surgery Training and Research Hospital, İzmir, Turkey

M. Turgut
Department of Neurosurgery, Aydın Adnan Menderes University School of Medicine, Aydın, Turkey

M. Turgut et al. (eds.), *Fungal Infections of the Central Nervous System*,
https://doi.org/10.1007/978-3-030-06088-6_29

of fungal infections of the CNS is necessary for accurate diagnosis because sometimes immune response is intact in immunocompromised patients (Khandelwal et al. 2011).

29.2 Fungal Infections

In contrast to other microorganisms, the term fungus is used for eukaryotic saprotrophic organisms with membrane-bound nuclei that derive nutrition from decomposition of organic matter (Shih and Koeller 2015). As a rule, the fungal infections of the CNS are caused by the systemic fungal pathogens via: (a) the hematogenous route; (b) direct extension from colonized sinuses or ear canal (sinonasal) (Fig. 29.1); or (c) direct inoculation during neurosurgical procedures (Chakrabarti 2007; Fockaert et al. 2014; Murthy 2007). In general, fungal infections of the CNS are opportunistic infections with hematogenous dissemination in susceptible subjects with immunodeficiency such as human immunodeficiency virus (HIV)/AIDS, systemic neoplasia, and organ transplantation (Shih and Koeller 2015). Fungi in the nature find a nidus in the human body and become pathogenic in hosts with immunocompromised states; thus, they increase the frequency of fungal infections (Shankar et al. 2007). Unlike tuberculosis, fungus is not transmitted from person to person by respiratory droplets but is acquired through inhalation of fungal spores from environment and soil (Shih and Koeller 2015). They reach to the CNS from pulmonary focus with hematogenous spreading.

Clinical manifestations of fungal infections of the CNS are related to the growth of the fungi, the antigenic feature of the capsule and the proteases secreted and may result in a clinical course ranging from acute fulminant course with significant morbidity and mortality to a chronic indolent form (Khandelwal et al. 2011; Shankar et al. 2007). Initial symptoms such as fever, nausea, vomiting, headache, seizures, lethargy, altered mental status, mass effect, or meningeal irritation findings are not specific and indistinguishable from other causes of meningoencephalitis. Rarely, it has been reported that some clinical syndromes are specific for some fungal infections: the rhinocerebral form in patients with zygomycosis, skull base syndromes in cases with sinocranial aspergillosis (Fig. 29.2), and meningitis in cases with cryptococcal infection (Borges 2005; Murthy 2007).

As a rule, the size of the size of the fungus is critical for the involvement of CNS because only small fungal pathogens may enter the circulatory system and then they cause meningitis and abscess formation, while hyphal forms produce ischemic or hemorrhagic infarcts by invading vessels (Shankar et al. 2007). Microbiologically, common causes of fungal acute and chronic meningitis are *Cryptococcus neoformans*, *Candida albicans*, *Coccidioides immitis*, and *Histoplasma capsulatum* (Chakrabarti 2007). However, *Aspergillus* spp., *Candida* spp., and *Zygomycetes* usually cause space-occupying lesions in the CNS (Chakrabarti 2007).

In this chapter, we will review radiological characteristics of fungal diseases involving the CNS, according to morphologic features of fungal pathogens: (a) yeast, (b) mold, and (c) dimorphic fungus (Mathur et al. 2012).

29.2.1 Yeasts

In fungal pathogens known as yeasts such as *Cryptococcus neoformans* and *Candida albicans*, only 1% of fungal species generally cause opportunistic infections in immunocompromised patients with HIV/AIDS with suppressed cell-mediated immunity (Shankar et al. 2007; Shih and Koeller 2015). On the other hand, *Cryptococcus gattii* may cause disseminated infections even in immunocompetent hosts (Suchitha et al. 2012). *Cryptococcus neoformans* is found in bird feces and transmitted by inhalation. It has a unique protective polysaccharide capsule that produces a characteristic halo with India ink stain (Shih and Koeller 2015). Cryptococcal meningitis is the most common fungal disease of the CNS, due to the presence of essential nutrients and the absence

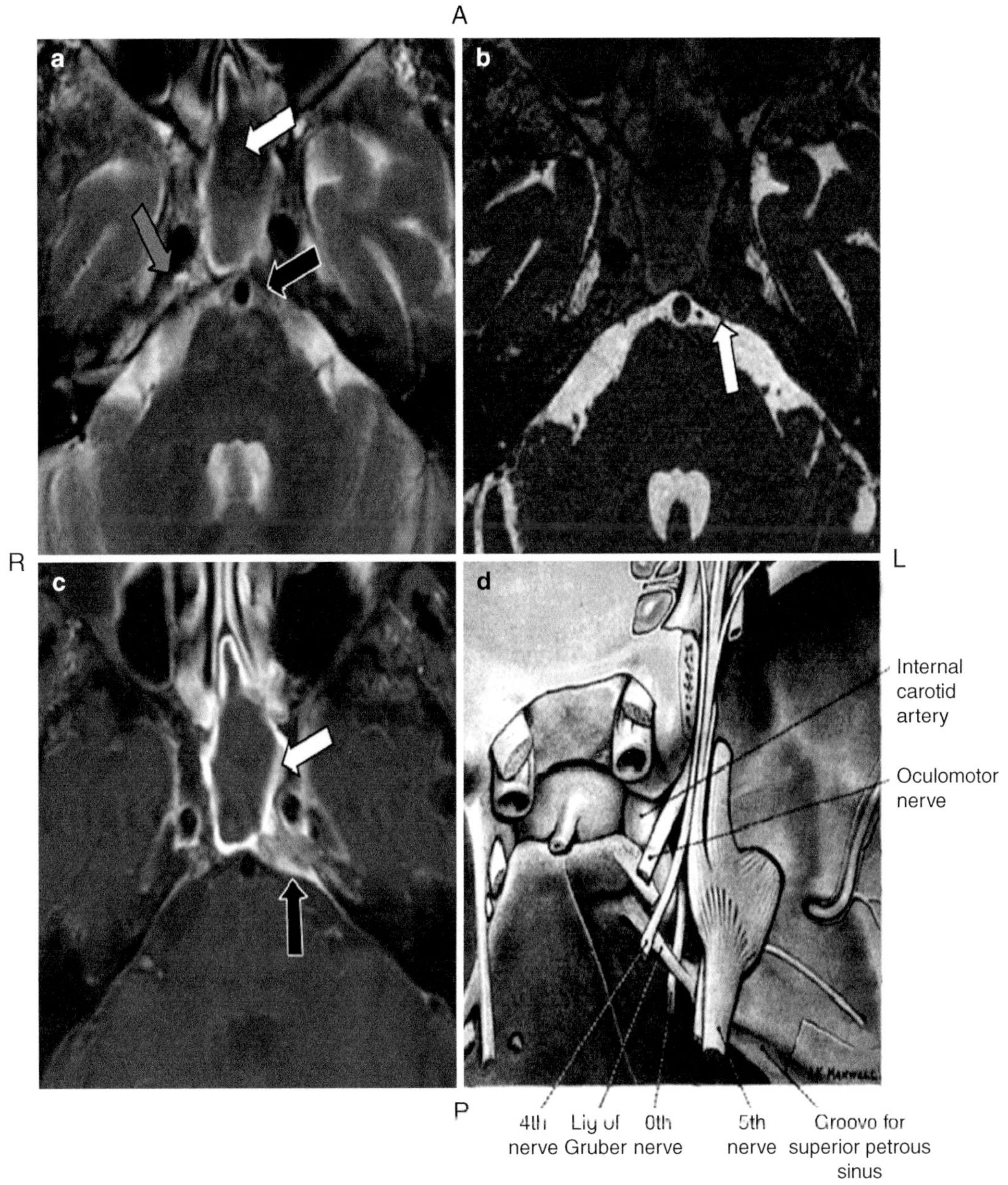

Fig. 29.1 (**a**) T2-weighted image at the level of Dorello's canal. The non-aerated sphenoid sinus has a very low signal intensity in the anterior part (white arrow), being compatible with fungal material. The fungus has invaded the clivus resulting in a low signal intensity replacing the normal marrow in the clivus on the left side, where the abducens nerve enters Dorello's canal (black arrow). The bone marrow on the right side has a normal high signal intensity (gray arrow). (**b**) 3D-balanced FFE image at the level of Dorello's canal. The clivus is slightly protruding in the prepontine cistern on the left side, and the signal intensity of the abducens nerve is slightly higher at the site where it is cutting the dura (arrow). (**c**) Gd-enhanced T1-weighted image with fat suppression. The invaded clivus on the left side protruding in the prepontine cistern is enhancing (black arrow). Non-aerated sphenoid sinus (white arrow). (**d**) Dorello's canal. The 6th cranial nerve enters the cavernous sinus at the Dorello's canal, formed by the petrous apex, the superolateral part of the clivus, and the petrosphenoidal ligament or Gruber's ligament (*A* anterior, *P* posterior, *L* left, *R* right) (from Fockaert et al. (2014), with permission)

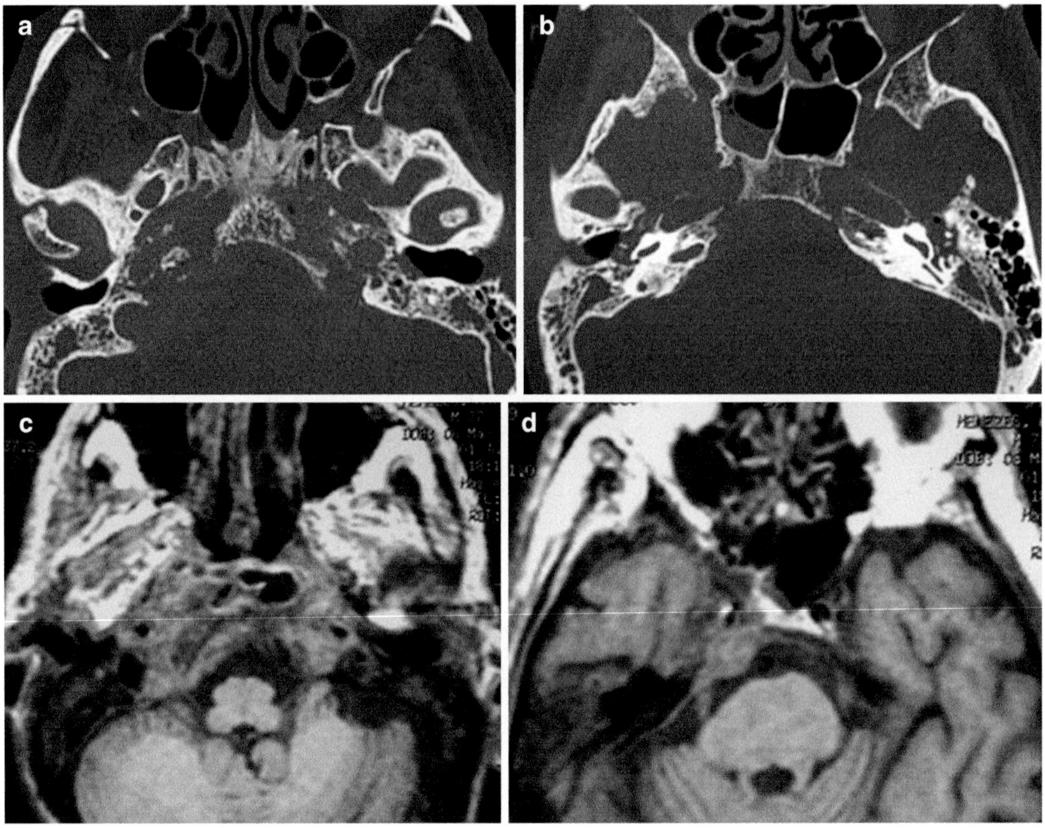

Fig. 29.2 (**a**, **b**) Axial computed tomography (CT) sections obtained through the skull base (bone algorithm) depicting bilateral opacification of the middle ear cavity and mastoid associated with bony destructive changes involving the petrous apices and central skull base. Note the destruction of the petrous carotid canals. (**c**, **d**) Axial SE T1W images revealing a soft tissue mass replacing the bone marrow of the central skull base, encasing the petrous carotid arteries bilaterally and infiltrating the left cavernous sinus. The abnormal thickening of the cisternal segment of the right trigeminal nerve and the soft tissue filling in Meckel's cave should be noted (skull base osteomyelitis, presumably of fungal etiology, in a diabetic patient presenting with Gradenigo's syndrome) (from Borges (2005), with permission)

of inhibitor substance in the CSF (Igel and Bolande 1966). This fungus can be seen worldwide, and not endemic. *Candida albicans* is found in the gut flora; candidiasis may manifest as invasive systemic disease (Shih and Koeller 2015).

Cryptococcus is small enough to enter the meningeal microcirculation through hematogenous dissemination (Shih and Koeller 2015). There are mainly three forms of this disease: meningitis, cryptococcomas, and gelatinous pseudocysts. The infection likes to involve the perivascular spaces. In meningitis form, nodular leptomeningeal enhancement is observed post-contrast T1-weighted images (Fig. 29.3) (Zhong et al. 2017). Neuroimaging findings include small or large cryptococcomas especially in midbrain or basal ganglia when infection passes through the brain parenchyma (Fig. 29.4) (George et al. 2009; Shih and Koeller 2015). Cryptococcomas have low signal in T1-weighted magnetic resonance images (MRIs) and high signal in T2-weighted MRIs and FLAIR. Contrast enhancement is variable. In some patients with cryptococcal infection involving the CNS, yeast typically produces "gelatinous pseudocysts" in the thalamus, midbrain, cerebellum, basal ganglia, and the regions adjacent to ventricular regions (Fig. 29.5) (Kovoor et al. 2002; Shih and Koeller 2015).

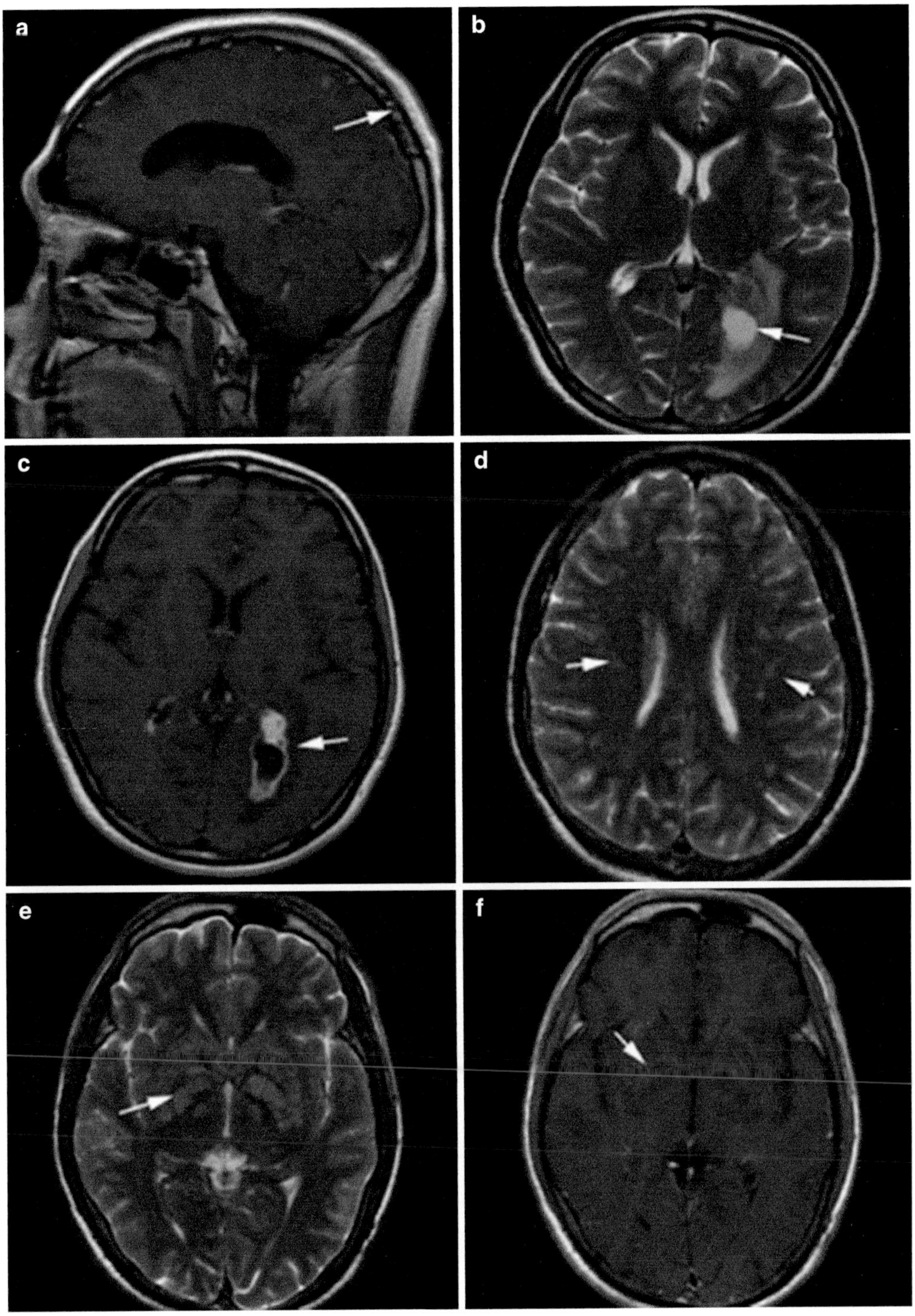

Fig. 29.3 The abnormal magnetic resonance findings in non-human immunodeficiency virus (HIV) patients with cryptococcal meningitis. (**a**) Sagittal T1-weighted post-gadolinium image showing apparent nodular meningeal enhancement. (**b**) Axial T2-weighted image depicting mass lesion in the white matter of the left lateral ventricle trigone. (**c**) Post-gadolinium MRI depicting remarkable ring enhancement of the mass lesion. (**d**) Axial T2-weighted image showing multiple dilated hyperintense Virchow-Robin spaces in bilateral centrum semiovale. (**e**) Axial T2 sequence revealing bilateral thick-walled, septated pseudocysts in the region of basal ganglia with a proteinaceous content. (**f**) Post-gadolinium MRI sequences (from Zhong et al. (2017), with permission)

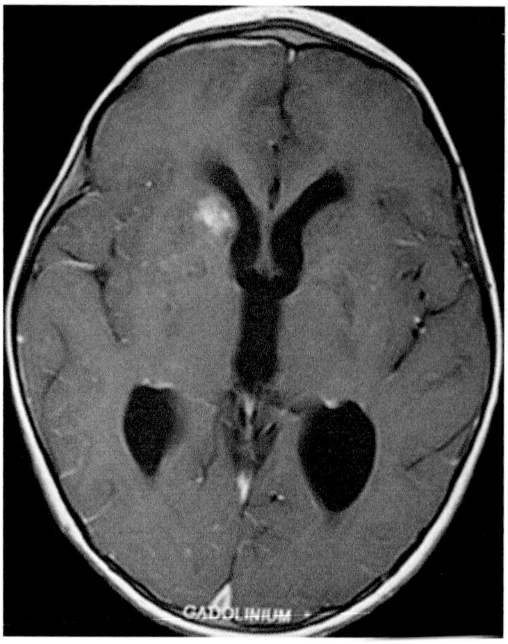

Fig. 29.4 Contrast-enhanced T1-W MRI showing an enhancing cryptococcus granuloma adjoining the right lateral ventricle (from George et al. (2009), with permission)

The mucin production may cause low signal intensity on T1-weighted MRI, high signal intensity on T2-weighted images, low signal intensity on FLAIR images, and restricted diffusion on DWI (Fig. 29.6). It can be seen typically like soap bubble. In all the three forms, one of the most common finding is hydrocephalus.

Cranial neuropathies including ophthalmoplegia are frequent complications of cryptococcal meningitis (Liyanage et al. 2014). It is known that the cranial nerve involvement (2nd, 3rd, 4th, 6th, 7th, and 8th cranial nerves) can be involved either in isolated or combined forms. This involvement may present with various symptoms depending on the cranial nerve that is affected. Ophthalmoplegia is a common form of presentation (Fig. 29.7). Direct invasion by the fungus may be the underlying mechanism for the involvement of the cranial nerves, whereas increased intracranial pressure may be the cause as in the cases with 6th nerve involvement.

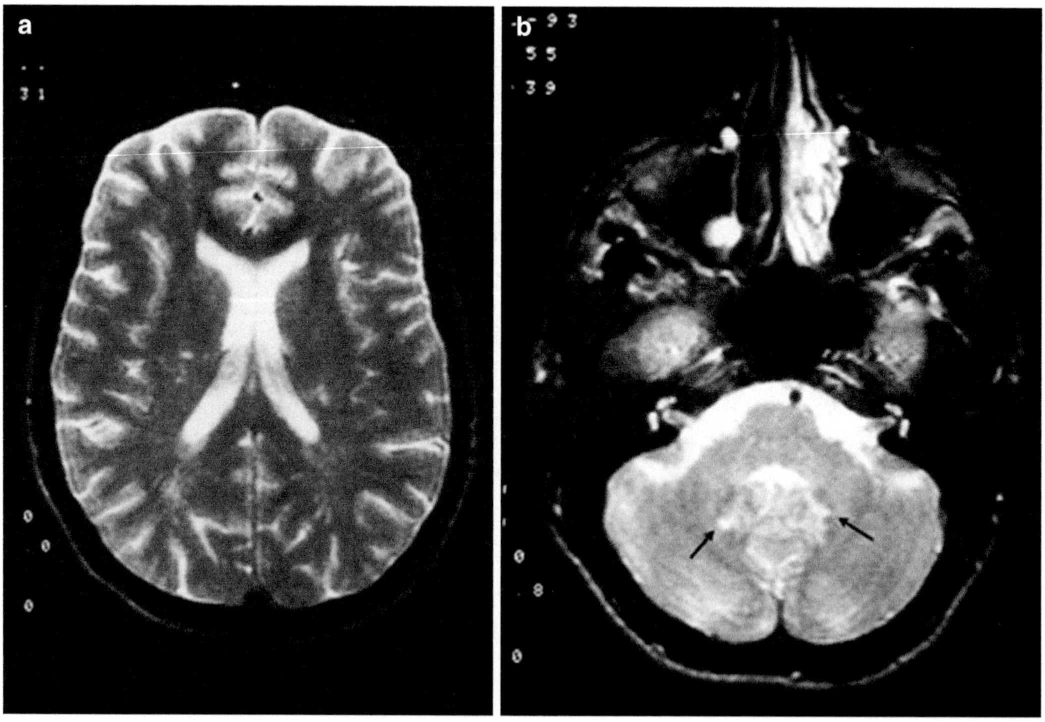

Fig. 29.5 (**a**) T2-weighted MRI showing dilated Virchow-Robin spaces in the central and periventricular parietal white matter. (**b**) Adjacent to the perivascular cerebrospinal fluid (CSF) spaces, small, CSF-isointense cyst-like lesions are seen in both cerebral and cerebellar hemispheres corresponding to focal dilatation of Virchow-Robin spaces or gelatinous pseudocysts. Note that no intraparenchymal lesions are detectable outside the CSF spaces (from Berkefeld et al. (1999), with permission)

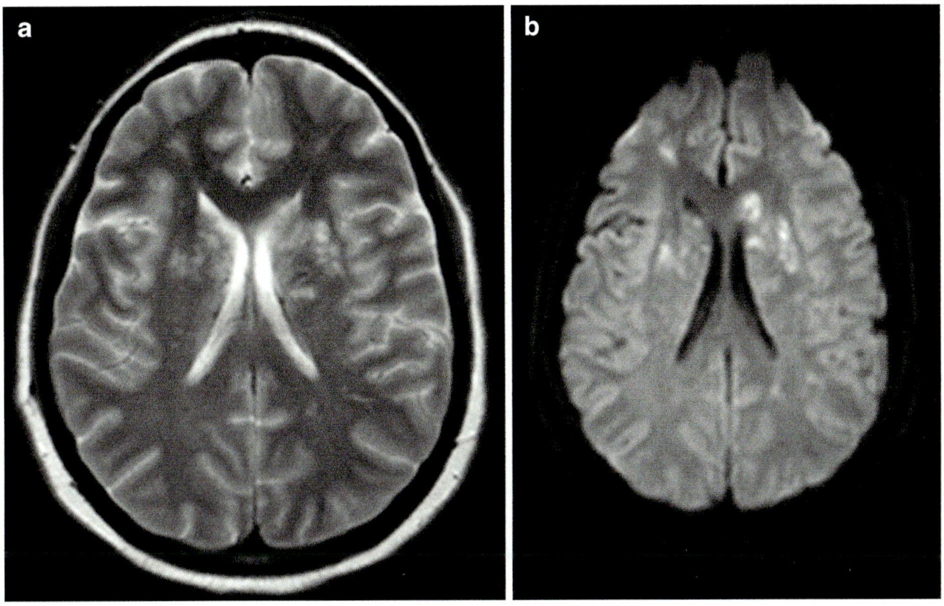

Fig. 29.6 Cryptococcosis: 36-year-old with axial T2 sequence (**a**) showing multiple hyperintense punctate lesions within the ganglia representing gelatinous pseudocysts. Diffusion-weighted imaging (DWI) (**b**) reveals areas of restricted diffusion correlating with the areas of signal abnormality (from Bhatia and Pruthi (2016), with permission)

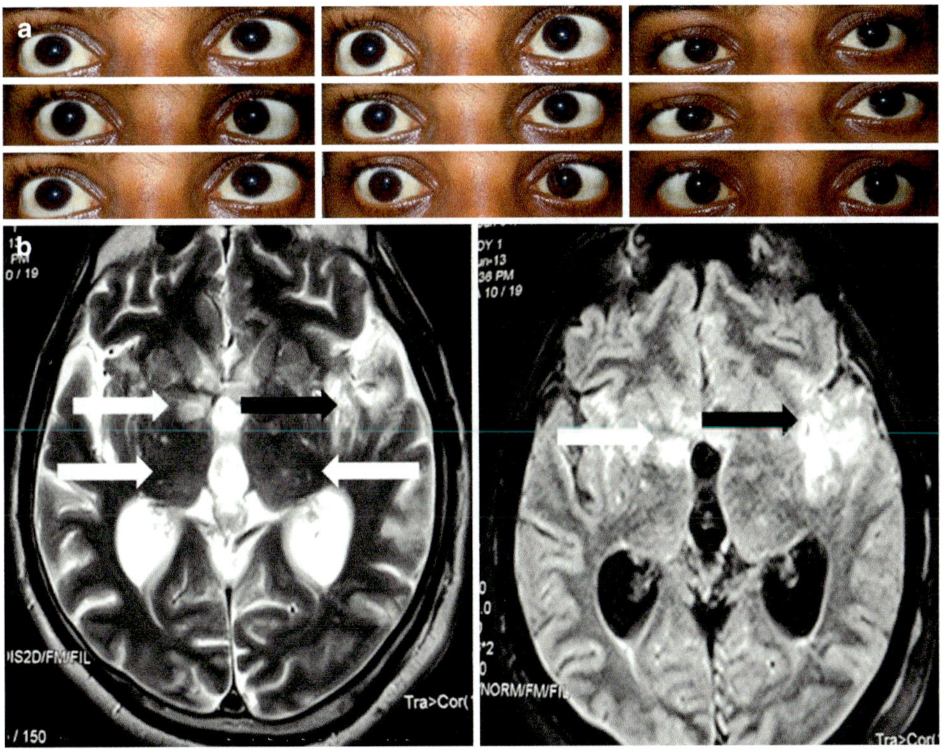

Fig. 29.7 (**a**) Eye movements. Bilateral symmetrical near-complete ophthalmoplegia. (**b**) Fluid-attenuated inversion recovery (FLAIR) (right) and T2-weighted (left) images of MRI of the brain. Bilateral multiple nodular lesions in basal ganglia and thalamus (white arrows). Ill-defined area of signal intensity change in the left temporoparietal region (black arrows) (from Liyanage et al. (2005), with permission)

In patients receiving immunosuppressive therapy or with indwelling catheters, *C. albicans* infection is the most common nosocomial fungal infection (Shih and Koeller 2015). *Candida* usually causes more invasive and disseminated parenchymal disease called a "pseudohyphal form" characterized by microabscesses, thrombosis, and hemorrhage, although macroabscesses, cerebral vasculitis, and meningitis are rarely seen (Shih and Koeller 2015; Tyc et al. 2014). *C. albicans* has small size, so it can pass microcirculation and leads to microabscesses which is typical for this disease (Fig. 29.8) (Starkey et al. 2014). They are less than 3 mm in size, multiple, and most commonly located at the gray-white matter junction, basal ganglia, and cerebellum. They have same imaging findings with other cause of abscesses. In addition, they can contain small hemorrhagic foci which is better seen on gradient-echo (GRE) or susceptibilityweighted imaging (SWI) MRIs. And also, because of hemorrhage, rim-like low signal is seen on T2-weighted MRIs. When infection affects leptomeninges, nonspecific enhancement may be seen, rarely. In differential diagnosis of candidal microabscesses, infections with *Staphylococcus aureus* and *Mycobacterium tuberculosis* infection, metastatic disease, and multiple sclerosis should be considered (Lai et al. 1997).

29.2.2 Molds

Molds grow as multicellular filaments called "hyphae" and then macroscopic networks called "mycelia" (Shih and Koeller 2015). Microbiologically, the most common pathogens producing hyphal forms are *Aspergillus* and *Zygomycetes* (Shankar et al. 2007). Some molds such as *Aspergillus* and *Mucorales* are pathogenic, although the vast majority of molds are beneficial (Shih and Koeller 2015). Molds are ubiquitous in the soil and can infect the respiratory tract after spore inhalation (Shih and Koeller 2015). They then can invade pulmonary arteries and access to systemic circulation and hematogenously spread to the CNS. Importantly, multicellular hyphae cause invasive parenchymal disease in immunocompromised patients because they are big pathogens for the meningeal microcirculation in contrast to yeasts (Shih and Koeller 2015).

Infections due to molds such as aspergillosis and mucormycosis involving the CNS may (a) originate from hematogenous dissemination from a distant pulmonary infection, (b) spread from a paranasal sinus or orbital infection known as "rhinocerebral disease" (Fig. 29.9), or (c) direct implantation during traumatic event (Fig. 29.10) (Dhirawani et al. 2015; McLean et al. 1996). It has been reported that aspergillosis frequently presents with ring-enhancing cerebral abscesses from hematogenous dissemination (Ashdown et al. 1994). In contrast to other abscesses caused by pyogenic organisms or *M. tuberculosis*, intracavitary hypointense projections on T2-weighted MRI and apparent diffusion coefficient MRI without associated enhancement are seen in fungal abscesses (Luthra et al. 2007). And also, they have peripheral low signal intensity on T2-weighted images which is better appreciated on GRE or SWI images, possibly due to hemorrhage (Fig. 29.11). They are often multiple and randomly localized (Starkey et al. 2014).

Aspergillosis may cause life-threatening cerebral infarction which is often multiple, present in a random distribution because of invasion to small or large blood vessels (Almutairi et al. 2009; Hurst et al. 2001; Negoro et al. 2013). Hemorrhage and mycotic aneurysms may accompany infarcts (Fig. 29.12).

The involvement of the cranial nerves in these localizations in the invasive disease caused by *Aspergillus* may cause the initial symptoms of the disease. Trigeminal neuralgia secondary to the involvement of the maxillary branch of the 5th cranial nerve may occur in invasive fungal

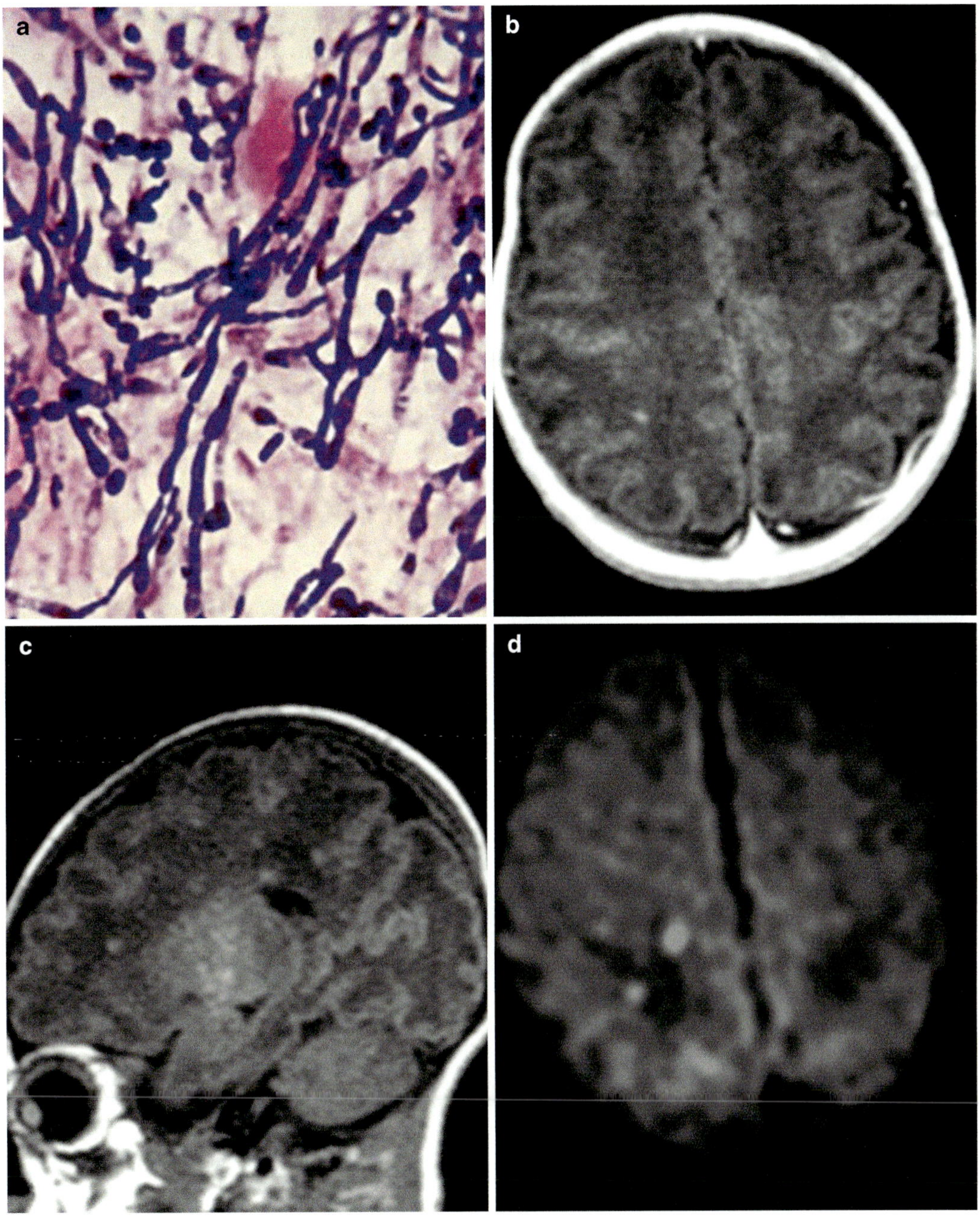

Fig. 29.8 Cerebral candidiasis in a 6-year-old boy with meconium ileus who developed lethargy. The entity usually presents as microabscesses measuring less than 3 mm. (**a**) Photomicrograph (original magnification, ×600; PAS stain) shows rounded bodies with some pseudohyphae typical of *Candida* species (courtesy of Centers for Disease Control (CDC)/Sherry Brinkman). (**b**, **c**) Axial and sagittal T1 post-gadolinium sequences show punctate subcortical foci of enhancement. (**d**) Axial DWI shows restricted diffusion of multiple lesions, including those that are not detectable on contrast-enhanced sequence (from Starkey et al. (2014), with permission)

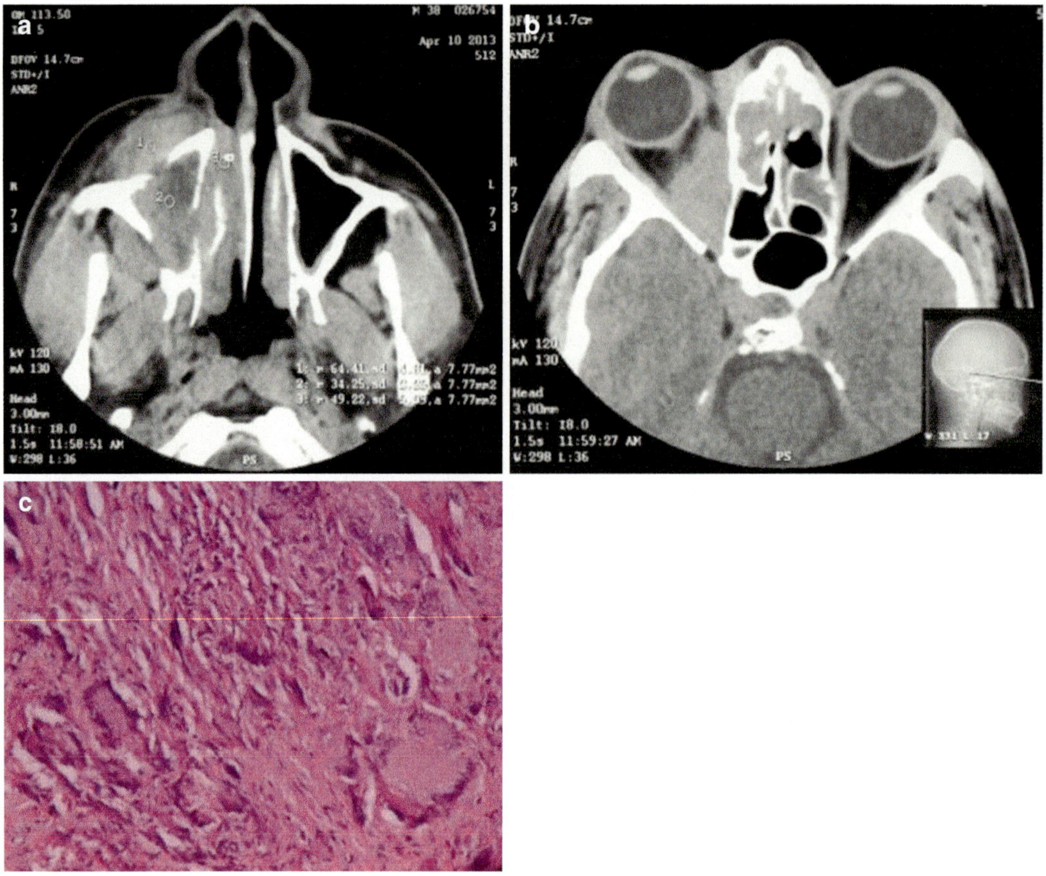

Fig. 29.9 (**a**) CT scan demonstrating a large heterogeneously enhancing mass lesion, invading the right maxillary sinus, eroding its medial and lateral walls and extending up to right pterygoid plate. (**b**) Extension of the lesion in retro-orbital planes engulfing the optic nerve leading to proptosis. (**c**) Histologic section confirmatory of Aspergillosis (from Dhirawani et al. (2004), with permission)

sinusitis (Fig. 29.13), whereas paralysis of 10th, 11th, and 12th cranial nerve may develop due to involvement of the skull base by invasive fungal osteomyelitis (Fig. 29.14) (Maschio et al. 2012; Ridder et al. 2015).

Mucormycosis is more likely to manifest as rhinocerebral disease in immunocompromised or diabetic patients because of a locally aggressive sino-orbital infection (Luthra et al. 2007).

In aggressive course, it may spread to the orbit and cranium in days and may result in death in turn. It may cause orbital apex syndrome secondary to multiple cranial nerve involvement (Fig. 29.15) and may be responsible for the symptoms associated with isolated involvement of the cranial nerves (Fig. 29.16) (Bakshi 2016; Jiang et al. 2016).

Osteomyelitis, local dural enhancement, and subdural empyema may also be present (Fig. 29.17) (Hassler et al. 2015). There is no doubt that early diagnosis, appropriate antifungal therapy, and surgical debridement are very important for these infections (Shih and Koeller 2015).

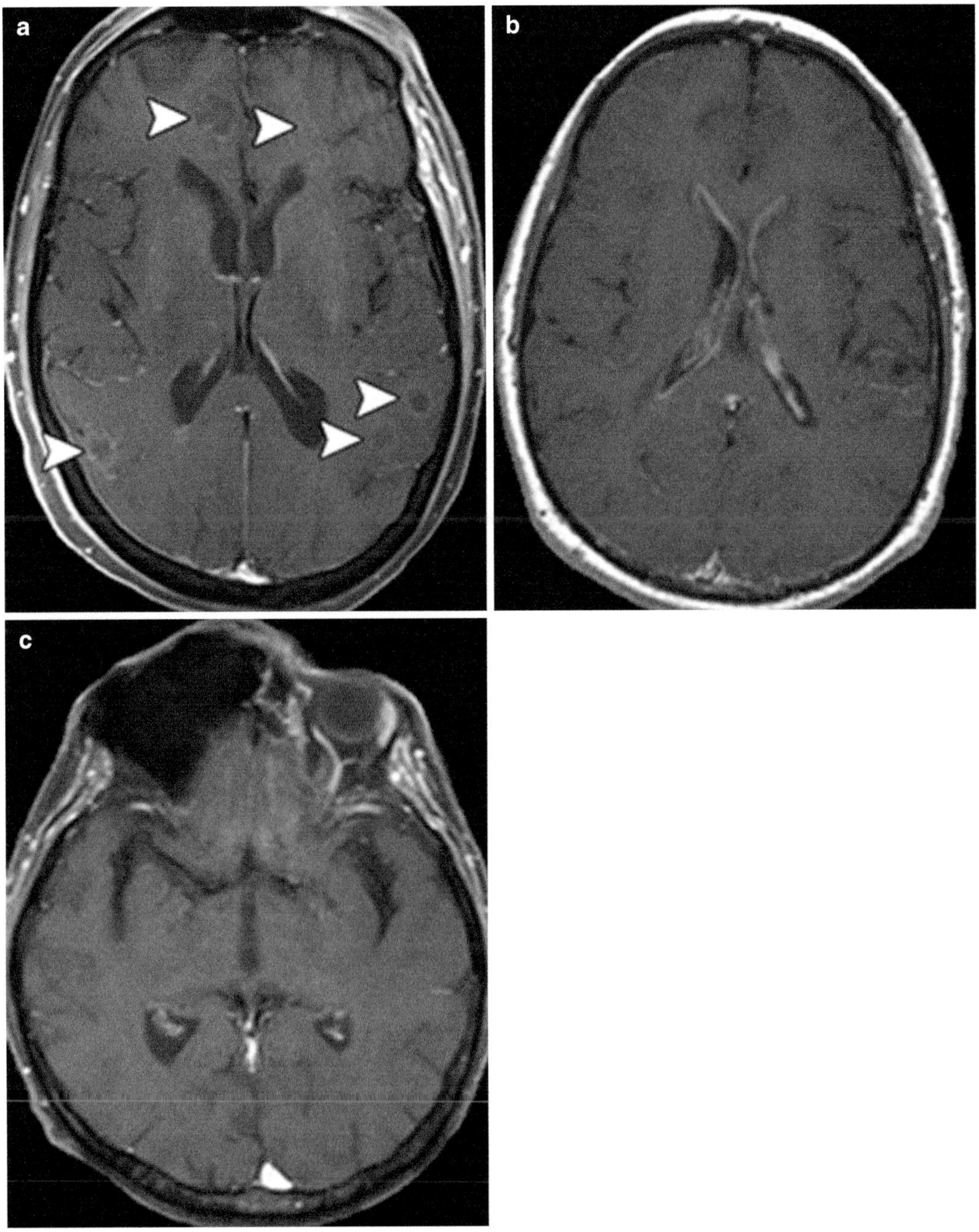

Fig. 29.10 Fungal central nervous system (CNS) infection may develop via hematogenous spread, CSF seeding, or direct extension. (**a**) Axial T1 post-gadolinium image shows typical lesions of multifocal angioinvasive aspergillosis at the gray-white junction (*arrowheads*). (**b**) Axial T1 post-gadolinium image reveals typical cryptococcal meningitis resulting in ventricular wall enhancement and subtle frontal and occipital leptomeningeal enhancement. (**c**) Axial T1 post-gadolinium image depicts mucormycosis with intracranial extension and enhancement at the inferior frontal lobe developing after a sinus infection (from Starkey et al. (2014), with permission)

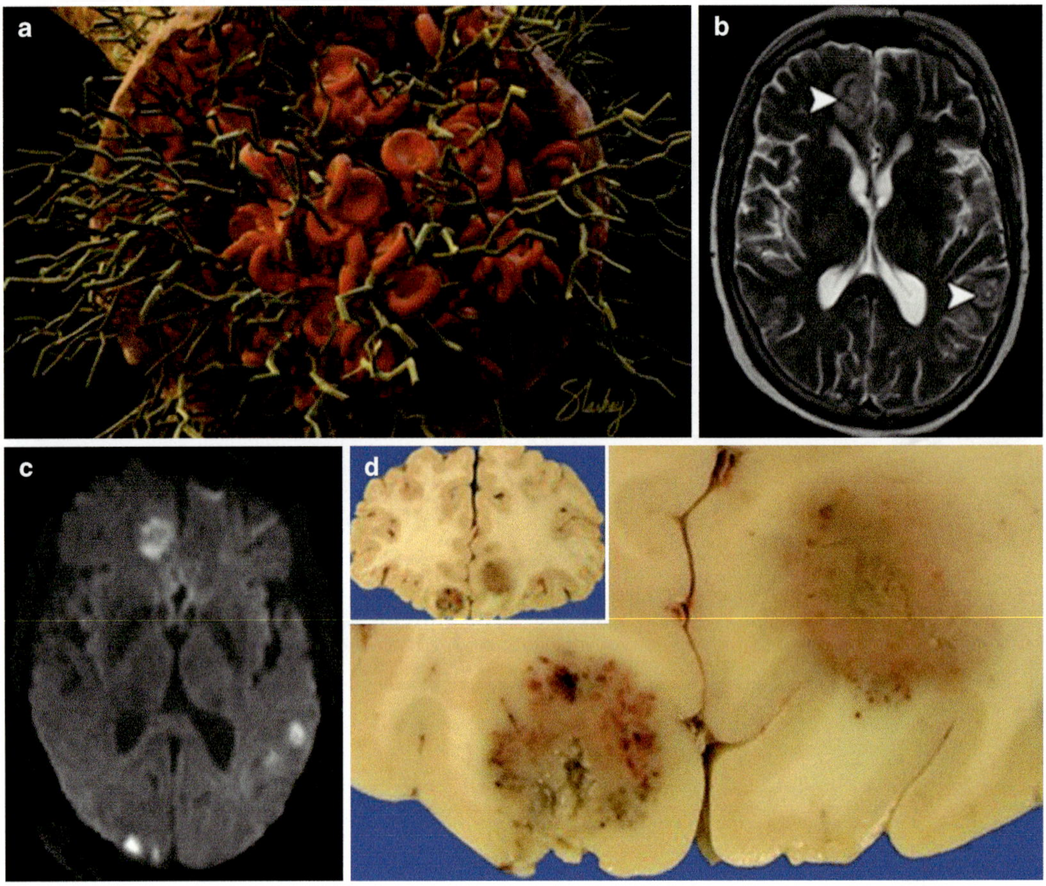

Fig. 29.11 *Aspergillus* species are usually angioinvasive, multiplying within blood vessels and producing artery-destroying elastases and resulting in microhemorrhage and infection of adjacent brain parenchyma in turn. Fungal elements clogging vessels cause downstream sterile infarction. (**a**) Illustration showing angioinvasive nature of *Aspergillus* with fungal elements in the vessel lumen and hyphae invading the vessel wall. (**b**) Axial T2 sequence shows characteristic peripheral low signal intensity (*arrowheads*), which may be secondary to hemorrhage and increased iron associated with fungal elements and hemorrhage. (**c**) Axial diffusion-weighted sequences show magnetic susceptibility artifact implying microhemorrhage and reduced diffusion representing infarction in the lesions located at the gray-white junction. (**d**) Gross pathologic examination shows corresponding lesion with peripheral hemorrhage and central necrosis. The patient was a 56-year-old woman with acute myelogenous leukemia who developed widely disseminated multiorgan aspergillosis (from Starkey et al. (2014), with permission)

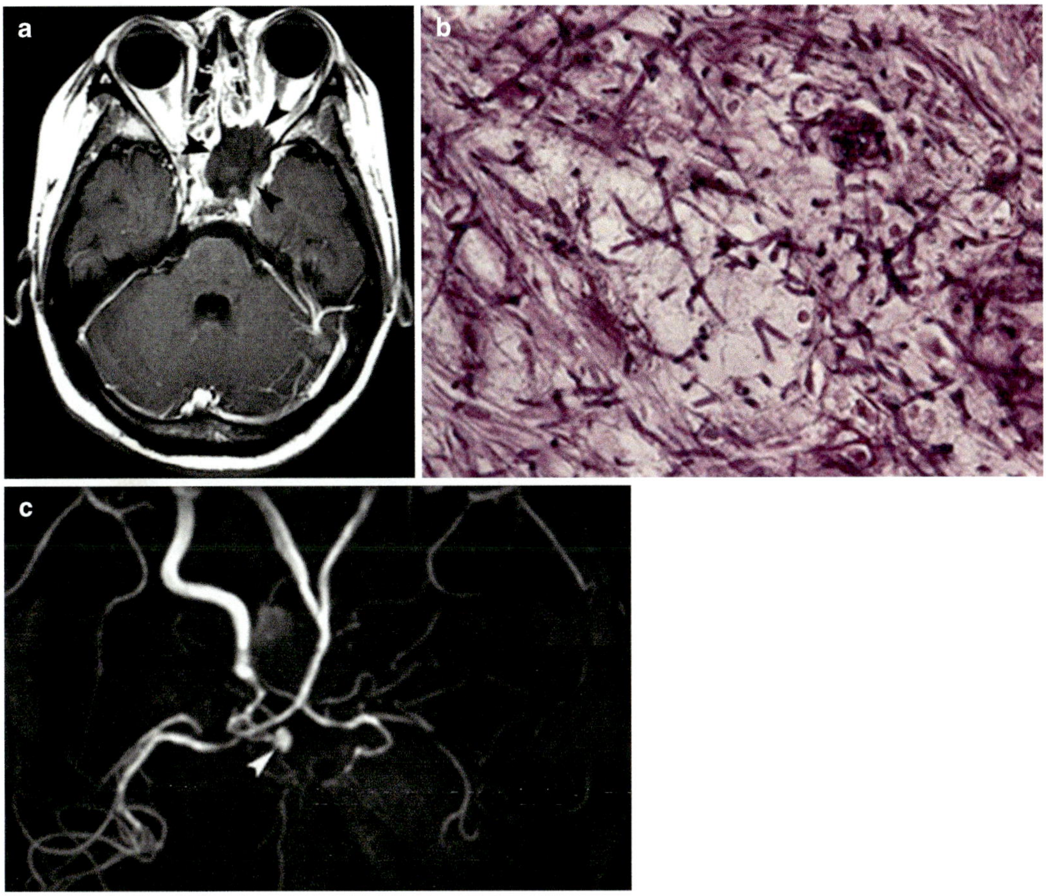

Fig. 29.12 (**a**) Gadolinium-enhanced T1-weighted MRI scans of the brain showing low intensity in the sphenoid sinus. (**b**) The fungus in the sphenoid sinus had a long uniformity and septate hyphae which had parallel contours and branched at 45°. *Aspergillus* species was suggested by microscopic morphology (periodic acid Schiff staining). (**c**) A mycotic aneurysm in the left anterior cerebral artery (from Negoro et al. (2013), with permission)

29.2.3 Dimorphic Fungi

Typically, dimorphic fungi have a conversion ability at fungal culture: they grow as mold at 25–30°C but as yeast at 35–37°C (Hughes et al. 2004; Shih and Koeller 2015). *Blastomyces dermatitidis*, *Coccidioides immitis*, and *Histoplasma capsulatum* are unicellular eukaryotes at body temperature (Shih and Koeller 2015). At room temperature, *Blastomyces dermatitidis*, *Coccidioides immitis*, and *Histoplasma capsulatum* are unicellular eukaryotes in the soil as

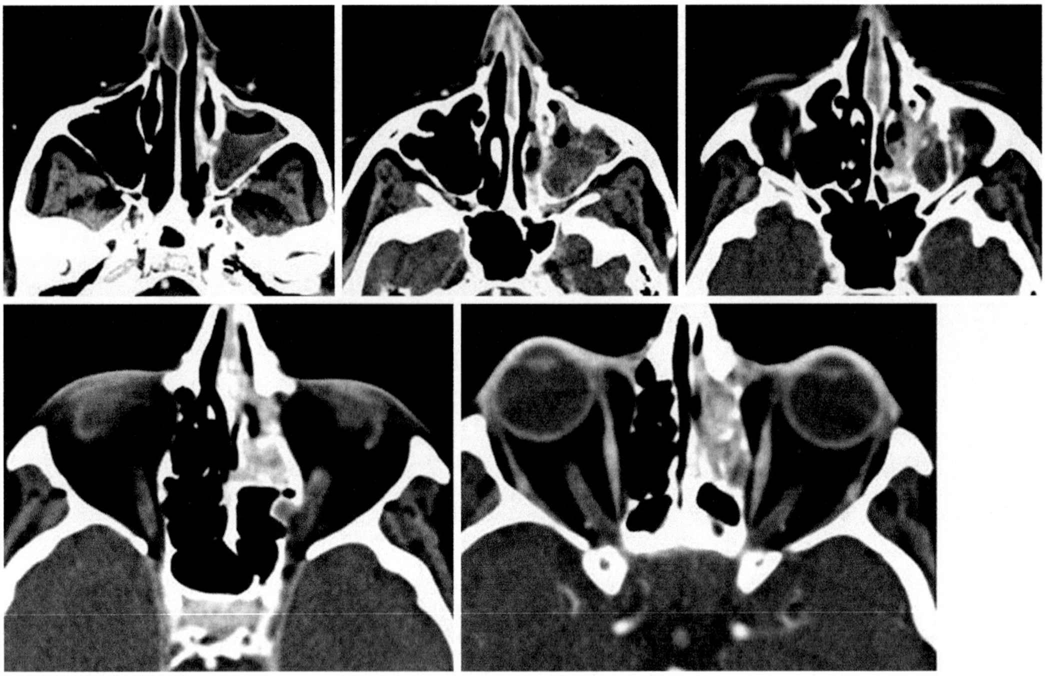

Fig. 29.13 CT scans show a hypodense tissue associated with an inflammatory disease in the left maxillary sinus with a fluid level and in the left ethmoid sinus, without bone erosion (from Maschio et al. (2012), with permission)

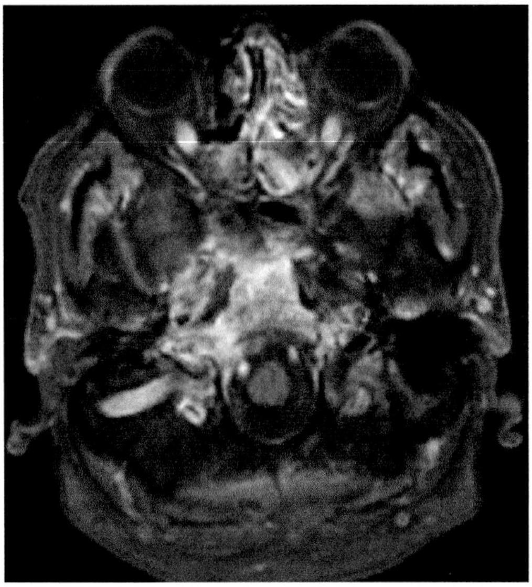

Fig. 29.14 MRI of a 69-year-old patient with pares is of the glossopharyngeal and the hypoglossal nerve showing central skull base osteomyelitis accentuated around the right-sided jugular foramen (from Ridder et al. 2015, with permission)

molds called "multicellular mycelia," and inhalation of spore released by these fungi may lead to acute or chronic pulmonary disease, nodular or disseminated, requiring antifungal therapy (Galgiani et al. 2005; Shih and Koeller 2015).

Coccidioidomycosis caused by *Coccidioides immitis* and *Coccidioides posadasii* has a high incidence in endemic regions of the world including the United States and Latin America if a wet season is followed by a dry season (Hirschmann 2007; Shih and Koeller 2015). The disease can occur in immunocompetent individuals, especially with repeated exposure, but the risk is more high in the immunocompromised.

In a patient with disseminated infection, release of endospores of fungal pathogens causing coccidioidomycosis, histoplasmosis, or blastomycosis results in fungal meningitis firstly and then parenchymal space-occupying lesions called granulomas or abscesses (Fig. 29.18) (Shih and Koeller 2015). Radiologically, the findings of

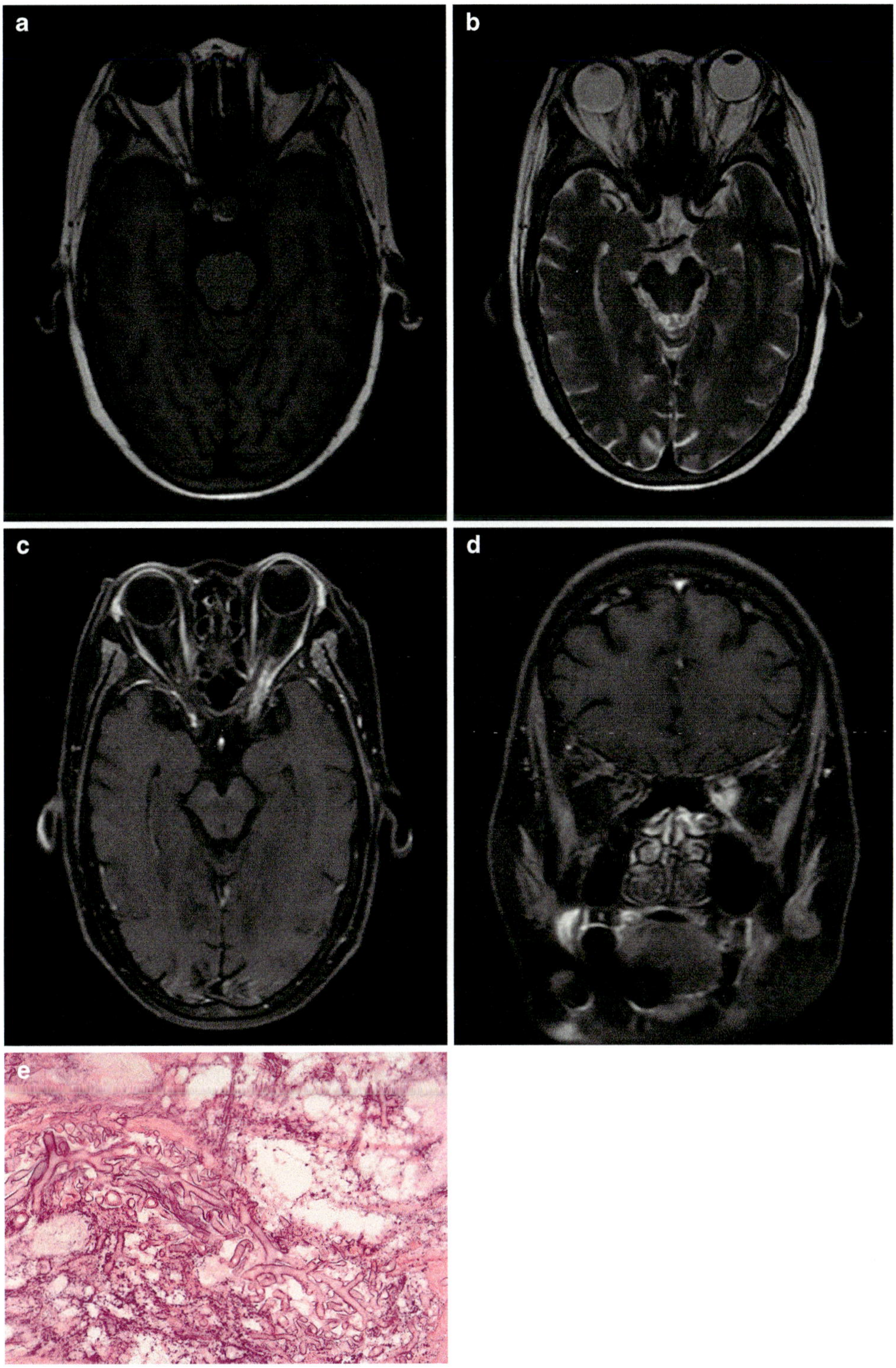

Fig. 29.15 MRI scans of mucormycosis presenting with orbital apex syndrome. (**a**) Axial T1WI MRI shows an isointense lesion in the left orbital apex; (**b**) axial T2WI MRI shows a lesion with low signal intensity lesion in the left orbital apex and high signal in the sphenoid sinus; (**c**) axial contrast-enhanced T1WI MRI shows an enhancing lesion in the left orbital apex; (**d**) coronal contrast-enhanced T1WI MRI shows an enhancing lesion in the left orbital apex. Nasal biopsy shows mycelial filaments of variable thickness and necrosis (PAS; ×200) (from Jiang et al. (2016), with permission)

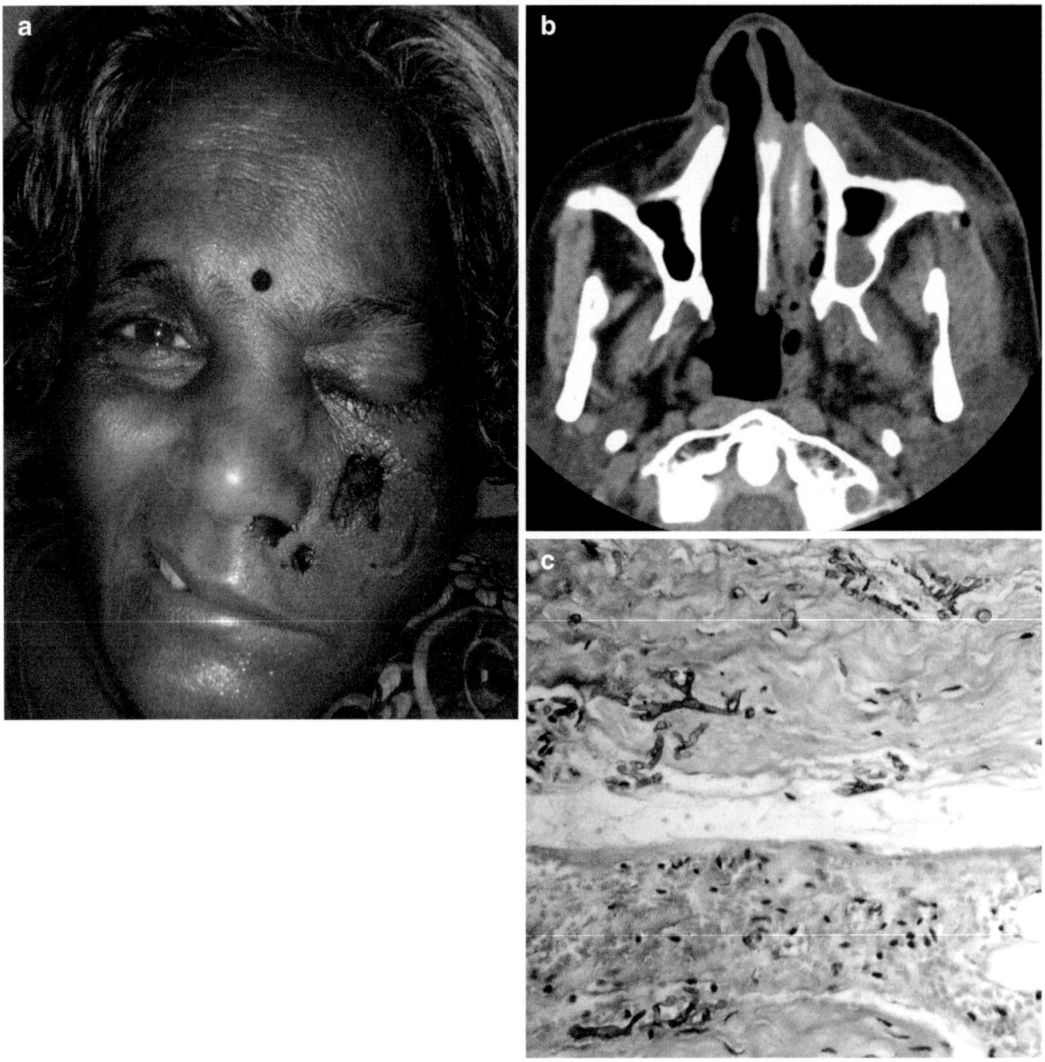

Fig. 29.16 (**a**) Female patient presenting with mucormycosis and ulcer over the left cheek and facial nerve palsy (L) side. (**b**) CT scan showing soft tissue opacification of the left nasal cavity with fluid collection in the left maxillary sinus and edema over left cheek. (**c**) Microscopic picture revealing broad, irregular, ribbon-like fungal hyphae which are aseptate with a background showing necrosis (HE, ×100) (from Bakshi (2016), with permission)

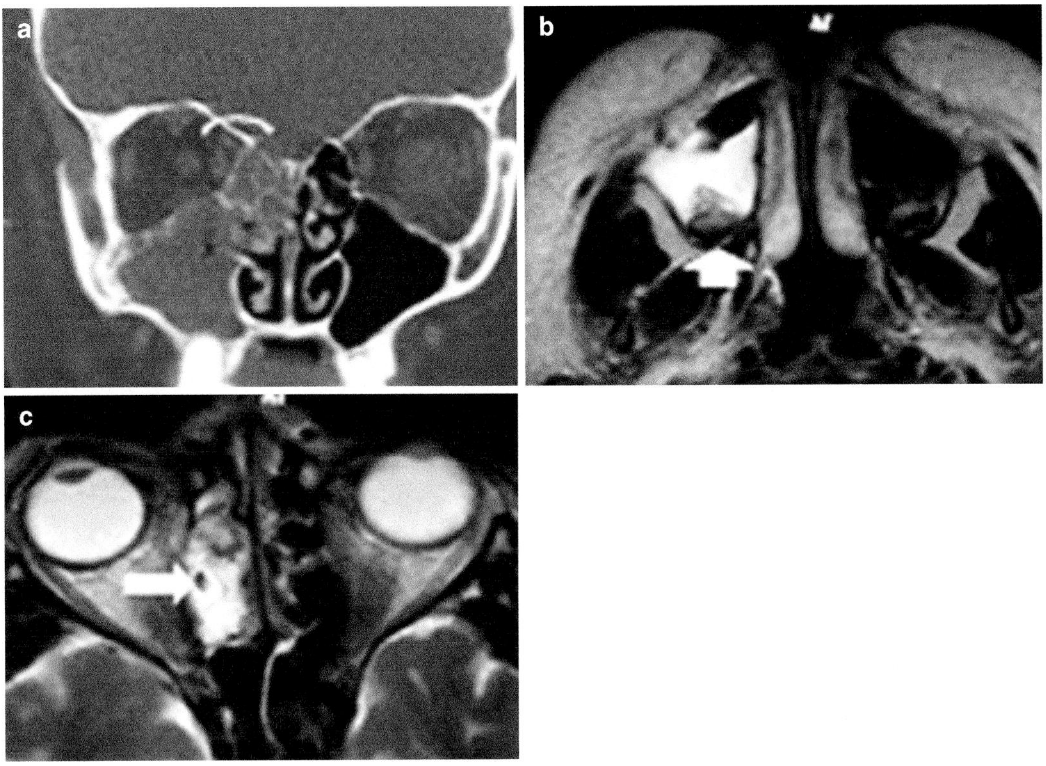

Fig. 29.17 10-year-old girl with aplastic anemia presenting with mucormycosis. (**a**) CT shows the destruction of the frontobasis in the area of the cribriform plate (curved arrow). (**b**, **c**) Axial T2-weighted images show areas of low signal intensity in the right maxillary and in the right ethmoidal sinus (straight arrows) (from Hassler et al. (2015), with permission)

coccidioidal meningitis are characterized by the presence of thick exudate and enhancement in subarachnoid space and basal cisterns. It can also extend to the spinal cord. Secondary communicating hydrocephalus often develops, but it may be absent early in the course. Basal cisterns are also affected in patients with neurotuberculosis; it must be considered in differential diagnosis (Shih and Koeller 2015). In some patients, vasculitis, infarction, cerebritis, abscesses, or subarachnoid hemorrhage may develop as a result of extension of granulomatous inflammation along large vessels or in perivascular spaces (Erly et al. 1999a; Zalduondo et al. 1996).

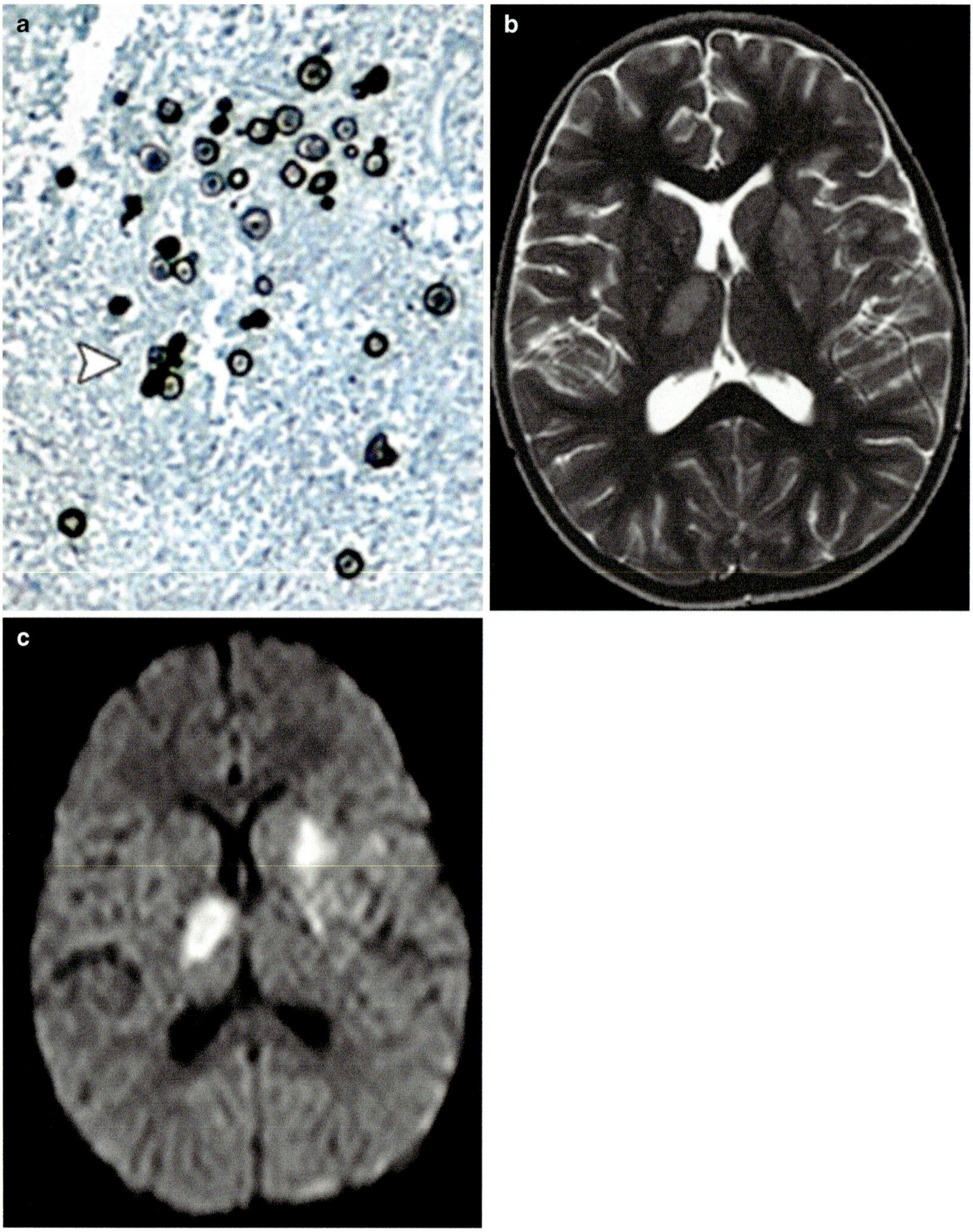

Fig. 29.18 The rare *Coccidioides* CNS infections generally occur only in endemic regions of the Southwestern United States. (**a**) Photomicrograph (original magnification, ×400; GMS stain) shows rounded spherules of *Coccidioides immitis* (*arrowhead*) (courtesy of CDC/Martin D. Hicklin). (**b**) Axial T2-weighted sequence reveals hyperintensity in the right globus pallidus and left putamen with mild narrowing of the left lateral ventricle. (**c**) Axial DWI shows reduced diffusion in a similar anatomical distribution. Contrast-enhanced imaging was not performed. The patient was a 4-year-old girl having a sudden onset of acute neurologic deficits following 3 days of nausea, vomiting, and dehydration with persistent headaches and "fuzzy" vision and had a history of recurrent rashes. The patient developed low-grade fevers. CSF fungal cultures grew *Coccidioides immitis*. The patient living in the Midwestern United States had no history of travel to endemic areas. Later she was diagnosed with hyper-IgE-related immunodeficiency, developed frank ventriculitis requiring shunt placement, and benefited from antifungal therapy (from Starkey et al. (2014), with permission)

29.3 Conclusion

Fungal pathogens involving the CNS, including the yeast *Cryptococcus* and the dimorphic fungi *Coccidioides*, *Histoplasma*, and *Blastomyces*, are important sources of morbidity and mortality worldwide, especially in immunocompromised patients in less developed countries. Today, it is well-known that they usually start with inhalation of spores, followed by hematogenous dissemination in susceptible individuals. Immunodeficient patients are at risk for parenchymal disease for aspergillosis and mucormycosis, whereas microabscesses are seen in invasive candidiasis. Radiologically, they have similar appearances to other granulomatous diseases, such as tuberculosis. Therefore, a high degree of suspicion is required for correct diagnosis and appropriate antifungal treatment in patients with fungal infections of the CNS. Computed tomography may show hydrocephalus, mass effect, and parenchymal or subarachnoid hemorrhage, but MRI is more diagnostic for early cerebritis, ventriculitis, and infarct. For hemorrhagic lesions, SWI or GRE can be preferred.

References

Almutairi BM, Nguyen TB, Jansen GH, Asseri AH. Invasive aspergillosis of the brain: radiologic-pathologic correlation. Radiographics. 2009;29:375–9.

Ashdown BC, Tien RD, Felsberg GJ. Aspergillosis of the brain and paranasal sinuses in immunocompromised patients: CT and MR imaging findings. AJR Am J Roentgenol. 1994;162:155–9.

Bakshi SS. An unusual cause for facial nerve palsy: mucormycosis. Int J Diabetes Dev Ctries. 2016;36:385–8.

Berkefeld J, Enzensberger W, Lanfermann H. Cryptococcus meningoencephalitis in AIDS: parenchymal and meningeal forms. Neuroradiology. 1999;41:129–33.

Bhatia A, Pruthi S. Imaging of pediatric infection within the central nervous system. Curr Radiol Reports. 2016;4:1–11.

Borges A. Trigeminal neuralgia and facial nerve paralysis. Eur Radiol. 2005;15:511–33.

Chakrabarti A. Epidemiology of central nervous system mycoses. Neurol India. 2007;55:191–7.

Dhirawani R, Asrani S, Pathak S, Sharma A. Facial translocation approach for management of invasive sinonasal aspergillosis. J Maxillofac Oral Surg. 2015;14:482–7.

Erly WK, Bellon RJ, Seeger JF, Carmody RF. MR imaging of acute coccidioidal meningitis. AJNR Am J Neuroradiol. 1999a;20:509–14.

Fockaert N, D'Hooghe L, Casselman J, Dycke AV. Sixth cranial nerve palsy in isolated sphenoid sinusitis: a case report. Acta Neurol Belg. 2014;114:335–7.

Galgiani JN, Ampel NM, Blair JE. Coccidioidomycosis. Clin Infect Dis. 2005;41:1217–23.

George R, Andronikou S, Plessis J, Plessis A, Toorn RV, Maydell A. Central nervous system manifestations of HIV infection in children. Pediatr Radiol. 2009;39:575–85.

Hassler A, Porto L, Lehrnbecher T. Cerebral fungal infection in pediatric cancer patients. Curr Fungal Infect Rep. 2015;9:6–14.

Hirschmann JV. The early history of coccidioidomycosis: 1892-1945. Clin Infect Dis. 2007;44:1202–7.

Hughes AD, Lorusso GD, Greer DL. Cost-effective method for identification of dimorphic fungi. J Clin Microbiol. 2004;42:4408–9.

Hurst RW, Judkins A, Bolger W, Chu A, Loevner LA. Mycotic aneurysm and cerebral infarction resulting from fungal sinusitis: imaging and pathologic correlation. AJNR Am J Neuroradiol. 2001;22:858–63.

Igel HJ, Bolande RP. Humoral defense mechanisms in cryptococcosis: substances in normal human serum, saliva, and cerebrospinal fluid affecting the growth of Cryptococcus neoformans. J Infect Dis. 1966;116:75–83.

Jiang N, Zhao G, Yang S, Lin J, Hu L, Che C, Wang Q, Xu Q. A retrospective analysis of eleven cases of invasive rhino-orbito-cerebral mucormycosis presented with orbital apex syndrome initially. BMC Ophthalmol. 2016;16:10. https://doi.org/10.1186/s12886-016-0189-1.

Khandelwal N, Gupta V, Singh P. Central nervous system fungal infections in tropics. Neuroimaging Clin N Am. 2011;21:859–66.

Kovoor JM, Mahadevan A, Narayan JP, Govindappa SS, Satishchandra P, Taly AV, Shankar SK. Cryptococcal choroid plexitis as a mass lesion: MR imaging and histopathologic correlation. AJNR Am J Neuroradiol. 2002;23:273–6.

Lai PH, Lin SM, Pan HB, Yang CF. Disseminated miliary cerebral candidiasis. AJNR Am J Neuroradiol. 1997;18:1303–6.

Liyanage DS, Pathberiya LPS, Gooneratne IK, Caldera MHPC, Perera PWS. Cryptococcal meningitis presenting with bilateral complete ophthalmoplegia: a case report. BMC Res Notes. 2014;7:328.

Luthra G, Parihar A, Nath K, Jaiswal S, Prasad KN, Husain N, Husain M, Singh S, Behari S, Gupta RK. Comparative evaluation of fungal, tubercular, and pyogenic brain abscesses with conventional and diffusion MR imaging and proton MR spectroscopy. AJNR Am J Neuroradiol. 2007;28:1332–8.

Maschio M, Mengarelli A, Girmenia C, Vidiri A, Kayal R, Gallo MT, Prignano G, Dessanti ML, D'Andrea M, Petti MC. Trigeminal neuralgia as unusual isolated symptom of fungal paranasal sinusitis in patients with haematological malignancies. Neurol Sci. 2012;33:647–52.

Mathur M, Johnson CE, Sze G. Fungal infections of the central nervous system. Neuroimaging Clin N Am. 2012;22:609–32.

McLean FM, Ginsberg LE, Stanton CA. Perineural spread of rhinocerebral mucormycosis. AJNR Am J Neuroradiol. 1996;17:114–6.

Murthy JM. Fungal infections of the central nervous system: the clinical syndromes. Neurol India. 2007;55:221–5.

Murthy JM, Sundaram C. Fungal infections of the central nervous system. Handb Clin Neurol. 2014;121:1383–401.

Negoro E, Morinaga K, Taga M, Kaizaki Y, Kawai Y. Mycotic aneurysm due to Aspergillus sinusitis. Int J Hematol. 2013;98:4–5.

Ridder GJ, Breunig C, Kaminsky J, Pfeiffer J. Central skull base osteomyelitis: new insights and implications for diagnosis and treatment. Eur Arch Otorhinolaryngol. 2015;272:1269–76.

Scully EP, Baden LR, Katz JT. Fungal brain infections. Curr Opin Neurol. 2008;21:347–52.

Shankar SK, Mahadevan A, Sundaram C, Sarkar C, Chacko G, Lanjewar DN, Santosh V, Yasha TC, Radhakrishnan VV. Pathobiology of fungal infections of the central nervous system with special reference to the Indian scenario. Neurol India. 2007;55: 198–215.

Shih RY, Koeller KK. Bacterial, fungal, and parasitic infections of the central nervous system: radiologic-Pathologic correlation and historical perspectives. Radiographics. 2015;35:1141–69.

Starkey J, Moritani T, Kirby P. MRI of CNS fungal infections: review of Aspergillosis to Histoplasmosis and everything in between. Clin Neuroradiol. 2014;24:217–30.

Suchitha S, Sheeladevi CS, Sunila R, Manjunath GV. Disseminated cryptococcosis in an immunocompetent patient: a case report. Case Rep Pathol. 2012;2012:652351.

Tyc KM, Kühn C, Wilson D, Klipp E. Assessing the advantage of morphological changes in Candida albicans: a game theoretical study. Front Microbiol. 2014;5:41.

Zalduondo FM, Provenzale JM, Hulette C, Gorecki JP. Meningitis, vasculitis, and cerebritis caused by CNS histoplasmosis: radiologic-pathologic correlation. AJR Am J Roentgenol. 1996;166:194–6.

Zhong Y, Zhou Z, Fang X, Peng F, Zhang W. Magnetic resonance imaging study of cryptococcal neuroradiological lesions in HIV-negative cryptococcal meningitis. Eur J Clin Microbiol Infect Dis. 2017;36:1367–72.

Imaging Findings of Fungal Infections of the Sinuses Extending into the Brain

30

Ahmed Abdel Khalek Abdel Razek

Abbreviations

CT Computed tomography
MR Magnetic resonance
PNS Paranasal sinuses

30.1 Introduction

Fungal infection of PNS represents a wide spectrum of disorders, including acute or chronic and invasive or noninvasive forms. Fungal infection of the PNS most often involves the maxillary or ethmoid sinuses, less commonly the sphenoid, and rarely the frontal sinus. Mucormycosis is the most common fungal species that extend into the adjacent tissue and is suspected when the clinical triad of ketoacidosis, meningoencephalitis, and naso-orbital infection is present (Aribandi et al. 2007; Bozeman et al. 2011; Velayudhan et al. 2017). The infection spreads from the nasal cavity to the PNS and, eventually, to the orbits and cavernous sinuses (Al-Swiahb and Al-Dousary 2011; Holbrook et al. 2014; Velayudhan et al. 2017).

Fungal sinusitis in immunosuppressed patient is associated with necrotizing vasculitis of the PNS and rapidly extends into the orbits, deep face, and cranial cavity. This results from perivascular, perineural, or direct soft tissue invasion by the fungi, causing vasculitis, thrombosis, and infarction. Patients often present acutely with headache, fever, facial swelling, sinusitis, and unilateral orbital apex syndrome. Neurologic deficits occur secondary to brain abscess and septic thrombosis of major intracranial vessels (Aribandi et al. 2007; Bozeman et al. 2011).

A. A. K. A. Razek (✉)
Department of Diagnostic Radiology, Mansoura Faculty of Medicine, Mansoura, Egypt
e-mail: arazek@mans.edu.eg

30.2 Classification

Fungal disease of the PNS is broadly categorized into either invasive or noninvasive forms. Invasive fungal sinusitis is classified into acute or chronic invasive and chronic granulomatous forms, and noninvasive fungal sinusitis is classified into allergic fungal sinusitis and fungus ball (Bozeman et al. 2011; Marfani et al. 2010).

30.3 Predisposing Factors

Invasive fungal sinusitis may develop in an immunocompromised or diabetic patient, whereas noninvasive fungal sinusitis should be considered in a chronic situation, resistant to antibiotics in immunocompetent patients. Allergic fungal sinusitis is related to hypersensitivity of the host to the fungus. In the noninvasive forms, surgical

M. Turgut et al. (eds.), *Fungal Infections of the Central Nervous System*,
https://doi.org/10.1007/978-3-030-06088-6_30

treatment is essential, sometimes combined with antifungal treatment. The invasive forms require aggressive course of antifungal treatment, combined with surgery in some forms, particularly mucormycosis (Raz et al. 2015; Velayudhan et al. 2017).

30.4 Methods of Examination

Non-contrast CT remains the initial imaging study of choice in the work-up of fungal sinusitis. In complicated cases especially invasive fungal sinusitis, contrast MR imaging can be performed for better evaluation (Abdel Razek et al. 2014; Aribandi et al. 2007; Bozeman et al. 2011).

30.4.1 CT

CT is the initial method of examination in patients with fungal sinusitis as it can depict sinus lesion and extension into the adjacent orbit and skull base. Axial contrast CT with reconstruction in the coronal and sagittal planes is recommended for better evaluation of the extent of fungal infection into the adjacent bony and soft tissues. Contrast CT can be used to quickly assess for intracranial complications, such as extra-axial collections and brain abscess (Ghegan et al. 2006; Stewart et al. 2011; Velayudhan et al. 2017)

30.4.2 MR

MR is more sensitive in the evaluation of orbital and intracranial complications of fungal sinusitis. Pre- and post-contrast MR imaging in three orthogonal planes are recommended. MR imaging is better at evaluating disease extension into the orbit, skull base, and the intracranial cavity. Contrast MR imaging helps to differentiate abscess from phlegmon and detect cavernous sinus invasion and intracranial collections and meningitis (Bozeman et al. 2011; Velayudhan et al. 2017). Diffusion-weighted MR imaging has a role in early detection of ischemic infarction of the brain, and MR angiography can detect stenosis and occlusion of carotid artery in the cavernous sinus (Abdel Razek et al. 2011; Razek et al. 2009).

30.5 Imaging Appearances of Fungal Sinusitis

Fungal sinusitis shows characteristic imaging appearances at CT and MR imaging that help to differentiate them from bacterial infection (Bozeman et al. 2011; Raz et al. 2015). At CT, fungal concretions appear as hyperdense due to deposition of calcium, magnesium salts, and fungus-infected mucin. At MR imaging, the lesion shows low signal intensity on T1- weighted images and low signal or signal void on T2-weighted images due to metabolic ions, high protein content, and low water content of inspissated secretions within the fungal lesions. This can mimic an aerated sinus (Raz et al. 2015; Velayudhan et al. 2017).

30.5.1 Allergic Fungal Sinusitis

Allergic fungal sinusitis is the most common form of fungal sinusitis that occurs in patients with asthma and allergic rhinitis. This disease is typically bilateral and involves multiple sinuses. The sinuses may be expanded with central high attenuation within the sinuses on CT (Fig. 30.1).

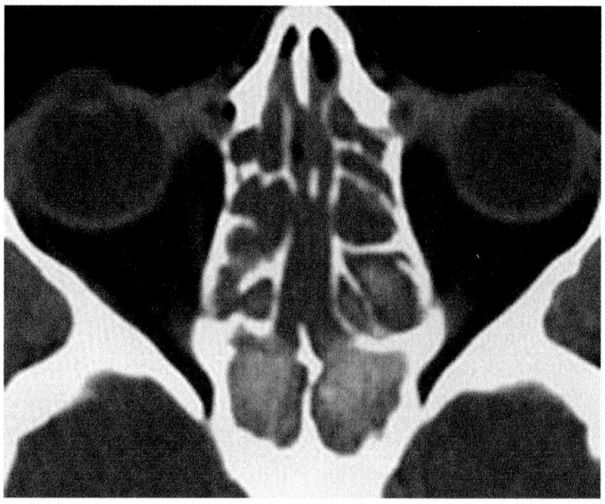

Fig. 30.1 Allergic fungal sinusitis: axial computed tomography (CT) scan shows hyperdense lesion within the ethmoid air cells and sphenoid sinus. Note expansion of ethmoid air cells

Chronic form of the disease may be associated with thinned and eroded sinus with intra-orbital and intracranial extension (Chan et al. 2000; Ghegan et al. 2006; Velayudhan et al. 2017).

30.5.2 Mycetomas

Mycetomas (fungus balls) typically involve one sinus, usually the maxillary sinus, and are hyperdense on CT with areas of calcifications (Fig. 30.2). The sinus walls may be thickened due to chronic infection or attenuated and eroded from the expansion or pressure necrosis from the mycetoma. On MR, the mycetoma shows marked decrease or no signal on T2-weighted images and variable T1 signal (Aribandi et al. 2007; Bozeman et al. 2011; Raz et al. 2015).

30.5.3 Acute (Fulminant) Invasive Fungal Sinusitis

Acute invasive fungal sinusitis is the most lethal form of fungal sinusitis with high mortality (50–80%) that is commonly reported in diabetic and immunocompromised patients. The ethmoid and sphenoid sinuses are more commonly involved. The disease progresses within a few days to invade the mucosa, submucosa, blood vessels, and bones with intracranial and orbital extension. Also, angioinvasion of the cavernous sinus and internal carotid artery may occur initially producing significant unilateral inflammatory changes and mucosal

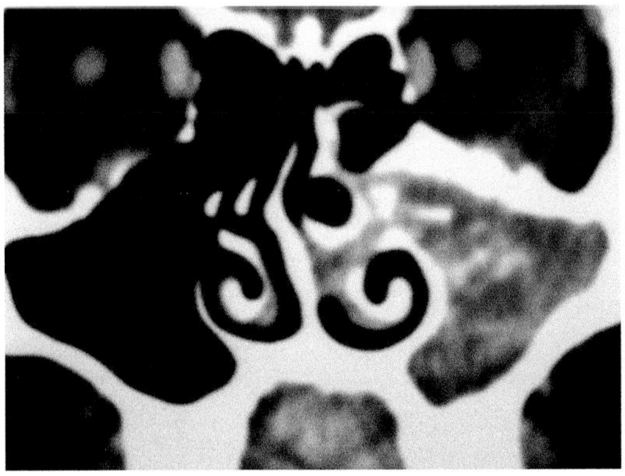

Fig. 30.2 Fungal ball: coronal CT scan shows calcified lesion in the left maxillary sinus

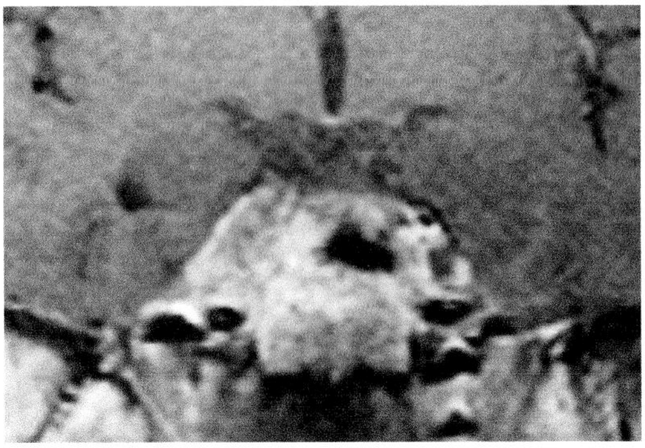

Fig. 30.3 Acute invasive fungal sinusitis with cavernous sinus invasion: coronal contrast T1-weighted magnetic resonance (MR) image shows enhancing lesion seen in the right cavernous sinus that extends from fungal infection of adjacent sphenoid sinus

edema in the nasal cavity. Disease progresses from the nasal cavity to the sinuses, orbits, and intracranial cavity to involve the cavernous sinuses, brain, and meninges. Sinus mucosal thickening may be subtle or mild. As the disease progresses, sinus opacification increases and bone destruction occurs (Fig. 30.3) (Aribandi et al. 2007; Bozeman et al. 2011; Velayudhan et al. 2017).

30.5.4 Chronic Invasive Fungal Sinusitis

Chronic invasive fungal sinusitis occurs in immunocompetent patients that is similar to the acute form but with progressive course over a long time. This disorder is primary reported in North Africa at Sudan. Chronic and granulomatous invasive fungal sinusitis can present with similar findings as advanced fulminant invasive disease. CT shows high attenuation material within the sinus with areas of calcification. The lesion appears as isointense to hypointense on T1-weighted images and is marked hypointense on T2-weighted images. Bony destruction or sclerosis may be present with extension beyond the sinus into the skull base, masticator space, and cranial cavity (Fig. 30.4). The mass-like appearance, bone destruction, and transpatial involvement of the chronic and granulomatous invasive fungal sinusitis may mimic tumors. The presence of calcifications, markedly diminished

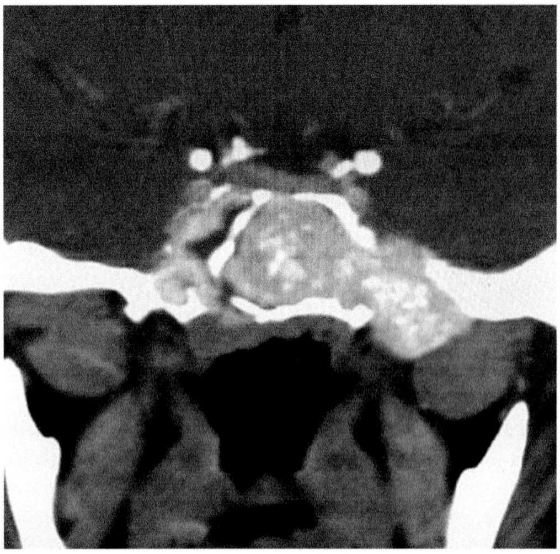

Fig. 30.4 Chronic invasive fungal sinusitis with skull base and intracranial extension: coronal CT scan shows expansile calcified lesion occupying the sphenoid sinus with erosion of skull base extension into the cranial cavity and into the deep spaces of the neck on the left side

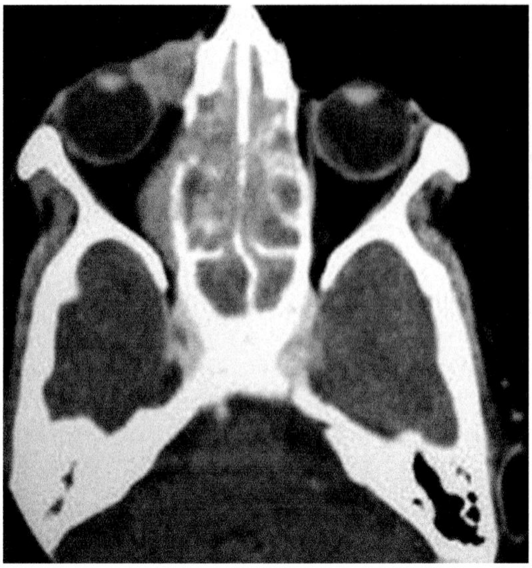

Fig. 30.5 Allergic fungal sinusitis with orbital invasion: axial CT scan shows hyperdense lesion seen in both ethmoid air cells with defect in the right orbital wall and extension into the extraconal space of the right orbit

T2 signal, and lack of enhancement favor the chronic invasive sinusitis over neoplastic lesion (Velayudhan et al. 2017).

Skull base involvement from invasive fungal infection usually occurs late in the course of the disease in spite of extensive deep soft tissue extension. This has been attributed to the angioinvasiveness of the fungi and their propensity to extend into the soft tissues of the orbit and deep face and into the intracranial cavity through the vessels penetrating through the skull base (Velayudhan et al. 2017).

30.6 Complications of Fungal Sinusitis

Complications of fungal sinusitis include orbital extension, skull base extension with bony erosion, cavernous venous invasion, perineural spread, intracranial vascular lesion, and intracranial infection (Bozeman et al. 2011; Marfani et al. 2010; Raz et al. 2015; Velayudhan et al. 2017).

30.6.1 Orbital Extension

Orbital extension of fungal infection has been reported in patients with allergic fungal sinusitis. There is expansion of ethmoid air cells with erosion of the medial orbital wall with extension of hyperdense fungal infection into the extraconal space of the orbit (Fig. 30.5) (Lafont et al. 2017; Marfani et al. 2010; Montone 2016). The infection may extend to involve the intraconal space and the optic nerve (Al-Radadi and Alnoury 2011; Thakar et al. 2011).

30.6.2 Skull Base Extension

Fungal infection of PNS may be associated with erosion of the skull base and extend into the skull base and masticator spaces (Fig. 30.4) (Al-Swiahb and Al-Dousary 2011; Asimakopoulos et al. 2013; Chan et al. 2000). Skull base involvement from sinonasal mucormycosis usually occurs late in the course of the disease (Ghegan et al. 2006; Holbrook et al. 2014; Lafont et al. 2017). This is attributed to the angioinvasiveness of the fungi and their propensity to extend into the soft tissues of the orbit and deep face and into the brain by way of vessels penetrating through partitions in the skull base (Marfani et al. 2010; Montone 2016; Stewart et al. 2011).

30.6.3 Cavernous Sinus Invasion

Acute invasive fungal infection of PNS commonly extends into the adjacent cavernous sinus. Contrast MR imaging is the beast imaging modality that can detect cavernous sinus invasion in fungal PNS infection (Fig. 30.3) (Brenet et al. 2016; Cheung et al. 2009; Mandava et al. 2001; Razek and Castillo 2009). Occlusion of the internal carotid arteries within the cavernous sinus is related to vasculitis. Flow-sensitive gradient-echo MR sequences and MR angiography are useful in documenting arterial occlusion (Fig. 30.6) (Brenet et al. 2016; Cheung et al. 2009; Mandava et al. 2001; Razek and Castillo 2009).

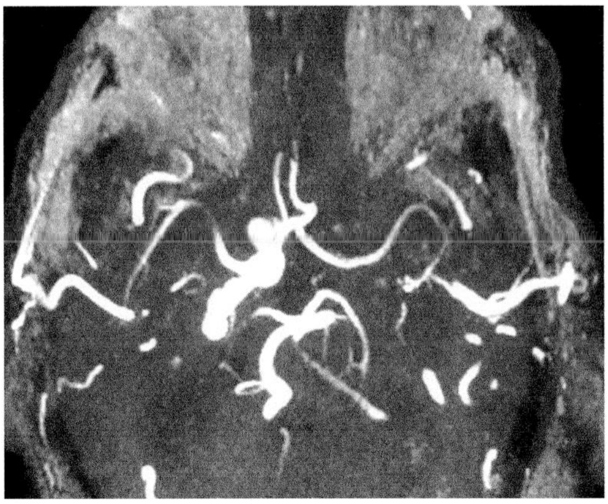

Fig. 30.6 Acute invasive fungal sinusitis with vascular invasion: MR angiography shows occlusion of left carotid artery within the left cavernous sinus

30.6.4 Perineural Spread

Rarely, invasive form of fungal infection of PNS that often progresses to the orbit and cavernous sinus may be complicated by perineural invasion and spread (Orguc et al. 2005).

30.6.5 Intracranial Vascular Spread

Angioinvasion of the blood vessels at the base of the skull is often associated with intracranial vascular complications such as ischemic infarction and mycotic emboli. Diffusion-weighted MR imaging is sensitive for early detection of ischemic infarction of the brain as restricted diffusion. Mycotic emboli appear as multiple hyperintense lesions on T2-weighted images, and mycotic aneurysm also has been reported in patients with fungal disease of PNS (Abdel Razek et al. 2014; Hurst et al. 2001).

30.6.6 Intracranial Infection

Fungal infection of PNS may extend intracranially with extradural fluid collection or brain abscess formation. The extradural fluid collection shows marginal enhancement at the skull base. The brain abscess typically shows marginal contrast enhancement and is commonly seen in the frontal region (Fig. 30.7). The abscess shows restricted diffusion at diffusion-weighted MR imaging (Asimakopoulos et al. 2013; Petkar et al. 2011; Stewart et al. 2011; Viola and Sutton 2010).

30.7 Conclusion

Cross-sectional imaging with CT and MR imaging is important for diagnosis and assessment of invasive and noninvasive forms of fungal infec-

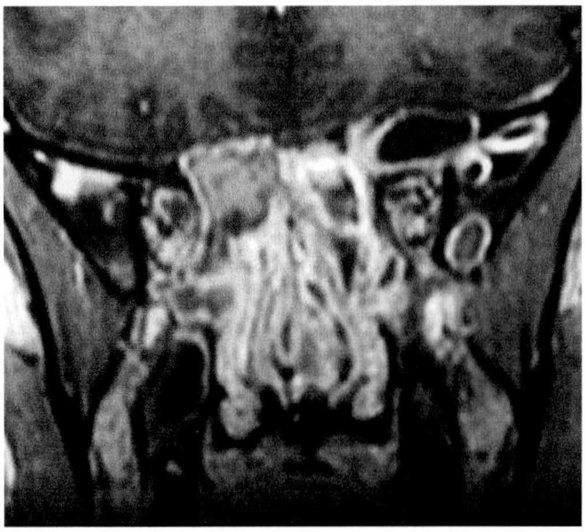

Fig. 30.7 Acute invasive fungal sinusitis with intracranial infection: contrast MR imaging shows enhanced lesion in both nasal cavity and the ethmoid air cell with localized marginally enhanced intracranial infected fluid collection on left side

tion of paranasal sinuses and its extension into the skull base, orbit, cavernous sinus, and cranial cavity.

References

Abdel Razek A, Mossad A, Ghonim M. Role of diffusion-weighted MR imaging in assessing malignant versus benign skull-base lesions. Radiol Med. 2011;116:125–32.

Abdel Razek AA, Alvarez H, Bagg S, Refaat S, Castillo M. Imaging spectrum of CNS vasculitis. Radiographics. 2014;34:873–94.

Al-Radadi AM, Alnoury KI. Optic chiasma involvement secondary to allergic fungal rhinosinusitis. J Pak Med Assoc. 2011;61:704–7.

Al-Swiahb JN, Al-Dousary SH. Bone erosions associated with allergic fungal sinusitis. Saudi Med J. 2011;32:417–9.

Aribandi M, McCoy V, Bazan C. Imaging features of invasive and noninvasive fungal sinusitis: a review. Radiographics. 2007;27:1283–96.

Asimakopoulos P, Supriya M, Kealey S, Vernham GA. A case-based discussion on a patient with non-otogenic fungal skull base osteomyelitis: pitfalls in diagnosis. J Laryngol Otol. 2013;18:1–5.

Bozeman S, deShazo R, Stringer S, Wright L. Complications of allergic fungal sinusitis. Am J Med. 2011;124:359–68.

Brenet E, Boulagnon-Rombi C, N'guyen Y, Litré CF. Cavernous sinus thrombosis secondary to aspergillus granuloma: a case report and review of the literature. Auris Nasus Larynx. 2016;43:566–9.

Chan LL, Singh S, Jones D, Diaz EM, Ginsberg L. Imaging of mucormycosis skull base osteomyelitis. AJNR Am J Neuroradiol. 2000;21:828–31.

Cheung EJ, Scurry WC, Isaacson JE, McGinn JD. Cavernous sinus thrombosis secondary to allergic fungal sinusitis. Rhinology. 2009;47:105–8.

Ghegan MD, Lee FS, Schlosser RJ. Incidence of skull base and orbital erosion in allergic fungal rhinosinusitis (AFRS) and non-AFRS. Otolaryngol Head Neck Surg. 2006;134:592–5.

Holbrook JF, Eastwood JD, Kilani RK. Intracranial abscess as a complication of allergic fungal sinusitis. J Neuroimaging. 2014;24:95–8.

Hurst RW, Judkins A, Bolger W, Chu A, Loevner LA. Mycotic aneurysm and cerebral infarction resulting from fungal sinusitis: imaging and pathological correlation. AJNR Am J Neuroradiol. 2001;22:858–63.

Lafont E, Aguilar C, Vironneau P, Kania R, Alanio A, Poirée S, Lortholary O, Lanternier F. Fungal sinusitis. Rev Mal Respir. 2017;34:672–92.

Mandava P, Chaljub G, Patterson K, Hollingsworth J. MR imaging of cavernous sinus invasion by mucormycosis: a case study. Clin Neurol Neurosurg. 2001;103:101–4.

Marfani MS, Jawaid MA, Shaikh SM, Thaheem K. Allergic fungal rhinosinusitis with skull base and orbital erosion. J Laryngol Otol. 2010;124:161–5.

Montone KT. Pathology of fungal rhinosinusitis: a review. Head Neck Pathol. 2016;10:40–6.

Orguc S, Vefa Yuceturk A, Demir MA, Goktan C. Rhinocerebral mucormycosis: perineural spread via the trigeminal nerve. J Clin Neurosci. 2005;12:484–6.

Petkar A, Rao L, Elizondo DR, Cutler J, Taillon D, Magone MT. Allergic fungal sinusitis with massive intracranial extension presenting with tearing. Ophthal Plast Reconstr Surg. 2011;27:e98–e100.

Raz E, Win W, Hagiwara M, Lui YW, Cohen B, Fatterpekar GM. Fungal Sinusitis. Neuroimaging Clin N Am. 2015;25:569–76.

Razek AA, Castillo M. Imaging lesions of the cavernous sinus. AJNR Am J Neuroradiol. 2009;30:444–52.

Razek AA, Sieza S, Maha B. Assessment of nasal and paranasal sinus masses by diffusion-weighted MR imaging. J Neuroradiol. 2009;36:206–11.

Stewart TA, Carter CS, Seiberling K. Temporal lobe abscess in a patient with isolated sphenoiditis. Allergy Rhinol. 2011;2:40–2.

Thakar A, Lal P, Dhiwakar M, Bahadur S. Optic nerve compression in allergic fungal sinusitis. J Laryngol Otol. 2011;125:381–5.

Velayudhan V, Chaudhry ZA, Smoker WRK, Shinder R, Reede DL. Imaging of intracranial and orbital complications of sinusitis and atypical sinus infection: what the radiologist needs to know. Curr Probl Diagn Radiol. 2017;46:441–51.

Viola GM, Sutton R. Allergic fungal sinusitis complicated by fungal brain mass. Int J Infect Dis. 2010;14(Suppl 3):e299–301.

Imaging Findings of Fungal Infections of Spine and Spinal Cord

31

Jitender Saini, Mudit Gupta, and Rakesh K. Gupta

Abbreviations

18F-FDG-PET	18F-fluorodeoxyglucose positron emission tomography
CSF	Cerebrospinal fluid
CT	Computed tomography
HIV	Human immunodeficiency virus
MRI	Magnetic resonance imaging
WI	Weighted image

31.1 Introduction

Fungal infections of the spine are relatively uncommon and were first described by Keating in 1932 (Keating 1932). Incidence of fungal infections is increasing, and similar trends are being observed for the spinal fungal infections. *Candida*, *Aspergillus*, *Cryptococcus*, *Coccidioides* and *Histoplasma* are some of the common fungi which affect the susceptible patients, and they gain access to the vascular system through intravenous lines, during implantation of prosthetic devices or during surgery (Kim et al. 2006). Spinal involvement is usually the result of haematogenous or direct spread of organisms from an initial pulmonary focus of infection. Immunosuppressed patients are at higher risk than immunocompetent patients (Frazier et al. 2001).

The vertebral body, posterior bony vertebral elements, epidural space and paraspinal soft tissues may be affected, and imaging typically demonstrates reduced disc space, paradiscal bony erosions, frank bone destruction, lytic bony vertebral lesions and epidural and perivertebral soft tissue mass formation that may be phlegmonous or due to frank abscess formation. Occasionally, like granulomatous infection (e.g. tuberculosis), the intervertebral disc may be relatively spared early in the infectious process (Kim et al. 2006).

The imaging findings are non-specific and may suggest infective rather than fungal etiology. We will describe the imaging finding of various specific fungal infections in this chapter with an emphasis on its early recognition and histopathology confirmation to obtain favourable response to specific treatment.

31.2 *Candida*

Incidence of candidiasis is on the increase, and it is often seen in association with factors such as central venous catheter, administration of antibiotics and parenteral nutrition, haemodialysis,

J. Saini
Department of Neuroimaging and Intervention Radiology, NIMHANS, Bangalore, India

M. Gupta
Department of Radiology, Saral Diagnostics Classic, Noida, India

R. K. Gupta (✉)
Fortis Memorial Research Institute, Gurgaon, India

Department of Radiology and Imaging, Fortis Memorial Research Institute, Gurgaon, Haryana, India

M. Turgut et al. (eds.), *Fungal Infections of the Central Nervous System*,
https://doi.org/10.1007/978-3-030-06088-6_31

human immunodeficiency virus (HIV) infection, injectable drug use, surgery, immunosuppression, debilitating disease and neutropenia. It can cause vertebral osteomyelitis, epidural abscess meningitis, spinal arachnoiditis and syringomyelia (Derkinderen et al. 2000; Phanthumchinda and Kaoropthum 1991; Miller and Mejicano 2001).

Candida infection reaches the spine most commonly through haematogenous route (Miller and Mejicano 2001). Infection is usually centred around the intervertebral disc space, leading to narrowing of the disc cartilage and destruction of the vertebral endplates and underlying vertebral bone (Gathe et al. 1987). The low virulence of the *Candida* species and the poor vascularization of the disc space result in a slowly progressive inflammatory destruction and thus a delay in the diagnosis (Ugarriza et al. 2004).

Typically, the patient presents with back pain, fever, focal tenderness and neurological deficits. However, the absence of fever does not rule out the diagnosis of candidal vertebral osteomyelitis (Hennequin et al. 1996). Presence of point tenderness over the affected area is the most useful clinical sign (Hennequin et al. 1996; Smith and Blaser 1991). Only 20% of the patients with candidal vertebral osteomyelitis develop neurological defects (Miller and Mejicano 2001).

Laboratory findings may show elevated erythrocyte sedimentation rate and C-reactive protein. Blood and urine cultures are rarely positive. Diagnosis of candidal vertebral osteomyelitis is a diagnostic problem due to the insidious progression of disease, the non-specific clinical and laboratory findings and the failure to recognize *Candida* as a potential pathogen (Ozdemir et al. 2008).

There are no typical radiological findings in candidal vertebral osteomyelitis (Ozdemir et al. 2008). Magnetic resonance imaging (MRI) is more sensitive, specific and accurate than radioisotope bone scan or computed tomography (CT) scan for early recognition and localization of infectious disease. MRI features include absence of disc hyperintensity and preservation of the internuclear cleft on T2-weighted images and enhancement on gadolinium-enhanced T1-weighted images (Williams et al. 1999). If the clinical suspicion is high and MRI features are not definitive, or if MRI is contraindicated, a bone scan can be combined with a Gallium-67 scan to improve the specificity for the diagnosis of osteomyelitis (Palestro 2015). 18fluorodeoxyglucose positron emission tomography (18F-FDG-PET) is especially helpful if the MRI is indeterminate due to degenerative disc disease (Palestro 2015).

Vertebral collapse and neurological deficits usually appear within 3–6 months from the onset of symptoms (Stumpe et al. 2002; Khazim et al. 2006). Neurological symptoms may result from spinal epidural abscess, vertebral collapse, spinal cord infarct or meningitis. Indications for surgical treatment are presence of neurological deficit, to provide a diagnosis, failure of medical therapy and presence of spinal instability (Ugarriza et al. 2004).

Spinal cord lesions in candidal spondylodiscitis are often caused by vertebral collapse and/or spinal cord infarct rather than by associated epidural abscess (Derkinderen et al. 2000). MRI is an excellent way of demonstrating the presence of epidural or paraspinal extension of the infection (Fig. 31.1) and thus may be useful for early diagnosis and starting early medical treatment (Torres-Ramos et al. 2004).

31.3 Aspergillosis

Aspergillus is the most common cause of skeletal mycosis, and the vertebral column is the most commonly involved bony structure in mycotic osteomyelitis. Infection spreads through haematogenous route; however, direct spread from the adjacent organ most commonly the lung and iatrogenic infection during spine surgery are other routes of infection. Haematogenous spread occurs from infections primarily located in pulmonary, gastrointestinal or cerebral locations. The most common causative species is *Aspergillus fumigatus* with *A. flavus*, *A. niger*, *A. nidulans* and *A. terreus* species being other rare causes (Kim et al. 2006).

On MRI, spinal aspergillosis shows relatively non-specific findings like vertebral marrow hypointensity on T1-weighted images (WIs) and iso- or minimal hyperintensity on T2-WIs with intervening disc involvement. Relative preservation of disc height, signal intensity and retained intranuclear cleft are features which may be seen in *Aspergillus* infection of the spine (Fig. 31.2).

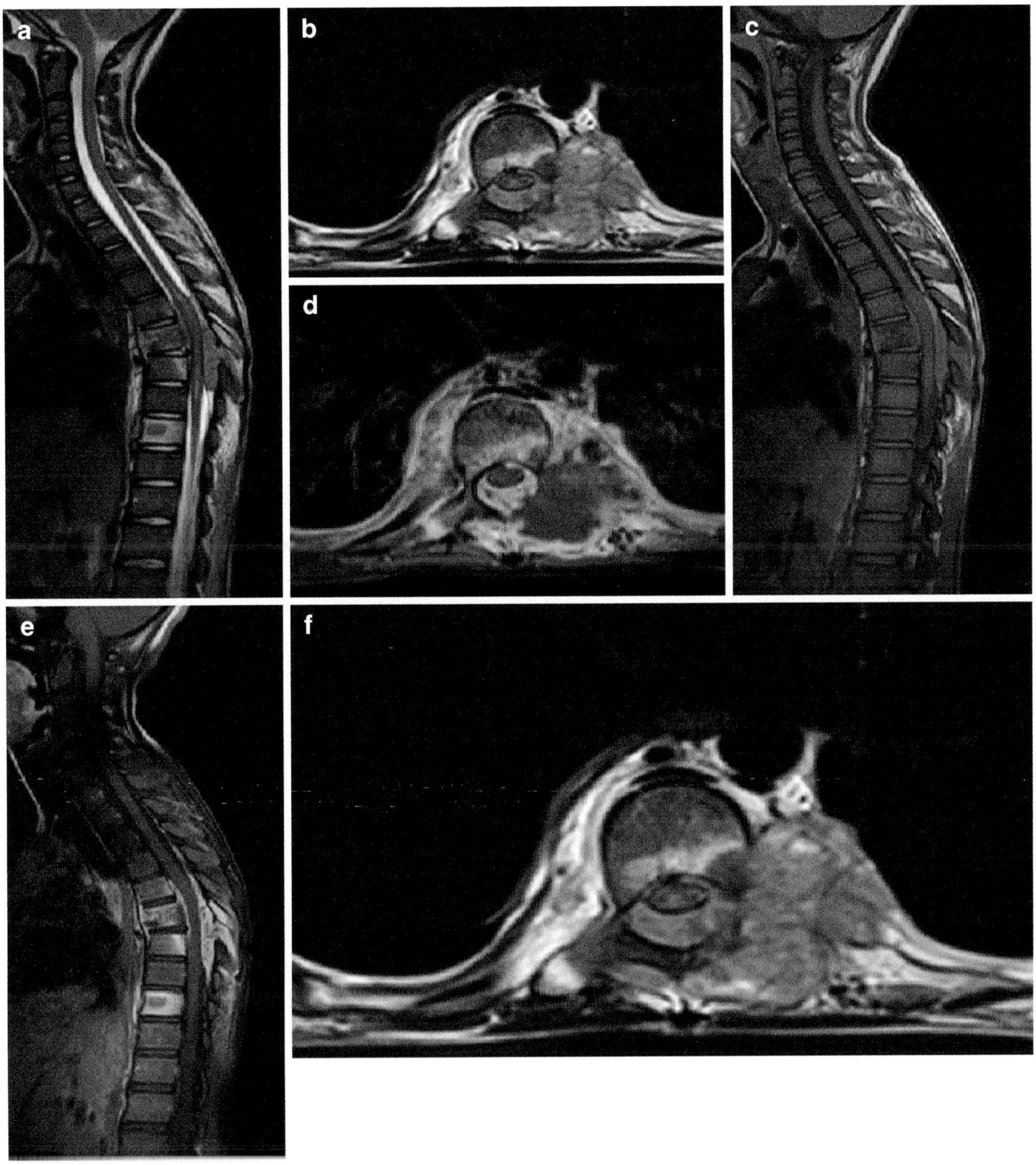

Fig. 31.1 *Candida* spondylitis. Sagittal and axial T2-weighted image (WI) and T1-WI show D5–7 vertebral body signal changes with relative preservation of intervertebral disc, posterior elements signal changes and large posterior epidural soft tissue (**a**–**d**). Sagittal and axial post-contrast T1-WI show heterogeneous enhancement with central necrotic area well (**e**, **f**)

Epidural and rarely intradural abscess may be seen in spinal *Aspergillus* infection (Kwon et al. 2011; Winterstein et al. 2010; McCaslin et al. 2015). Paraspinal inflammation is minimal to moderate in comparison to the vertebral destruction which is a hallmark of tubercular disease in which large paraspinal abscesses are seen. Minimal disc changes despite fungal disc invasion may be due to a blunted immune response in immunocompromised patients. Factors intrinsic to fungi like presence of paramagnetic and ferromagnetic elements within fungi may contribute to an absence of disc hyperintensity on T2-WIs. Similar mechanism for T2 hypointensity in fungal sinusitis has been proposed previously (Winterstein et al. 2010).

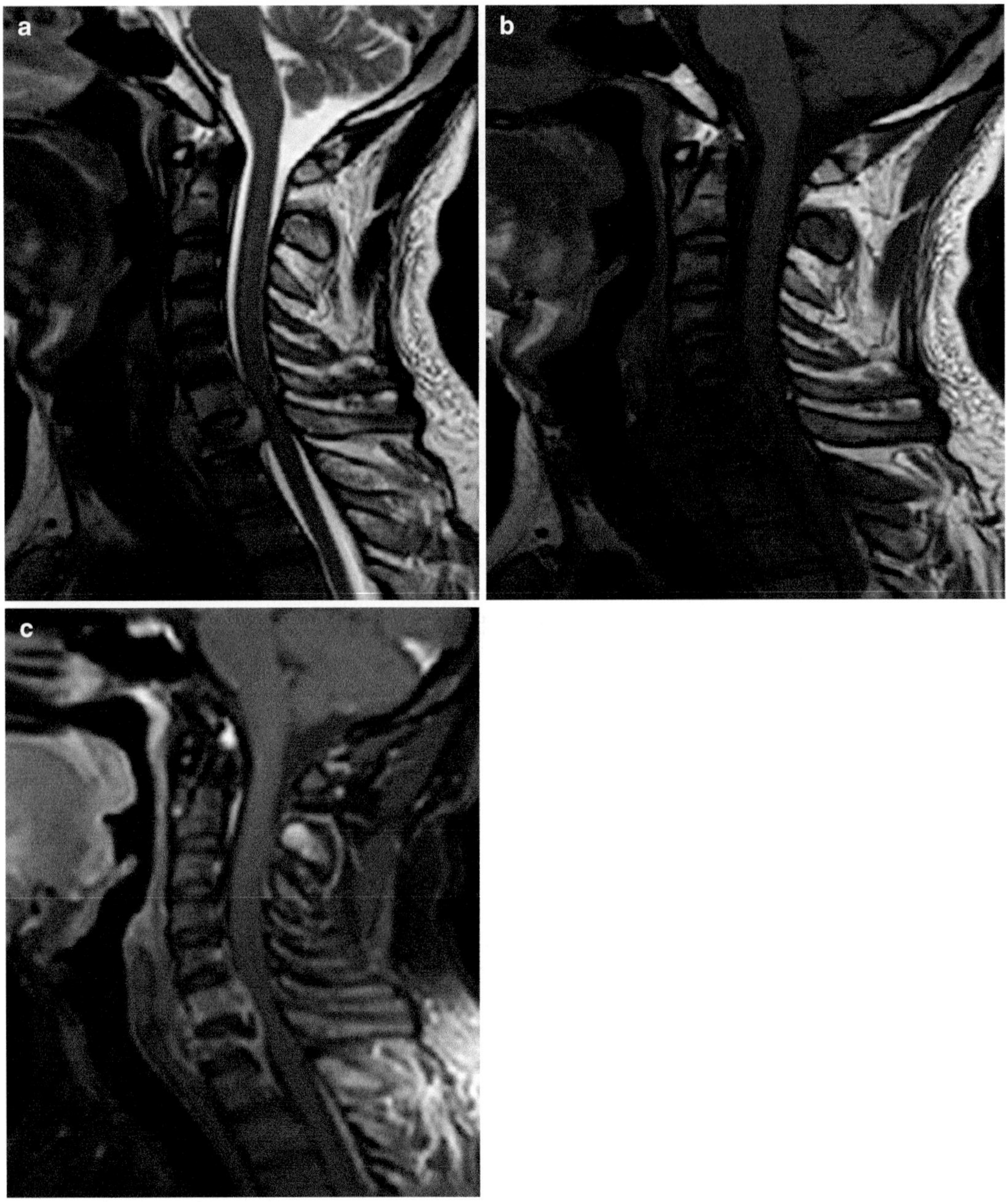

Fig. 31.2 *Aspergillus spondylitis*: Sagittal T2-WI, T1-WI and post contrast T1-WI of the cervical spine show destructive lesion involving C6 and C7 vertebral bodies with large prevertebral and epidural soft tissue (**a** and **b**). Post contrast T1-WI shows heterogenous enhancement within the abnormal soft tissue and relative preservation of the intervertebral disc (**c**)

Mollahoseini et al. described a case of cerebral aspergillosis in an immunocompetent patient who was treated successfully for *Aspergillus* infection of the brain (Mollahoseini and Nikoobakht 2011). Brain lesion resolved after antifungal therapy that was confirmed by follow-up contrast-enhanced brain MRI. One month later the patient developed features of spinal cord involvement, and MRI showed T2 hyperintensity involving the entire cord with no significant enhancement to suggest myelitis. Brain MRI was unremarkable at this time to suggest postinfective demyelination of the spinal cord. The patient was treated with corticosteroids and showed complete recovery to suggest post-*Aspergillus* infection demyelination.

31.4 Cryptococcosis

Spinal cord disease is a rare presentation of cryptococcosis. Bony involvement is seen in 5% of disseminated cryptococcosis. The neuroimaging findings are remarkable, although not specific, and are characterized by involvement of the vertebral body with involvement of the posterior elements and paraspinal and perivertebral soft tissues with relative preservation of the disc. The vertebral body may show osteolytic lesions with discrete margins, absent surrounding sclerosis and periosteal reaction (Wang et al. 2014). Meningoradiculitis (Fig. 31.3) and spinal cryptococcal granulomas are other rare forms of spinal involvement seen in cryptococcal infection (Grosse et al. 2001; Deus-Silva et al. 2004). Diffusion-weighted MRI in a case of spinal *Cryptococcus* infection shows hyperintensity of involved vertebral body, epidural space and posterior elements (Chhem et al. 2001).

Asanuma et al. described an unusual case of isolated extradural cryptococcoma involving the left S1 and S2 roots (Asanuma et al. 2014). MRI showed enhancing extradural mass with enhancement of the right S2 nerve sheath. On surgery fibrous tissue was removed and S1 and S2 nerve roots were decompressed and histopathology and microbial examination showed cryptococcosis.

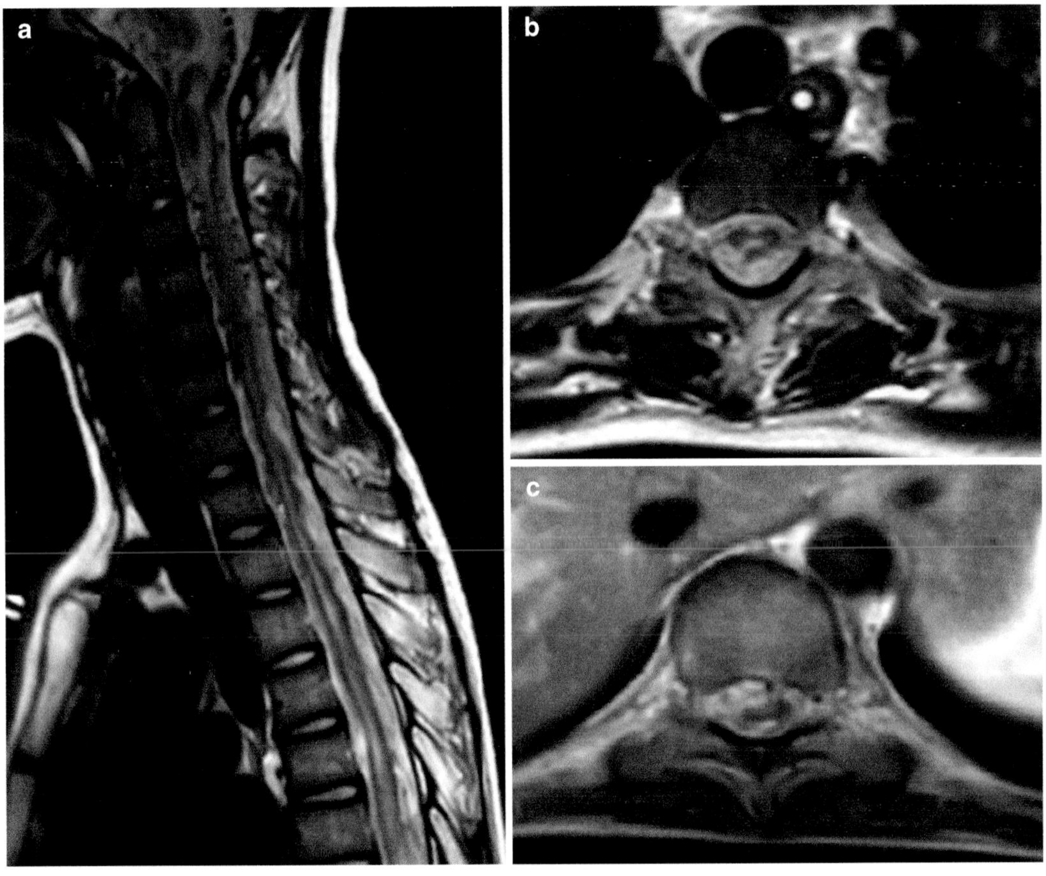

Fig. 31.3 Cryptococcal myelitis with arachnoiditis. Sagittal and axial T2-WI of the cervical spine show hyperintense signal in the spinal cord with irregular margins (**a**, **b**). Axial post-contrast T1-WI shows leptomeningeal enhancement (**c**). Cerebrospinal fluid (CSF) was positive for *Cryptococcus neoformans* (Courtesy of Dr. Aruna Pallewatta, Radiologist, Hemas Hospital, Thalawathugoda Sri Lanka)

31.5 Coccidioidomycosis

Skeletal coccidioidomycosis is frequently multicentric and may involve almost any bone. The axial skeleton is the most common site of involvement. Spinal involvement is seen in approximately 25% of patients with disseminated disease. Spinal lesions are usually well demarcated but may present with an ill-defined border and permeative type of bone destruction. The typical imaging findings are disc signal abnormalities, heterogeneous marrow signal alteration and extensive extraosseous involvement with relative lack of bony destruction (Olson et al. 1998). On MRI, involved structures show hyperintense signal on T2- and hypointense signal on T1-WIs with heterogeneous enhancement on post-contrast images. Other imaging features include phlegmonous, enhancing, non-liquefactive soft tissue abnormalities, cord compression and nerve root impingement. As the disease is multifocal in nature, MRI screening of the entire vertebral column often reveals occult areas of involvement. The extensive soft tissue and marrow abnormalities with relative lack of bony abnormalities help to differentiate coccidioidomycosis from other causes of infective spondylitis. However, the MRI features of coccidioidomycosis spinal infection are non-specific, and biopsy with culture is required to establish the diagnosis (Olson et al. 1998).

31.6 Blastomycosis

Bone is one of the frequent sites of infection in patients with blastomycosis, and vertebral column is most commonly affected with predilection for lower thoracic or lumbar regions. MRI and CT are valuable in determining the presence and extent of involvement by the granulomatous disease. Most lesions are hyperintense on T2-WIs and show post-contrast enhancement (Fig. 31.4). The anterior aspect of the vertebral body usually is affected initially followed by bone destruction leading to vertebral compression fractures and spread to adjacent vertebral bodies through the discs. Noncongruent vertebral bodies also can be affected by the spread of infection along the anterior longitudinal ligament. Psoas or paravertebral abscesses may also be formed along with cutaneous sinuses, and gross deformity of the spine may also be seen (Saccente et al. 1998).

The clinical and imaging picture can be confused with other destructive bone lesions caused by other fungal organisms, tuberculosis, bacterial infections and metastatic carcinomas. In blastomycosis, as in coccidioidomycosis and tuberculosis, there is a severe destruction of the vertebral bodies. However, in tuberculosis the posterior elements of the vertebral body are relatively spared, whereas in coccidioidomycosis and blastomycosis, all the bone elements of the spine may be affected. In coccidioidomycosis, bony destruction may be less, and disc may be relatively spared, whereas in blastomycosis, disc space may be involved in the early stages of the disease (Hadjipavlou et al. 1998). Blastomycosis can rarely present as an isolated intramedullary lesion with non-specific appearance on MRI (Parr and Fewer 2004).

Treatment of fungal spondylitis is often delayed because of difficulty in the diagnosis. Delay in the diagnosis leads to poorer results in terms of neurologic recovery. Performing fungal cultures whenever a spinal infection is suspected might hasten the diagnosis. Patients should be given a guarded prognosis and informed of the many possible complications of the disease.

31.7 Miscellaneous Fungal Infections

Many rare fungal infections of the spine have been described in the literature. Some of these rare entities described in the literature are discussed below. A case of *Scedosporium prolificans* in an immunocompetent patient described in the literature (Carod-Artal et al. 2009) underwent spinal MRI which showed a thoracic and

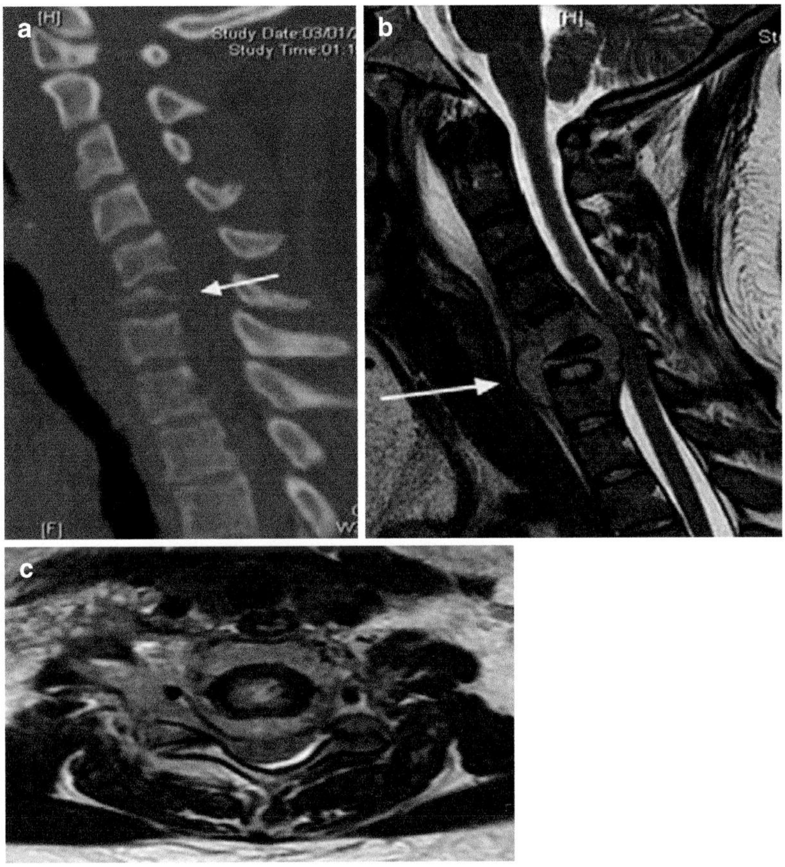

Fig. 31.4 Cervical blastomycosis: Sagittal section of computed tomography shows near-complete destruction of C6 vertebral body (arrow) (**a**). Sagittal and axial T2WI at the C6 level show C6 osteomyelitis with significant vertebral body destruction (arrow) and vertebral abscess at C6 and C7 levels with posterior sub-ligamentous extension into the spinal canal including mild posterior displacement and compression of cervical spinal cord (**b**, **c**). In addition, extensive prevertebral collection noted extension from the D1 vertebral level to the skull base level. (With permission Patel KR et al. Journal of Medical Case Reports (2015) 9:271)

lumbar epidural lesion heterogeneously enhancing on contrast-enhanced T1-WI. In addition, enlargement and edema of the thoracolumbar spinal cord appeared as intramedullary hyperintensity and showed intramedullary and leptomeningeal enhancement on post-contrast T1-WIs. Histopathologic examination of the obtained contents showed marked chronic inflammatory process and fibrosis. Culture of the material obtained from the epidural inflammatory collection revealed infection by *S. prolificans*.

We observed a case with multiple thoracic vertebral involvements with sparing of the disc in a 63-year-old female patient who was found to have *Triadelphia pulvinata* on culture. MRI showed T2 hyperintense lesion involving the thoracic vertebrae with paravertebral soft tissue that is enhanced on post-contrast study (Fig. 31.5). The galactomannan and (1,3)-β-d-glucan antigen assays were both negative in the serum. Review of the literature suggested that involvement of the spine due to *Triadelphia pulvinata* has not been previously reported. There are only two reported cases of human infection involving the skin and blood in the patient of acute myeloid leukaemia on autologous bone marrow transplant (Edathodu et al. 2013).

31.8 Iatrogenic Fungal Infections of the Spine

Postoperative fungal spondylodiscitis: Postoperative fungal spondylodiscitis is a rare cause of infection. In the literature, 14 cases of postoperative fungal spondylodiscitis have been

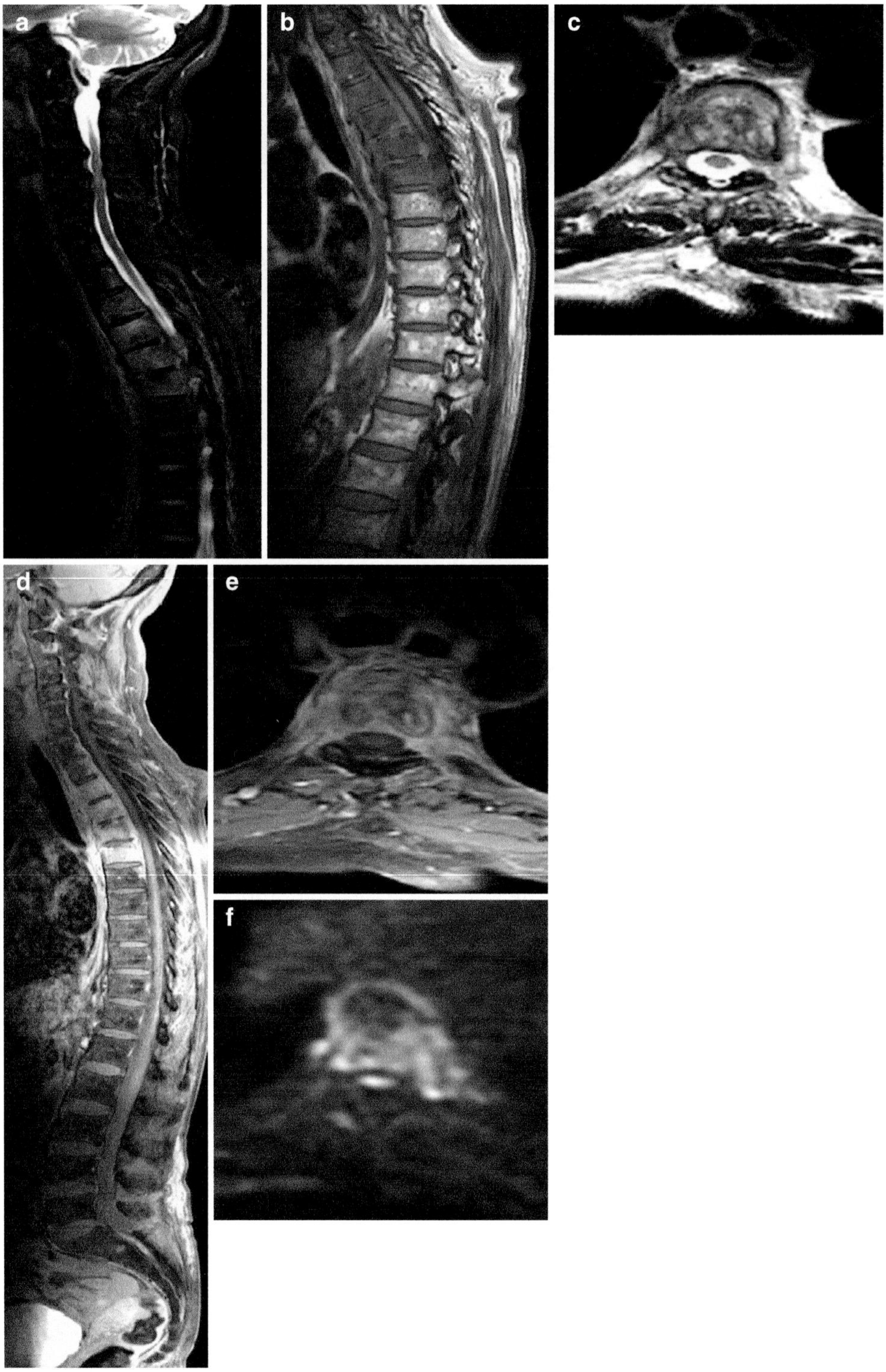

Fig. 31.5 *Triadelphia pulvinata* fungal infection. A 60-year-old female presented with pain in the cervicodorsal region. MRI of the cervicodorsal region shows T2 hyperintense signal from D2 to D6 vertebral bodies which appear hypointense on T1-WI with sparing of intervertebral discs (**a**, **b**). Axial T2-WI, sagittal and axial post-contrast T1-WI and diffusion imaging through the D4 vertebra show abnormal signal of the vertebra with no compression of the spinal cord, diffuse enhancement of the vertebral body with perivertebral soft tissue enhancement and restricted diffusion (**c**–**f**). Biopsy from vertebral body revealed non-specific infective etiology. The tissue culture revealed *Triadelphia pulvinata* fungal infection

described (Gerometta et al. 2012), nine caused by molds and five by *Candida* species. The most common organism was *Aspergillus* spp followed by *Candida* and *Scedosporium prolificans*, *Rhizopus rhizopodoformis* and *Trichosporon asahii*. All the cases have been reported in lumbosacral region. The most common symptom was back pain followed by fever, while neurological deficits were seen in two patients. Onset of symptoms was delayed, and the first symptom appeared average 6 weeks after the primary procedure (Gerometta et al. 2012). MRI showed osteomyelitis and/or discitis in all cases, complicated by paravertebral abscess in three cases and by epidural abscess in four cases. All patients received antifungal drugs.

MRI remains the most sensitive and specific imaging modality for the diagnosis of postoperative spondylodiscitis (Kim et al. 2006; Gerometta et al. 2012). MRI findings of postoperative discitis include decreased signal intensity on T1-WIs and increased signal intensity on T2-WIs in the disc space, secondary to inflammation and infection. Post-gadolinium T1-WIs showed disc and adjacent bone marrow enhancement.

In 2011, Li et al. (Li et al. 2011) reported radiographic findings in 34 patients with postoperative intervertebral discitis and found disc space narrowing in 29 patients and destructive and sclerotic vertebral body changes in 14 patients. Nielsen et al. (Nielsen et al. 1990) reported disc space loss and vertebral fusion in 17% of patients following postoperative discitis. In the study of Hsieh et al. (Hsieh et al. 2011), all patients were found to have loosening of the pedicle screws. Kulkarni et al. (Kulkarni and Hee 2006) reported a case of adjacent-level discitis after anterior cervical discectomy and fusion, and the radiographs showed segmental kyphosis, decreased disc height, erosion of endplates, halo around the screws and enlarged prevertebral soft tissue shadow. MRI showed discitis with prevertebral and epidural abscesses. Ohtori et al. (Ohtori et al. 2010) who analysed the utility of the 18F-FDG-PET for patients with suspected spondylitis showing Modic change concluded that the rate of detecting spondylodiscitis infection was very high if FDG-PET was used along with other diagnostic methods. FDG-PET can successfully distinguish between common Modic change and spinal infection.

Contamination of the steroid with Exserohilum rostratum resulting in infections: Moudgal et al. reported a large series of patients who received methylprednisolone epidural injection for pain and who developed pain and/or spinal/paraspinal infection following treatment and underwent at least one MRI study (Moudgal et al. 2014). Abnormalities were most often noted in the lumbosacral region which was the site of injection of contaminated methylprednisolone (New England Compounding Center, Framingham, Massachusetts). In few patients noncontiguous sites of involvement were also noted. Initial study was able to identify infection in majority of patients; however, in approximately 15% of patients, additional follow-up MRI was needed to identify the presence of infection. The imaging findings included an epidural or paraspinal abscess or phlegmon, arachnoiditis and osteomyelitis (Fig. 31.6).

31.9 Conclusion

Fungal infections of the spine are rare and are usually diagnosed late due to slow onset of the disease and should be evaluated with MRI even if the imaging features are non-specific. Once the lesion is detected on MRI, it should be immediately biopsied to confirm the diagnosis using culture and histopathology which should result in early institution of antifungal treatment. Delay in diagnosis results in poor prognosis.

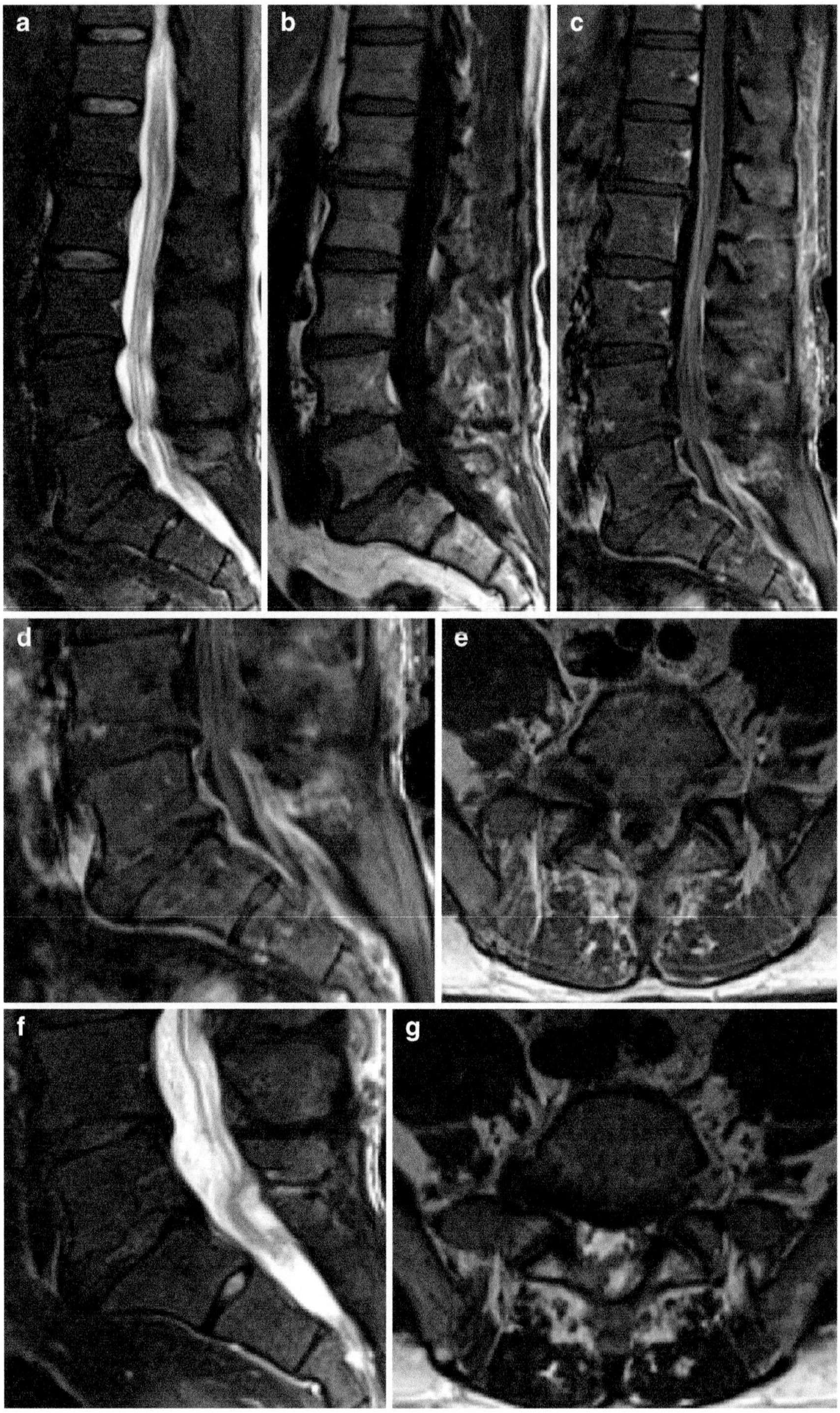

Fig. 31.6 *Exserohilum rostratum* fungal meningitis after epidural injection of methyl prednisone from New England Compounding Center, Framingham, Massachusetts. Sagittal T2-WI, T1-WI and post-contrast T1-WI of the lumbosacral spine show enhancement and clumping of the nerve roots with CSF loculation (**a**–**c**). Repeat study following treatment with antifungal agent shows interval decrease in the amount of enhancement within the spinal canal with decreased dural and leptomeningeal enhancement, decreased size of enhancing multiloculated fluid collection in the left posterior epidural space at the S1 level and continued clumping and waviness of the cauda equina, in keeping with arachnoiditis (**d**–**g**) (Courtesy: Dr. Suyash Mohan, Department of Neuroradiology, University of Pennsylvania, USA)

References

Asanuma Y, Fujimoto H, Nakabayashi H, Akeda K, Asanuma K, Tanaka M, et al. Extradural cryptococcoma at the sacral spine without bone involvement in an immunocompetent patient. J Orthop Sci. 2014;19(6):1040–5.

Carod-Artal FJ, Ferreira-Coral L, Mauro-Couto J, Gomes E, de Agassiz-Vasques M. Chronic spinal epidural abscess caused by Scedosporium prolificans in an immunocompetent patient. Spine. 2009;34(9):E330–2.

Chhem RK, Wang S, Jaovisidha S, Schmit P, Friedman L, Bureau NJ, et al. Imaging of fungal, viral, and parasitic musculoskeletal and spinal diseases. Radiol Clin North Am. 2001;39(2):357–78.

Derkinderen P, Bruneel F, Bouchaud O, Regnier B. Spondylodiscitis and epidural abscess due to Candida albicans. Eur Spine J. 2000;9(1):72–4.

Deus-Silva L, Costa AE, Bevilacqua JM, Assis DB, Ferraz CA, Oliveira ACP, et al. Meningoradiculitis due to Cryptococcus neofermans in an immunocompetent patient. Arq Neuropsiquiatr. 2004;62(1):147–9.

Edathodu J, Al-Abdely HM, Althawadi S, Wickes BL, Thompson EH, Wiederhold NP, et al. Invasive fungal infection due to Triadelphia pulvinata in a patient with acute myeloid leukemia. J Clin Microbiol. 2013;51(10):3426–9.

Frazier DD, Campbell DR, Garvey TA, Wiesel S, Bohlman HH, Eismont FJ. Fungal infections of the spine. Report of eleven patients with long-term follow-up. J Bone Joint Surg Am. 2001;83-A(4):560–5.

Gathe JC, Harris RL, Garland B, Bradshaw MW, Williams TW. Candida osteomyelitis. Report of five cases and review of the literature. Am J Med. 1987;82(5):927–37.

Gerometta A, Bittan F, Rodriguez Olaverri JC. Postoperative spondilodiscitis. Int Orthop. 2012;36(2):433–8.

Grosse P, Tintelnot K, Söllner O, Schmitz B. Encephalomyelitis due to Cryptococcus neoformans var gattii presenting as spinal tumour: case report and review of the literature. J Neurol Neurosurg Psychiatry. 2001;70(1):113–6.

Hadjipavlou AG, Mader JT, Nauta HJ, Necessary JT, Chaljub G, Adesokan A. Blastomycosis of the lumbar spine: case report and review of the literature, with emphasis on diagnostic laboratory tools and management. Eur Spine J. 1998;7(5):416–21.

Hennequin C, Bourée P, Hiesse C, Dupont B, Charpentier B. Spondylodiskitis due to Candida albicans: report of two patients who were successfully treated with fluconazole and review of the literature. Clin Infect. 1996;23(1):176–8.

Hsieh M-K, Chen L-H, Niu C-C, Fu T-S, Lai P-L, Chen W-J. Postoperative anterior spondylodiscitis after posterior pedicle screw instrumentation. Spine J. 2011;11(1):24–9.

Keating PM. Fungus infection of bone and joint. South Med J. 1932;25(10):1072–9.

Khazim RM, Debnath UK, Fares Y. Candida albicans osteomyelitis of the spine: progressive clinical and radiological features and surgical management in three cases. Eur Spine J. 2006;15(9):1404–10.

Kim CW, Perry A, Currier B, Yaszemski M, Garfin SR. Fungal infections of the spine. Clin Orthop. 2006;444:92–9.

Kulkarni AG, Hee HT. Adjacent level discitis after anterior cervical discectomy and fusion (ACDF): a case report. Eur Spine J. 2006;15(Suppl 5):559–63.

Kwon JW, Hong SH, Choi S-H, Yoon YC, Lee SH. MRI findings of *Aspergillus* spondylitis. Am J Roentgenol. 2011;197(5):W919–23.

Li J, Yan D, Duan L, Zhang Z, Zhu H, Zhang Z. Percutaneous discectomy and drainage for postoperative intervertebral discitis. Arch Orthop Trauma Surg. 2011;131(2):173–8.

McCaslin AF, Lall RR, Wong AP, Lall RR, Sugrue PA, Koski TR. Thoracic spinal cord intramedullary aspergillus invasion and abscess. J Clin Neurosci. 2015;22(2):404–6.

Miller DJ, Mejicano GC. Vertebral osteomyelitis due to Candida species: case report and literature review. Clin Infect Dis. 2001;33(4):523–30.

Mollahoseini R, Nikoobakht M. Diffuse myelitis after treatment of cerebral aspergillosis in an immune competent patient. Acta Med Iran. 2011;49(6):402–6.

Moudgal V, Singal B, Kauffman CA, Brodkey JA, Malani AN, Olmsted RN, et al. Spinal and paraspinal fungal infections associated with contaminated methylprednisolone injections. Open Forum Infect Dis. 2014;1(1):ofu022.

Nielsen VA, Iversen E, Ahlgren P. Postoperative discitis. Radiology of progress and healing. Acta Radiol. 1990;31(6):559–63.

Ohtori S, Suzuki M, Koshi T, Yamashita M, Yamauchi K, Inoue G, et al. 18F-fluorodeoxyglucose-PET for patients with suspected spondylitis showing Modic change. Spine. 2010;35(26):E1599–603.

Olson EM, Duberg AC, Herron LD, Kissel P, Smilovitz D. Coccidioidal spondylitis: MR findings in 15 patients. AJR Am J Roentgenol. 1998;171(3):785–9.

Ozdemir N, Celik L, Oğuzoğlu S, Yildirim L, Bezircioğlu H. Cervical vertebral osteomyelitis and epidural abscess caused by Candida albicans in a patient with chronic renal failure. Turk Neurosurg. 2008;18(2):207–10.

Palestro CJ. Radionuclide imaging of osteomyelitis. Semin Nucl Med. 2015;45(1):32–46.

Parr AM, Fewer D. Intramedullary blastomycosis in a child: case report. Can J Neurol Sci. 2004;31(2):282–5.

Phanthumchinda K, Kaoropthum S. Syringomyelia associated with post-meningitic spinal arachnoiditis due to Candida tropicalis. Postgrad Med J. 1991;67(790):767–9.

Saccente M, Abernathy RS, Pappas PG, Shah HR, Bradsher RW. Vertebral blastomycosis with paravertebral abscess: report of eight cases and review of the literature. Clin Infect Dis. 1998;26(2):413–8.

Smith AS, Blaser SI. Infectious and inflammatory processes of the spine. Radiol Clin North Am. 1991;29(4):809–27.
Stumpe KDM, Zanetti M, Weishaupt D, Hodler J, Boos N, Von Schulthess GK. FDG positron emission tomography for differentiation of degenerative and infectious endplate abnormalities in the lumbar spine detected on MR imaging. AJR Am J Roentgenol. 2002;179(5):1151–7.
Torres-Ramos FM, Botwin K, Shah CP. Candida spondylodiscitis: an unusual case of thoracolumbar pain with review of imaging findings and description of the clinical condition. Pain Physician. 2004;7(2):257–60.
Ugarriza LF, Cabezudo JM, Lorenzana LM, Rodríguez-Sánchez JA. Candida albicans spondylodiscitis. Br J Neurosurg. 2004;18(2):189–92.
Wang C, Jia N, Zhang L, Liu K, Liu H, Yu H. Imaging findings of cryptococcal infection of the thoracic spine. Int J Infect Dis. 2014;29:162–5. Available from: https://www.ncbi.nlm.nih.gov/pubmed/25449251
Williams RL, Fukui MB, Meltzer CC, Swarnkar A, Johnson DW, Welch W. Fungal spinal osteomyelitis in the immunocompromised patient: MR findings in three cases. AJNR Am J Neuroradiol. 1999;20(3):381–5.
Winterstein AR, Bohndorf K, Vollert K, Wagner T, Gnekow A, Roemer FW. Invasive aspergillosis osteomyelitis in children—a case report and review of the literature. Skeletal Radiol. 2010;39(8):827–31.

Part V

Therapy of Fungal Infections Involving Central Nervous System and Its Coverings

Surgical Therapy

32

Mehmet Turgut

Abbreviations

AIDS	Acquired immunodeficiency syndrome
BBB	Blood-brain barrier
CNS	Central nervous system
HIV	Human immunodeficiency virus
IICP	Increased intracranial pressure
MRI	Magnetic resonance imaging

32.1 Introduction

Despite the introduction of new antifungal agents, improved imaging technology, and intensive care facilities, fungal infections involving the central nervous system (CNS) are still a major source of morbidity and mortality, possibly due to lack of immune system of unique structures such as the brain and spinal cord, and they are extremely rare in the general population (Muzumdar 2011). In clinical practice, fungal infections of CNS are frequently seen in immunocompromised patients, including those with acquired immunodeficiency syndrome (AIDS), transplanted organ or bone marrow, steroid therapy, and drug resistance (Menon et al. 2008). Accordingly, Perfect et al. (2010) reported that there are three important risk groups for cryptococcal meningoencephalitis including human immunodeficiency virus (HIV)-infected subjects, recipients of organ transplant, and non-HIV-infected or nontransplanted individuals. Moreover, there are also various recommendations for other risk groups including children and pregnant women in the current literature.

In this chapter, various surgical therapy options for fungal granulomas and abscesses involving the CNS are described in detail together with brief review of fungal pathogens, clinical and imaging findings, differential diagnosis, antifungal chemotherapy, and outcome.

32.2 Causative Fungal Pathogens

Fungal granulomas and abscesses involving the CNS are caused by yeast (e.g., *Cryptococcus* spp., *Candida* spp.), dimorphic fungi (e.g., *Coccidioides* spp., *Histoplasma* spp., *Blastomyces* spp.), and molds (e.g., *Rhizopus*, *Aspergillus* spp.) in immunocompromised patients as a result of long-term use of some immunosuppressive agents (Menon et al. 2008; Kaczorowska et al. 2007) (Fig. 32.1). It is also interesting to note that, fungal infections may be also seen in immunocompetent humans with normal immune function. In general, fungal infections are opportunistic, and fungal agents exist in the airway passages of healthy humans, but they are not

M. Turgut (✉)
Department of Neurosurgery, Aydın Adnan Menderes University School of Medicine, Aydın, Turkey

M. Turgut et al. (eds.), *Fungal Infections of the Central Nervous System*,
https://doi.org/10.1007/978-3-030-06088-6_32

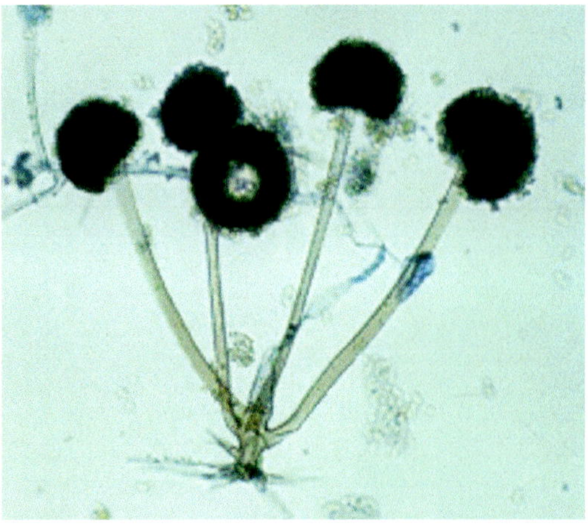

Fig. 32.1 Nonseptate hyphae with short sporangiophores bearing terminal round dark sporangia filled with spores. Rhizoids seen arising at the node: *Rhizopus* species. Lactophenol cotton blue mount 40× (courtesy of L. Vemu, M.D.)

pathogenic. In clinical practice, meningitis or meningoencephalitis caused by *Cryptococcus* spp. is most frequently encountered fungal infection of the CNS, followed by those caused by aspergillosis and candidiasis, though any kind of fungus may cause infection involving the CNS (Muzumdar 2011). In particular, aspergillosis among fungal infections involving the CNS is very resistant to antifungal therapy with AmB preparations, with high mortality and morbidity rates (Kural et al. 2018; Turgut et al. 2008). In recent years, however, uncommon space-occupying fungal lesions of the CNS, called granuloma or abscesses, have an increasing surgical importance for neurosurgeons in the world.

32.3 Clinical Presentation and Imaging Findings

Even today, it is not easy to diagnose fungal infections involving the CNS because clinical symptoms and signs are very similar to space-occupying neoplastic lesions of CNS. Basically, there are different clinical presentations including epilepsy, fever, cranial nerve deficits, and focal motor and/or sensory deficits (Rajshekhar 2007). In fungal lesions caused by *Aspergillus* species, microhemorrhage and sterile infarction are typical findings because of their angioinvasive nature and clogging of vessels by fungal elements (Fig. 32.2) (Starkey et al. 2014). Magnetic resonance imaging (MRI) is the gold standard for radiological diagnosis of fungal lesions involving the CNS; they are usually iso-hypointense in T1-weighted MRIs and hypo-hyperintense in T2-weighted MRIs, with peripheral enhancement in post-contrast images (Figs. 32.2 and 32.3) (Kural et al. 2018; Starkey et al. 2014). On MRI, these lesions are demonstrated as mass lesions with/without ring-shaped cystic component, although histopathological examination of the lesion is imperative for definitive diagnosis of the lesion (Figs. 32.2 and 32.3) (Muzumdar 2011; Starkey et al. 2014; Li et al. 2010; Mazumder and Cleveland 2010).

32.4 Differential Diagnosis

Recently, Starkey et al. (2014) suggested that involvement of gyrus rectus is characteristic finding in cases with CNS infections caused by mucormycosis (Fig. 32.3) (Starkey et al. 2014). However, neuroradiological findings are often nonspecific, and differential diagnosis of deep-situated space-occupying fungal lesions, granulomas, or abscesses is difficult from primary or metastatic tumors and pyogenic abscesses involving the CNS (Muzumdar 2011). In recent years, various fungal infections involving the CNS are encountered more frequently, possibly owing to increased incidence of AIDS, and HIV, in spite of introduction of advanced diagnostic methods in microbiology and new neuroradiological techniques (Muzumdar 2011).

32.5 Medical Therapy

Nowadays, the treatment of patients with fungal lesions involving the CNS usually consists of a combination of surgical removal of the lesion(s)

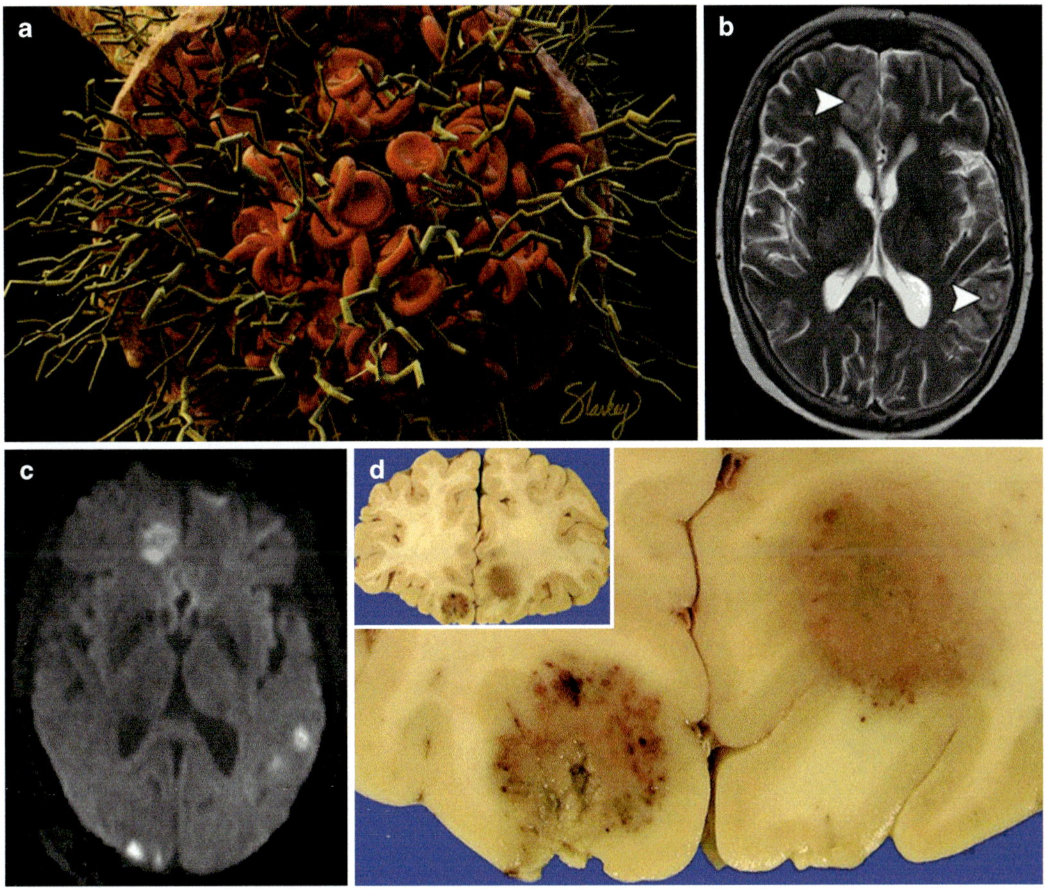

Fig. 32.2 (**a**) Photograph illustrating angioinvasive feature of *Aspergillus* with fungal elements in the lumen of the vessel, with hyphae involving the vessel wall. (**b**) Axial T2-weighted magnetic resonance imaging (MRI) demonstrating typical peripheral hypointensity (*arrowheads*) owing to high iron caused by hemorrhage and fungal elements. (**c**) Axial diffusion-weighted MRI showing microhemorrhage and reduced diffusion caused by infarction in the lesions at the gray–white junction region. (**d**) Gross specimen photograph illustrating hemorrhage with central necrosis caused by fungi (from Starkey et al. (2014), with permission)

together with medical treatment, in addition to removal of immunosuppressive agents, if possible (Kural et al. 2018). In patients with fungal infections involving the CNS, duration of systemic antifungal agents and morbidity/mortality of fungal diseases treated without oral or intravenous antifungal agents, including liposomal amphotericin B, fluconazole, and voriconazole, however, are still among unsolved questions in neurosurgery (Turgut et al. 2008). Based on experience from our case of multiple fungal granulomas involving the brain due to aspergillosis, which was treated by long-term antifungal treatment, it has been suggested that only medical therapy with conventional AmB or combination of liposomal AmB and oral itraconazole is the choice of treatment for this infection, even if complete surgical excision of the multiple mass lesions, granulomas, or abscesses is not possible in complicated cases (Turgut et al. 2008). In cases with meningoencephalitis caused by fungi, induction therapy including fungicidal regimens with flucytosine and then suppressive regimens with fluconazole are advised, while surgery may be necessary in the most of the patients

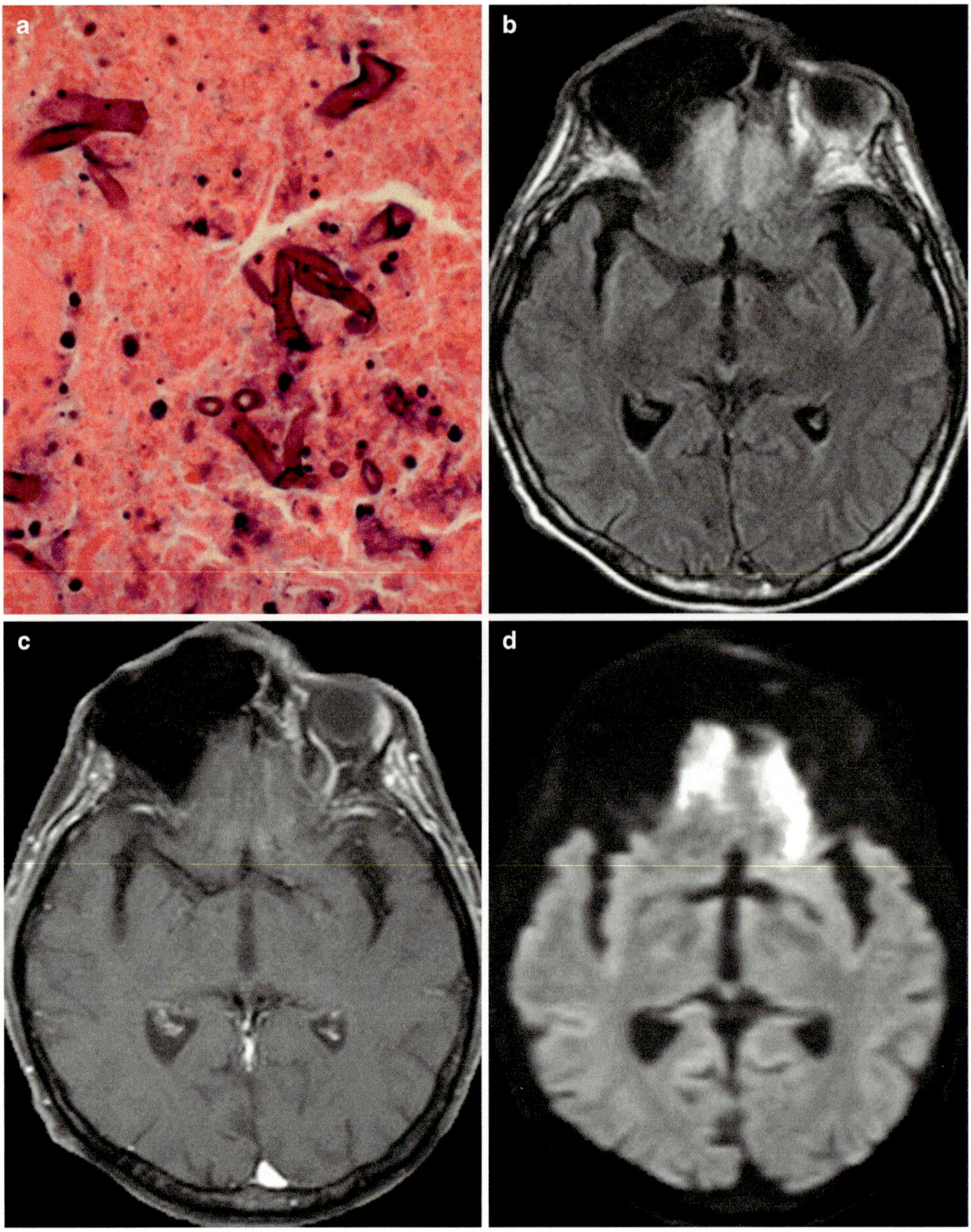

Fig. 32.3 (**a**) Photographs demonstrating fungal forms with broad, pleomorphic hyphae within a necrotic brain tissue (original magnification, 400×; PAS stain). (**b**) Axial FLAIR image demonstrating hyperintensity areas involving both gyrus rectus. (**c**) Axial T1 MRI following gadolinium administration demonstrating presence of enhancement. (**d**) Axial diffusion-weighted MRI revealing a reduced diffusion (from Starkey et al. (2014), with permission)

with fungal granulomas and abscesses involving the CNS (Muzumdar 2011). Furthermore, amphotericin B regimens with lipid formulations may be used as an alternative agent in patients with renal disease (Muzumdar 2011). Moreover, in some cases with refractory infections, use of adjunctive recombinant cytokine, growth factor, or corticosteroid may be used as an alternative approach (Panackal and Williamson 2015).

32.6 Surgical Intervention

Classically, total excision of the space-occupying compressive fungal mass lesions, either granulomas or abscesses, via open surgical craniotomy/laminectomy, in addition to systemic antifungal drugs, is the treatment of choice in patients with fungal infections of the CNS (Rajshekhar 2007; Li et al. 2010; Mazumder and Cleveland 2010). In these patients, surgical intervention provides definitive diagnosis, but early diagnosis before surgery is also important for both prevention of the spread of fungi and treatment of increased intracranial pressure (IICP) in cases with infections of the CNS. Therefore, a high index of suspicion for a fungal etiology is necessary for microbiological diagnosis and histopathological confirmation in cases with space-occupying lesions within the CNS (Rajshekhar 2007). Today, minimal invasive stereotactic procedures versus open surgical craniotomy/laminectomy for total excision of the fungal granulomas and abscesses is one of the controversial topics in neurosurgical practice (Li et al. 2010; Thurnher and Olatunji 2016). In addition, issues of optimal treatment for hydrocephalus, aneurysm of the intracranial arteries, and involvement of paranasal sinuses in patients with fungal infections involving the CNS need further clinical studies, as mentioned below in detail.

32.6.1 Open Surgical Craniotomy/Laminectomy Procedure

In patients with large or compressive fungal mass lesions such as granulomas and abscesses which are located in accessible regions of the brain or spinal cord, it has been reported that complete/incomplete excision of space-occupying lesions via open surgical craniotomy/laminectomy is a feasible and safe procedure, as mentioned above. On the other hand, open surgical craniotomy/laminectomy procedure is also performed in the presence of a suspected fungal granuloma and abscess (Rajshekhar 2007; Panackal and Williamson 2015; Thurnher and Olatunji 2016).

32.6.1.1 Complete/Incomplete Excision of Fungal Granuloma/Abscess

Importantly, it has been suggested that complete or incomplete removal of the fungal granulomas and abscesses and reduction of IICP may provide penetration of systemic antifungal drugs into the infected tissue such as the brain and spinal cord (Sharma et al. 1997). Today, it is generally accepted that outcome of patients with fungal infections of the CNS, granuloma or abscess, is good if complete resection of the mass lesion is done (Rajshekhar 2007; Panackal and Williamson 2015; Thurnher and Olatunji 2016; Sharma et al. 1997; Coleman et al. 1995; Dubey et al. 2005; Haran and Chandy 1993; Jamjoom et al. 1995; Middelhof et al. 2005; Nadkarni and Goel 2005; Salama et al. 1997; Young et al. 1985). However, it is not possible for space-occupying lesions in eloquent critical areas of the brain and brain stem, especially in patients with poor general condition (Rajshekhar 2007). Siddiqui et al. (2004) suggested that aggressive surgical approaches are not appropriate in the management of the fungal granulomas and abscesses of the CNS because of risks of high morbidity and mortality. At present, however, a radical approach without additional neurological deficits is advised based on the current literature, although there is no data that total excision of the mass lesions improves outcome of the patients with fungal granulomas and abscesses. Some authors reported that repeated craniotomies/laminectomies in same patient may be necessary for residual or recurrent fungal granulomas and abscesses involving the brain and spinal cord (Panackal and Williamson 2015;

Thurnher and Olatunji 2016; Sharma et al. 1997).

32.6.1.2 Local/Intracavitary Antifungal Adjuvant Therapy After Surgical Excision

Interestingly, it has also been reported that local antifungal therapy with amphotericin B has been used in patients with incomplete removal of the fungal granulomas and abscesses during open surgery craniotomy procedure in a previous study (Langmayr et al. 1993). Most recently, it has been suggested that intracavitary amphotericin B therapy may be given as an adjunct following the surgical excision of granuloma or abscess in patients with intracranial aspergillosis because the administration of antifungal drugs through the blood brain barrier (BBB) is limited, with aim of the regression of mass lesion or avoid from the recurrence (Kural et al. 2018).

32.6.2 Minimal Invasive Stereotactic Procedure

As expected, minimal invasive stereotactic surgery procedure is less invasive than open surgical craniotomy procedure, and it can be performed even in patients with poor general condition, in contrast to that of open craniotomy procedure, as an alternative.

32.6.2.1 Stereotactic Biopsy and Aspiration

Minimal invasive stereotactic biopsy and aspiration procedure for the fungal mass lesions of brain such as granuloma and abscess is used if the lesions are multiple or located in deep or eloquent brain regions such as brain stem, basal ganglion, thalamus, motor strip, or Broca and Wernicke areas (Rajshekhar 2007). Using a minimal invasive procedure, it is possible to obtain infected tissue or pus for microbiological examination for definitive diagnosis (Rajshekhar 2007). However, some authors suggested that minimal invasive stereotactic biopsy and aspiration procedures, in addition to systemic antifungal therapy, provide a good outcome in patients with fungal infections involving the CNS (Salama et al. 1997; Arunkumar et al. 2000; Casey et al. 1994; Goodman and Coffey 1989; Kerkmann et al. 1994). In patients whose general health condition is not good for open surgery, minimal invasive stereotactic procedures may be used for total excision of the fungal granulomas and abscesses, even under local anesthesia (Rajshekhar 2007). Importantly, Siddiqui et al. (2004) suggested that the periphery of the mass lesions, granuloma, or abscess, in addition to its center, should be targeted because the fungal hyphae are frequently located in the periphery region of the lesion.

32.6.2.2 Stereotactic Craniotomy

To reduce the morbidity and mortality of an open surgery with craniotomy, stereotactic craniotomy may be used in some patients with fungal granulomas and abscesses of the CNS (Rajshekhar 2007; Middelhof et al. 2005).

32.6.2.3 Placement of Ommaya Reservoir

Surgically, stereotactic placement of Ommaya reservoir may be used for the injection of amphotericin B into fungal granulomas or abscesses involving the CNS (Rajshekhar 2007; Young et al. 1985). In a previous study, Camarata et al. (1992) reported that intracavitary drug administration of amphotericin B for fungal infections involving the CNS, granuloma or abscess, provide a better outcome in selected cases. Then, it has been suggested that such therapy avoids high systemic toxicity of the antifungal agents by bypassing the BBB (Jamjoom et al. 1995; Siddiqui et al. 2004).

32.6.3 Other Surgical Procedures

32.6.3.1 Ventriculoperitoneal Shunt for Hydrocephalus

In some patients with fungal mass lesions involving the CNS, such as granuloma and abscess, a communicating type of hydrocephalus may develop due to blockage of cerebrospinal fluid flow as a result of arachnoiditis of the basal cisterns, and they may require the surgical placement of a ventriculoperitoneal shunt either in the early period as a primary procedure or in late period as a secondary procedure during medical therapy (Rajshekhar 2007; Sharma et al. 1997; Dubey et al. 2005; Jamjoom et al. 1995; Young et al. 1985; Siddiqui et al. 2004; Mehta et al. 1985).

32.6.3.2 Clipping or Coiling for Fungal Aneurysms

In the literature, there are several reports of obliteration of fungal aneurysms with surgical clipping (Sharma et al. 1997; Dubey et al. 2005) or minimal invasive endovascular techniques such as stenting and coiling (Hurst et al. 2001). Unfortunately, however, it has been reported that outcome of these patients is poor (Hurst et al. 2001).

32.6.3.3 Surgery for Involvement of Paranasal Sinuses

In the presence of fungal granulomas and abscesses within the paranasal sinuses, complete surgical excision of the diseased fungal tissue using functional endoscopic sinus surgery technique is required (Rajshekhar 2007; Siddiqui et al. 2004).

32.7 Outcome

In general, the outcome of fungal infections of the CNS is poor, although surgical decompression for fungal mass lesions such as granuloma and abscess may provide a transient improvement related with reduction in the IICP of the patients (Menon et al. 2008; Kaczorowska et al. 2007). Importantly, it should be kept in mind that some complications such as IICP and drug resistance may be encountered in the management of fungal infections involving the CNS (Muzumdar 2011). In particular, cryptococcosis among many fungal infections is one of the most important mycoses with significant morbidity and mortality. However, it is a treatable disease when correct diagnosis is made early and appropriate treatment is given to control the underlying disease without delay (Perfect et al. 2010). There is no doubt that the prognosis of patients with the fungal space-occupying lesions of the CNS, granuloma or abscess, is determined by their anatomic location within the CNS (Muzumdar 2011).

32.8 Conclusion

In conclusion, fungal infections of the CNS are still one of major problems in developing countries in spite of introduction of new antifungal agents and current developments in surgical techniques. Early and appropriate local/systemic antifungal therapy and surgical drainage/excision of fungal granulomas and abscesses should be performed to decrease neurological deficits and mortality rates in these patients.

References

Arunkumar MJ, Rajshekhar V, Chandy MJ, Thomas PP, Jacob CK. Management and outcome of brain abscess in renal transplant recipients. Postgrad Med J. 2000;76:207–11.

Camarata PJ, Dunn DL, Farney AC, Parker RG, Seljeskog EL. Continual intracavitary administration of amphotericin B as an adjunct in the treatment of aspergillus brain abscess: case report and review of the literature. Neurosurgery. 1992;31:575–9.

Casey AT, Wilkins P, Uttley D. Aspergillosis infection in neurosurgical practice. Br J Neurosurg. 1994;8:31–9.

Coleman JM, Hogg GG, Rosenfeld JV, Waters KD. Invasive central nervous system aspergillosis: cure with liposomal amphotericin B, itraconazole and radical surgery-case report and review of the literature. Neurosurgery. 1995;36:858–63.

Dubey A, Patwardhan RV, Sampath S, Santosh V, Kolluri S, Nanda A. Intracranial fungal granuloma: analysis of 40 patients and review of the literature. Surg Neurol. 2005;63:254–60.

Goodman ML, Coffey RJ. Stereotactic drainage of Aspergillus brain abscess with long-term survival: case report and review. Neurosurgery. 1989;24:96–9.

Haran RP, Chandy MJ. Intracranial aspergillus granuloma. Br J Neurosurg. 1993;7:383–8.

Hurst RW, Judkins A, Bolger W, Chu A, Loevner LA. Mycotic aneurysm and cerebral infarction resulting from fungal sinusitis: imaging and pathological correlation. AJNR Am J Neuroradiol. 2001;22:858–63.

Jamjoom AB, al-Hedaithy SA, Jamjoom ZA, al-Hedaithy M, el-Watidy SF, Rahman N, al-Moallem M. Intracranial mycotic infections in neurosurgical practice. Acta Neurochir. 1995;137:78–84.

Kaczorowska B, Chmielewski H, Pawełczyk M, Przybyła M, Błaszczyk B, Chudzik W. The case of multiple brain abscesses conservatively treated (in Polish). Pol Merkur Lekarski. 2007;22:150–3.

Kerkmann ML, Blaschke-Hellmessen R, Mikulin HD. Successful treatment of cerebral aspergillosis by stereotactic operation and antifungal therapy. Mycoses. 1994;37:123–6.

Kural C, Ozer MI, Ezgu MC, Mehtiyev R, Yasar S, Kutlay AM, Daneyemez MK, Onguru O, Erdogan E, Izci Y. Intracavitary amphotericin B in the treatment of intracranial aspergillosis. J Clin Neurosci. 2018;51:75–9. https://doi.org/10.1016/j.jocn.2018.02.018.

Langmayr JJ, Schwarz A, Buchberger W, Hochleitner W, Twerdy K. Local amphotericin for fungal brain abscess. Lancet. 1993;342:123.

Li Q, You C, Liu Q, Liu Y. Central nervous system cryptococcoma in immunocompetent patients: a short review illustrated by a new case. Acta Neurochir. 2010;152:129–36.

Mazumder SA, Cleveland KO. Cryptococcal meningitis after neurosurgery. Am J Med Sci. 2010;339:582–3.

Mehta VS, Bhatia R, Mahapatra LN, Banerji AK. Intracranial mycotic infection in non-immunocompromised individuals. J Indian Med Assoc. 1985;83:185–8.

Menon S, Bharadwaj R, Chowdhary A, Kaundinya DV, Palande DA. Current epidemiology of intracranial abscesses: a prospective 5 year study. J Med Microbiol. 2008;57:1259–68.

Middelhof CA, Loudon WG, Muhonen MD, Xavier C, Greene CS Jr. Improved survival in central nervous system aspergillosis: A series of immunocompromised children with leukemia undergoing stereotactic resection of aspergillomas. Report of four cases. J Neurosurg. 2005;103:374–8.

Muzumdar D. Central nervous system infections and the neurosurgeon: a perspective. Int J Surg. 2011;9:113–6.

Nadkarni T, Goel A. Aspergilloma of the brain: an overview. J Postgrad Med. 2005;51:37–41.

Panackal AA, Williamson PR. Fungal infections of the central nervous system. Continuum (Minneap Minn). 2015;21(6 Neuroinfectious Disease):1662–78. https://doi.org/10.1212/CON.0000000000000241.

Perfect JR, Dismukes WE, Dromer F, Goldman DL, Graybill JR, Hamill RJ, Harrison TS, Larsen RA, Lortholary O, Nguyen MH, Pappas PG, Powderly WG, Singh N, Sobel JD, Sorrell TC. Clinical practice guidelines for the management of cryptococcal disease: 2010 update by the infectious diseases society of America. Clin Infect Dis. 2010;50:291–322.

Rajshekhar V. Surgical management of intracranial fungal masses. Neurol India. 2007;55:267–73.

Salama AD, Rogers T, Lord GM, Lechler RI, Mason PD. Multiple Cladosporium brain abscesses in a renal transplant patient: aggressive management improves outcome. Transplantation. 1997;63:160–2.

Sharma BS, Khosla VK, Kak VK, Banerjee AK, Vasishtha RK, Prasad KS, Sharma SC, Mathuriya SN, Tewari MK, Pathak A. Intracranial fungal granuloma. Surg Neurol. 1997;47:489–97.

Siddiqui AA, Shah AA, Bashir SH. Craniocerebral aspergillosis of sinonasal origin in immunocompetent patients: clinical spectrum and outcome in 25 cases. Neurosurgery. 2004;55:602–13.

Starkey J, Moritani T, Kirby P. MRI of CNS fungal infections: review of aspergillosis to histoplasmosis and everything in between. Clin Neuroradiol. 2014;24:217–30.

Thurnher MM, Olatunji RB. Infections of the spine and spinal cord. Handb Clin Neurol. 2016;136:717–31.

Turgut M, Ozsunar Y, Oncü S, Akyüz O, Ertuğrul MB, Tekin C, Gültekin B, Sakarya S. Invasive fungal granuloma of the brain caused by Aspergillus fumigatus: a case report and review of the literature. Surg Neurol. 2008;69:169–74.

Young RF, Gade G, Grinnell V. Surgical treatment for fungal infections in the central nervous system. J Neurosurg. 1985;63:371–81.

Prognosis of Fungal Infections Involving the Central Nervous System and Its Coverings

33

Kartik Munta and Jay Dip Ray Chaudhuri

Abbreviations

AIDS	Acquired immunodeficiency syndrome
CNS	Central nervous system
CSF	Cerebrospinal fluid
HIV	Human immunodeficiency virus

33.1 Introduction

Over 1.5 million fungal species have been known to be existing. There has been description of only 70,000 species reported in literature. Out of the described species, 300 have been suspected to show signs of virulence in humans. Amongst them 10–15% affect the central nervous system (CNS) in human beings (Köhler et al. 2015). Fungal organisms encountered in the CNS can be classified into *yeasts* (*Candida* and *Cryptococcus* species), *moniliaceous (hyaline or lightly pigmented) molds* (*Aspergillus* spp., *Fusarium* spp., *Pseudallescheria/Scedosporium* spp.), *Zygomycetes* (*Mucor* spp., *Rhizopus* spp.) *dimorphic fungi* (*Blastomyces*, *Coccidioides*, *Histoplasma* species) and dematiaceous fungi.

Recent therapeutic advancements, increase in the number of patients receiving chemotherapy and patients undergoing solid organ transplantation has led to significant rise in the number of immunocompromised subjects who are at a risk of acquiring invasive fungal infections (Marr et al. 2002; Banerjee et al. 2001). Human immunodeficiency virus (HIV)-affected patients also form a significant number of patients with opportunistic infections of the CNS (Collazos 2003).

CNS fungal infections can be categorized as parenchymal (granulomas, cerebritis, abscess), extra-axial (meningitis), and vascular (vasculitis) (Mathur et al. 2012).

CNS fungal infections are associated with high mortality and morbidity. The cure rate in immunocompetent patients receiving antifungal therapy for cryptococcal meningitis is 75% and is only 25% for CNS aspergillosis and mucormycosis (Johnson and Perfect 2010). Henceforth fungal infections of CNS requires prompt diagnosis and early appropriate medical as well as surgical management in improving the outcomes (Raman Sharma 2010). Fungal infections can be observed in otherwise immunocompetent individuals. Most of the patients with CNS aspergillosis reported from the Indian subcontinent are immunocompetent (Santosh et al. 1996; Sharma et al. 1997a; Kartik et al. 2017).

Prognosis of fungal meningitis or meningoencephalitis varies with the type of organism involved (molds or yeasts) and extent of involvement of neuraxis (whether involving meninges, parameningeal spaces, the cortex, or subcortical basal ganglia involving blood vessels in the brain causing vasculitis, etc. Prognosis also depends upon the host, whether the patient is immunocompromised due to

K. Munta (✉) · J. D. R. Chaudhuri
Yashoda Superspeciality Hospital, Hyderabad, India

M. Turgut et al. (eds.), *Fungal Infections of the Central Nervous System*,
https://doi.org/10.1007/978-3-030-06088-6_33

acquired immunodeficiency syndrome (AIDS), malignancy, immunological defects (which might arise due to hereditary factors), organ transplant recipients, or patients receiving immunosuppressive medications. (Gavito-Higuera et al. 2016).

33.2 *Candida* Species

Candida infection in the CNS is usually uncommon. Autopsy studies in patients of proven candidemia who succumbed due to invasive candidiasis have shown disseminated spread of infection in the CNS (Thorn et al. 2010). *C. albicans* is the most frequent cause of meningitis and abscess of the brain among *Candida* species. Other less common species are *C. tropicalis*, *C. parapsilosis*, *C. lusitaniae*, *C. glabrata*, and *C. krusei*. Incidence rate of candida meningitis is higher in infants than in older patients (Arsenault and Bliss 2015).

The progression of disease in the brain due to *Candida* infections is dependent upon factors which control the local proliferation of the organism. Neutropenia is one of the most important risk factors for developing CNS candidiasis and it usually carries poor prognosis. Autosomal recessive caspase recruitment domain–containing protein 9 immunodeficiency may lead to recurrent candida meningoencephalitis occurrence (Lanternier et al. 2015). Candida ophthalmitis is frequently seen in patients with candida meningitis and it should be detected early. Presence of endophthalmitis usually has been associated with prolonged course of therapy and increased morbidity (Hassan et al. 2012).

Hydrocephalus can be seen in cases of CNS candida, more often leading to performing a ventriculostomy. Candida forms biofilms over ventriculoperitoneal shunt and harbors as source of infection leading to untimely removal of these shunts. CNS candidiasis can lead to brain abscess and mycotic aneurysms causing ruptures leading to subrachnoid hemorrhage. Posterior circulation stroke due to basilar artery thrombosis has been reported in these patients (Jamjoom et al. 1992).

Prognosis of candida meningitis depends mainly on the risk group involved. The mortality rates may range around 10% for neurosurgical patients, whereas it increased up to 30% in HIV-infected patients (Nguyen and Yu 1995; Casado et al. 1997). Candida meningitis in premature infants has a higher rate of mortality and is associated with neurodevelopmental abnormalities (Lee et al. 1998).

33.3 *Aspergillus* Species

Aspergillus fumigatus is the most frequent species among pathogenic fungi known to cause invasive infections. Abscesses of the brain are more common in disseminated aspergillosis, whereas meningitis occurrence is rare (Dupont 2003).

A. flavus contributes to major part of infections in paranasal sinuses (Chakrabarti and Sharma 2000). Cerebral and spinal aspergilloses occur in 10–20% of patients with aspergillosis in rhinosinopulmonary infections. CNS presentation of invasive aspergillosis varies from occurrence of meningitis, cerebral abscess, myelitis, ophthalmoplegia, and vasculitis to anterior and middle cerebrovascular strokes and venous thrombosis (Schwartz 2010; Fasciano et al. 1999).

The invasion to CNS occurs due to direct inoculation into a region anatomically nearer to the brain or by hematogenous seeding. The hematogenous dissemination is also initiated by direct inoculation into bloodstream via the middle ear, paranasal sinuses, eye, and mastoid infections or as a consequence of open-heart surgery.

Extended periods of neutropenia and use of high-dose corticosteroids are the main predisposing factors for occurrence of aspergillus infections (Dupont 2003; Ribaud et al. 1999). Immunocompetent host can develop aspergillosis, but spread is limited by a fibrous capsule developed by host around the abscess/granulomas. Dihydrorhodamine flow cytometry-based assay helps in determining functionality of neutrophils, thereby predicting the prognosis of infection (Richardson et al. 1998). CNS aspergillosis presenting with signs like ophthalmoplegia, ptosis, proptosis and cavernous sinus thrombosis or stroke syndrome fare poorly than other individuals.

Aspergillus spp. is the commonest causative fungal pathogen accounting for 56–69% of the intracranial fungal mass lesions (Sharma et al. 1997b; Dubey et al. 2005). Early institution of voriconazole therapy, immunosuppressive therapy, transfusion of granulocytes, and hyperbaric oxygen may improve outcomes in these patients (Mattiuzzi and Giles 2005; Antinori et al. 2013).

33.4 *Cryptococcus neoformans*

The two varieties of *C. neoformans* are var. *neoformans* (serotypes A and D) and var. *gattii* (serotypes B and C). The most prevalent agent causing chronic fungal meningitis is *C. neoformans* var. *neoformans*, and 90% of infections happen in immunocompromised patients (Speed and Dunt 1995). Cryptococcus incidence is higher among AIDS survivors in Africa and Southeast Asia than in the population of the west (Levitz 1991). Both cryptococcal species *neoformans*- and *gattii*-related meningitis outcomes remained the same. But a non-outbreak *gattii*-related CNS infection seemed to produce worse outcome when compared to outbreak-related *gattii* infections (Lockhart et al. 2012).

Important markers of poor prognosis in HIV-associated cryptococcal meningitis include altered mental status at presentation and high organism load, (as determined by cerebrospinal fluid (CSF) culture or CSF antigen titer) (Brouwer et al. 2004). Low CSF white cell count, high CSF lactate, and raised CSF opening pressure are associated with a poor outcome. Mortality in non-HIV-associated cryptococcal meningitis is associated with factors like chronic renal failure, liver failure, hematological malignancy, absence of headache, and altered mental status (Pappas et al. 2001). 10-week mortality rates due to cryptococcal meningitis remain high at around 10%. Few have reported higher rates, up to 26% in selected groups. Studies from Africa and Asia have shown between 20% and 40% where amphotericin B therapy has been available (Kambugu et al. 2003; Imwidthaya and Poungvarin 2000). Cryptococcal meningitis has been the leading cause of death in HIV-infected patients in Thailand, Uganda, Malawi, and South Africa, with an estimated mortality risk of 17% at 2 weeks and 34% at 10 weeks (Jarvis et al. 2014). Chronic neuropsychiatric sequelae and altered brain imaging are common after cryptococcal meningitis (Lu et al. 2011).

Patient treated with amphotericin B and flucytosine carried better prognosis than those who received only amphotericin B (Perfect et al. 2010). Development of an apparent paradoxical immune response (immune reconstitution inflammatory syndrome) while on treatment was associated with cerebral edema and worsening of neurological symptoms. Many of these patients required treatment with steroids and it leads to increased morbidity and prolonged hospitalization (Singh et al. 2005). Acetazolamide and mannitol therapy for increased intracranial pressure was also associated with poor outcomes (Newton et al. 2002).

Cryptococcoma or brain mass lesions because of *C. neoformans* are less frequently seen in comparison to meningitis caused by serotypes A and D. In contrast, serotype B, commonly seen in non-immunocompromised hosts, frequently causes a pseudotumor mass in the brain. Rarely does such a mass lesion occur without meningitis (Kovoor et al. 2002).

33.5 Dimorphic Fungi

Coccidioides immitis and Histoplasma capsulatum are the commonest organisms of this class causing infections of the CNS. The most frequent cause of meningitis among both organisms is *C. immitis* which is geographically limited to Southwest United States and South America countries (Dupont 2003; Singh and Husain 2001). *Coccidioides* meningitis occurs in 30–50% of patients with disseminated infection. HIV-positive individuals, solid organ transplant recipients treated with steroids, and pregnant patients are at a high risk of dissemination and developing CNS infections. Prognosis depends on the host response. The disease may cause unique symptoms among HIV-positive patients. Patients who developed hydrocephalus, infarcts due to vasculitis generally had poorer outcomes. Despite advances in antifungal therapy, the morbidity and mortality associated with Coccidioides meningitis remain high, with a current mortality rate at around 30%. Due to high risk of relapse if therapy is stopped, treatment should be given lifelong in these individuals (Dewsnup et al. 1996).

Histoplasmosis caused by *H. capsulatum* is endemic in the United States, South America, Southeast Asia, and Africa. This fungus can cause meningitis in 5–25% of AIDS patients which is similar to its incidence in non-AIDS patients (Wheat et al. 1990). Occasionally, brain abscesses are caused due to *Histoplasma* (Venger et al. 1987). Approximately 20–40% of these patients who fail initial therapy may have relapse (Wheat et al. 2005).

33.6 Dematiaceous Fungi

These pigmented soil-based fungi are known to cause CNS infections in both immunocompromised and immunocompetent individual. Hematogenous spread of this fungus is known to cause brain abscesses. Mortality is not dependent on host immune status. Outbreak of *Exserohilum rostratum* infection was reported after contamination of methyl prednisolone containers in 2013 which had reported 9% mortality (White and Barnes 2014). Various types of CNS pathologies including meningitis, abscess, stroke, epidural abscess, and cauda equina syndrome have been documented (Larone and Walsh 2013). Patients who had cauda equina syndrome or posterior circulation stroke secondary to infection had worst outcomes. Low CSF sugars are seen universally in these infections. Complete resection of mass lesion surgically was associated with better outcomes than partial resection (Katragkou et al. 2014).

Scedosporium apiospermum affects individuals in drowning and near-drowning situations (Munta et al. 2015). It can cause brain abscess, meningitis, vasculitis, and stroke secondary to infection. Spinal cord involvement in these fungal infections is uncommon. It also may follow penetrating traumatic brain injury leading to CNS infections. Outcome may not be influenced by host immune status in scedosporium infections. Prognosis depends upon early diagnosis, early surgical resection of the abscess, and early use of voriconazole (Gopinath et al. 2010). Concomitant usage of terbinafine with voriconazole has shown to improve outcomes in CNS infections caused by *Scedosporium prolificans* (Cooley et al. 2007).

33.6.1 Melanized Fungi

Exophiala dermatitidis, *Ramichloridium mackenziei*, and *Cladosporium bantiana* mainly cause the primary cerebral infections. *E. dermatitidis* has been described as the major neurotropic fungi of East Asia though it is isolated worldwide in environment. An uncommon presentation of brain involvement is formation of abscess without meningitis. Otherwise, meningitis can be the only manifestation (Middleton et al. 1976).

33.7 *Zygomycetes*

CNS zygomycosis is a worldwide fungal infection caused by class *Zygomycetes*. *Zygomycetes* class includes genera *Rhizopus*, *Rhizomucor*, *Absidia*, *Mucor*, *Cunninghamella*, *Apophysomyces*, and *Saksenaea*. *Zygomycetes* thrive in a highly acid condition that has rich carbohydrate. Therefore a diabetic ketoacidosis person has a more risk due to defective phagocyte function and offers an environment for quick invasion (Chakrabarti et al. 2006). *Zygomycetes* proliferate in neutropenic patients whose serum iron concentration is increased by deferoxamine (Pagano et al. 1997).

33.8 Conclusion

Fungal neuroinfections are known to be associated with high morbidity and mortality. More than other pathogens involving the CNS, fungal ones require timely diagnosis and early appropriate treatment in improving the outcomes.

Prognosis will also depend on the host, the underlying disease, the virulence of the fungal pathogen implicated, the extent of infection, and the response to treatment.

References

Antinori S, Corbellino M, Meroni L, et al. Aspergillus meningitis: a rare clinical manifestation of central nervous system aspergillosis - case report and review of 92 cases. J Infect. 2013;66(3):218–38.

Arsenault AB, Bliss JM. Neonatal candidiasis: new insights into an old problem at a unique host-pathogen interface. Curr Fungal Infect Rep. 2015;9(4):246–52.

Banerjee U, Datta K, Majumdar T, Gupta K. Cryptococcosis in India: the awakening of a giant? Med Mycol. 2001;39:51–67.5.

Brouwer AE, Rajanuwong A, Chierakul W, et al. Combination antifungal therapies for HIV-associated cryptococcal meningitis: a randomised trial. Lancet. 2004;363(9423):1764–7.

Casado JL, Quereda C, Oliva J, et al. Candidal meningitis in HIV-infected patients: analysis of 14 cases. Clin Infect Dis. 1997;25(3):673–6.

Chakrabarti A, Sharma SC. Paranasal sinus mycoses. Indian J Chest Dis Allied Sci. 2000;42:293–304.

Chakrabarti A, Das A, Mandal J, et al. The rising trend of invasive zygomycosis in patients with uncontrolled diabetes mellitus. Med Mycol. 2006;44(4):335–42.

Collazos J. Opportunistic infections of the CNS in patients with AIDS: diagnosis and management. CNS Drugs. 2003;17(12):869–87.

Cooley L, Spelman D, Thursky K, et al. Infection with Scedosporium apiospermum and S. prolificans, Australia. Emerg Infect Dis. 2007;13(8):1170.

Dewsnup DH, Galgiani JN, Graybill JR, et al. Is it ever safe to stop azole therapy for Coccidioides immitis meningitis? Ann Intern Med. 1996;124(3):305–10.

Dubey A, Patwardhan RV, Sampth S, Santosh V, Kolluri S, Nanda A. Intracranial fungal granuloma: analysis of 40 patients and review of the literature. Surg Neurol. 2005;63(3):254–60.

Dupont B. Fungal infections of the central nervous system. In: Anaissie EJ, McGinnis MR, Pfaller MA, editors. Clinical mycology. 1st ed. New York: Churchill Livinstone; 2003. p. 539–53.

Fasciano JW, Ripple MG, Suarez JI, Bhardwaj A. Central nervous system Aspergillosis: a case report and literature review. Hosp Physician. 1999;1:63–7.

Gavito-Higuera J, Mullins CB, Ramos-Duran L, Olivas Chacon CI, Hakim N, Palacios E. Fungal infections of the central nervous system: a pictorial review. J Clin Imaging Sci. 2016;6:24.

Gopinath M, Cherian A, Baheti NN, Das A, Antonty M, Sarada C. An elusive diagnosis: Scedosporium apiospermum infection after near-drowning. Ann Indian Acad Neurol. 2010;13:213–5.

Hassan A, Poon W, Baker M, Linton C, Mühlschlegel FA. Confirmed Candida albicans endogenous fungal endophthalmitis in a patient with chronic candidiasis. Med Mycol Case Rep. 2012;1(1):42–4.

Imwidthaya P, Poungvarin N. Cryptococcosis in AIDS. Postgrad Med J. 2000;76(892):85–8.

Jamjoom A, al-Abedeen Jamjoom Z, al-Hedaithy S, Jamali A, Naim-Ur-Rahman MT. Ventriculitis and hydrocephalus caused by Candida albicans successfully treated by antimycotic therapy and cerebrospinal fluid shunting. Br J Neurosurg. 1992;6(5):501–4.

Jarvis JN, Bicanic T, Loyse A, et al. Determinants of mortality in a combined cohort of 501 patients with HIV-associated cryptococcal meningitis: implications for improving outcomes. Clin Infect Dis. 2014;58(5):736–45.

Johnson MD, Perfect JR. Use of antifungal combination therapy: agents, order, and timing. Curr Fungal Infect Rep. 2010 May 1;4(2):87–95.

Kambugu AD, Kamya M, Mayanja-Kizza H, et al. The high mortality of HIV associated Cryptococcal meningitis despite high dose amphotericin B therapy in Uganda. 41st Annual Meeting of The Infectious Diseases Society of America. San Diego, 2003.

Kartik M, Kanala A, Sunilnadikuda RSM, Prakasham PS. Invasive mediastinal Aspergillosis in immunocompetent male with invasion of left atrium and hilar structures. Indian J Crit Care Med. 2017;21:408–11.

Katragkou A, Pana ZD, Perlin DS, Kontoyiannis DP, Walsh TJ, Roilides E. Exserohilum infections: review of 48 cases before the 2012 United States outbreak. Med Mycol. 2014;52(4):376–86.

Köhler JR, Casadevall A, Perfect J. The spectrum of fungi that infects humans. Cold Spring Herb Perspect Med. 2015;5:a019273. https://doi.org/10.1101/cshperspecte.0.019273.

Kovoor JM, Mahadevan A, Narayan JP, et al. Cryptococcal choroid plexitis as a mass lesion: MR imaging and histopathologic correlation. AJNR Am J Neuroradiol. 2002;23(2):273–6.

Lanternier F, Mahdaviani SA, Barbati E, et al. Inherited CARD9 deficiency in otherwise healthy children and adults with meningo-encephalitis and/or colitis caused by Candida. J Allergy Clin Immunol. 2015;135(6):1558–68.

Larone DH, Walsh TJ. Exserohilumrostratum: anatomy of a national outbreak of fungal meningitis. Clin Microbiol Newsl. 2013;35(23):185–93.

Lee BE, Cheung PY, Robinson JL, et al. Comparative study of mortality and morbidity in premature infants with candidaemia or candidal meningitis. Clin Infect Dis. 1998;27(3):559–65.

Levitz SM. The ecology of Cryptococcus neoformans and the epidemiology of cryptococcosis. Rev Infect Dis. 1991;13:1164–9.

Lockhart SR, Iqbal N, Bolden CB, DeBess EE, Marsden-Haug N, Worhle R, Thakur R, Harris JR, Cryptococcus gattii PNW Public Health Working Group. Epidemiologic cutoff values for triazole drugs in Cryptococcus gattii: correlation of molecular type and in vitro susceptibility. Diagn Microbiol Infect Dis. 2012;73:144–8.

Lu CH, Chen HL, Chang WN, et al. Assessing the chronic neuropsychologic sequelae of human immunodeficiency virus-negative cryptococcal meningitis by using diffusion tensor imaging. AJNR Am J Neuroradiol. 2011;32(7):1333–9.

Marr KA, Carter RA, Crippa F, Wald A, Corey L. Epidemiology and outcome of mold infections in hematopoietic stem cell transplant recipient. Clin Infect Dis. 2002;34:909–17. 4.

Mathur M, Johnson CE, Sze G. Fungal infections of the central nervous system. Neuroimaging Clin N Am. 2012;22(4):609–32.

Mattiuzzi G, Giles FJ. Management of intracranial fungal infections in patients with haematological malignancies. Br J Haematol. 2005;131:287–300.

Middleton FG, Jurgenson PF, Utz JP, Shadomy S, Shadomy J. Brain abscess caused by Cladosporium trichoides. Ann Int Med. 1976;136:444–8.

Munta K, Gopal PB, Vigg A. Invasive aspergillosis in near drowning nonneutropenic patient. Indian J Crit Care Med. 2015;19:739–42.

Newton PN, Thai LH, LH TNQ, Short JM, Chierakul W, Rajanuwong A, Pitisuttithum P, Chasombat S, Phonrat B, Maek-A-Nantawat W, Teaunadi R, Lalloo DG, White NJ. A randomized, double-blind, placebo-controlled trial of acetazolamide for the treatment of elevated intracranial pressure in cryptococcal meningitis. Clin Infect Dis. 2002;35:769–72.

Nguyen MH, Yu VL. Meningitis caused by Candida species: an emerging problem in neurosurgical patients. Clin Infect Dis. 1995;21(2):323–7.

Pagano L, Ricci P, Tonso A, et al. Mucormycosis in patients with haematological malignancies: a retrospective clinical study of 37 cases. Br J Haematol. 1997;99(2):331–6.

Pappas PG, Perfect JR, Cloud GA, et al. Cryptococcosis in human immunodeficiency virus-negative patients in the era of effective azole therapy. Clin Infect Dis. 2001;33(5):690–9.

Perfect JR, Dismukes WE, Dromer F, Goldman DL, Graybill JR, Hamill RJ, Harrison TS, Larsen RA, Lortholary O, Nguyen MH, Pappas PG, Powderly WG, Singh N, Sobel JD, Sorrell TC. Clinical practice guidelines for the management of cryptococcal disease: 2010 update by the infectious diseases society of America. Clin Infect Dis. 2010;50:291–322.

Raman Sharma R. Fungal infections of the nervous system: current perspective and controversies in management. Int J Surg. 2010;8(8):591–601.

Ribaud P, Chastang C, Latgé JP, et al. Survival and prognostic factors of invasive aspergillosis after allogeneic bone marrow transplantation. Clin Infect Dis. 1999;28(2):322–30.

Richardson MP, Ayliffe MJ, Helbert M, Davies EG. A simple flow cytometry assay using dihydrorhodamine for the measurement of the neutrophil respiratory burst in whole blood: comparison with the quantitative nitrobluetetrazolium test. J Immunol Methods. 1998;219(1):187–93.

Santosh V, Yasha TC, Khanna N. Fungal infections of the nervous system - a pathological study. Neurol Infect Epidemiol. 1996;1:69–79.

Schwartz S. Cerebral aspergillus infections and meningitis. Aspergillosis: from diagnosis to prevention. Dordrecht: Springer; 2010.

Sharma BS, Khosla VK, Kak VK, Banerjee AK, Vasishtha RK, Prasad KS, et al. Intracranial fungal granuloma. Surg Neurol. 1997a;47:48997.

Sharma BS, Prasad KSM, Banerjee AK, et al. Intracranial fungal granuloma. Surg Neurol. 1997b;47(5):489–97.

Singh N, Husain S. Infections of the central nervous system in transplant recipients. Transpl Infect Dis. 2001;2:101–11.

Singh N, Lortholary O, Alexander BD, Gupta KL, John GT, Pursell K, Munoz P, Klintmalm GB, Stosor V, del Busto R, Limaye AP, Somani J, Lyon M, Houston S, House AA, Pruett TL, Orloff S, Humar A, Dowdy L, Garcia-Diaz J, Kalil AC, Fisher RA, Husain S, Cryptococcal Collaborative Transplant Study Group. An immune reconstitution syndrome-like illness associated with Cryptococcus neoformans infection in organ transplant recipients. Clin Infect Dis. 2005;40:1756–61.

Speed B, Dunt D. Clinical and host differences between infections with the two varieties of Cryptococcus neoformans. Clin Infect Dis. 1995;21(1):28–36.

Thorn JL, Gilchrist KB, Sobonya RE, Gaur NK, Lipke PN, Klotz SAK. Postmortem candidemia: marker of disseminated disease. J Clin Pathol. 2010;63(4):337–40.

Venger BH, Landon G, Rose JE. Solitary Histoplasmoma of the thalamus: case report and literature review. Neurosurgery. 1987;20(5):784–7.

Wheat LJ, Batteiger BE, Sathapatayavongs B. Histoplasma capsulatum infections of the central nervous system, a clinical review. Medicine. 1990;69:244–60.

Wheat LJ, Musial CE, Jenny-Avital E. Diagnosis and management of central nervous system histoplasmosis. Clin Infect Dis. 2005;40(6):844–52.

White P, Barnes R. Not over yet: fungal infections following methyl prednisolone injections smoulder on. J Clin Microbiol. 2014;52(9):3506.

Part VI

Further Insights into Fungal Infections

Fungal Infections of the Spine Mimicking Tuberculosis

34

Turan C. Dülgeroğlu and Mehmet Turgut

Abbreviations

AIDS Acquired immunodeficiency syndrome
ATT Antitubercular therapy
CSF Cerebrospinal fluid
CT Computerized tomography
FNAB Fine-needle aspiration biopsy
HIV Human immunodeficiency virus
IVD Intervertebral disc
MRI Magnetic resonance imaging

34.1 Introduction

The infections involving soft tissues, ligaments and intervertebral disc (IVD), and bony structures of the spine are frequently caused by bacteria, called pyogenic (spondylo)discitis or osteomyelitis, but tuberculous and fungal infections involving the spine, known as non-pyogenic granulomas, are the less common etiologies (Aagaard et al. 2013; Caldera et al. 2016; Clamp and Grevitt 2009; Duarte and Vaccaro 2013; Kim et al. 2006). *Mycobacterium tuberculosis* is the main pathogen responsible for non-pyogenic infections of the spine, known as Pott's disease, in underdeveloped countries (Caldera et al. 2016; Kim et al. 2006), while fungal infections have also become more common in susceptible patients living in specific geographic regions of the world (Caldera et al. 2016; Clamp and Grevitt 2009; Kim et al. 2006; Sugrue and Koski 2011; Sundaram and Doshi 2016). It should be noted that both of them have a devastating potential in terms of destruction of the vertebra, fracture-dislocation with spinal instability, and spinal cord compression, and ultimately irreversible neurological compromise, although they are less common than bacterial pathogens in the etiology of spine infections (Sugrue and Koski 2011).

Recently, there has been a considerable rise in the incidence of fungal infections due to extensive use of immunosuppressive drugs and indwelling catheters, prolonged use of broad-spectrum antibacterial antibiotics, and the rising prevalence of acquired immunodeficiency syndrome (AIDS) in the world (Caldera et al. 2016; Duarte and Vaccaro 2013; Broner et al. 1996; Kulcheski et al. 2015; Schmiedel and Zimmerli 2016). The fungal infections involving the spine have insidious clinical picture and nonspecific symptoms, although early diagnosis and treatment of both tuberculous and fungal spine infections are vital (Oksi et al. 2013; Pahlavan and Bhatia 2016). Unfortunately, the diagnostic delay is common in fungal infections involving the

T. C. Dülgeroğlu (✉)
Department of Orthopaedics and Traumatology, Kütahya Health Sciences University School of Medicine, Kütahya, Turkey

M. Turgut
Department of Neurosurgery, Aydın Adnan Menderes University School of Medicine, Aydın, Turkey

M. Turgut et al. (eds.), *Fungal Infections of the Central Nervous System*,
https://doi.org/10.1007/978-3-030-06088-6_34

spine due to difficulty of cultivating the microorganisms in the culture (Clamp and Grevitt 2009; Sugrue and Koski 2011; Frazier et al. 2001; Hannallah et al. 2002). This necessitates a high index of suspicion that the clinical picture of fungal infections involving the spine may mimic tubercular spinal infections (Sharma 2010).

In this chapter, we will review the fungal infections involving the spine mimicking tuberculosis, in terms of epidemiology, clinical presentation, imaging findings, differential diagnosis, treatment modalities, and prognosis.

34.2 Epidemiology

Fungal infections of the spine are considered as uncommon clinical entity, comprising only 1% of all spinal infections, and they occur more frequently in the fifth decade of life and in the immunosuppressed patients with history of immune disorders, diabetes, surgical intervention, malignancy, solid organ transplantation, use of immunosuppressive drugs, parenteral nutrition, prolonged intravenous access, or travel to any endemic regions of the world (Caldera et al. 2016; Kim et al. 2006; Schmiedel and Zimmerli 2016; Pahlavan and Bhatia 2016; Gouliouris et al. 2010).

Today, spinal tuberculosis is seen in up to 5% of all cases with tuberculosis (Weinberg and Silber 2004) being more frequently in the first three decades of life, particularly in the underdeveloped countries, as a result of various predisposing factors such as immunocompromised status, poor nutrition, social deprivation, AIDS, renal failure, and increased immigration (Clamp and Grevitt 2009; Sugrue and Koski 2011; James and Davies 2006; Moorthy and Prabhu 2002). In particular, *M. tuberculosis* is the main pathogen responsible for tuberculous spine infections in human immunodeficiency virus (HIV)-positive patients (Duarte and Vaccaro 2013; Sugrue and Koski 2011). On the other hand, the risk of spinal infections from fungi such as *Aspergillus* species, *Candida* species, and *Mucor* species (Fig. 34.1) is higher in immunocompromised patients, but *Coccidioides* species, *Blastomyces dermatitidis*, and *Histoplasma capsulatum* have regional predilections, and thus they may affect immunocompetent patients with the proper exposure history (Sundaram and Doshi 2016).

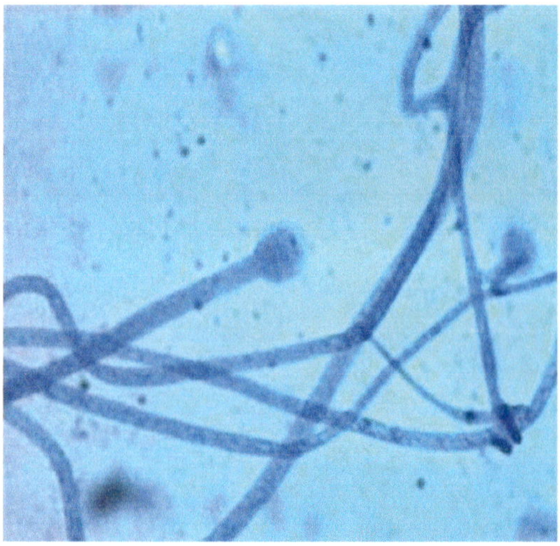

Fig. 34.1 Nonseptate hyphae with long branched sporangiophores bearing terminal round sporangia filled with spores. Rhizoids absent—*Mucor* species. Lactophenol cotton blue mount 40× (courtesy of L. Vemu, M.D.)

34.3 Clinical Findings

In both fungal and tuberculous infections of the spine, the most frequent initial symptom is limitation of the motion of the spinal column and localized pain in contrast to pyogenic infections of the spine, though nonspecific symptoms such as night sweating, weight loss, fever, and malaise may be seen in some patients (Sugrue and Koski 2011; Sundaram and Doshi 2016; Pahlavan and Bhatia 2016). As a general rule, a detailed history and physical examination are very important for diagnosis (Sugrue and Koski 2011). Furthermore, existence of predisposing factors such as existence of immunosuppression or travel history should raise the index of suspicion for various infections, fungal or tubercular, involving the spine (Sugrue and Koski 2011). Recently, Caldera et al. (2016) suggested that presence of weight loss and dermal sequelae of disease suggests a fungal infection in an older patient. On the other hand, tuberculous infections involving the spine have a predilection for the thoracic spine in a younger age (Sundaram and Doshi 2016). Nonetheless, fungal infections of the spine may mimic tuberculous infections involving the spine, thus complicating the differential diagnosis (Hali 2004).

34.4 Imaging Findings

In conventional radiographs and computerized tomography (CT) of the spine, vertebral body involvement with severe kyphotic angulation (gibbus deformity) is frequently seen in advanced cases of both tuberculous and fungal spine infections (Sundaram and Doshi 2016). Specifically, however, fungal infections have a predilection for paraspinal encroachment involving the adjacent ribs with a typical intervertebral disc sparing (Sundaram and Doshi 2016).

In the differential diagnosis of fungal and tuberculous infections of the spine from pyogenic infections caused by bacteria, the sparing of the intervertebral disc tissue on magnetic resonance imaging (MRI), affection of the posterior spinal elements, and the formation of paraspinal masses are important findings (Sundaram and Doshi 2016; Sharma 2010). From two different kinds of infections involving the spine, fungal ones produce destructive lesions affecting "middle/center" of the vertebral bodies of the entire spine, while tuberculous ones involve "anterior" of the vertebral body in the thoracic spine (Sundaram and Doshi 2016; Sharma 2010).

Radiologically, the thoracic part of the spinal column is the most frequently affected part in cases with Pott's disease (Duarte and Vaccaro 2013; Sundaram and Doshi 2016; Acharya and Gibbs 2016; Rankine 2004). In cases with tuberculous infections involving the spine, there is a heterogeneous enhancement of the corpus of the vertebra and a "large" paraspinal abscess demonstrating rim enhancement (thin and/or smooth) on MRI (Duarte and Vaccaro 2013; Sundaram and Doshi 2016; Acharya and Gibbs 2016; Rankine 2004). Also, involvement of intervertebral space ranges from IVD sparing with lack of T2 hyperintensity up to severe destruction, while an extensive loss of vertebral body height with severe kyphotic angulation, called "gibbus deformity," may be observed in very advanced cases of tuberculosis (Duarte and Vaccaro 2013; Sundaram and Doshi 2016; Acharya and Gibbs 2016; Rankine 2004). Moreover, "skip lesions" with multiple level involvement is also a feature of tuberculous infections of the spine (Duarte and Vaccaro 2013; Sundaram and Doshi 2016; Acharya and Gibbs 2016; Rankine 2004). Nevertheless, tendency for sparing of the IVD and existence of "skip lesions" with multiple level involvement are also common imaging features of fungal infections involving the spine (Duarte and Vaccaro 2013; Sundaram and Doshi 2016; Acharya and Gibbs 2016; Rankine 2004). It has been reported that fungal infections involving the spine tend to show more subtle changes on MRI compared to those in cases with tuberculous spondylodiscitis (Duarte and Vaccaro 2013; Sundaram and Doshi 2016; Acharya and Gibbs 2016; Rankine 2004). In contrast, fungal infections of the spine also include a "small" paraspinal abscess demonstrating thick and irregular rim enhancement, and they have a tendency to involve posterior elements and adjacent ribs (Duarte and Vaccaro 2013; Sundaram and Doshi 2016; Acharya and Gibbs 2016; Rankine 2004) (Table 34.1).

Interestingly, it should be noted that certain imaging findings in patients with fungal infections of the spine suggest certain fungal causative agents as follows: (1) swelling of the paravertebral soft tissue and affection of the posterior elements of the spine with *Coccidioides* infections (Fig. 34.2); (2) the vertebral body lytic lesions with *Cryptococcus* and *Coccidioides* infections (Fig. 34.3); (3) vertebral body collapse and gibbus formation with *Blastomyces* infections (Fig. 34.4); and (4) the presence of high T2 signal vertebral body microabscesses or vertebral, paravertebral macro-abscess with *Candida* infections (Fig. 34.5) (Sugrue and Koski 2011; Sundaram and Doshi 2016; Hali 2004; Chen et al. 2013; Chemm et al. 2001; Hadjipavlou et al. 1998; Kathuria and Gupta 2001; Lai et al. 2017; Lindner et al. 1995).

Table 34.1 Differential diagnosis of fungal vs. tuberculous infections involving the spine according to imaging findings[a]

	Imaging features	
	Tuberculous spinal infection	Fungal spinal infection
Spine region	Thoracic	Lumbar
Vertebral body	Early stage: anterior part of vertebral body Late stage: T1 variable intensity with bone healing	Serrated margins of CEPs without severe destruction of vertebral body
Involvement of IVD	Variable: from IVD sparing up to severe destruction	Typically spared; lack of T2 hyperintensity
Involvement of paraspinal/epidural space	"Large" paraspinal abscesses and thin/smooth rim enhancement	"Small" paraspinal abscesses and thick and irregular rim enhancement
Posterior elements	May be involved	May be involved
Spread to anterior subligamentous structures	May be more extensive than vertebral involvement	Common
Involvement of adjacent vertebral levels	High bone destruction	Uncommon
Multi-level involvement (skip lesions)	Common	Common

IVD intervertebral disc, *CEP* cartilage end plates

[a]Adapted from: Eur Spine J. 2013;22(12):2787–99. https://doi:10.1007/s00586-013-2850-1 (Duarte and Vaccaro 2013)

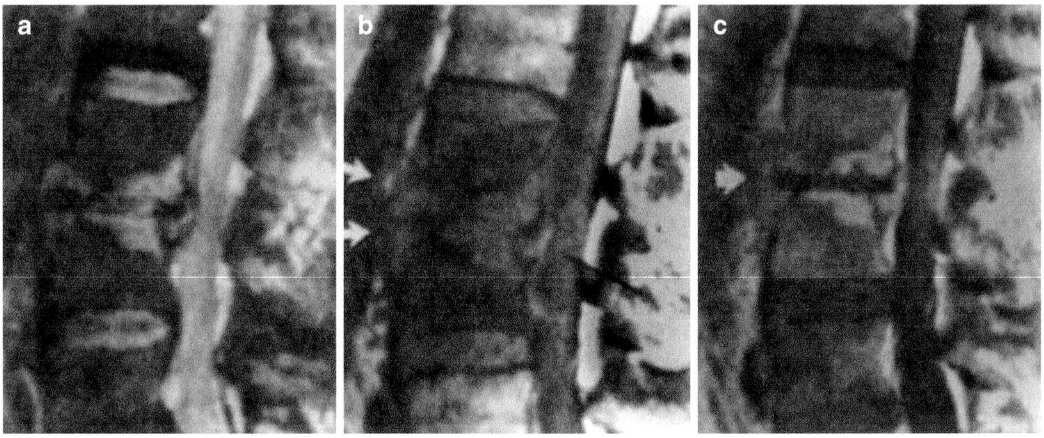

Fig. 34.2 Spondylitis caused by coccidioidomycosis. (**a**) Sagittal T1-weighted magnetic resonance imaging (MRI) shows hyperintensity within intervertebral disc (IVD) and adjacent cartilage end plates (CEPs) with bone marrow edema in the vertebral bodies of L3 and L4, with involvement of anterior and posterior ligamentous structures. (**b**) Sagittal T2-weighted MRI demonstrates hyperintensity within the IVD and adjacent CEPs with narrowing of the spaces and prevertebral region (white arrows). (**c**) Postcontrast T1-weighted sagittal MRI demonstrates mild enhancement of the diseased vertebrae and prevertebral region near to IVD (white arrow) (from Kathuria and Gupta (2001), with permission)

34.5 Differential Diagnosis

In cases with fungal spine lesions mimicking lesions of mycobacterial infections, differential diagnosis between the fungal and tuberculous lesions is not easy based on clinical presentation and/or imaging findings. Therefore, several diagnostic markers and methods, including scintigraphy, fungal antibody tests, carbohydrate assimilation test for *Candida*, phenol oxidase reaction for *Cryptococcus*, tuberculin skin testing, and nonspecific serum markers such as white blood cell count, erythrocyte sedimentation rate, and C-reactive protein level, have been introduced for differential diagnosis between fungal infections and tuberculous lesions (Sugrue and Koski 2011).

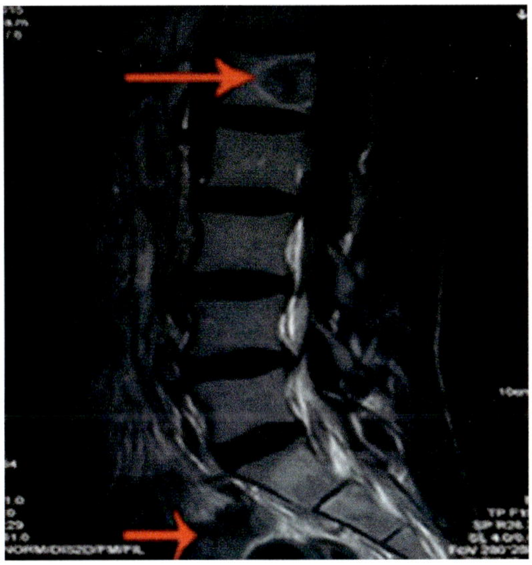

Fig. 34.3 Preoperative sagittal MRI demonstrates presence of bone destruction and vertebral abnormalities in L1 (upper red arrow), S1, and S2 (lower red arrow) levels (From Lai et al. (2017), with permission)

There is no doubt that microscopic identification of the organism by histopathologic examination of the surgical specimen is essential for correct diagnosis and definite treatment of fungal infections involving the spine (Sugrue and Koski 2011; Gupta et al. 2003; Prapruttam et al. 2014). Accordingly, a high index of suspicion is of utmost importance in differential diagnosis of fungal infections from tuberculous ones and timely starting of appropriate medical therapy for fungi to reduce the rates of mortality and morbidity (Sugrue and Koski 2011; Gupta et al. 2003; Prapruttam et al. 2014). Unfortunately, in cases with fungal infections of spine misdiagnosed as tuberculous spine infection, the delay in diagnosis of fungal etiology results with a high mortality rate (Gupta et al. 2003, 2012; Houda et al. 2011; Jain et al. 1999).

In a previous report, Jain et al. (1999) reported a case of cryptococcosis involving T6 vertebra mimicking tuberculosis in an old diabetic patient with diagnosis of *Cryptococcus neoformans* based on a CT-guided fine-needle aspiration biopsy (FNAB). Gupta et al. (2003) reported a young patient presented with cervical

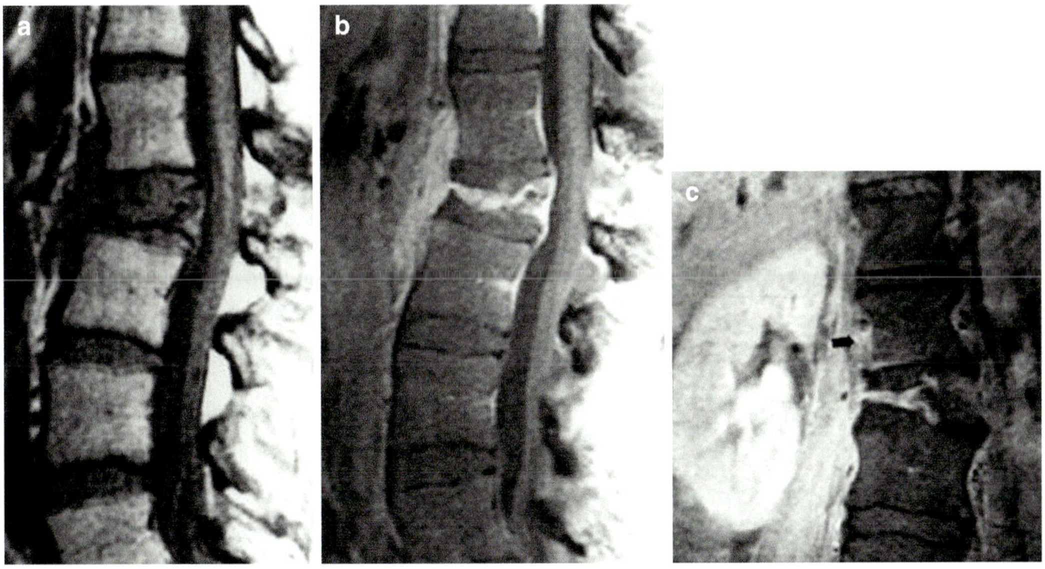

Fig. 34.4 (**a**) Sagittal T1-weighted MRI shows replacement of the normal fatty signal of L2 vertebra. (**b** and **c**) Following gadolinium administration with fat saturation sagittal and coronal MRIs sections demonstrate abnormal enhancement of the L2 vertebra spreading to right and left psoas muscles. The IVDs are spared with involvement of the L1 vertebra (black arrow) (from Hadjipavlou et al. (1998), with permission)

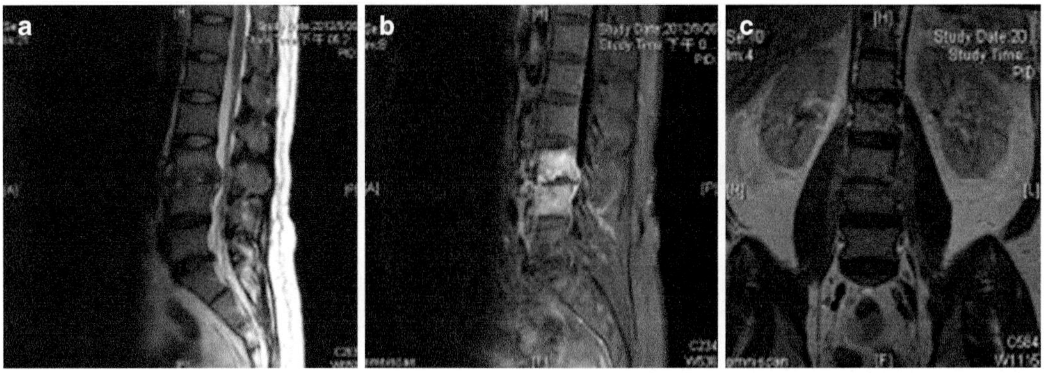

Fig. 34.5 MRI of the lumbar spine reveals presence of erosion of the CEP and diffuse bone marrow infiltration at L3 and L4 levels, which is characterized by enhancement in affected vertebrae and paravertebral regions following gadolinium administration (from Chen et al. (2013), with permission)

lymphadenopathy, with a definitive diagnosis of tuberculosis by FNAB, and received antitubercular therapy (ATT) for 5 months; a rapidly progressive paraparesis developed because of presence of spinal cord compression by a destructive osseous lesion involving T2–3 associated with a paraspinal abscess, and then antifungal therapy was started with definitive diagnosis of cryptococcosis on histopathological examination, but the patient passed away 2 weeks after surgery (Gupta et al. 2003). Afterward, Houda et al. (2011) reported a case of vertebral cryptococcosis mimicking tuberculosis of the spine with findings of destructive lesions of the vertebral bodies associated with a paraspinal abscess and then treatment with antifungal agents following isolation of *C. neoformans* in cerebrospinal fluid (CSF) culture provided a good prognosis (Houda et al. 2011). Based on their experience in a 30-year-old patient with immunocompetent disseminated cryptococcosis, who was diagnosed with tubercular spondylodiscitis and treated with 4 months of ATT, Gupta et al. (2012) suggested that antigen detection in the blood and CSF as an adjunct to direct microscopy and fungal culture can be used for isolation of causative pathogens (Gupta et al. 2012). In another interesting case report, Wang et al. (2014) reported a case of cryptococcosis involving the thoracic spinal column with a lytic irregular lesion at T2–T3 as surrounded by reactive bony sclerosis and mimicking Pott's disease (Wang et al. 2014).

34.6 Treatment

Medical management with antifungal drugs including polyenes (e.g., amphotericin B, amphotericin B with lipid formulation), triazole drugs (e.g., fluconazole, itraconazole, posaconazole, and voriconazole), and echinocandins (caspofungin, anidulafungin, micafungin) is the first approach for the treatment of fungal infections involving the spine (Caldera et al. 2016; Duarte and Vaccaro 2013; Pahlavan and Bhatia 2016; Sharma 2010). Although use of protocol consisting of amphotericin B for 2–3 weeks and then fluconazole for 6–12 months has become the mainstay first-line treatment, several other options, albeit controversies remain regarding to their selection and clinical use, have become available with introduction of novel drugs such as the lipid-based formulations of the amphotericin B, echinocandins, and triazoles in recent years (Caldera et al. 2016; Sharma 2010).

Persistence of infection despite medical treatment, presence of neurologic involvement, collapsed vertebrae or instability, and rapidly progressive disease are indications for wide surgical debridement of the infected tissues followed by reconstruction of the diseased segments and mechanical stabilization by posterior approach (Caldera et al. 2016; Duarte and Vaccaro 2013; Pahlavan and Bhatia 2016). Currently open surgery is considered to be the gold standard, while minimally invasive techniques have increasingly been used even in more severe cases (Caldera et al. 2016; Pahlavan and Bhatia 2016). The necessity and safety of using instrumentation in the surgical treatment of fungal infections involving the spine still remains inconclusive (Caldera et al. 2016).

34.7 Outcome

The long-term prognosis after medical therapy in fungal spine infections in terms of functional recovery and pain relief remains uncertain (Caldera et al. 2016). However, the frequently observed delay in the treatment due to challenges in diagnosis has been considered as the main risk factor for poor neurological outcome (Caldera et al. 2016; Duarte and Vaccaro 2013; Pahlavan and Bhatia 2016). In addition to the delayed diagnosis, presence of comorbidities predisposing immunocompromised status, older age, cervical/thoracic location, and presentation with paralysis or bowel/bladder dysfunction are also considered among the poor prognostic factors associated with increased risk of a permanent neurological deficit (Clamp and Grevitt 2009; Pahlavan and Bhatia 2016).

Provision of medical management by a multidisciplinary approach with careful consideration of appropriate duration of therapy, resistance to drugs, and medical compliance alongside timely implementation of surgery in the presence of clear indications are considered critical for favorable prognosis (Caldera et al. 2016; Martinez-Del-Campo et al. 2017).

34.8 Conclusion

Nowadays, incidence of spinal infections, fungal and tubercular, involving the spine is increasing worldwide due to considerable rise in the number of immunosuppressed patients. It is well-known that fungal lesions closely may mimic mycobacterial infections and microscopic identification of the organism is very important for definite diagnosis of fungal infection. Therefore, a high index of suspicion is of utmost importance in differentiating fungal infections from tuberculous ones to reduce the rates of mortality and morbidity. To make a correct diagnosis, it is necessary to do a detailed investigation by microscopy, culture of the specimen, and antigen detection for fungal agents.

References

Aagaard T, Roed C, Dragsted C, Skinhøj P. Microbiological and therapeutic challenges in infectious spondylodiscitis: a cohort study of 100cases, 2006-2011. Scand J Infect Dis. 2013;45:417–24.

Acharya J, Gibbs WN. Imaging spinal infection. Radiol Infect Dis. 2016;3:84–91.

Broner FA, Garland DE, Zigler JE. Spinal infections in the immunocompromised host. Orthop Clin North Am. 1996;2:37–46.

Caldera G, Cahueque M, Cobar A, Gómez G, Rodríguez O. Fungal spondylodiscitis: review. J Spine. 2016; 5:2–6.

Chemm RK, Wang S, Jaovisidha S, Schmit P, Frieedman L, Bureau NJ, Cardinal E. Imaging of fungal, viral, and parasitic musculoskeletal and spinal diseases. Radiol Clin N Am. 2001;39:357–78.

Chen CH, Chen WL, Yen HC. Candida albicans lumbar spondylodiscitis in an intravenous drug user: a case report. BMC Res Notes. 2013;6:529.

Clamp JA, Grevitt MP. Spinal infections. Surgery. 2009;27:306–10.

Duarte RM, Vaccaro AR. Spinal infection: state of the art and management algorithm. Eur Spine J. 2013; 22:2787–99.

Frazier DD, Campbell DR, Garvey TA, Wiesel S, Bohlman HH, Eismont FJ. Fungal infections of the spine. Report of eleven patients with long-term follow-up. J Bone Joint Surg Am. 2001;83:560–5.

Gouliouris T, Aliyu SH, Brown NM. Spondylodiscitis: update on diagnosis and management. J Antimicrob Chemother. 2010;65(suppl 3):11–24.

Gupta SK, Chhabra R, Sharma BS, Das A, Khosla VK. Vertebral cryptococcosis simulating tuberculosis. Br J Neurosurg. 2003;17:556–9.

Gupta R, Kushwaha S, Behera S, Jaiswal A, Thakur R. Vertebro-cerebral cryptococcosis mimicking tuberculosis: a diagnostic dilemma in countries with high burden of tuberculosis. Indian J Med Microbiol. 2012;30:245–8.

Hadjipavlou AG, Mader JT, Nauta HJ, Necessary JT, Chaljub G, Adesokan A. Blastomycosis of the lumbar spine: case report and review of the literature, with emphasis on diagnostic laboratory tools and management. Eur Spine J. 1998;7:416–21.

Hali T. Spinal infections. Eur J Radiol. 2004;50:120–33.

Hannallah D, Altman D, Kang J. Infections in the spine. Oper Tech Orthop. 2002;12:310–4.

Houda B, Wafa A, Zoubida TM, Mohamed A, Mohamed A, Hicham H. Vertebral cryptococcosis in an immunocompetent patient—a case report. Pan Afr Med J. 2011;8:42.

Jain M, Sharma S, Jain TS. Cryptococcosis of thoracic vertebra simulating tuberculosis: diagnosis by fine-needle aspiration biopsy cytology-a case report. Diagn Cytopathol. 1999;20:385–6.

James SL, Davies AM. Imaging of infectious spinal disorders in children and adults. Eur J Radiol. 2006;58:27–40.

Kathuria MK, Gupta RK. Fungal infections. In: Gupta RK, Lufkin RB, editors. MR imaging and spectroscopy of central nervous system infections. New York: Kluwer Press; 2001. p. 177–203.

Kim CW, Perry A, Currier B, Yaszemski M, Garfin SR. Fungal infections of the spine. Clin Orthop Relat Res. 2006;444:92–9.

Kulcheski ÁL, Graells XS, Benato ML, Santoro PG, Sebben AL. Fungal spondylodiscitis due to Candida albicans: an atypical case and review of the literature. Rev Bras Ortop. 2015;50:739–42.

Lai Q, Liu Y, Yu X, Lv X, Wang Q, Zhou Y, Guo R, Zhang B. Diagnosis and treatment of nonadjacent cryptococcal infections at the L1 and S1 vertebrae. Orthopade. 2017;46:85–9.

Lindner A, Becker G, Warmuth-Metz M, Schalke BC, Bogdahn U, Toyka KV. MRI findings of spinal intramedullary abscess caused by Candida albicans: a case report. Neurosurgery. 1995;36:411–3.

Martinez-Del-Campo E, Kalb S, Rangel-Castilla L, Moon K, Moran A, Gonzalez O, Soriano-Baron H, Theodore N. Spinal coccidioidomycosis: a current review of diagnosis and management. World Neurosurg. 2017;108:69–75.

Moorthy S, Prabhu NK. Spectrum of MR imaging findings in spinal tuberculosis. AJR Am J Roentgenol. 2002;179:979–83.

Oksi J, Finnilä T, Hohenthal U, Rantakokko-Jalava K. Candida dubliniensis spondylodiscitis in an immunocompetent patient. Case report and review of the literature. Med Mycol Case Rep. 2013;3:4–7.

Pahlavan S, Bhatia NN. Fungal spine. Semin Spine Surg. 2016;28:163–72.

Prapruttam D, Hedgire SS, Mani SE, Chandramohan A, Shyamkumar NK, Harisinghani M. Tuberculosis-the great mimicker. Semin Ultrasound CT MR. 2014;35:195–214.

Rankine JJ. MRI of spinal infection. Curr Orthop. 2004;18:426–33.

Schmiedel Y, Zimmerli S. Common invasive fungal diseases: an overview of invasive candidiasis, aspergillosis, cryptococcosis, and pneumocystis pneumonia. Swiss Med Wkly. 2016;146:w14281.

Sharma R. Fungal infections of the nervous system: current perspective and controversies in management. Int J Surg. 2010;8:591–601.

Sugrue PA, Koski TR. Fungal and tubercular infections of the spine. In: Winn RH, editor. Youmans neurological surgery. 6th ed. Philadelphia, PA: Saunders; 2011. p. 2848–58.

Sundaram VK, Doshi A. Infections of the spine: a review of clinical and imaging findings. Appl Radiol. 2016;45:10–20.

Wang C, Jia N, Zhang L, Liu K, Liu H, Yu H. Imaging findings of cryptococcal infection of the thoracic spine. Int J Infect Dis. 2014;29:162–5.

Weinberg J, Silber JS. Infections of the spine: what the orthopedist needs to know. Am J Orthop. 2004;33:13–7.

Fungal Infections in Cancer Patients

35

Yaşar Barış Turgut, Gökhan Sargın, and Özgür Tanrıverdi

Abbreviations

CNS Central nervous system
MRI Magnetic resonance imaging

35.1 Introduction

Cytotoxic agents such as chemotherapy and radiation destroy cancer cells, but they also suppress the hematopoietic system, limiting the doses of chemotherapeutic drugs that can be tolerated as well as impairing host protective mechanisms, which can increase incidence of development of various fungal infections (Crawford et al. 2004). Theoretically, fungal infection of central nervous system (CNS) may occur due to spread from blood stream, seeding by cerebrospinal fluid, or direct extension from infection involving the neighboring anatomical structures (Fig. 35.1) (Starkey et al. 2014). The most serious hematologic toxicity with a reduction in white blood cell count, known as "neutropenia," has a risk of life-threatening infections, reduction of doses of chemotherapeutic agents, and delay of treatment; thus, it results in an unfavorable outcome (Crawford et al. 2004). Neutropenic complications related with myelosuppressive chemotherapy are well-known cause of morbidity and mortality in spite of recent advances in antimicrobial drug development (Crawford et al. 2004). Even today, topic of fungal infections involving the CNS remains a challenge in spite of advances in approach for the diagnosis and management of the cancer patients (Krishnan 2016; Mcneil 2001).

In this chapter, we will briefly review the recent literature to give an update on research in chemotherapeutical agent-induced neutropenic complications, including febrile neutropenia, and fungal infections as a serious complication of cancer patients who are treated with myelosuppressive chemotherapy.

Y. B. Turgut
Department of Internal Medicine, Muğla Sıtkı Koçman University School of Medicine, Muğla, Turkey

G. Sargın
Department of Internal Medicine, Aydın Adnan Menderes University School of Medicine, Aydın, Turkey

Ö. Tanrıverdi (✉)
Division of Medical Oncology, Muğla Sıtkı Koçman University School of Medicine, Muğla, Turkey

35.2 Epidemiology and Incidence

In the past, *Candida* and *Aspergillus* spp. were responsible for the majority of yeast and mold infections in immunocompromised patients with cancer. Nevertheless, there has been an increased incidence of non-*Candida* yeast, non-fumigatus *Aspergillus* spp., *Fusarium spp., Scedosporium*

M. Turgut et al. (eds.), *Fungal Infections of the Central Nervous System*,
https://doi.org/10.1007/978-3-030-06088-6_35

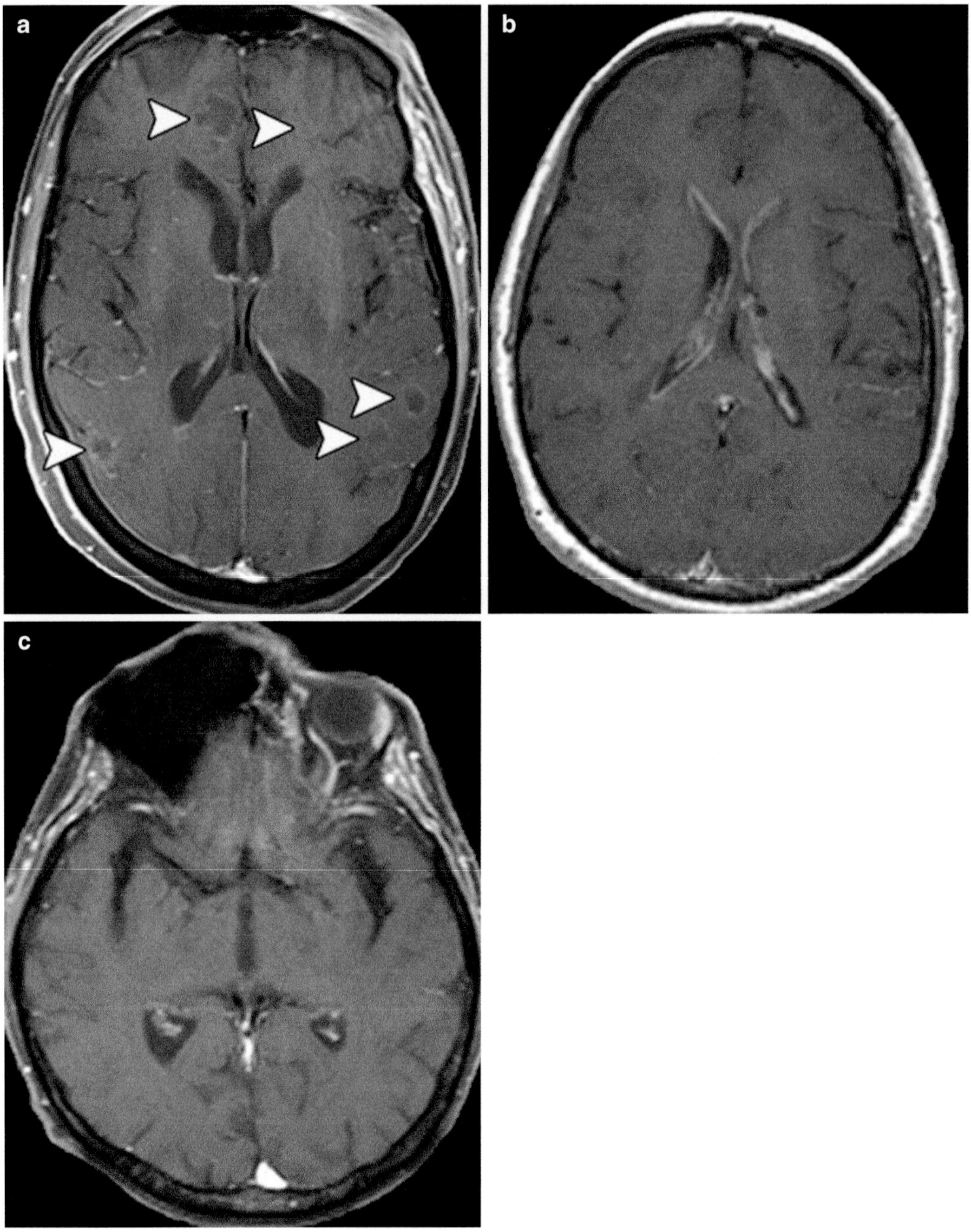

Fig. 35.1 (**a**) Axial T1-weighted magnetic resonance imaging (MRI) after administration of gadolinium showing typical lesions of aspergillosis localized in the junction of gray–white junction (*arrowheads*). (**b**) Axial T1-weighted MRI after administration of gadolinium showing enhancement of ventricular wall, frontal, and occipital leptomeninges in a case with cryptococcal meningitis. (**c**) Axial T1-weighted MRI after administration of gadolinium showing mucormycosis with intracranial extension involving the inferior frontal lobe (from Starkey et al. (2014), with permission)

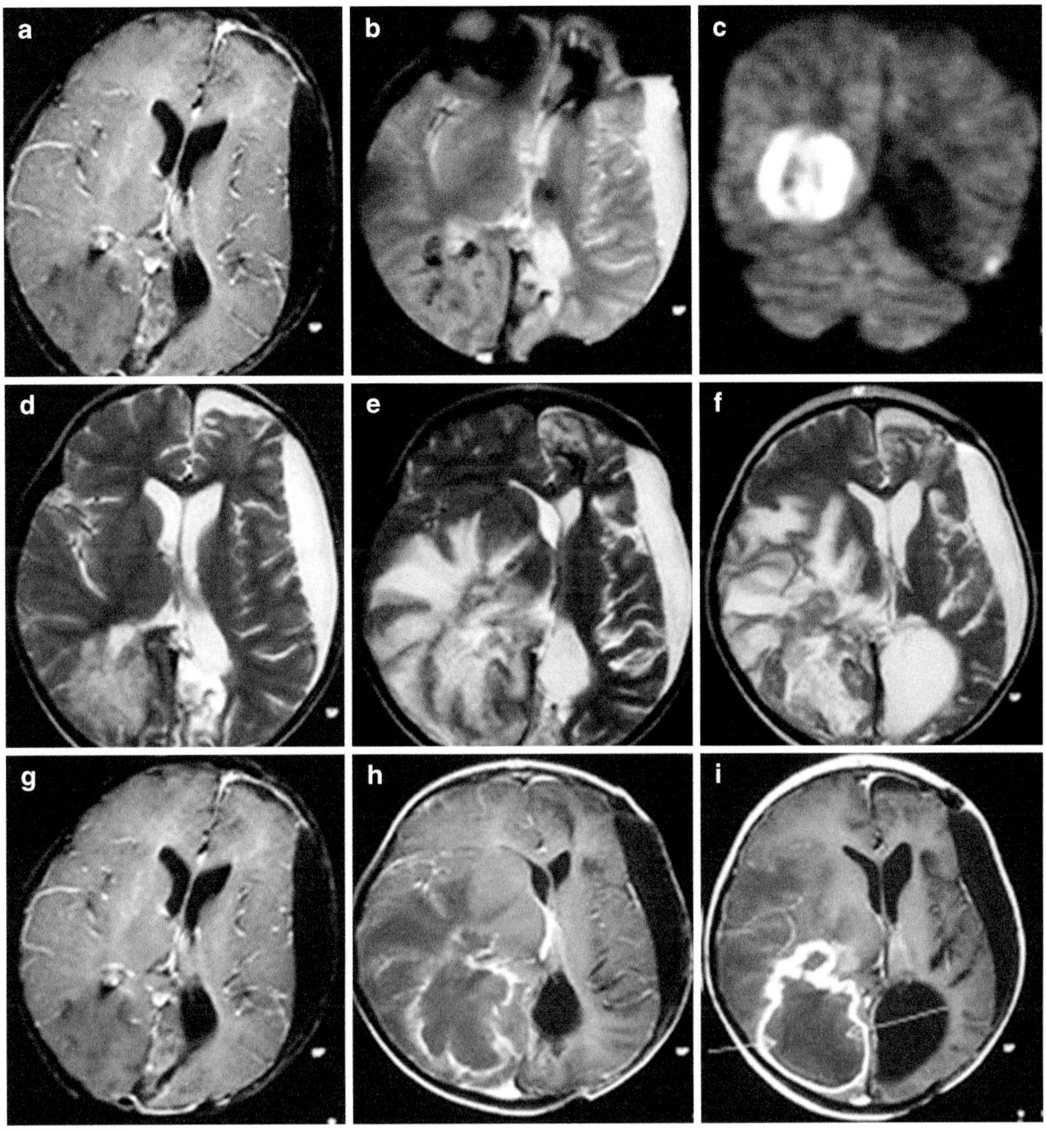

Fig. 35.2 (a–c) Axial T1-weighted MRI following contrast demonstrating a heterogeneous lesion in the right parieto-occipital region of the brain in a 7-year-old girl patient with acute lymphoblastic leukemia complicated with cerebral aspergillosis (**a**). The fungal lesion is hypointense on T2-weighted MRI (**b**). Diffusion-weighted MRIs demonstrating a hyperintensity lesion with restricted diffusion in the cavity of the lesion (**c**). T2-weighted MRI demonstrating a heterogeneous lesion in the right parieto-occipital region with surrounding edema (**d**, **f**). Follow-up post-contrast MRIs demonstrating a lesion as an isointense mass (**g**) and an abscess formation having peripheral contrast enhancement (*arrows*) (**h** and **i**) (from Haßler et al. (2015), with permission)

spp., and Zygomycetes from different hospitals over the world during the last decade (Fig. 35.2) (Chitasombat et al. 2012; Douglas et al. 2016; Haßler et al. 2015; Malani and Kauffman 2007; Pfaller et al. 2006; Peghin et al. 2016). On the other hand, incidence of fungal infections of the CNS in immunocompromised patients with cancer has a different distribution in some parts of the world owing to various geographical and meteorological factors affecting the spread of fungal spores, in addition to the lack of appropriate health conditions in the hospitals (Chamilos et al.

2006). Today, an increasing incidence of invasive fungal infections of the CNS in immunocompromised cancer patients has also been observed, possibly due to an increased use of antifungal prophylaxis and new chemotherapeutic agents, an increased use of new chemotherapeutic and immunosuppressive agents, an increase in the numbers of rare fungal pathogens, and prolonged survival of immunocompromised cancer patients (Krishnan 2016).

35.3 Cancer Types

In general, it is well-known that the frequency of fungal infections among cancer patients is high. In particular, stem cell and solid organ transplanted patients or those who have a hematologic malignancy such as lymphoma, myeloma, or leukemia are at high risk for development of fungal infections than individuals with other types of cancer (Fig. 35.2) (Haßler et al. 2015; Bodey et al. 1992; Pagano et al. 2011). In a previous study, fungal infections were diagnosed in approximately 25% of leukemic patients and transplant recipients for each, respectively (Bodey et al. 1992).

35.4 Chemotherapy Protocols

Risk of infection may be different according to the strength of chemotherapy protocol of the patient. Some types of cancer may need stronger chemotherapy protocol, known as "aggressive chemotherapy," than others, especially the blood cancers. In particular, such chemotherapy protocol weakens the immune system seriously and may increase the risk for development of a fungal infection (Ribaud 1997).

35.5 Severity of Neutropenia

Recent studies revealed that "neutropenia" has a serious problem associated with a high rate of morbidity, mortality, and cost (Crawford et al. 2004). As a rule, a reduced low white blood cell count called "neutropenia" as a toxicity of chemotherapy, which is limiting the dose, may result in a high risk of infection (Infectious Diseases Working Party (AGIHO) of the German Society of Hematology and Oncology (DGHO) et al. 2009). Recently, Stanzani et al. (2016) suggested various patterns of invasive fungal disease with different radiographic findings in patients with neutropenia (Fig. 35.3). Even today, end results of "neutropenia" and its effects still remain unknown (Crawford et al. 2004). Considering the presenting signs and symptoms, neutropenic patients are usually categorized as those at "high risk" or "low risk" for infection, underlying cancer, form of therapy, and associated comorbidities (Freifeld et al. 2011).

35.6 Types of Fungal Infections

Invasive fungal infections are common causes of high rates of mortality and morbidity in immunocompromised patients with cancer, especially in patients with leukemia, receiving various chemotherapeutical agents (Bodey et al. 1992; Pagano et al. 2011; Infectious Diseases Working Party (AGIHO) of the German Society of Hematology and Oncology (DGHO) et al. 2009; CDC et al. 2001; Center for International Blood and Marrow Transplant Research (CIBMTR) et al. 2009). From a clinical perspective, there are different forms of fungal infections, ranging from mild to severe forms, and they mimic many bacterial or viral infections. Despite appropriate therapy, rare but important fungal pathogens causing invasive fungal infections of the CNS in immunocompromised cancer patients are as follows: yeast-like fungi (*Trichosporon* spp., *Rhodotorula* spp., *Malassezia furfur*, *Geotrichum capitatum*), mold filamentous fungi (*Aspergillus* spp., *Scedosporium* spp., *Fusarium* spp., *Zygomycetes*), and phaeohyphomycetes (cryptococcus) (Figs. 35.2, 35.4, 35.5 and 35.6) (Haßler et al. 2015; Kappagoda et al. 2017). Among these fungal pathogens, in particular, some fungi including *Aspergillus* spp., *Candida* spp., and molds (e.g., *Zygomycetes* and *Fusarium* spp.) are the most important fungal pathogens infecting susceptible individuals who

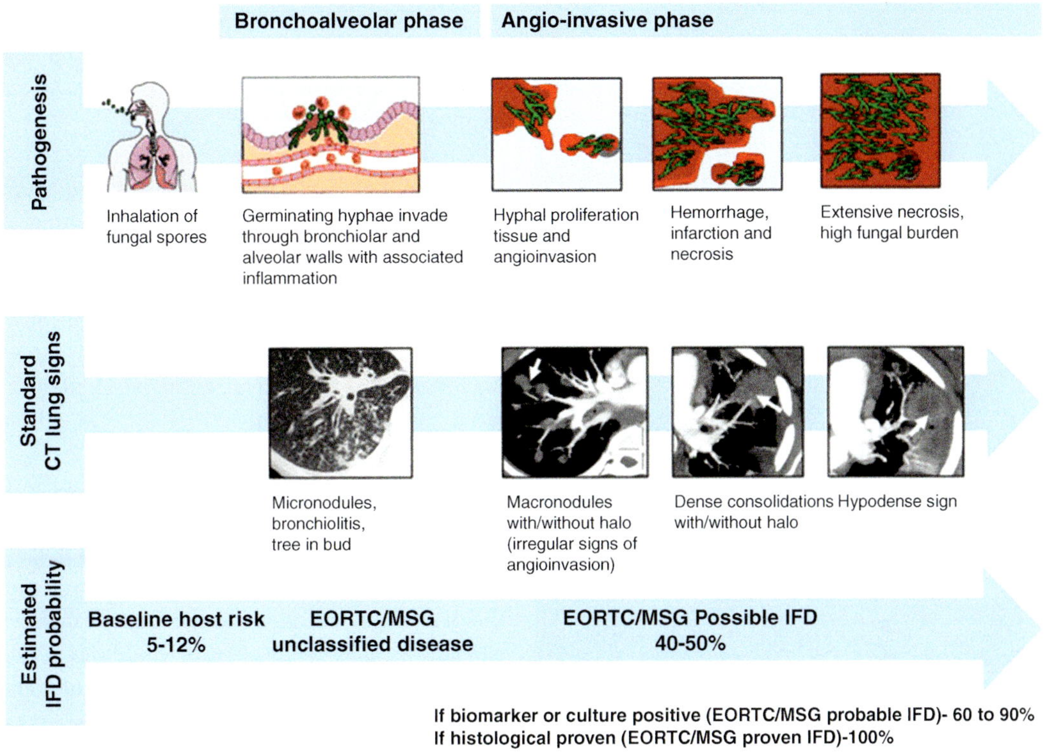

Fig. 35.3 Various forms of invasive fungal disease and their typical radiographic features in severe neutropenic patients (from Stanzani et al. (2016), with permission)

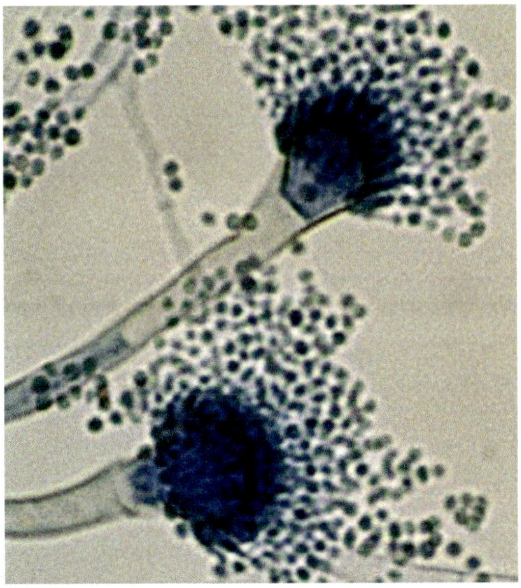

Fig. 35.4 Reproductive structures: conidiophore, conidiogenous cells and conidia: *Aspergillus* species. Lactophenol cotton blue mount 40× (courtesy of L. Vemu, M.D.)

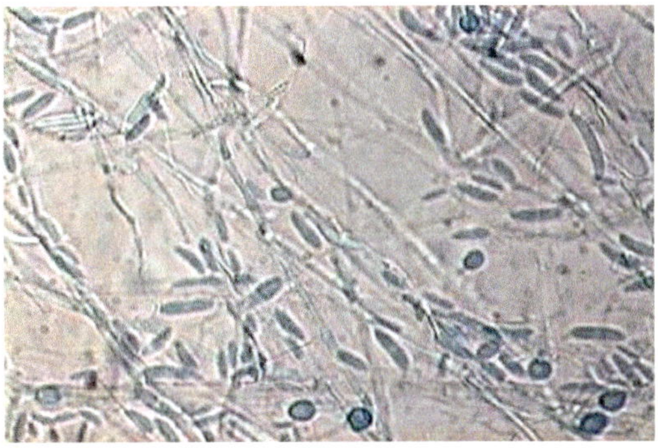

Fig. 35.5 Multi-celled, sickle-form macroconidia of *Fusarium* species. Lactophenol cotton blue mount 40× (courtesy of L. Vemu, M.D.)

are associated with a high incidence of morbidity and mortality (Pagano et al. 2011). It has been reported that 58% of fungal infections as a complication was caused by *Candida* spp. (Fig. 35.7) and 30% by *Aspergillus* spp. (Fig. 35.4) (Bodey et al. 1992). Interestingly, some molds are quite

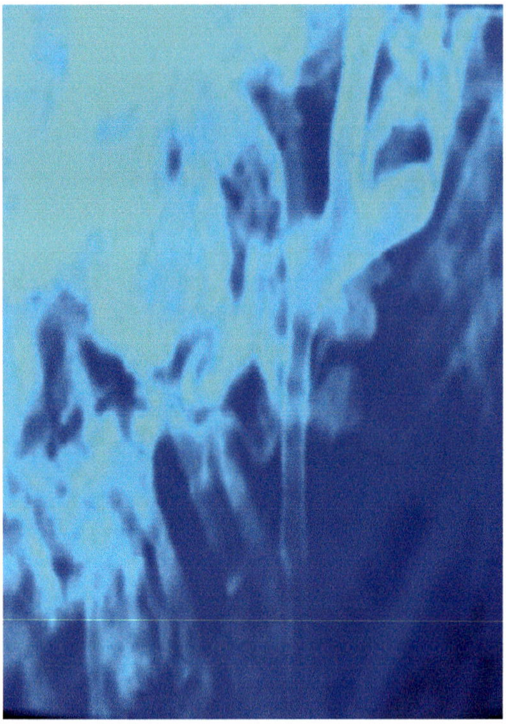

Fig. 35.6 Broad aseptate hyphae with wide-angled branching of *Zygomycetes* (courtesy of L. Vemu, M.D.)

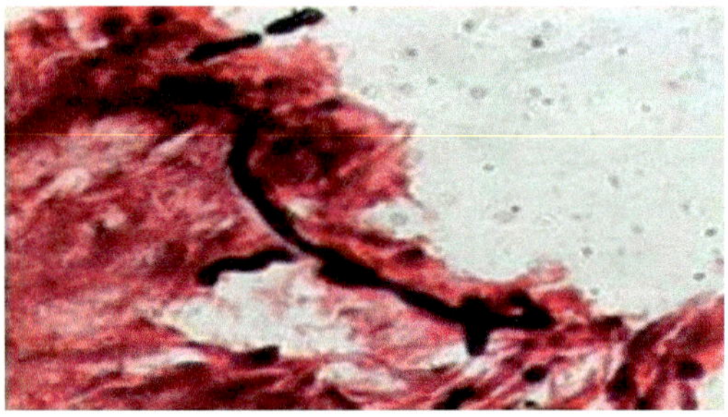

Fig. 35.7 Budding yeasts with pseudo hyphae of *Candida* species. Gram's stain 100× (courtesy of L. Vemu, M.D.)

frequent among all forms of patients with cancer, although others are limited to certain patients, like allogeneic hematopoietic stem cell or solid organ-transplanted recipients (Pagano et al. 2011).

In immunocompromised subjects, it has been reported that a group of pathogens called *Emmonsia*-like fungi can cause disseminated disease (Schwartz et al. 2015). In 1970, among these, *E. helica* was first reported in Canada, in a fatal case of encephalitis and pneumonia (Sekhon et al. 1982), and then another fatal patient of *Emmonsia* infection was reported from the USA in a new case following a liver transplant (Kappagoda et al. 2017).

Clinically, certain fungal infections are mild skin rashes, while others are life-threating, such as fungal pneumonia. Therefore, it is important to recognize the symptoms early to prevent development of a serious illness. Also, it is vital to treat the patient without delay to avoid fungal infections, because almost all patients with cancer may benefit with prophylactic antiviral, antibacterial, and antifungal drugs (Freifeld et al. 2011).

35.7 Predisposing Risk Factors

This clearly shows that predisposing risk factors for fungal infections, especially for invasive candidiasis, may be associated with the host and the hospital. Chronic disorders such as solid and hematological malignancies, neutropenia, prior immunosuppressive drugs, renal failure, or diabetes mellitus are host-related factors, while surgery, mechanical ventilation, parental nutrition, duration of hospital stay, and catheter placement are among the hospital-related factors (Wang et al. 2014). Bloodstream fungal infections are uncommon in pediatric patients with cancer but significantly associated with neutropenia as a risk factor (Calton et al. 2014). There are some differences in risk factors for infections caused by *Candida albicans* and *Candida non-albicans* species. When both groups are compared with each other, solid malignancies, older age, and hypoproteinemia are prominent risk factors for *Candida albicans*, while length of hospital stay, chemotherapy, neutropenia, hematologic malignancies, and the usage of glycopeptides and corticosteroids for nonalbicans species (Pu et al. 2017).

35.7.1 Duration of Hospital Stay

Hospitalization for a long time after transplantation and increase number of procedures can increase the chance of development of a fungal infection.

35.7.2 Geographical Area and Travelers

As a corresponding agent of disease, some fungi are more frequent in some regions of the world (Lortholary et al. 2013). As a result of this fact, there was an important variability in the frequency of fungal infections in different countries of the world (Bodey et al. 1992). Interestingly, some environmental conditions are closely related to the impairment of the immune system (Pagano et al. 2011).

In addition to patients with neutropenia, the risk of fungal infections is high when immunocompromised patients with human immunodeficiency virus infection and transplant recipients travel to another geographical region for business or tourism. Therefore, specialists of internal medicine should be aware of all clinical pictures of various fungal infections and risk factors related with the geographical region visited in the world (Lortholary et al. 2013). Recently, it has been suggested that almost all patients with signs of fever and neutropenia should be managed with appropriate broad-spectrum antibiotics to overcome both gram-positive and negative pathogens (Freifeld et al. 2011).

35.8 Differential Diagnosis

Fungal infections often resemble other illnesses. Differential diagnosis is very important because faster diagnosis may prevent serious illness.

35.9 Medical Treatment

To date, many studies investigated patients who are at high-risk groups, and they investigated ways to prevent the fungal infections of the CNS (Infectious Diseases Working Party (AGIHO) of the German Society of Hematology and Oncology (DGHO) et al. 2009; Freifeld et al. 2011; CDC et al. 2001; Center for International Blood and Marrow Transplant Research (CIBMTR) et al. 2009). In these patients, early and appropriate antifungal regimen is necessary to prevent fungal infections and to improve their survival (Infectious Diseases Working Party (AGIHO) of the German Society of Hematology and Oncology (DGHO) et al. 2009; CDC et al. 2001; Center for International Blood and Marrow Transplant Research (CIBMTR) et al. 2009). Today, a number of more effective, albeit expensive, antifungal chemotherapeutic agents, in contrast to the previous gold standard amphotericin B deoxycholate, are available (Infectious Diseases Working Party (AGIHO) of the German Society of Hematology and Oncology (DGHO) et al. 2009; CDC et al. 2001; Center for International Blood and Marrow Transplant Research (CIBMTR) et al. 2009). Recently, it has been reported that voriconazole treatment increases survival of patients with invasive aspergillosis in allogeneic hematopoietic stem cell transplant recipients (Salmeron et al. 2012).

Nowadays, the best choice drugs for the treatment for invasive *Candida* infections are voriconazole, amphotericin B, fluconazole, and lipid formulations of amphotericin B (Infectious Diseases Working Party (AGIHO) of the German Society of Hematology and Oncology (DGHO) et al. 2009), while voriconazole, amphotericin B, and its lipid formulations, caspofungin, itraconazole, and posaconazole are well-known drug options in patients with invasive aspergillosis (Infectious Diseases Working Party (AGIHO) of the German Society of Hematology and Oncology (DGHO) et al. 2009; CDC et al. 2001; Center for International Blood and Marrow Transplant Research (CIBMTR) et al. 2009). However, optimal antifungal therapy algorithms for use of empirical or preemptive are still evolving (Freifeld et al. 2011). In addition to antifungal drugs, other alternative procedures such as surgical intervention, immunotherapy, and granulocyte transfusion may be used in these patients (Infectious Diseases Working Party (AGIHO) of the German Society of Hematology and Oncology (DGHO) et al. 2009).

35.10 Prognosis of Fungal Infections in Cancer Patients

Prognosis of patients with invasive aspergillosis following stem cell transplantation has dramatically improved after the use of voriconazole

(Salmeron et al. 2012). Mortality due to fungal infection is lower in febrile neutropenic patients treated with various forms of amphotericin B (conventional, lipid complex, liposomal amphotericin B), itraconazole, and voriconazole compared to the antifungal-free group. Despite recent advances in medical drug technology, the mortality rates exceed 30% in patients with invasive fungal infections (Chen et al. 2017). Empirical antifungal therapy improves the outcome of invasive fungal infection, but no significant difference was found on overall mortality. It was reported that most effective agents for empiric treatment seem to be echinocandins in patients with febrile neutropenia based on mortality (Chen et al. 2017). However, the patients with cancer are not at the same risk of death associated with fungal infection due to their nonhomogeneity.

35.11 Prevention Strategies

To avoid from fungi—which usually live on plants and trees or in soil in the outside of the house, is difficult since they are a natural environmental component. Furthermore, fungi are on many indoor surfaces and on the skin of the humans. Nevertheless, there may be different precautions to lower the chances of development of a severe fungal infection as follows: (1) to avoid environment having dust or bird to avoid disease-causing fungi, (2) to wear gloves when handling materials, and (3) to wear long dress and shoes during activities outside (Crawford et al. 2004). Lastly, it is very important to note that these precautions have not been confirmed to avoid fungal infections, although these actions are recommended. Today, it is obvious that new studies investigating the risks of neutropenic complications may provide identification of patients at greater risk with appropriate preventive precautions including "antifungal prophylaxis," thereby minimizing the healthcare costs in the near future (Crawford et al. 2004).

35.12 Conclusion

Nowadays, a high incidence of invasive fungal infections of the CNS in immunocompromised patients with cancer has been reported in spite of advances in approach for both the diagnosis and management of these patients. In some geographical and meteorological conditions, the diagnosis of fungal infection involving the CNS should be considered in any cancer patient with mild to severe neutropenia. There is no doubt that early diagnosis and proper treatment will improve prognosis, and this will result in reduced mortality and morbidity rates.

References

Bodey G, Bueltmann B, Duguid W, Gibbs D, Hanak H, Hotchi M, Mall G, Martino P, Meunier F, Milliken S, Naoe S, Okudaira M, Scevola D, van't Wout J. Fungal infections in cancer patients: an international autopsy survey. Eur J Clin Microbiol Infect Dis. 1992;11:99–109.

Calton EA, Le Doaré K, Appleby G, Chisholm JC, Sharland M, Ladhani SN, CABIN Participants. Invasive bacterial and fungal infections in paediatric patients with cancer: incidence, risk factors, aetiology and outcomes in a UK regional cohort 2009-2011. Pediatr Blood Cancer. 2014;61:1239–45.

CDC, Infectious Disease Society of America, the American Society of Blood and Marrow Transplantation. Guidelines for preventing opportunistic infections among hematopoietic stem cell transplant recipients. Recommendations of CDC, the Infectious Disease Society of America, and the American Society of Blood and Marrow Transplantation. Cytotherapy. 2001;3:41–54.

Center for International Blood and Marrow Transplant Research (CIBMTR), National Marrow Donor Program (NMDP), European Blood and Marrow TransplantGroup (EBMT), American Society of Blood and Marrow Transplantation (ASBMT), Canadian Blood and Marrow Transplant Group (CBMTG), Infectious Disease Society of America (IDSA), Society for Healthcare Epidemiology of America (SHEA), Association of Medical Microbiology and Infectious Diseases Canada (AMMI), Centers for Disease Control and Prevention (CDC). Guidelines for preventing infectious complications among hematopoietic cell transplant recipients: a global perspective. Bone Marrow Transplant. 2009;44:453–8.

Chamilos G, Luna M, Lewis RE, Bodey GP, Chemaly R, Tarrand JJ, Safdar A, Raad II, Kontoyiannis DP. Invasive fungal infections in patients with hematologic malignancies in a tertiary care cancer center: an autopsy study over a 15-year period (1989–2003). Haematologica. 2006;91:986–9.

Chen K, Wang Q, Pleasants RA, Ge L, Liu W, Peng K, Zhai S. Empiric treatment against invasive fungal diseases in febrile neutropenic patients: a systematic review and network meta-analysis. BMC Infect Dis. 2017;17:159.

Chitasombat MN, Kofteridis DP, Jiang Y, Tarrand J, Lewis RE, Kontoyiannis DP. Rare opportunistic (non-Candida, non-Cryptococcus) yeast bloodstream infections in patients with cancer. J Infect. 2012;64:68–75.

Crawford J, Dale DC, Lyman GH. Chemotherapy-induced neutropenia: risks, consequences, and new directions for its management. Cancer. 2004;100:228–37.

Douglas AP, Chen SC, Slavin MA. Emerging infections caused by non-Aspergillus filamentous fungi. Clin Microbiol Infect. 2016;22:670–80.

Freifeld AG, Bow EJ, Sepkowitz KA, Boeckh MJ, Ito JI, Mullen CA, Raad II, Rolston KV, Young JA, Wingard JR, Infectious Diseases Society of America. Clinical practice guideline for the use of antimicrobial agents in neutropenic patients with cancer: 2010 update by the Infectious Diseases Society of America. Clin Infect Dis. 2011;52:e56–93.

Haßler A, Porto L, Lehrnbecher T. Cerebral fungal infection in pediatric cancer patients. Curr Fungal Infect Rep. 2015;9:6–14.

Infectious Diseases Working Party (AGIHO) of the German Society of Hematology and Oncology (DGHO), Böhme A, Ruhnke M, Buchheidt D, Cornely OA, Einsele H, Enzensberger R, Hebart H, Heinz W, Junghanss C, Karthaus M, Krüger W, Krug U, Kubin T, Penack O, Reichert D, Reuter S, Silling G, Südhoff T, Ullmann AJ, Maschmeyer G. Treatment of invasive fungal infections in cancer patients—recommendations of the Infectious Diseases Working Party (AGIHO) of the German Society of Hematology and Oncology (DGHO). Ann Hematol. 2009;88:97–110.

Kappagoda S, Adams JY, Luo R, Banaei N, Concepcion W, Ho DY. Fatal *Emmonsia* sp. infection and fungemia after orthotopic liver transplantation. Emerg Infect Dis. 2017;23:346–9.

Krishnan NS. Emerging fungal infections in cancer patients- a brief overview. Med Mycol. 2016;2:16. https://doi.org/10.21767/2471-8521.100016.

Lortholary O, Charlier C, Lebeaux D, Lecuit M, Consigny PH. Fungal infections in immunocompromised travelers. Clin Infect Dis. 2013;56:861–9.

Malani AN, Kauffman CA. Changing epidemiology of rare mold infections: implications for therapy. Drugs. 2007;67(13):1803–12.

Mcneil MM. Trends in mortality due to invasive aspergillosis in the United States 1980-1997. Clin Infect Dis. 2001;33:641–7.

Pagano L, Akova M, Dimopoulos G, Herbrecht R, Drgona L, Blijlevens N. Risk assessment and prognostic factors for mould-related diseases in immunocompromised patients. J Antimicrob Chemother. 2011;66(Suppl 1):i5–14.

Peghin M, Monforte V, Martin-Gomez MT. Epidemiology of invasive respiratory disease caused by emerging non-Aspergillus molds in lung transplant recipients. Transpl Infect Dis. 2016;18:70–8.

Pfaller MA, Pappas PG, Wingard JR. Invasive fungal pathogens: current epidemiological trends. Clin Infect Dis. 2006;43:S3–S14.

Pu S, Niu S, Zhang C, Xu X, Qin M, Huang S, Zhang L. Epidemiology, antifungal susceptibilities, and risk factors for invasive candidiasis from 2011 to 2013 in a teaching hospital in southwest China. J Microbiol Immunol Infect. 2017;50:97–103.

Ribaud P. Fungal infections and the cancer patient. Eur J Cancer. 1997;33(suppl 4):S50–4.

Salmeron G, Porcher R, Bergeron A, Robin M, Peffault de Latour R, Ferry C, Rocha V, Petropoulou A, Xhaard A, Lacroix C, Sulahian A, Socié G, Ribaud P. Persistent poor long-term prognosis of allogeneic hematopoietic stem cell transplant recipients surviving invasive aspergillosis. Haematologica. 2012;97:1357–63.

Schwartz IS, Kenyon C, Feng P, Govender NP, Dukik K, Sigler L, Jiang Y, Stielow JB, Muñoz JF, Cuomo CA, Botha A, Stchigel AM, de Hoog GS. 50 years of *Emmonsia* disease in humans: the dramatic emergence of a cluster of novel fungal pathogens. PLoS Pathog. 2015;11:e1005198.

Sekhon AS, Jackson FL, Jacobs HJ. Blastomycosis: report of the first case from Alberta, Canada. Mycopathologia. 1982;79:65–9.

Stanzani M, Sassi C, Battista G, Cavo M, Lewis RE. Improved radiographic imaging of invasive fungal disease: the cornerstone to antifungal stewardship in the hematology units? Curr Fungal Infect Rep. 2016;10:78–86.

Starkey J, Moritani T, Kirby P. MRI of CNS fungal infections: review of aspergillosis to histoplasmosis and everything in between. Clin Neuroradiol. 2014;24:217–30.

Wang H, Liu N, Yin M, Han H, Yue J, Zhang F, Shan T, Guo H, Wu D. The epidemiology, antifungal use and risk factors of death in elderly patients with candidemia: a multicentre retrospective study. BMC Infect Dis. 2014;14:609.

Invasive Fungal Infections in Patients with Hematologic Malignancies

36

Yaşar Barış Turgut, Gökhan Sargın, and Gökhan Pektaş

Abbreviations

AHSCT	Allogeneic hematopoietic stem cell transplantation
AML	Acute myeloid leukemia
CNS	Central nervous system
IFI	Invasive fungal infection
MRI	Magnetic resonance imaging

36.1 Introduction

Hematological malignancies are defined as the most high risk group in terms of invasive fungal infections (IFIs), as the duration of neutropenia is longer than that of solid organ tumors (Pagano et al. 2006, 2010a, b). It is aimed to increase survival in hematologic malignancies with newly developed treatment modalities. With the introduction of new treatments, patients have begun to develop long-term myelosuppression, and have been made more risky for IFIs (Lass-Flörl 2009; Sainz et al. 2007; Viscoli et al. 2005). Nowadays, new diagnostic methods and new antifungal agents are used to reduce this risk, but the most important issue in the reduction of morbidity and mortality in IFIs is early diagnosis and early onset of treatment (Jahagirdar and Morrison 2002; Somboonwit and Greene 2002). It is very important to identify risky groups nowadays where definite diagnostic parameters cannot be determined for IFIs. In particular, acute myeloid leukemia, allogeneic hematopoietic stem cell transplantation (AHSCT) recipients, and treated non-Hodgkin's lymphoma patients are the highest-risk community (Pagano et al. 2006, 2010a, b; Montagna et al. 2012). The right choice of patients who will receive prophylactic, empiric-preemptive, or targeted antifungal therapy is the main principle of IFIs treatment (Cordonnier et al. 2009). In this chapter, we will review IFIs in hematologic malignancies with current literature.

36.2 Epidemiology and Incidence

The epidemiology of IFIs in patients with hematological malignancies has changed among different nations of the world in recent years (Montagna et al. 2012; Chamilos et al. 2006; Pagano et al. 2007). Geographically, different distributions of fungal pathogens, unavailability of appropriate conditions in the hospitals, some negative meteorological features, and vari-

Y. B. Turgut
Department of Internal Medicine, Muğla Sıtkı Koçman University School of Medicine, Muğla, Turkey

G. Sargın (✉)
Department of Internal Medicine, Aydın Adnan Menderes University School of Medicine, Aydın, Turkey

G. Pektaş
Division of Hematology, Muğla Sıtkı Koçman University Hospital, Muğla, Turkey

M. Turgut et al. (eds.), *Fungal Infections of the Central Nervous System*,
https://doi.org/10.1007/978-3-030-06088-6_36

ous factors affecting the spread of fungal spores have an important role in the incidence of IFIs in patients (Chamilos et al. 2006). During the last half-century, the incidence of IFIs in patients with hematologic malignancies was underestimated due to non-specific clinical manifestations, difficulty in diagnosis from biological samples, and it has increased from 3% to 30% (Hsiao et al. 2006; Martino and Girmenia 1999).

Unfortunately, the incidence of invasive mycoses has increased in the early period of the hematologic diseases, due to various difficulties in the clinical and therapeutic approach (Martino and Girmenia 1999). Thus, even today, IFIs are frequent causes of morbidity and mortality in these patients.

36.3 Pathogenesis

Majority of IFIs are caused by *Aspergillus* (Fig. 36.1) and *Candida* species but unusual fungal pathogens such as *Zygomycetes*, *Trichosporon*, *Fusarium*, and *Scedosporium* species, and other rare molds or yeasts may be observed as a cause of infection in these patients (Pagano et al. 2010a, b; Jahagirdar and Morrison 2002; Ruhnke and Maschmeyer 2002; Segal et al. 2002). From mycological view of point, various fungal pathogens such as *Fusarium*, *Scedosporium*, *Zygomycetes*, *Trichosporon*, *Malassezia*, *Penicillium*, and *Paecilomyces* are well-known causative agents in these patients (Jahagirdar and Morrison 2002).

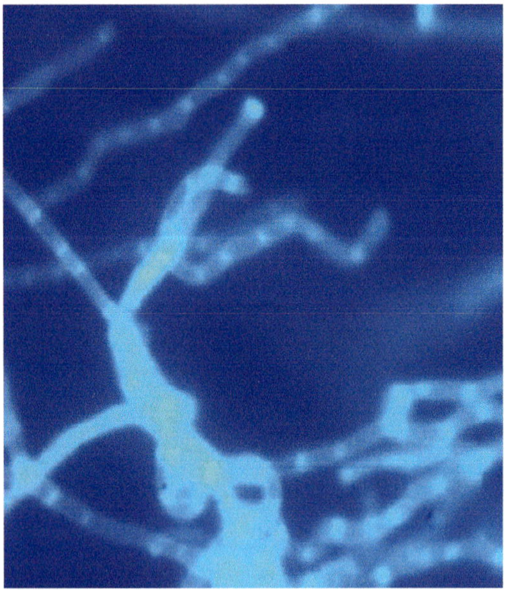

Fig. 36.1 Thin frequently septate hyphae with acute angled branching of *Aspergillus* species (courtesy of L. Vemu, M.D.)

Candida albicans among yeasts is an important pathogen, while other *Candida* species such as *C. glabrata*, *C. guilliermondii*, *C. parapsilosis*, *C. tropicalis*, and *C. krusei* have also been described (Pagano et al. 2006; Montagna et al. 2012; Caggiano et al. 2008; Girmenia et al. 2006; Marr 2004; Neofytos et al. 2009). On the other hand, *Aspergillus* spp. among molds is a serious mortal complication in cases with hematological malignancies, while other molds, including *Zygomycetes* and *Fusarium* spp. have also been previously reported (Montagna et al. 2012). Moreover, infections of other filamentous fungi are also rarely seen (Pagano et al. 2006). In clinical practice, the IFIs in patients with hematological malignancies are caused by yeasts than by filamentous fungi (Montagna et al. 2012).

Risk factors for fungal infections involving the central nervous system (CNS) are neutropenia for patients with underlying acute myeloid leukemia (AML), use of steroid or cytarabine, use of various medicines), advanced age, genetic predisposition, and other systemic comorbidities (Lass-Flörl 2009; Sainz et al. 2007; Viscoli et al. 2005). Importantly, it has been reported that *Cryptococcus neoformans* and *Pneumocystis carinii* may produce serious infections in patients with severe T-cell suppression (Segal et al. 2002) (Fig. 36.2).

Nowadays, the patients are classified into three groups depending on the risk for IFIs: (a) high-risk group, (b) intermediate-risk group, and (c) low-risk group (Rambaldi et al. 2017). In particular, patients with AML those treated with an allogeneic HSCT and some conditions like neutropenia and use of steroids at high doses are classified as high risk for developing IFI (Rambaldi et al. 2017).

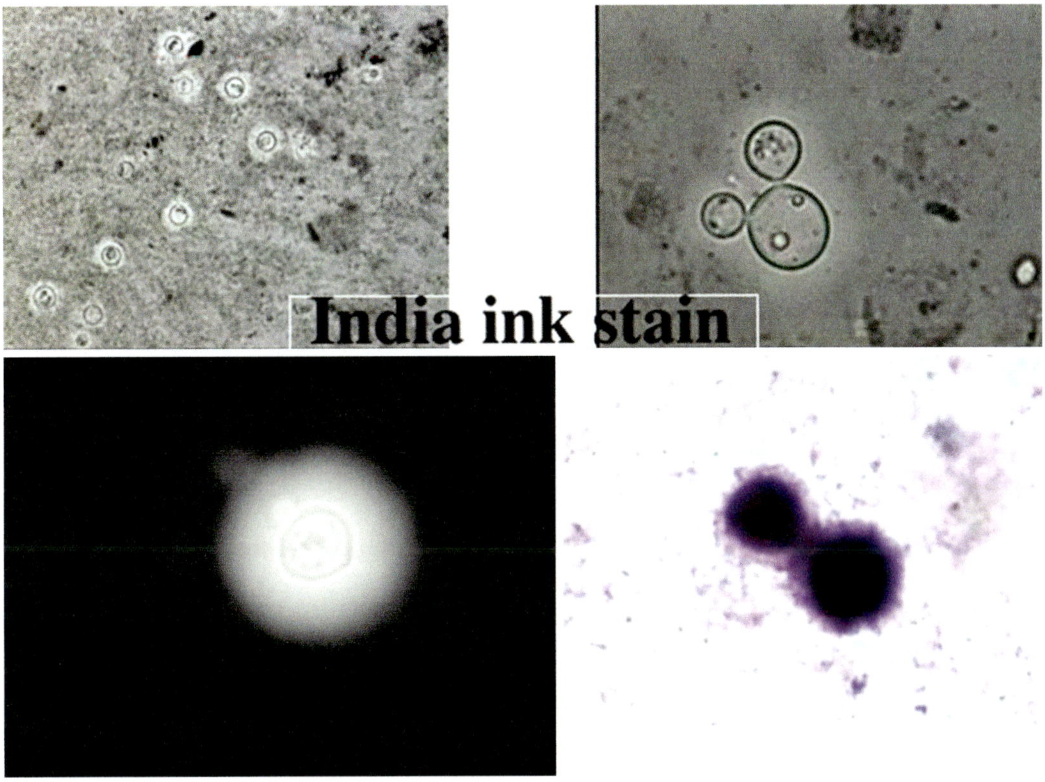

Fig. 36.2 Capsulated, narrow-based budding yeast—*Cryptococcus neoformans* (courtesy of L. Vemu, M.D.)

36.4 Hematological Malignancies

In addition to patients with aplastic anemia (Fig. 36.3) (Haßler et al. 2015), and patients with allogeneic HSCTs the hematological malignancies including AML or non-Hodgkin's lymphoma are at highest risk of development of various fungal infections (Pagano et al. 2006; Montagna et al. 2012). In particular, among patients with AML and those who receive HSCT, IFIs are frequent with prolonged neutropenia and/or fever, unresponsiveness to broad-spectrum antibacterial therapy in cases with chronic lymphocytic leukemia (30%) compared to those with AML (1.5%), possibly due to the wide use of monoclonal antibodies therapy and presence of severe immunosuppression (Pagano et al. 2010a, b). Some authors reported that the incidence of IFIs due to molds increases following an immunosuppressive therapy (Pagano et al. 2010a, b). In addition to *Aspergillus* species, other molds such as *Zygomycetes* and *Fusarium* are encountered increasingly in clinical practice, possibly due to the use of aggressive chemotherapy protocols in recent years (Pagano et al. 2006).

36.5 Clinical Manifestations

Clinically, many of fungal infections involving the CNS have a characteristic clinical disease spectrum (Jahagirdar and Morrison 2002). The clinical findings are usually non-specific and symptoms are seen late in the course of the infection (Chen et al. 2017). Clinical features of chronic pulmonary aspergillosis include prolonged and recurrent cough, shortness of breath, and hemoptysis. The most common

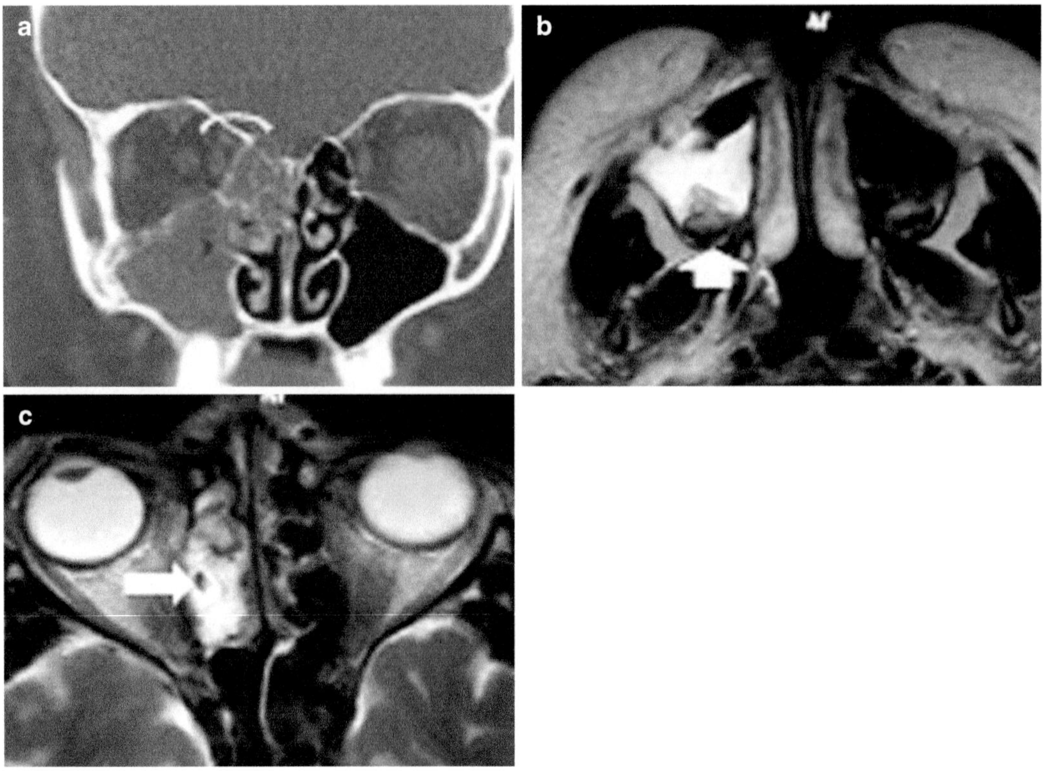

Fig. 36.3 (**a**) Computerized tomography of a 10-year-old girl with aplastic anemia suffering from mucormycosis demonstrating the destruction of the anterior skull base near the cribriform plate (*curved arrow*). (**b**, **c**) Axial T2-weighted magnetic resonance imaging (MRI) demonstrating hypointensity areas in the maxillary and ethmoidal sinus on the right side (*straight arrows*) (from Haßler et al. (2015), with permission)

symptoms reported were cough in 92.8%, hemoptysis in 63.8%, sputum production, fever, shortness of breath, and chest pain in decreasing frequency, respectively. Asymptomatic cases constitute only 5.8% (Hou et al. 2017). Saprophytic aspergillosis is usually asymptomatic, and hemoptysis is the most frequent symptom. In patients with semi-invasive pulmonary aspergillosis, the clinical pictures are non-specific, and 15% of patients may have hemoptysis. The fever, cough, recurrent wheezing, recurrent pneumonia, mucoid plugs due to excessive mucus production, and sputum are common in patients with chronic allergic bronchopulmonary aspergillosis. Patients with airway-invasive aspergillosis may present with more serious clinical findings such as hypoxia (Franquet et al. 2001).

36.6 Diagnostic Evaluation

Use of correct imaging studies and diagnostic techniques allow for early diagnosis and appropriate treatment of fungal infections (Somboonwit and Greene 2002). Despite novel diagnostic modalities, however, early identification of IFIs still remains challenging (Sinkó et al. 2008). Montagna et al. (2012) reported that the diagnosis was made by the detection of the circulating antigens galactomannan and (1,3)-β-D-glucan in 6 of the 10 patients with suspected aspergillosis. Mycologically, the time period between the first and last blood cultures with positive result is called as "duration of fungemia," and the persistence of positive blood cultures from the time of the first positive blood culture for more than 2 days is also defined as "persistent fungemia"

(Montagna et al. 2012). In general, the detection of the (1,3)-β-D-glucan antigen is made using calorimetric methods (Montagna et al. 2012). Morphologically, fungi are diagnosed with standard techniques based on their macroscopic and microscopic features (de Hoog et al. 2009).

36.7 Differential Diagnosis

There are many granulomatous diseases such as tuberculosis, brucellosis, and sarcoidosis that share similar histological features with fungal infection. Histoplasmosis and coccidioidomycosis may lead to a clinical picture that resembles tuberculosis (Fig. 36.4). The difference between tuberculosis, sarcoidosis, and coccidioidomycosis (an infection caused by the fungus *Coccidioides*) is important. Fungal infections of the CNS caused by *Coccidioides* occur in the southwestern regions of USA in the world (Fig. 36.5) (Starkey et al. 2014). Bronchopulmonary disease, lymphadenitis, abscesses of skin, and soft tissue are clinical manifestations of tuberculosis. The diagnosis of brucellosis depends on clinical features, serological, and histopathologic findings (Zumla and James 1996). It is widely accepted that IFI is a frequent com-

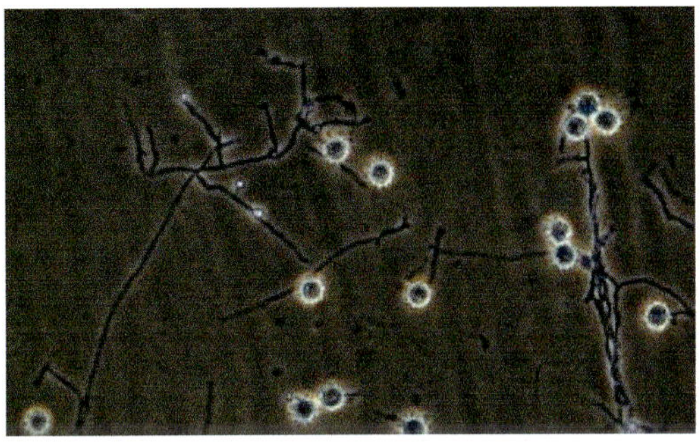

Fig. 36.4 Large, rounded, single-celled, tuberculate macroconidia and small, pyriform-shaped microconidia of *Histoplasma capsulatum*. Lactophenol cotton blue mount 40× (courtesy of L. Vemu, M.D.)

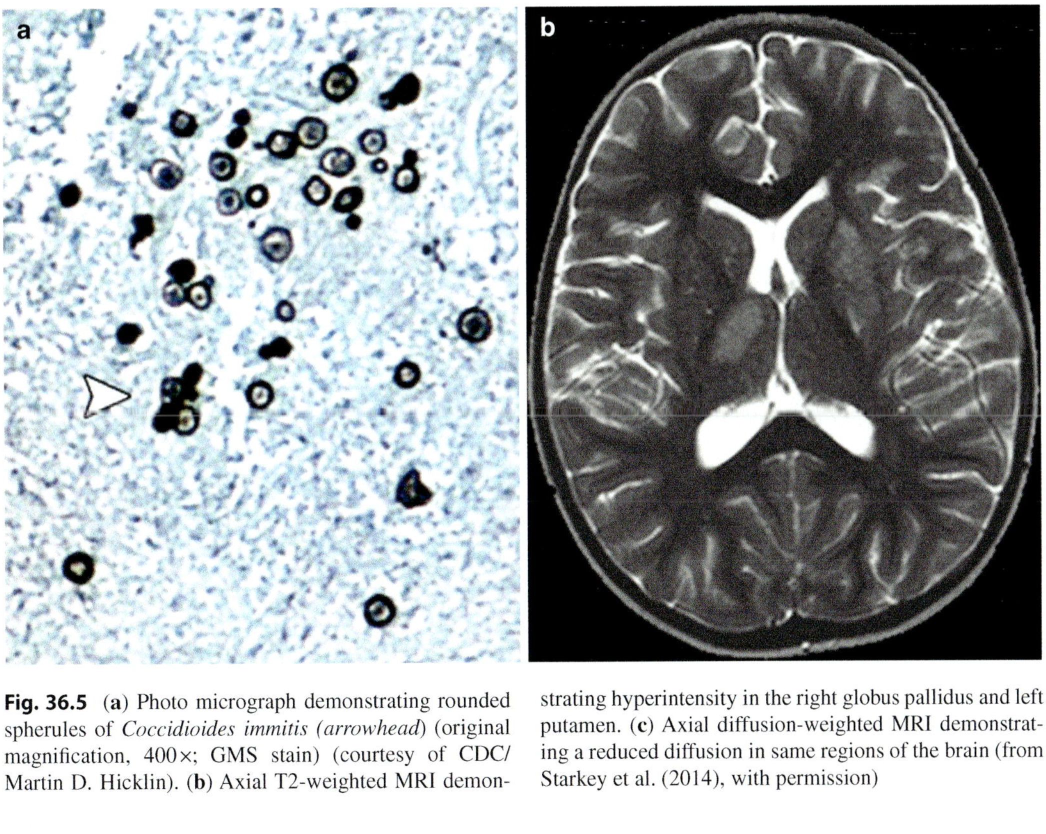

Fig. 36.5 (**a**) Photo micrograph demonstrating rounded spherules of *Coccidioides immitis (arrowhead)* (original magnification, 400×; GMS stain) (courtesy of CDC/Martin D. Hicklin). (**b**) Axial T2-weighted MRI demonstrating hyperintensity in the right globus pallidus and left putamen. (**c**) Axial diffusion-weighted MRI demonstrating a reduced diffusion in same regions of the brain (from Starkey et al. (2014), with permission)

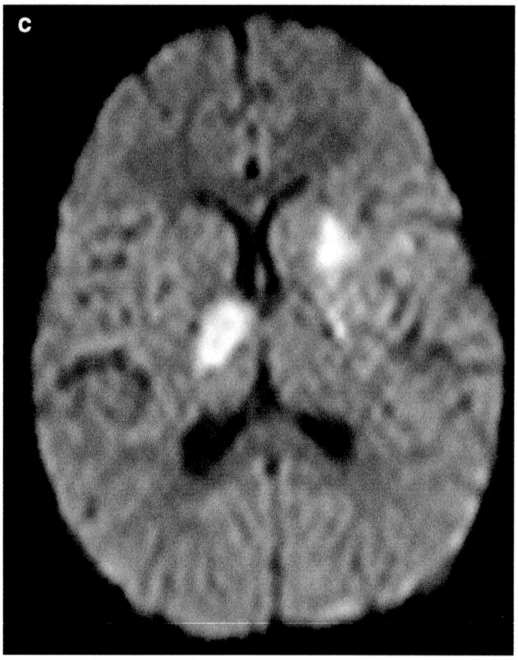

Fig. 36.5 (continued)

plication in allogeneic HSCT recipients, and the most commonly detected agent in these cases is *Aspergillus* spp (Pagano et al. 2007). Differential diagnosis is very important in patients of proven or probable invasive aspergillosis because faster diagnosis may prevent serious illness.

36.8 Medical Treatment

In the last few years, many new antifungal agents such as liposomal amphotericin B, voriconazole, caspofungin, and posaconazole have been suggested to improve outcomes of these patients with IFIs caused by major fungal pathogens, and these new agents provide a major advance in the pharmacological management of patients with hematological malignancies (Martino and Girmenia 1999). In general, the pharmacological treatment of the hematological adult patient is made according to European Conference on Infections in Leukemia (ECIL) 2007 and Infectious Diseases Guidelines of America (IDSA) 2008 guidelines (Maertens et al. 2007; Walsh et al. 2008). At present, there are two antifungal treatment approaches for patients with hematological malignancies: (1) empirical or preemptive antifungal therapy and (2) targeted antifungal therapy.

36.8.1 Empirical Antifungal Therapy Modality

Empirical or preemptive antifungal therapy is an early treatment for occult fungal infections with hematological malignancies before microbiological identification of a fungal pathogen or development of radiological signs such as pneumonia, sinusitis, etc. develop (Cordonnier et al. 2009). Unfortunately, there is no standard protocol upon preemptive antifungal treatment at present, while many guidelines have been described for empirical therapy for patients with febrile neutropenia with high-risk to date.

In clinical practice, empirical and preemptive antifungal therapy is given as soon as signs and symptoms like fever begin in neutropenic patients with hematological malignancies because of the difficulty in diagnosing IFIs and high mortality rates in cases of delayed therapy (Cordonnier et al. 2009). In general, empirical antifungal therapy is associated with a lower rate of IFI. In a previous study, it has been reported that various empirical and preemptive antifungal strategies provide similar survival rates in the fungal infections (Cordonnier et al. 2009).

Nowadays, it is widely accepted that empirical or preemptive antifungal therapy is a satisfactory management option in the majority of neutropenic patients with hematological malignancies. In particular, empirical antifungal treatment should be an option for induction of remission in patients with AML. It has been reported that empirical treatment improved the survival rates in patients with AML receiving induction chemotherapy (Cordonnier et al. 2009).

36.8.2 Targeted Antifungal Therapy Modality

Targeted antifungal therapy, administering an agent which is effective against the fungal pathogen, is used in patients with clear evidence of a certain fungal microorganism. As expected, it reduces the overuse or more than enough of antifungal agents, compared with the empirical approach, but it has some disadvantages such as delayed diagnosis and development of thrombocytopenia in these patients with hematologic malignancies and may cause difficulty in histological diagnosis. Today, targeted therapy is suggested for the majority of mold and yeast infections. Echinocandin drugs are more effective against *Candida* in nonneutropenic patients with hematologic malignancies. Furthermore, voriconazole among anti-*Aspergillus* treatments is widely accepted as the gold standard. Moreover, treatment with liposomal amphotericin B or posaconazole improves the prognosis of patients with zygomycosis, a rare fungal infection.

36.9 Prognosis

As a general rule, early diagnosis and prompt treatment of IFIs in patients with hematological malignancies is the key to a successful outcome (Jahagirdar and Morrison 2002; Somboonwit and Greene 2002). Furthermore, it has been reported that the length of duration of neutropenia in these patients is an important prognostic factor (Görük et al. 2015). Despite progress in the past years, survival of patients with IFIs has increased in the treatment of patients with hematological malignancies, but they are still one of the factors causing to morbidity and mortality in cases with cancer (Somboonwit and Greene 2002; Ruhnke and Maschmeyer 2002; Segal et al. 2002; Sinkó et al. 2008). In particular, in addition to patients with aspergillosis, patients with AML and those who have undergone HSCT are at especially high risk and high mortality rate (Pagano et al. 2010a, b, 2007). Among various fungal agents, *Aspergillus* and *Candida* species, *Zygomycetes*, or other rare molds or yeasts are responsible for opportunistic fungal infections in patients with hematological malignancies (Pagano et al. 2010a, b; Segal et al. 2002). Nowadays, prognosis of patients with hematological malignancies has improved as a result of development of new diagnostic procedures and therapeutic progresses (Martino and Girmenia 1999).

36.10 Prophylaxis for Fungal Infections

Currently, a number of new prophylactic antifungal agents have been suggested for patients at high risk for infection for prolonged periods. However, it is difficult to identify patients at high-risk period, and there are limitations of broad-spectrum antifungal prophylaxis, including drug interactions, drug resistance, and toxicity related to fungal infection. Nowadays, many authors reported that the usage of prophylactic antifungal treatment in patients with hematologic malignancies reduced the incidence of IFIs including mycoses, resulting in a decrease in mortality rate. Based on the literature data, Pagano et al. (2010a, b) suggested the following guideline for these patients at high risk: (1) antifungal therapy is indicated in patients at high risk for IFIs; (2) as a general rule, any antifungal agent used should provide a protection against either molds or yeasts; and (3) today, successful management of adult patients with fungal infections was performed with fluconazole (Pagano et al. 2010a, b; Montagna et al. 2012). In adult patients, who are unresponsive to broad-spectrum antibiotic therapy, an empiric antifungal therapy (caspofungin or amphotericin B) is used (Montagna et al. 2012). It has been reported that voriconazole or caspofungin or amphotericin B are also appropriate in the presence of microbiological evidence (Montagna et al. 2012). In the pediatric patients, however, antifungal prophylaxis with fluconazole is used for patients with severe neutropenia, but an empiric antifungal therapy with caspofungin or amphotericin B is administered in cases who are unresponsive to an antibiotic therapy (Montagna et al. 2012).

36.11 Conclusion

The risk of IFI is high in the presence of neutropenia and high-dose steroid use in patients treated with AML or allogeneic HSCT. Early imaging of fungal infections is facilitated by accurate imaging methods. An effective antifungal prophylaxis in high risk patients is important in reducucing mortality and morbidity. However, it is concluded that both diagnostic procedures and therapeutic modalities are still suboptimal for the successful management of IFIs in patients with HSCT (Sinkó et al. 2008).

References

Caggiano G, Iatta R, Laneve A, Manca F, Montagna MT. Observational study on candidaemia at a university hospital in southern Italy from 1998 to 2004. Mycoses. 2008;51:123–8.

Chamilos G, Luna M, Lewis RE, Bodey GP, Chemaly R, Tarrand JJ, Safdar A, Raad II, Kontoyiannis DP. Invasive fungal infections in patients with hematologic malignancies in a tertiary care cancer center: an autopsy study over a 15-year period (1989–2003). Haematologica. 2006;91:986–9.

Chen K, Wang Q, Pleasants RA, Ge L, Liu W, Peng K, Zhai S. Empiric treatment against invasive fungal diseases in febrile neutropenic patients: a systematic review and network meta-analysis. BMC Infect Dis. 2017;17:159.

Cordonnier C, Pautas C, Maury S, Vekhoff A, Farhat H, Suarez F, Dhédin N, Isnard F, Ades L, Kuhnowski F, Foulet F, Kuentz M, Maison P, Bretagne S, Schwarzinger M. Empirical versus preemptive antifungal therapy for high-risk, febrile, neutropenic patients: a randomized, controlled trial. Clin Infect Dis. 2009;15(48):1042–51.

Franquet T, Müller NL, Giménez A, Guembe P, de La Torre J, Bagué S. Spectrum of pulmonary aspergillosis: histologic, clinical, and radiologic findings. Radiographics. 2001;21:825–37.

Girmenia C, Pizzarelli G, Cristini F, Barchiesi F, Spreghini E, Scalise G, Martino P. *Candida guilliermondii* fungemia in patients with hematologic malignancies. J Clin Microbiol. 2006;44:2458–64.

Görük M, Dal MS, Dal T, Karakus A, Tekin R, Özcan N, Ayyildiz O. Evaluation of febrile neutropenic patients hospitalized in a hematology clinic. Asian Pac J Trop Biomed. 2015;5(12):1051–4.

Haßler A, Porto L, Lehrnbecher T. Cerebral fungal infection in pediatric cancer patients. Curr Fungal Infect Rep. 2015;9:6–14.

de Hoog GS, Guarro J, Gené J, Figueras MJ. Atlas of clinical fungi. 3rd ed. Utrecht: Centraalbureau voor Schimmelcultures (CBS); 2009.

Hou X, Zhang H, Kou L, Lv W, Lu J, Li J. Clinical features and diagnosis of chronic pulmonary aspergillosis in Chinese patients. Medicine (Baltimore). 2017;96:e8315.

Hsiao HH, Tsai HJ, Liu YC, Tseng YT, Lu PL, Yang WC, Liu TC, Lin SF. Invasive fungal infections in patients with acute leukemia. Kaohsiung J Med Sci. 2006;22:217–22.

Jahagirdar BN, Morrison VA. Emerging fungal pathogens in patients with hematologic malignancies and marrow/stem-cell transplant recipients. Semin Respir Infect. 2002;17:113–20.

Lass-Flörl C. The changing face of epidemiology of invasive fungal disease in Europe. Mycoses. 2009;52:197–205.

Maertens JA, Frere P, Lass-Florl C, Heinz W, Cornely OA. Primary antifungal prophylaxis in leukaemia patients. Eur J Cancer. 2007;5:43–8.

Marr KA. Invasive Candida infections: the changing epidemiology. Oncology. 2004;18:9–14.

Martino P, Girmenia C. Mycoses and their treatment in malignant hemopathies (in Italian). Recenti Prog Med. 1999;90:160–8.

Montagna MT, De Giglio O, Napoli C, Lovero G, Caggiano G, Delia M, Pastore D, Santoro N, Specchia G. Invasive fungal infections in patients with hematologic malignancies (Aurora project): lights and shadows during 18-months surveillance. Int J Mol Sci. 2012;13:774–87.

Neofytos D, Horn D, Anaissie E, Steinbach W, Olyaei A, Fishman J, Pfaller M, Chang C, Webster K, Marr K. Epidemiology and outcome of invasive fungal infection in adult hematopoietic stem cell transplant recipients: analysis of Multicenter Prospective Antifungal Therapy (PATH) Alliance registry. Clin Infect Dis. 2009;48:265–73.

Pagano L, Caira M, Candoni A, Offidani M, Fianchi L, Martino B, Pastore D, Picardi M, Bonini A, Chierichini A, et al. The epidemiology of fungal infections in patients with hematologic malignancies: the SEIFEM-2004 study. Haematologica. 2006;91:1068–75.

Pagano L, Caira M, Nosari A, Van Lint MT, Candoni A, Offidani M, Aloisi T, Irrera G, Bonini A, Picardi M, Caramatti C, Invernizzi R, Mattei D, Melillo L, de Waure C, Reddiconto G, Fianchi L, Valentini CG, Girmenia C, Leone G, Aversa F. Fungal infections in recipients of hematopoietic stem cell transplants: results of the SEIFEM B-2004 study—Sorveglianza

Epidemiologica Infezioni Fungine Nelle Emopatie Maligne. Clin Infect Dis. 2007;45:1161–70.

Pagano L, Caira M, Candoni A, Offidani M, Martino B, Specchia G, Pastore D, Stanzani M, Cattaneo C, Fanci R, Caramatti C, Rossini F, Luppi M, Potenza L, Ferrara F, Mitra ME, Fadda RM, Invernizzi R, Aloisi T, Picardi M, Bonini A, Vacca A, Chierichini A, Melillo L, de Waure C, Fianchi L, Riva M, Leone G, Aversa F, Nosari A. Invasive aspergillosis in patients with acute myeloid leukemia: a SEIFEM-2008 registry study. Haematologica. 2010a;95:644–50.

Pagano L, Caira M, Valentini CG, Posteraro B, Fianchi L. Current therapeutic approaches to fungal infections in immunocompromised hematological patients. Blood Rev. 2010b;24:51–61.

Rambaldi B, Russo D, Pagano L. Defining invasive fungal infection risk in hematological malignancies: a new tool for clinical practice. Mediterr J Hematol Infect Dis. 2017;9(1):e2017012.

Ruhnke M, Maschmeyer G. Management of mycoses in patients with hematologic disease and cancer- review of the literature. Eur J Med Res. 2002;7:227–35.

Sainz J, Pérez E, Hassan L, Moratalla A, Romero A, Collado MD, Jurado M. Variable number of tandem repeats of TNF receptor type 2 promoter as genetic biomarker of susceptibility to develop invasive pulmonary aspergillosis. Hum Immunol. 2007;68:41–50.

Segal BH, Bow EJ, Menichetti F. Fungal infections in nontransplant patients with hematologic malignancies. Infect Dis Clin N Am. 2002;16:935–64.

Sinkó J, Csomor J, Nikolova R, Lueff S, Kriván G, Reményi P, Bátai A, Masszi T. Invasive fungal disease in allogeneic hematopoietic stem cell transplant recipients: an autopsy-driven survey. Transpl Infect Dis. 2008;10:106–9.

Somboonwit C, Greene JN. Diagnostic methodologies for invasive fungal infections in hematopoietic stem-cell transplant recipients. Semin Respir Infect. 2002;17:151–7.

Starkey J, Moritani T, Kirby P. MRI of CNS fungal infections: review of aspergillosis to histoplasmosis and everything in between. Clin Neuroradiol. 2014;24:217–30.

Viscoli C, Varnier O, Machetti M. Infections in patients with febrile neutropenia: epidemiology, microbiology, and risk stratification. Clin Infect Dis. 2005;40:240–5.

Walsh TJ, Anaissie EJ, Denning DW, Herbrecht R, Kontoyiannis DP, Marr KA, Morrison VA, Segal BH, Steinbach WJ, Stevens DA, et al. Treatment of aspergillosis: clinical practice guidelines of the infectious diseases society of America. Clin Infect Dis. 2008;46:327–60.

Zumla A, James G. Granulomatous infections: etiology and classification. Clin Infect Dis. 1996;23:146–58.

37 Fungal Infections of Central Nervous System and Their Relationship to Neuropsychiatric Disorders

Onur Gökçen, Nermin Gündüz,
and Mehmet Turgut

Abbreviations

AIDS	Acquired immunodeficiency syndrome
CNM	Cryptococcus neoformans meningitis
CNS	Central nervous system
CT	Computed tomography
EPS	Extrapyramidal symptoms
HAART	Highly active antiretroviral therapy
HIV	Human immunodeficiency virus
IV	Intravenous
MRI	Magnetic resonance imaging

37.1 Introduction

Nowadays, there has been a considerable rise in the incidence of fungal infections, possibly owing to prolonged use of broad-spectrum antibacterial antibiotics and immunosuppressive drugs, and increased prevalence of acquired immunodeficiency syndrome (AIDS) in the world (Chen et al. 2018). Unfortunately, clinical picture of fungal infections involving the central nervous system (CNS), spine and brain, is insidious, and the symptomatology is non-specific, and hence the diagnostic delay is common; however, early diagnosis and treatment of fungal infections are vital. Therefore, a high index of suspicion is necessary for the diagnosis of fungal infections involving the CNS.

In this chapter, we will review relationships between the fungal infections of the CNS and psychiatric disorders, in terms of neuropsychiatric manifestations of fungal infections, fungal infections in drug abusers, and dermatological fungal infections in neuropsychiatric disorders.

37.2 Neuropsychiatric Manifestations of Cryptococcus Neoformans Meningitis

There are cases in medical literature that includes *Cryptococcus neoformans* meningitis (CNM) with central fungal infection presented with psychiatric symptoms. CNM has been determined as a prominent cause of morbidity and mortality due to infectious disease in AIDS patients, and it is the second opportunistic infection involving the CNS (Jacob et al. 2013). Cryptococcal meningitis may appear in other immune deficiency condi-

O. Gökçen (✉)
Psychiatry Clinic, Kütahya Health Sciences University School of Medicine, Kütahya, Turkey

N. Gündüz
Department of Psychiatry, Kütahya Health Sciences University School of Medicine, Kütahya, Turkey

M. Turgut
Department of Neurosurgery, Aydın Adnan Menderes University School of Medicine, Aydın, Turkey

M. Turgut et al. (eds.), *Fungal Infections of the Central Nervous System*,
https://doi.org/10.1007/978-3-030-06088-6_37

tions other than AIDS such as diabetes mellitus, cancer, hematological malignancy, solid organ transplantation, autoimmune hemolytic anemia, sarcoidosis, and chronic steroid treatment (Kumar et al. 2011; Satishchandra et al. 2007). It often presents with chronic or subacute meningitis symptoms. Clinical picture including headache and fever is a characteristic in these patients. In addition, altered sensorium has been noted in the vast majority of these patients (Satishchandra et al. 2007).

The most frequent neuropsychiatric symptoms of CNM in the literature are manic episodes, and it is followed by delirium (Satishchandra et al. 2007; Johannessen and Wilson 1988; Johnson and Naraqi 1993; Spiegel et al. 2011; Tang et al. 2005). The retrospective study of 142 patients who meet the diagnostic criteria of cryptococcal meningitis and severe immunosuppression (CD4, b100 cells/mm^3) has defined the neuropsychiatric symptoms of the disease (Ibanez-Valdes et al. 2005). Delirium (47%) and manic episode (33%), followed by depression and anxiety (19% and 16%) have been determined in this series, and no dementia was determined (Ibanez-Valdes et al. 2005). Approximately 25% of women and 20% of men were determined to have mania (Ibanez-Valdes et al. 2005). Manic symptoms identified in CNM are elated and decreased need for sleep, irritable mood, flights of ideas, increased libido, impulsive behavior, grandiose delusions, persecution delusions, and various hallucinations (auditory and/or visual ones) (Tang et al. 2005; Ibanez-Valdes et al. 2005). Although lower than delirium and mania, a number of cases have been reported with acute psychosis symptoms such as persecution delusions, suspiciousness, and hallucinations, auditory or visual, without elated mood (Jacob et al. 2013; Kumar et al. 2011).

A summary of literature data upon neuropsychiatric manifestations of fungal infections of the CNS from several selected publications are given in Table 37.1 (Jacob et al. 2013; Kumar et al. 2011; Johannessen and Wilson 1988; Johnson and Naraqi 1993; Spiegel et al. 2011; Tang et al. 2005; Thienhaus and Khosla 1984; Sa'adah et al. 1995; Goeb et al. 2007; Prakash and Sugandhi 2009; Holikatti and Kar 2012; Chou et al. 2016). Some of these cases are human immunodeficiency virus (HIV) positive. In association with the pathophysiology of brain infection, HIV has been reported in literature for mania secondary to AIDS (Holikatti and Kar 2012). From a clinical aspect, HIV-positive patients with secondary mania at first episode have severe mania and psychosis symptoms, severe cognitive dysfunction, and serious immunosuppression (Nakimuli-Mpungu et al. 2008). However, a relation was determined between psychiatric symptoms and CNM with the cases, and patients have responded to CNM treatment (Table 37.1) (Jacob et al. 2013; Kumar et al. 2011; Johannessen and Wilson 1988; Johnson and Naraqi 1993; Spiegel et al. 2011; Tang et al. 2005; Thienhaus and Khosla 1984; Sa'adah et al. 1995; Goeb et al. 2007; Prakash and Sugandhi 2009; Holikatti and Kar 2012; Chou et al. 2016).

Another controversial topic is the time of initiating highly active antiretroviral therapy (HAART) in AIDS patients who have developed CNM. When an AIDS patient who has not received HAART develops CNM, HAART is required for long-term survival. Early administration may promote immune reconstitution inflammatory syndrome; however, delay in starting therapy has been associated with significant mortality in the developing world (Sloan et al. 2009). Nevertheless, other studies suggest that the reason of immune reconstitution inflammatory syndrome may be organism load rather than time of starting HAART (Bicanic et al. 2010). There is a need for more studies on the time of starting HAART in AIDS patients with CNM.

In general, infectious factors were not considered at first because most of the patients did not have symptoms such as fever and headache at the beginning (Table 37.1) (Jacob et al. 2013; Kumar et al. 2011; Johannessen and Wilson 1988; Johnson and Naraqi 1993; Spiegel et al. 2011; Tang et al. 2005; Thienhaus and Khosla

Table 37.1 Summary of selected case series from the current literature regarding fungal infections and their relationship to neuropsychiatric disorders[a]

Author(s), year	Age, gender, country	Psychiatric symptoms	Medical condition and neurological symptoms	Treatment and follow-up
Thienhaus and Khosla (1984)	63, male, USA	Restless, irritable, agitation, social disinhibition, insomnia	No fever and stiff neck. Occasional urinary incontinence over the past months	Chlorpromazine and lithium carbonate were started first. Amphotericin B was started after cryptococcus meningitis diagnosis
Johannessen and Wilson (1988)	35, male, USA	Insomnia, grandiose delusion, hyperactive, hypersexual	HIV positive Fever	Mania symptoms disappeared, then paranoia and disorientation. Patient died due to respiratory arrest after 3 months
	32, male, USA	Paranoid delusions, auditory and visual hallucinations, combative, trouble concentrating, insomnia	HIV positive	Positive response to haloperidol treatment
Johnson and Naraqi (1993)	38, male, Papua New Guinea	Restless, auditory and visual hallucinations, aggressiveness, distractibility, logorrhea, grandiose delusion, elated mood	No immune deficiency. Facial weakness, blindness, convulsions	Mental state improved, but patient died due to meningitis in a follow-up of 1 year
Sa'adah et al. (1995)	22, male, Kuwait	Psychosis symptoms	Confusion	Recovery with amphotericin B and 5-fluorocytosine
Tang et al. (2005)	25, female, China	Manic symptoms, grandiose delusions and disrupted orientation	HIV negative. Weight loss, fever, chills, rigor, bone pain, insomnia, lack of appetite	Olanzapine, clonazepam, and sodium valproate treatment was started first Amphotericin B was started after CNM diagnosis. Lithium carbonate was added to treatment. With the decrease of manic symptoms, patient was discharged. After 6 months, all psychotropic drugs were stopped with disappearance of all manic symptoms
Goeb et al. (2007)	27, male, France	Confusion, psychosis, affective disorder, but not hallucination or delusion. Social withdrawal suggesting schizophrenia	HIV negative. He was a sarcoid patient Fever, disrupted orientation in the follow-up	Amphotericin and 5-fluorocytosine; recovered
Prakash and Sugandhi (2009)	28, female, India	Insomnia, irritability, confusion, psychosis, disrupted reality	She had no immune deficiency. Fever	Olanzapine treatment was started first. Amphotericin B was started after CNM. Psychotropic treatment was stopped. She recovered after the 12-week treatment. Psychosis did not recur in the 1-year follow-up

(continued)

Table 37.1 (continued)

Author(s), year	Age, gender, country	Psychiatric symptoms	Medical condition and neurological symptoms	Treatment and follow-up
Kumar et al. (2011)	49, male, India	Psychosis symptoms	A case with hemolytic anemia with positive direct Coombs test. HIV negative. Headache for 2 months, and no fever	Olanzapine and clonazepam treatment was started. IV amphotericin B was started after CNM. Treatment was changed to oral fluconazole. Psychotropic drugs were stopped at discharge. There were no psychiatric signs in the 7-month follow-up
Spiegel et al. (2011)	53, male, USA	He had signs of mania, thoughts with grandiose content, lack of attention and concentration	HIV-positive patient	Manic symptoms have decreased with 14-day azole treatment and 10 mg olanzapine, and olanzapine treatment was stopped, and HAART was started at discharge
Jacob et al. (2013)	30, male, Singapore	Hallucination and acute psychosis symptoms	History of severe headache, high fever during monitoring	Firstly, 5 mg olanzapine was started and after HIV-positive result was determined during monitoring, CNM was diagnosed IV amphotericin and oral flucytosine treatment was initiated, and later treatment was changed to oral fluconazole. Antipsychotic treatment was stopped. Clinical status has recovered, and psychotic symptoms have disappeared
Holikatti and Kar (2012)	28, male, India	Manic symptoms, cognitive symptoms, persecution delusions, nihilistic delusions, hostility and insomnia	HIV-positive patient. Fever, headache, blurred vision, cognitive dysfunction	Divalproex, trifluoperazine, escitalopram, venlafaxine, and quetiapine treatments were used in the follow-up. After being diagnosed with CNM, amphotericin B treatment was administered, and then cognitive disruption was decreased, and suspiciousness was reduced, but auditory hallucinations persisted. Quetiapine treatment was continued
Chou et al. (2016)	78, male, China	Manic symptoms and grandiose delusions	Oriented at first, but then impaired consciousness. HIV-positive patient. Fever	Manic symptoms decreased after start of 2 weeks treatment with quetiapine and lorazepam. After CNM diagnosis at fourth week, psychotropic drugs were stopped, and amphotericin B and HAART were started. Manic symptoms have subsided, but he was infected with pneumocystis carinii at eighth week and died due to sepsis associated with pneumonia

CNM Cryptococcus neoformans meningitis, *HAART* highly active antiretroviral therapy, *HIV* human immunodeficiency virus, *IV* intravenous

[a]Adapted from: Gen Hosp Psychiatry. 2005;27:301–3. doi: 10.1016/j.genhosppsych.2005.03.003 (Tang et al. 2005) and Cases J. 2009;2:9084. doi: 10.1186/1757-1626-2-9084 (Prakash and Sugandhi 2009)

1984; Sa'adah et al. 1995; Goeb et al. 2007; Prakash and Sugandhi 2009; Holikatti and Kar 2012; Chou et al. 2016). It has been reported that psychiatric symptoms decreased with the use of various psychotropic drugs even before the initiation of antifungal treatment in CNM (Spiegel et al. 2011; Tang et al. 2005). Therefore, a positive response to treatment does not exclude the presence of underlying infection. Underlying infection can be recurring and fatal as a result of delayed diagnosis, though psychiatric symptoms generally respond to treatment (Spiegel et al. 2011; Tang et al. 2005). Due to lack of neurological symptoms and symptoms suggesting infectious factors such as fever, most cases in literature have been misdiagnosed due to psychiatric symptoms at first, and they were treated with psychotropic drugs which extend the disease course further. It has been reported that CNM is a fatal disease resulting in death in 83% of patients without neuropsychiatric symptoms and 76% of patients with neuropsychiatric symptoms, if appropriate treatment is not started without delay (Kumar et al. 2011; Ibanez-Valdes et al. 2005).

So far, olanzapine was preferred for treatment in most of the cases (Table 37.1). This was attributed to the limitations in the use of conventional mood regulators in HIV-infected patients (Spiegel et al. 2011). Furthermore, treatment of patients infected with HIV using dopamine receptor-2 antagonists may cause development of various extrapyramidal symptoms (EPS) since HIV causes neuronal damage in basal ganglia (Aylward et al. 1993). Risperidone, ziprasidone, and olanzapine were used safely in patients with AIDS in the previous case reports and series (Spiegel et al. 2011; Rummel-Kluge et al. 2012). Nevertheless, olanzapine was preferred among these antipsychotics since it was recognized that it poses lower risk of EPS (Spiegel et al. 2011). Likewise, quetiapine was preferred in a case due to low risk of EPS (Chou et al. 2016).

Case reports of patients with CNM, who have applied with acute psychosis, are very rare (Jacob et al. 2013; Kumar et al. 2011). If there are risk factors for identifying opportunistic infections and early treatment particularly in patients without premorbid history for family history and psychosis, HIV test is important for patients presenting with acute psychosis. Another neuropsychiatric manifestation in CNM is delirium. It may appear especially in elderly people and young individuals with disrupted metabolic picture (Satishchandra et al. 2007; Ibanez-Valdes et al. 2005). Delirium may appear due to many reasons disrupting metabolic picture. Different from psychosis and mania, place, time, and person orientation is disrupted, and there is impaired consciousness. There may be distractibility, sensory disorder, and agitation. These symptoms may show fluctuations within the day. While delirium may be the first symptom of CNM, it may be due to other neuro-AIDS factors like HIV encephalopathy, progressive multifocal leukoencephalopathy, herpes or cytomegalovirus encephalitis, neurosyphilis, toxoplasmosis, or lymphoma (Ibanez-Valdes et al. 2005). It was indicated in a case in literature that CNM was identified a 70-year-old male with treatment-resistant endogen depression 10 months following administration of antidepressant drugs and that his depressive symptoms were significantly recovered following successful treatment of infection of the CNS (Hsueh and Lin 2010).

In brief, CNM may manifest with mania, delirium, and acute psychosis without any other neurological symptoms or signs favoring infection. Caution should be exercised in risk groups, and this should be considered upon signs indicating CNM in the follow-up.

37.3 Fungal Infections in Drug Abusers

Systemic fungal infections like infections of the CNS and fulminant infective endocarditis may cause a high mortality, although occurrence of fungal infections in drug users is infrequent in comparison with bacterial and viral infections (Badiee and Hashemizadeh 2014).

There are some predisposing factors related with encountering microbial pathogens. Some of them are associated with substance use itself such as using unsterile needles or syringes, contaminated drug paraphernalia, and drug adulterants (Kaushik et al. 2011). In addition, substance use especially cannabis sativa or marijuana, opiates, cocaine, morphine, and heroin adversely affects the patient's immune system and nutrition. Patient gets prone to infectious diseases due to immune deficiencies and malnutrition (Kaushik et al. 2011; Friedman et al. 2006). On the other hand, some predisposing factors are directly associated with preparation of the drug; For example, dilution of black tar heroin, which is a form of raw and impure opium derivative (Bucardo et al. 2005), with farina, lidocaine, and even shoe-polish-saturated paper (Kaushik et al. 2011); addition of levamisole, which can cause infectious contaminations leading to reversible neutropenia, to cocaine for enhancing the cocaine's euphoric effects and using colored methamphetamines obtained by adding adulterants to increase their effects (Lee et al. 2012; Strathdee et al. 2008).

Drugs are generally dissolved within mild acids, like tartaric or citric acid, to increase tissue degradation on the injection site. One of the fruit juice used for dissolving heroin or cocaine before the injection is preserved lemon juice. Unfortunately, it is known to be a good culture medium for endogenous endophthalmitis caused by *Candida albicans* (Albini et al. 2007). Lemon juice is often used to dissolve solid brown heroin which is not only used after heating and inhaling but also used for injection (Melnychuk and Sole 2017). Sometimes the drug users put a tablet in their mouth and lick the injection syringe to facilitate the dissolving process. It may result as a potential source of *Candida inoculum* (Deutscher and Perlman 2008). Also, severe damage to the nasal epithelium during the inhalation of the drugs or damages on the skin during injection might play a predisposing role for infection (Kernt and Kampik 2010).

Several clinical manifestations of fungal infections such as endophthalmitis and chorioretinitis; infections of the CNS such as cerebral microabscesses, meningitis, and cerebral macroabscesses; vascular complications; and infective endocarditis may be observed as a result of intravenous (IV) drug use (Kaushik et al. 2011; Melnychuk and Sole 2017; Kernt and Kampik 2010; Aboltins et al. 2005; Hirst et al. 2005; Keyashian and Malani 2007; Zhou et al. 2016).

37.3.1 Endophthalmitis and Keratitis

Endogenous form of endophthalmitis is usually related to IV drug use. Hematogenous dissemination of the fungus especially *Candida* and *Aspergillus* species to the eye may result in endogenous endophthalmitis (Melnychuk and Sole 2017; Kernt and Kampik 2010; Keyashian and Malani 2007). There are some informative endogenous Candida endophthalmitis cases caused by injection of cocaine mixed with lemon juice in the related literature (Melnychuk and Sole 2017; Keyashian and Malani 2007). One of them was reported by Melnychuk and Sole (2017). This 23-year-old male patient with the history of IV brown heroin use reported to the Department of Emergency with the complaints of visual disturbances and left-sided visual loss. Fundoscopic examination of the patient was reported to be suggestive of possible *Candida* endophthalmitis (Melnychuk and Sole 2017). Another interesting and rarely reported endogenous *Candida* endophthalmitis case as a result of the use of buprenorphine was presented by Aboltins et al. (2005). Authors suggested that endophthalmitis could be associated with IV injection after sublingual diversion of the drug from the oropharyngeal cavity following its dispensation (Aboltins et al. 2005).

Aspergillus endophthalmitis and *Candida* endophthalmitis have also been reported among IV drug users associated with preparation of the drug such as using unsterile injection needles or syringes, dissolving solid drugs in impure tap water and/or or filtering the mix through cigarette filters (Hirst et al. 2005). While evaluating the literature, we noticed a rare case presenting as bilateral keratitis because of *Rhizopus* infection in a crack cocaine user, reported by Zhou et al. (2016). This 33-year-old male patient with the history of regularly using crack cocaine presented to the Department of Emergency with significant eye pain, redness, and progressively decreased vision in the right eye. He had been treated with antibiotics with no improvement. After culture results had been found to be positive for *Rhizopus* species and starting antifungal treatment, significant clinical improvement had been observed (Zhou et al. 2016).

In a case series including a total of 14 patients with crack cocaine-related corneal symptoms such as corneal ulcer or infectious keratitis, a total of 10 patients were defined to have both bacterial and fungal corneal ulcers (Sachs et al. 1993). One of the possible predisposing causes may be the anesthetic properties of cocaine causing the decreased corneal sensation and weakened blink reflex (Mantelli et al. 2015). Also the alkaline character of crack cocaine fumes can increase the risk of minimal chemical burns and can facilitate fungal infection on the corneal epithelial defects by promoting rubbing the eyes (Sachs et al. 1993).

Endogenous endophthalmitis and keratitis should be kept in mind by the psychiatrists because of its high morbidity and mortality among IV drug users. Once any visual change among these patients is noticed, because of early diagnosis and treatment's importance, ophthalmology consultation should be requested immediately. Second it is important to consider the fungal agents especially with a lack of clinical recovery after initial treatment with broad-spectrum antibiotics.

37.3.2 Infections Involving the Central Nervous System

Unfortunately, fungal infections of CNS can often be underdiagnosed or overlooked among IV drug users because of the lack of specific clinical symptoms for these populations. These patients were usually diagnosed after death (Kaushik et al. 2011).

Several clinical presentations of candidiasis such as cerebral micro- or macroabscesses, meningitis, and vascular complications can be seen as result of fungal infections of the CNS after systemic candidiasis (Henao and Vagner 2011). There are no "specific clinical manifestations" of CNS candidiasis especially for cerebral microabscesses which is defined as non-specific diffuse encephalopathy (Kaushik et al. 2011; Henao and Vagner 2011; Neves et al. 2014; Sánchez-Portocarrero et al. 2000). Although cerebral microabscesses are frequently diagnosed only after death of the patient because of being clinically silent, cerebral macroabscesses may be diagnosed easily with patient's clinical manifestations like fever, headache, diminished consciousness, and focal neurological signs and regarding neuroimaging studies such as computed tomography (CT) and magnetic resonance imaging (MRI) and also with culture of cerebrospinal fluid (Neves et al. 2014; Sánchez-Portocarrero et al. 2000). Vascular complications of fungal infections of the CNS can be observed as cerebral infarction, subarachnoid hemorrhage with or without mycotic aneurysms caused by *Candida* endocarditis (Sánchez-Portocarrero et al. 2000). Unfortunately, there is no specific diagnostic indication tool for fungal infections of the CNS regarding laboratory tests, serologic tests, and hematologic parameters. So, it is important to suspect fungal infections (Badiee and Hashemizadeh 2014).

In a review conducted by Kim et al. (1993), it was reported that drug addiction is one of the predisposing factors for cerebral aspergillosis. The cerebral infections, which are less frequent than candidiasis, were also reported with *Aspergillus* species among drug users (Hadley et al. 2017; Morrow et al. 1983). It has been reported that in immunocompromised patients with aspergillosis of the CNS, CT and MRI may reveal multiple septic infarcts involving the basal ganglia, internal capsule, and corpus callosum (Hadley et al. 2017). Also one of the less frequent but high mortal fungal infection among IV drug users is cerebral mucormycosis which is known to particularly affect the basal ganglia (Roden et al. 2005).

37.3.3 Infective Endocarditis

In a review conducted by Yuan (2014), it has been suggested that approximately in one-third of the patients with right-sided infective endocarditis, drug abuse was shown to be predisposing factor (Yuan 2014). IV drug user patients with infective endocarditis are frequently males and younger than non-drug user infective endocarditis (Colville et al. 2016). Also the most common fungal agent is *Candida albicans* (Ellis et al. 2001).

It has been suggested that drug paraphernalia and drug adulterants used for preparing the substance can impair the endocardium particularly on the right side and the tricuspid valve (Cole et al. 2011). One of the predisposing factors for infective endocarditis due to drug particularly cocaine is causing damage of the tissues or skin by vasoconstriction (Wurcel et al. 2015). Clinicians must be aware of infective endocarditis among IV drug users because of its high morbidity and mortality (Colville et al. 2016).

37.4 Dermatological Fungal Infections in Neuropsychiatric Disorders

It is well-known that psychiatric patients have various comorbid somatic conditions and a high death rate compared to general population (Dalmau et al. 1998). These may be due to many reasons such as insufficient self-care, side effects of psychotropic medications, alcohol and substance abuse, unhealthy eating habits, and immobile lifestyle (Brown et al. 1999; Weber et al. 2009). All these conditions are risk factors for metabolic disorders such as cardiovascular diseases, diabetes, and infectious diseases (Hennekens et al. 2005; Kernt and Kampik 2010; Weber et al. 2009). Among all of these comorbid conditions, skin disorders and fungal infections are relatively understudied subjects (Mookhoek et al. 2011). However, skin disorders are important for psychiatric disorders. This is because patients who have denied their psychiatric disease and seek no help may reach out for their dermatological disorders (Kuruvila et al. 2004). Indeed, it is expected that effective management of 1/3 of the patients who presented to Department of Dermatology is dependent on the recognition of emotional factors to some degree (Gupta and Gupta 1996).

Fungal infections involving the CNS have been included in the small number of investigations upon the various skin disorders in patients with psychiatric disorders. A high rate of skin disorders was determined in psychiatric patients in a study performed in the Netherlands and published on 2010, and higher rate of infectious skin disorders has been determined in psychiatric patients with diabetes and overweight psychiatric patients (Mookhoek et al. 2010). However, high prevalence of fungal infections in this study was determined to be similar with general European population (Mookhoek et al. 2010). Mookhoek et al. reported that fungal infections of the CNS may be more severe in patients with psychiatric disorders, and there may still be a significant difference between populations, because the severity of fungal infections has not been described in previous studies (Mookhoek et al. 2010). In a study of the same group on hospitalized psychiatric patients, dermatological problems were determined to be high in hospitalized psychiatric patients, infectious skin disorders were also determined to be high in diabetes patients, and prevalence of fungal infections was also determined to be similar with general European population (Mookhoek et al. 2011). In this study, fungal foot infections were determined to be higher in men (Mookhoek et al. 2011). In another study investigating the prevalence of dermatological disorders in subjects with psychiatric disorders, pityriasis versicolor, and dermatophyte infections were determined to be higher in male psychiatric patients (Kuruvila et al. 2004). In this study, pityriasis versicolor was determined to be significantly higher in psychiatric patients compared to control group (Kuruvila et al. 2004).

In a retrospective study performed in Japan (Kawai et al. 2014), tinea pedis was determined in 46.1% and tinea unguium was determined in 23.7% of 317 psychiatric inpatients. Tinea unguium was determined in 48.6% of patients with tinea pedis, and no statistically significant difference was observed between both sexes (men and women) or schizophrenic patients and depression patients in tinea pedis or tinea unguium rates (Kawai et al. 2014). The authors, suggesting that patients hospitalized in a psychiatric hospital may face difficulties in providing sufficient self-care including daily foot care due to various reasons such as apathy or lack of interest, and this may worsen the state of the foot in a psychiatric patient with tinea pedis, state that schizophrenia, and resistant depression should be recognized as important risk factors for tinea pedis and tinea unguium, like diabetes and HIV infections (Kawai et al. 2014).

In a previous study, a total of 337 patients with schizophrenia and healthy population were compared, and it was found that fungal infections were the most common skin disorder in schizophrenic patients in this study (Wu et al. 2014). While fungal infections are determined to be more common in obese patients, risk of fungal infections was determined to be lower in patients using clozapine compared to patients using typical antipsychotics (Wu et al. 2014). The authors attributed this to the fact that clozapine shows an immunomodulator effect by inducing several cytokines such as interleukin-6 and tumor necrosis factor-α, and they have indicated that this immunomodulator effect may alter the immune response of the patient against the fungal infection, and thus it may form a protective effect (Wu et al. 2014). Skin disorders were also determined to be much higher in schizophrenic patients compared to general population in this study (Wu et al. 2014).

Today, there are studies which determined an increased risk of fungal infections and other infectious skin disorders in subjects with schizophrenia and other psychiatric disorders. According to studies, this risk is higher particularly in patients with obesity and diabetes. This may be due to several different reasons. To begin with, metabolic syndrome and diabetes are common comorbid disorders in schizophrenia and some psychiatric disorders by the effect of the nature of psychiatric disorders, lifestyle of patients, and psychotropic medications used. Considering the predisposition of diabetes patients toward infectious diseases, this relation may be secondary (Mookhoek et al. 2010, 2011).

Another reason of the increased risk in schizophrenic patients may be related to immune response. In addition to decreased levels of natural killer cytotoxicity/lymphocyte proliferation in some psychiatric patients, disruption of monocytic system in schizophrenic patients may increase sensitivity toward infectious skin disorders (Cohen et al. 2001; Krause et al. 2012).

Another reason may be the disruption of self-care and decreased seeking of medical care due to symptoms such as cognitive impairment, apathy, anergy, and lack of interest in schizophrenia and some psychiatric disorders (Moftah et al. 2013; Mohamed et al. 1999). Inability of patients to perform daily cleaning routines increases the risk of fungal infections and other infectious skin disorders (Moftah et al. 2013; Mercan and Kivac Altunay 2006). Some of patients may even be unaware of these disorders due to negative symptoms (Wu et al. 2014). Moreover, there are studies showing that schizophrenic patients have higher pain threshold, and this may prevent them from seeking help until their symptoms become severe (Jeste et al. 1996). Fungal infections of the CNS may cause secondary acute bacterial cellulitis and increase morbidity in this patient group, if they are undetected and untreated in early period (Bristow and Spruce 2009).

Similar to the fact that psychiatric disorders increase the risk of infectious skin disorders and some fungal infections, some fungal infections may have an effect on the mental state (Chacon et al. 2013). Psychological and social parameters affect function, well-being, and quality of life. Chacon et al. suggested that the prevalence of major depression is increased in patients with onychomycosis due to negative psychosocial reasons such as shame, low self-esteem and social withdrawal (Chacon et al. 2013). Accordingly, in a study performed in 258 patients with onychomycosis in 1998, 74% of patients have reported they are ashamed of their state (Drake et al. 1998). Also, it has been stated that the mental health of onychomycosis patients is under higher risk compared to normal population due to reasons such as appearance anxiety and disrupted social functionality (Chacon et al. 2013; Lubeck et al. 1993).

37.5 Conclusion

In recent years, an increased incidence of fungal infections involving the CNS is worldwide due to considerable rise in the number of immunosuppressed patients. In some cases, fungal lesions may present with various neuropsychiatric symptoms; therefore microscopic identification of the organism is very important for definite diagnosis of fungal infection in these cases. We stress that a high index of suspicion is of utmost importance in differentiating fungal infections from certain neuropsychiatric disorders to reduce the rates of mortality and morbidity.

References

Aboltins CA, Allen P, Daffy JR. Fungal endophthalmitis in intravenous drug users injecting buprenorphine contaminated with oral Candida species. Med J Aust. 2005;182:427.

Albini TA, Sun RL, Holz ER, Khurana RN, Rao NA. Lemon juice and candida endophthalmitis in crack-cocaine misuse. Br J Ophthalmol. 2007;91:702–3.

Aylward EH, Henderer JD, McArthur JC, Brettschneider PD, Harris GJ, Barta PE, Pearlson GD. Reduced basal ganglia volume in HIV-1-associated dementia: results from quantitative neuroimaging. Neurology. 1993;43:2099.

Badiee P, Hashemizadeh Z. Opportunistic invasive fungal infections: diagnosis & clinical management. Indian J Med Res. 2014;139:195–204.

Bicanic T, Jarvis JN, Muzoora C, Harrison TS. Should antiretroviral therapy be delayed for 10 weeks for patients treated with fluconazole with cryptococcal meningitis? Clin Infect Dis. 2010;51:986–7.

Bristow IR, Spruce MC. Fungal foot infection, cellulitis and diabetes: a review. Diabet Med. 2009;26:548–51.

Brown S, Birtwistle J, Roe L, et al. The unhealthy lifestyle of people with schizophrenia. Psychol Med. 1999;29:697–701.

Bucardo J, Brouwer KC, Magis-Rodríguez C, Ramos R, Fraga M, Perez SG, Patterson TL, Strathdee SA. Historical trends in the production and consumption of illicit drugs in Mexico: implications for the prevention of blood borne infections. Drug Alcohol Depend. 2005;79:281–93.

Chacon A, Franca K, Fernandez A, Nouri K. Psychosocial impact of onychomycosis: a review. Int J Dermatol. 2013;52:1300–7.

Chen M, Xu Y, Hong N, Yang Y, Lei W, Du L, Zhao J, Lei X, Xiong L, Cai L, Xu H, Pan W, Liao W. Epidemiology of fungal infections in China. Front Med. 2018;12:58–75.

Chou PH, Ouyang WC, Lan TH, Chan CH. Secondary mania due to AIDS and cryptococcal meningitis in a 78-year-old patient. Psychogeriatrics. 2016;16: 135–8.

Cohen S, Miller GE, Rabin BS. Psychological stress and antibody response to immunization: a critical review of the human literature. Psychosom Med. 2001; 63:7–18.

Cole C, Jones L, McVeigh J, Kicman A, Syed Q, Bellis M. Adulterants in illicit drugs: a review of empirical evidence. Drug Test Anal. 2011;3:89–96.

Colville T, Sharma V, Albouaini K. Infective endocarditis in intravenous drug users: a review article. Postgrad Med J. 2016;92:105–11.

Dalmau AB, Berman BK, Brismar BG. Somatic morbidity among patients diagnosed with affective psychosis and paranoid disorders. Psychosomatics. 1998;39:253–62.

Deutscher M, Perlman DC. Why some injection drug users lick their needles: a preliminary survey. Int J Drug Policy. 2008;19:342–5.

Drake LA, Scher RK, Smith EB, Faich GA, Smith SL, Hong JJ, Stiller MJ. Effect of onychomycosis on quality of life. J Am Acad Dermatol. 1998;38:702–4.

Ellis ME, Al-Abdely H, Sandridge A, Greer W, Ventura W. Fungal endocarditis: evidence in the world literature, 1965–1995. Clin Infect Dis. 2001;32:50–62.

Friedman H, Pross S, Klein TW. Addictive drugs and their relationship with infectious diseases. FEMS Immunol Med Microbiol. 2006;47:330–42.

Goeb JL, Leon V, Kechid G. Cryptococcal meningitis with acute psychotic confusion in a sarcoid patient. Prim Care Companion J Clin Psychiatry. 2007;9:393–4.

Gupta MA, Gupta AK. Psychodermatology: an update. J Am Acad Dermatol. 1996;34:1030–46.

Hadley C, Mohamed AWH, Singhal A. Central nervous system fungal infection in a young male with a history of intravenous drug abuse and hepatitis C. Radiol Case Rep. 2017;13(12):590–6.

Henao NA, Vagner B. Infections of the central nervous system by Candida. J Infect Dis Immun. 2011;3:79–81.

Hennekens CH, Hennekens AR, Hollar D, Casey DE. Schizophrenia and increased risks of cardiovascular disease. Am Heart J. 2005;150:1115–21.

Hirst LW, Thomas JV, Green WR. Endophthalmitis. In: Mandell GL, Bennett JE, Dolin R, editors. Mandell, Douglas, and Bennett's principles and practice of infectious diseases. Philadelphia, PA: Churchill Livingstone; 2005. p. 760–7.

Holikatti PC, Kar N. Psychiatric manifestations in a patient with HIV-associated neurocognitive symptoms and cryptococcal meningitis. Indian J Psychol Med. 2012;34:381–2.

Hsueh KL, Lin PY. Treatment-resistant depression prior to the diagnosis of cryptococcal meningitis: a case report. Gen Hosp Psychiatry. 2010;32:560.e9–10.

Ibanez-Valdes L, Foyaca-Sibat H, Mfenyana K, Chandia J, Gonzalez-Aguilera H. Neuropsychiatry manifestations in patients presenting cryptococcal meningitis. Int J Neurol. 2005;5(1)

Jacob R, Zhimin Z, Rayapureddy S, Isaacs RT. Cryptococcal meningitis presenting as acute psychosis in a HIV positive patient. Asian J Psychiatr. 2013;6:624–5.

Jeste DV, Gladsjo JA, Lindamer LA, Lacro JP. Medical comorbidity in schizophrenia. Schizophr Bull. 1996;22:413–30.

Johannessen DJ, Wilson LG. Mania with cryptococcal meningitis in two AIDS patients. J Clin Psychiatry. 1988;49:200–1.

Johnson FY, Naraqi S. Manic episode secondary to cryptococcal meningitis in a previously healthy adult. P N G Med J. 1993;36:59–62.

Kaushik KS, Kapila K, Praharaj AK. Shooting up: the interface of microbial infections and drug abuse. J Med Microbiol. 2011;60:408–22.

Kawai M, Suzuki T, Hiruma M, Ikeda S. A retrospective cohort study of tinea pedis and tinea unguium in inpatients in a psychiatric hospital. Med Mycol J. 2014;55:E35–41.

Kernt M, Kampik A. Endophthalmitis: pathogenesis, clinical presentation, management, and perspectives. Clin Ophthalmol. 2010;4:121–35.

Keyashian K, Malani PN. Endophthalmitis associated with intravenous drug use. South Med J. 2007;100:1219–20.

Kim DG, Hong SC, Kim HJ, Chi JG, Han MH, Choi KS, Han DH. Cerebral aspergillosis in immunologically competent patients. Surg Neurol. 1993;40:326e31.

Krause DL, Wagner JK, Wildenauer A, Matz J, Weidinger E, Riedel M, Obermeier M, Gruber R, Schwarz M, Müller N. Intracellular monocytic cytokine levels in schizophrenia show an alteration of IL-6. Eur Arch Psychiatry Clin Neurosci. 2012;262:393–401.

Kumar A, Gopinath S, Dinesh KR, Karim S. Infectious psychosis: cryptococcal meningitis presenting as a neuropsychiatry disorder. Neurol India. 2011;59:909–11.

Kuruvila M, Gahalaut P, Zacharia A. A study of skin disorders in patients with primary psychiatric conditions. Indian J Dermatol Venereol Leprol. 2004;70:292–5.

Lee KC, Ladizinski B, Federman DG. Complications associated with use of levamisole-contaminated cocaine: an emerging public health challenge. Mayo Clin Proc. 2012;87:581–6.

Lubeck DP, Patrick DL, McNulty P, Fifer SK, Birnbaum J. Quality of life of persons with onychomycosis. Qual Life Res. 1993;2:341–3.

Mantelli F, Lambiase A, Sacchetti M, Orlandi V, Rosa A, Casella P, Bonini S. Cocaine snorting may induce ocular surface damage through corneal sensitivity impairment. Graefes Arch Clin Exp Ophthalmol. 2015;253:765–72.

Melnychuk EM, Sole DP. A rare central nervous system fungal infection resulting from brown heroin. J Emerg Med. 2017;52:314–7.

Mercan S, Kivac Altunay I. Psychodermatology: collaboration between psychiatry and dermatology. Turk Psikiyatri Derq. 2006;17:305–13.

Moftah NH, Kamel AM, Attia HM, El-Baz MZ, Abd El-Moty HM. Skin diseases in patients with primary psychiatric conditions: a hospital based study. J Epidemiol Glob Health. 2013;3:131–8.

Mohamed S, Paulsen JS, O'Leary D, Arndt S, Andreasen N. Generalized cognitive deficits in schizophrenia: a study of first-episode patients. Arch Gen Psychiatry. 1999;56:749–54.

Mookhoek EJ, Van De Kerkhof PC, Hovens JE, Brouwers JR, Loonen AJ. Skin disorders in chronic psychiatric illness. J Eur Acad Dermatol Venereol. 2010;24:1151–6.

Mookhoek EJ, van de Kerkhof PC, Hovens JE, Brouwers JR, Loonen AJ. Substantial skin disorders in psychiatric illness coincide with diabetes and addiction. J Eur Acad Dermatol Venereol. 2011;25:392–7.

Morrow R, Wong B, Finkelstein WE, Sternberg SS, Armstrong D. Aspergillosis of the cerebral ventricles in a heroin abuser. Case report and review of the literature. Arch Intern Med. 1983;143:161–4.

Nakimuli-Mpungu E, Musisi S, Kiwuwa Mpungu S, Katabira E. Early-onset versus late-onset HIV-related secondary mania in Uganda. Psychosomatics. 2008;49:530–4.

Neves N, Santos L, Reis C, Sarmento A. Candida albicans brain abscesses in an injection drug user patient: a case report. BMC Res Notes. 2014;7:837.

Prakash PY, Sugandhi RP. Neuropsychiatric manifestation of confusional psychosis due to Cryptococcus neoformans var. grubii in an apparently immunocompetent host: a case report. Cases J. 2009;2:9084.

Roden MM, Zaoutis TE, Buchanan WL, Knudsen TA, Sarkisova TA, Schaufele RL, Sein M, Sein T, Chiou CC, Chu JH, Kontoyiannis DP, Walsh TJ. Epidemiology and outcome of Zygomycosis: a review of 929 reported cases. CID. 2005;4:634–53.

Rummel-Kluge C, Komossa K, Schwarz S, Hunger H, Schmid F, Kissling W, Davis JM, Leucht S. Second-generation antipsychotic drugs and extrapyramidal side effects: a systematic review and meta-analysis of head-to-head comparisons. Schizophr Bull. 2012;38:167–77.

Sa'adah MA, Araj GF, Diab SM, Nazzal M. Cryptococcal meningitis and confusional psychosis: a case report and literature review. Trop Geogr Med. 1995;47:224–6.

Sachs R, Zagelbaum BM, Hersh PS. Corneal complications associated with the use of crack cocaine. Ophthalmology. 1993;100:187–91.

Sánchez-Portocarrero J, Pérez-Cecilia E, Corral O, Romero-Vivas J, Picazob JJ. The central nervous system and infection by Candida species. Diagn Microbiol Infect Dis. 2000;37:169–79.

Satishchandra P, Mathew T, Gadre G, Nagarathna S, Chandramukhi A, Mahadevan A, Shankar SK. Cryptococcal meningitis: clinical, diagnostic and therapeutic overviews. Neurol India. 2007;55:226–32.

Sloan D, Dedicoat MJ, Lalloo DG. Treatment of cryptococcal meningitis in resource limited settings. Curr Opin Infect Dis. 2009;22:455–63.

Spiegel DR, Bayne CE, Wilcox L, Somova M. A case of mania due to cryptococcal meningitis, successfully treated with adjunctive olanzapine, in a patient with acquired immunodeficiency syndrome. Gen Hosp Psychiatry. 2011;33:301.e3–6.

Strathdee SA, Case P, Lozada R, Mantsios A, Alvelais J, Pu M, Brouwer KC, Miller CL, Patterson TL. The color of meth: is it related to adverse health outcomes? An exploratory study in Tijuana, Mexico. Am J Addict. 2008;17:111–5.

Tang WK, Hui M, Ungvari GS, Leung CM. Cryptococcal meningitis mimicking primary mania in a young female. Gen Hosp Psychiatry. 2005;27:301–3.

Thienhaus OJ, Khosla N. Meningeal cryptococcosis misdiagnosed as a manic episode. Am J Psychiatry. 1984;141:1459–60.

Weber NS, Cowan DN, Millikan AM, Niebuhr DW. Psychiatric and general medical conditions comorbid with schizophrenia in the National Hospital Discharge Survey. Psychiatr Serv. 2009;60:1059–67.

Wu BY, Wu BJ, Lee SM, Sun HJ, Chang YT, Lin MW. Prevalence and associated factors of comorbid skin diseases in patients with schizophrenia: a clinical survey and national health database study. Gen Hosp Psychiatry. 2014;36:415–21.

Wurcel AG, Merchant EA, Clark RP, Stone DR. Emerging and underrecognized complications of illicit drug use. Clin Infect Dis. 2015;15(61):1840–9.

Yuan SM. Right-sided infective endocarditis: recent epidemiologic changes. Int J Clin Exp Med. 2014;7:199–218.

Zhou M, Farooq AV, Andreoli MT, Ali M, Traish AS. Bilateral Rhizopus keratitis in a cocaine user. Can J Ophthalmol. 2016;51:e21–3.

Real-Time PCR: Advanced Technologies and Applications

38

Güliz Uyar Güleç and Yaşar Barış Turgut

Abbreviations

CNS	Central nervous system
CSF	Cerebrospinal fluid
dsDNA	Double-stranded DNA
FRET	Fluorescence resonance energy transfer
HIV	Human immunodeficiency virus
ITS	Internal transcribed spacer
PCR	Polymerase chain reaction
rDNA	Ribosomal DNA

38.1 Introduction

Fungal infections of central nervous system (CNS) are uncommon clinical situations (Panackal and Williamson 2015; Sharma 2010). But clinical presentations are variable and subtle, diagnosis is difficult, and the therapy has challenges (Sharma 2010; Sheikh and Amr 2010). Unfortunately, the incidence of fungal infections of CNS has greatly increased especially in the immunocompromised person even in the pediatric population in recent times (Sharma 2010; McCarthy et al. 2017). Granulocytopenia, cellular- and humoral-mediated immune dysfunctions because of organ transplants, chemotherapies, human immunodeficiency virus (HIV) infections, and the widespread use of antibacterial agents are the factors that increase the number of at risk group (Sheikh and Amr 2010; Schwartz et al. 2018). Furthermore, immunocompetent subjects may be infected through inoculation during neurosurgical procedures, contaminated devices, or drug preparations including intravenous drug misuse or following heavy exposure in endemic areas (Schwartz et al. 2018).

The fungal infections of CNS may cause different clinical syndromes as discussed in earlier chapters, such as fungal meningoencephalitis, granuloma or abscess formation, communicating or obstructive hydrocephalus, cerebral infarction, arterial aneurysm, and various spinal syndromes (Panackal and Williamson 2015; McCarthy et al. 2017; Schwartz et al. 2018). These infections are life-threatening and have high morbidity and mortality (Panackal and Williamson 2015; Sheikh and Amr 2010). The early recognition of clinical syndromes with implementation of efficacious management is essential (Panackal and Williamson 2015). Laboratory diagnosis of fungal CNS infection is based on culture, histopathological examination, and serological testing. Because of limitations of these methods, molecular techniques such as polymerase chain reaction

G. U. Güleç (✉)
Deparment of Infectious Diseases and Clinical Microbiology, Aydın Adnan Menderes University School of Medicine, Aydın, Turkey
e-mail: guliz.uyar@adu.edu.tr

Y. B. Turgut
Department of Internal Medicine, Muğla Sıtkı Koçman University School of Medicine, Muğla, Turkey

M. Turgut et al. (eds.), *Fungal Infections of the Central Nervous System*,
https://doi.org/10.1007/978-3-030-06088-6_38

(PCR) techniques could facilitate diagnostic confirmation (Schwartz et al. 2018). Real-time PCR has emerged as a suitable and faster technique for identification and quantification of fungal agents.

In this chapter we aim to discuss general characteristics and clinical applications of real-time PCR technique based on clinical trials.

38.2 General Characteristics of Real-Time PCR

The PCR assay has found extensive use in microbiology laboratories since its introduction in 1983. Improvements in technology and chemistry developed PCR methods in time (Stephenson 2016). Firstly, as quoted by Kaltenboeck and Wang (2005) Higuchi et al. introduced real-time PCR by to analyze the kinetics of PCR by constructing a system for detection of PCR products in the amplification process. The most prominent feature of real-time PCR assays is that products of a reaction are measured in "real time," as the PCR reaction is being performed, rather than following the completion of the reaction (Loftis and Reeves 2012).

In real-time PCR, two general chemistries are available for amplicon detection. These are DNA-binding dyes and fluorescent probes (Arya et al. 2005). The assays using DNA-binding dyes are simple and cost-effective. Ethidium bromide was used in the earliest form of real-time PCR. SYBR Green 1, less toxic and sensitive dye, binds to only double-stranded DNA (dsDNA) (Loftis and Reeves 2012; Arya et al. 2005). The progress of PCR amplification may be followed in real time by measuring the fluorescence of sample during each stage of amplification reaction cycle (Kaltenboeck and Wang 2005; Loftis and Reeves 2012).

The other one uses fluorescently labeled oligonucleotide probe that anneals to one of the template strands. Specific hybridization between probe and template generates signal. Among the probe formats, the most common are fluorescence resonance energy transfer (FRET), TaqMan or 5′ nuclease, scorpions, and molecular beacons (Stephenson 2016; Arya et al. 2005; Espy et al. 2006). After hybridization of the oligonucleotide to the amplicon, the light emission of a fluorescent dye coupled to an oligonucleotide changes. This is the basis for the amplicon-specific detection of fluorescence (Kaltenboeck and Wang 2005). In real-time PCR, several examples of amplicon detection methods are shown in Fig. 38.1 (Yadav and Singh 2017).

In the conventional PCR, qualitative information may be obtained by detection of a specific dsDNA product using gel electrophoresis at the end of amplification (Kaltenboeck and Wang 2005). In real-time PCR, however, quantitative information may be obtained by plotting the intensity of the fluorescence signal versus cycle number (Kaltenboeck and Wang 2005).

Melting curve analysis is performed to understand whether the obtained fluorescence is achieved by amplification of the desired target region or is a nonspecific product (Loftis and Reeves 2012). After the amplification is complete, samples are cooled and then slowly heated, while fluorescence is monitored to determine the temperature at which the dsDNA-binding dye is released (Loftis and Reeves 2012). In Fig. 38.2, an example of melting curve analysis is shown (Buil et al. 2017).

As filamentous fungi have complex cell wall that is difficult to disrupt, rigorous extraction methods are required. It has been reported that the most important factors for the sensitivity of any PCR assay are complete lysis of fungal cells from various biological samples and purification of DNA without inhibitors (Espy et al. 2006; Francesconi et al. 2008). There are manual and automated or semiautomated extraction methods. The use of a standardized, efficient, and rapid DNA extraction method is a main component for both the optimization and reproducibility of quantitative PCR assays (Espy et al. 2006; Francesconi et al. 2008).

The PCR primer must be highly efficient and specific for the target primer sequences in the specimen of interest (Espy et al. 2006). For molecular identification of fungi, the DNA-coding sequences appear as an excellent target for PCR amplification, while RNA is very rarely used (Somogyvari et al. 2012). The vast majority of assays target the ribosomal DNA (rDNA)

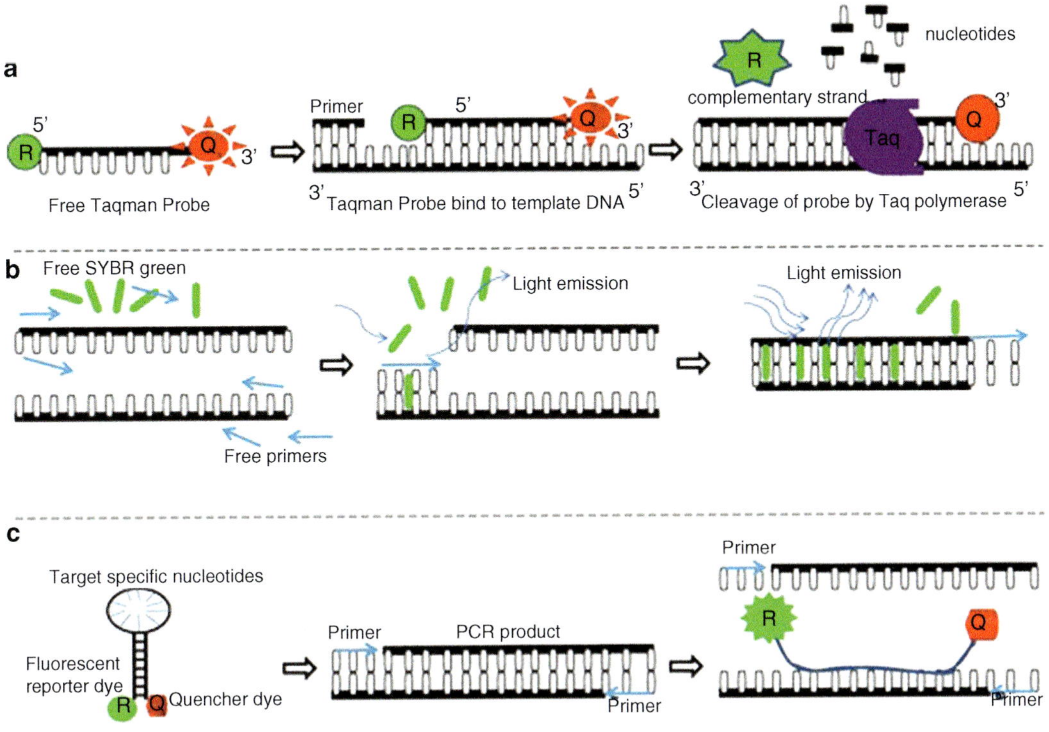

Fig. 38.1 Three representative examples of amplicon detection methods in real-time polymerase chain reaction (PCR). (**a**) TaqMan probe, (**b**) SYBR Green 1 dye method, (**c**) Molecular beacon method (Reproduced, with permission, from Yadav and Singh: Molecular Markers in Mycology. Fungal Biology. Springer, Cham, 2017)

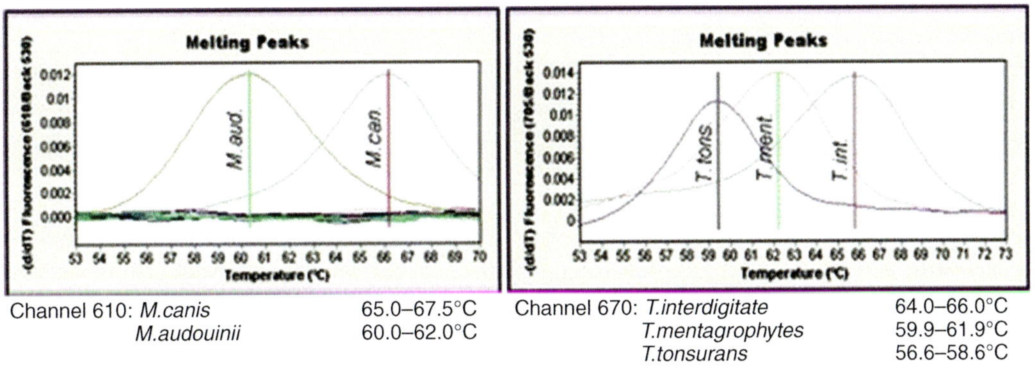

Fig. 38.2 A representative example of melting curve analysis (Reproduced, with permission, from Buil et al.: Molecular Diagnostics. Springer, Singapore, 2017)

genes 18S, 28S, and 5.8S and the intervening internal transcribed spacer (ITS) regions (ITS1 and ITS2) on rDNA (Lau et al. 2007). Owing to the presence of multicopy genes, they have universal fungal primers and contain highly variable regions for identification of species (Lau et al. 2007). In addition, the ITS sequences may be used as reference standards for the validation of some methods such as repetitive-sequence PCR (Somogyvari et al. 2012). Studies regarding identification of fungi showed that the most useful targets are the ITS1 are the ITS2 regions which are followed by the D1 and D2 regions of the 28S rDNA (Lau et al. 2007).

Significant application areas of real-time PCR are detecting and quantifying DNA and RNA of microorganism, genotyping and following treatment efficacy, monitoring the transcription of genes, and typing of genetic polymorphisms (Kaltenboeck and Wang 2005; Espy et al. 2006; Bretagne 2003). The fast turnaround time of less than 2 h and minimal false-positive results because of no postamplification handling are advantages of real-time PCR for routine mycology laboratory (Bretagne 2003).

Nevertheless, there are some disadvantages of real-time PCR assays: (1) false-negative results due to their excess sensitivity to various inhibitors in the environment, (2) lack of any information about infectivity of pathogen because the assays give only number of total pathogens, and (3) the presence of inconsistent results from variable assay designs for same samples (Johnson et al. 2012).

38.3 Clinical Applications of Real-Time PCR

Fungi are important as emerging pathogens. The diagnostic approach for invasive fungal infections is to detect the strain as early as possible (Liu et al. 2012). To date, many real-time PCR protocols have been suggested for *Aspergillus* and *Candida* species, but there are also protocols for other less frequent species (Klingspor and Jalal 2006; Schabereiter-Gurtner et al. 2007). It may be difficult to obtain CNS samples due to the poor conditions of the patients. Samples are valuable and may be small in amount.

Morton et al. (Morton et al. 2011) used real-time PCR in blood, brain, cerebrospinal fluid (CSF), and spinal cord samples for detection of *A. fumigatus* in neutropenic mice; fungal DNA was detected at highest concentrations in the brain (96%) and spinal cord (92%). Their extraction protocol allowed PCR detection of fungal DNA from small sample volumes (10 μl CSF, 200 μl blood) (Morton et al. 2011). In another study, CSF samples and sera from patients suspected of fungal meningitis were evaluated for *Aspergillus* and *Candida* DNA by real-time PCR (Badiee and Alborzi 2011). In this study, a total 152 samples from 38 patients were examined; 10 patients had positive real-time PCR result in CSF samples; and 4 of them had positive serum results for *Aspergillus* or *Candida* spp (Badiee and Alborzi 2011).

A study from Sweden evaluated clinical applicability of real-time PCR targeting 18S rRNA in the detection of *Candida* spp. and *Aspergillus* spp., using a total of 1330 blood samples, 295 samples of other body fluids, and 25 samples of biopsy specimen (Klingspor and Jalal 2006). In this study, a positive result for *Candida* spp was obtained in only 4 of 24 CSF samples (17%) (Klingspor and Jalal 2006). However, it has been reported that the technique used identified fungal DNA in various samples with a high sensitivity and specificity in a short time (Klingspor and Jalal 2006).

Cultural isolation of fungus is time-consuming and not always possible. PCR-based diagnostic approaches may be considered for formalin-fixed, paraffin-embedded material if there is no alternative sample material available. Nowadays, many studies have underlined the advantages of PCR technology for identification of fungal pathogens, viable or nonviable, in different biopsy samples. However, sample age and environmental contaminants are important factors to be considered in these studies (Frickmann et al. 2015).

In a retrospective study, a total of 151 biopsy specimens including lung, skin, liver, and brain samples were examined; fresh (n = 92) and paraffin-embedded (n = 52) tissues were analyzed, and a total of 28 different fungal species were detected: *Aspergillus* spp. (47%), endemic mycoses (21%), *Mucormycetes* (10%), *Candida* spp. (8%), and other rare species. (14%) (Buitrago et al. 2014). In another study, the ability of a quantitative real-time PCR assay targeting the ITS region of rDNA of *Aspergillus*, *Fusarium*, *Scedosporium*, and *Mucormycetes* was retrospectively evaluated in a total of 102 paraffin-embedded tissue specimens following formalin fixation (Salehi et al. 2016). It has been confirmed that real-time PCR assay is useful for rapid and accurate identification of various fungal pathogens (Salehi et al. 2016).

A real-time PCR that could simultaneously detect bacteria and fungi in same CSF by one

PCR reaction was designed. Among 137 CSF specimens, 20 bacterial strains and 7 fungal strains were detected with higher sensitivity than conventional methods. The authors concluded that this TaqMan probe-based real-time PCR can be applied to other biological fluids as well as CSF (Han et al. 2014).

When the clinical picture does not point out a specific agent, the utility of species-specific approaches remains limited. Therefore, fungal PCR assays with a broad range as an alternative method have been developed to overcome this problem. Landlinger et al. (Landlinger et al. 2010) introduced a real-time PCR with panfungal range for detection of more than 80 pathogenic fungi. In this study, more than 600 peripheral blood specimens, 11 CSF, and 2 lung biopsies were investigated (Landlinger et al. 2010). They found the sensitivity of the assay as 96% (95% CI, 82–99%) and the specificity as 77% (95% CI, 66–85%), while the negative and positive predictive values were 98% (95% CI, 90–100%) and 62% (95% CI, 47–75%), respectively (Landlinger et al. 2010). A real-time PCR assay with panfungal range using the combination of a DNA-binding dye and specific molecular beacon probes following by a melting curve analysis was designed by Valero et al. (2016). In this study, a total of 44 fresh or paraffin-embedded biopsy specimens, 8 respiratory samples, 5 CSF, 1 aqueous humor, and 1 nail sample were tested, with a sensitivity of 83.3% (Valero et al. 2016).

Specifically, a fast identification is of great importance for effective treatment for mucorales (Spellberg et al. 2009). Therefore, a real-time PCR assay using the FRET probes was developed for detection of mucorales, and the sensitivity of the PCR assay using samples from culture and fresh tissue was 100%, in contrast to lower values at 57% from samples from paraffin-embedded tissues following formalin fixation (Hata et al. 2008). No cross-reactivity demonstrated with the species of other fungi and bacteria (Hata et al. 2008). The authors concluded that use of real-time PCR in the diagnosis of mucormycosis reduced the duration of diagnosis from days to hours (Hata et al. 2008). Moreover, 18S rDNA-specific real-time PCR was evaluated in a study using serum and tissue samples from patients with invasive mucormycosis because biopsy procedure in a patient may cause various complications. This PCR-based method has a high sensitivity (91%) in paraffin-embedded tissue samples, and more importantly *Mucorales* DNA was detected in the sera of all probable/proven patients (100%), with an earlier diagnosis than tissue samples (Springer et al. 2016).

Cryptococcal disease has become a major infection, especially in HIV-infected individuals. Conventional nested and real-time PCR were compared in murine model of cryptococcal meningitis. Real-time PCR was found more sensitive and rapid method (Bialek et al. 2002). For endemic mycosis the role of real-time PCR is unclear and limited in clinical experience or remains investigational (McCarthy et al. 2017).

38.4 Conclusion

Real-time PCR is highly sensitive and rapid technique for fungal identification. Quantification of fungal burden is one of the important steps for management of fungal infections of CNS. With developments in molecular technologies, real-time PCR methodology is improving. Nucleic acid extraction method, primers, targets, and PCR detection chemistries must carefully be chosen for reliable results. Usefulness of real-time PCR in clinical laboratory should strengthen with prospective clinical trials.

References

Arya M, Shergill IS, Williamson M, Gommersal L, Arya N, Patel HRH. Basic principles of real-time quantitative PCR. Expert Rev Mol Diagn. 2005;5(2):209–19.

Badiee P, Alborzi A. Assessment of a real-time PCR method to detect human non-cryptococcal fungal meningitis. Arch Iran Med. 2011;14(6):381–4.

Bialek R, Weiss M, Bekure-Nemariam K, Najvar LK, Alberdi MB, Graybill JR, Reischl U. Detection of Cryptococcus neoformans DNA in tissue samples by nested and real-time PCR assays. Clin Diagn Lab Immunol. 2002;9(2):461–9.

Bretagne S. Molecular diagnostics in clinical parasitology and mycology: limits of the current polymerase chain reaction (PCR) assays and interest of the real-time PCR assays. Clin Microbiol Infect. 2003;9:505–11.

Buil JB, Zoll J, Verweij PE, Melchers WJ, Bergmans A. Mycology. In: van Pelt-Verkuil E, van Leeuwen W, te Witt R, editors. Molecular diagnostics. Singapore: Springer; 2017.

Buitrago MJ, Bernal-Martinez L, Castelli MV, Rodriguez-Tudela JL, Cuenca-Estrella M. Performance of panfungal- and specific-PCR-based procedures for etiological diagnosis of invasive fungal diseases on tissue biopsy specimens with proven infection: a 7-year retrospective analysis from a reference laboratory. J Clin Microbiol. 2014;52(5):1737–40.

Espy MJ, Uhl JR, Sloan LM, Buckwalter SP, Jones MF, Vetter EA, Yao JDC, Wengenack NL, Rosenblatt JE, Cockerill FR, Smith TF. Real-time PCR in clinical microbiology: applications for routine laboratory testing. Clin Microbiol Rev. 2006;19(1):165–256.

Francesconi A, Kasai M, Harrington SM, Beveridge MG, Petraitiene R, Petraitis V, Schaufele RL, Walsh TJ. Automated and manual methods of DNA extraction for *Aspergillus fumigatus* and *Rhizopus oryzae* analyzed by quantitative real-time PCR. J Clin Microbiol. 2008;46(6):1978–84.

Frickmann H, Loderstaedt U, Racz P, Tenner-Racz K, Eggert P, Haeupler A, Bialek R, Hagen RM. Detection of tropical fungi in formalin-fixed, paraffin-embedded tissue: still an indication for microscopy in times of sequence-based diagnosis? Biomed Res Int. 2015;2015:938721.

Han H, Hu Z, Sun S, Yao F, Yan X, Zhang X, Wu B. Simultaneous detection and identification of bacteria and fungi in cerebrospinal fluid by TaqMan probe-based real-time PCR. Clin Lab. 2014;60:1287–93.

Hata DJ, Buckwalter SP, Pritt BS, Roberts GD, Wengenack NL. Real-time PCR method for detection of zygomycetes. J Clin Microbiol. 2008;46(7):2353–8.

Johnson GL, Bibby DF, Wong S, Agrawal SG, Bustin SA. A MIQE-compliant real-time PCR assay for Aspergillus detection. PLoS One. 2012;7(7):e40022.

Kaltenboeck B, Wang C. Advances in real-time PCR: application to clinical laboratory diagnostics. Adv Clin Chem. 2005;40:219–59.

Klingspor L, Jalal S. Molecular detection and identification of Candida and Aspergillus spp. from clinical samples using real-time PCR. Clin Microbiol Infect. 2006;12(8):745–53.

Landlinger C, Preuner S, Bašková L, van Grotel M, Hartwig NG, Dworzak M, Mann G, Attarbaschi A, Kager L, Peters C, Matthes-Martin S, Lawitschka A, van den Heuvel-Eibrink MM, Lion T. Diagnosis of invasive fungal infections by a real-time panfungal PCR assay in immunocompromised pediatric patients. Leukemia. 2010;24(12):2032–8.

Lau A, Chen S, Sorrell T, Carter D, Malik R, Martin P, Halliday C. Development and clinical application of a panfungal PCR assay to detect and identify fungal DNA in tissue specimens. J Clin Microbiol. 2007;45(2):380–5.

Liu CM, Kachur S, Dwan MG, Abraham AG, Aziz M, Hsueh P, Huang Y, Busch JD, Lamit LJ, Gehring CA, Keim P, Price LB. FungiQuant: a broad-coverage fungal quantitative real-time PCR assay. BMC Microbiol. 2012;12:255.

Loftis AD, Reeves WK. Principles of real- time PCR. In: Wang C, Kaltenboeck B, Freeman MD, editors. Veterinary PCR diagnostics: Bentham ebooks; 2012. p. 3–17.

McCarthy MW, Kalasauskas D, Petraitis V, Petraitiene R, Walsh TJ. Fungal infections of the central nervous system in children. J Pediatric Infect Dis Soc. 2017;6(3):e123–e33.

Morton CO, Clemons KV, Springer J, Mueller JG, Rogers TR, Stevens DA, Kurzai O, Einsele H, Loeffler J, Real-time PCR. Quantitative culture for monitoring of experimental *Aspergillus fumigatus* intracranial infection in neutropenic mice. J Med Microbiol. 2011;60(Pt7):913–9.

Panackal AA, Williamson PR. Fungal infections of the central nervous system. Continuum (Minneap Minn). 2015;21(6):1662–78.

Salehi E, Hedayati MT, Zoll J, Rafati H, Ghasemi M, Doroudinia A, Abastabar M, Tolooe A, Snelders E, van der Lee HA, Rijs AJ, Verweij PE, Seyedmousavi S, Melchers WJ. Discrimination of aspergillosis, mucormycosis, fusariosis, and scedosporiosis in formalin-fixed paraffin-embedded tissue specimens by use of multiple real-time quantitative PCR assays. J Clin Microbiol. 2016;54(11):2798–803.

Schabereiter-Gurtner C, Selitsch B, Rotter ML, Hirschl AM, Willinger B. Development of novel real-time PCR assays for detection and differentiation of eleven medically important Aspergillus and Candida species in clinical specimens. J Clin Microbiol. 2007;45(3):906–14.

Schwartz S, Kontoyiannis DP, Harrison T, Ruhnke M. Advances in the diagnosis and treatment of fungal infections of the CNS. Lancet Neurol. 2018;17:362–72.

Sharma RR. Fungal infections of the nervous system: current perspective and controversies in management. Int J Surg. 2010;8:591–601.

Sheikh SS, Amr SS. Fungal infections of the central nervous system. In: Rai M, Kövics G, editors. Progress in mycology. India: Scientific Publishers; 2010. p. 141–80.

Somogyvari F, Horvath A, Serly J, Majoros H, Vagvolgyi C, Peto Z. Detection of invasive fungal pathogens by real-time PCR and high-resolution melting analysis. In Vivo. 2012;26:979–84.

Spellberg B, Walsh TJ, Kontoyiannis DP, Edwards J Jr, Ibrahim AS. Recent advances in the management of mucormycosis: from bench to bedside. Clin Infect Dis. 2009;48(12):1743–51.

Springer J, Lackner M, Ensinger C, Risslegger B, Morton CO, Nachbaur D, Lass-Flörl C, Einsele H, Heinz WJ, Loeffler J. Clinical evaluation of a Mucorales-specific real-time PCR assay in tissue and serum samples. J Med Microbiol. 2016;65:1414–21.

Stephenson FH. Real-time PCR. In: Stephenson F, editor. Calculations for molecular biology and biotechnology. 3rd ed. London: Elsevier; 2016. p. 215–320.

Valero C, de la Cruz-Villar L, Zaragoza Ó, Buitrago MJ. New panfungal real-time PCR assay for diagnosis of invasive fungal infections. J Clin Microbiol. 2016;54:2910–8.

Yadav MK, Singh BP. Real-time polymerase chain reaction (PCR) based identification and detection of fungi belongs to genus *Fusarium*. In: Singh B, Gupta V, editors. Molecular markers in mycology. Cham: Fungal Biology. Springer; 2017.

39 Next-Generation Sequencing: Current Technologies and Applications

Dwarakanath Srinivas and Harsh Deora

Abbreviations

ALS	Amyotrophic lateral sclerosis
CNS	Central nervous system
HMP	Human Microbiome Project
ITS	Internal transcribed spacer
MetaHIT	Metagenomics of the Human Intestinal Tract
NGS	Next-generation sequencing
SNP	Single-nucleotide polymorphism

39.1 Introduction

The human body, apart from human cells, is composed of microbial flora, which plays an important role in various physiological processes, called as the *human microbiome* (Zoll et al. 2016). Population-scale projects such as the Human Microbiome Project (HMP) and the Metagenomics of the Human Intestinal Tract (MetaHIT) project have provided a glimpse into the microbial composition of different mucosa, like the skin, the gastrointestinal tract, the respiratory tract, and the urogenital tract (The NIH HMP Working Group et al. 2009; Huttenhower et al. 2012). Although fungi contribute less than 0.1% of the total microbiome, they contribute a major role in the various physiological and pathological processes of the body.

More importantly, etiological diagnosis of inflammatory disorders of the central nervous system (CNS) is a major challenge, with more than 50% cases going undiagnosed (Glaser et al. 2006). Next-generation sequencing (NGS) and metagenomics provide information regarding not only the transcriptome of the human tissue but also of the microbiome that resides in it (Salzberg et al. 2016). 16s rRNA gene-based pathogen identification is exclusive to prokaryotes, and hence deep sequencing of the total DNA or RNA has been utilized to detect even the rarest pathogens present in the microbiome (Wylie et al. 2013).

39.2 Current Technologies

NGS involves sequencing of the entire microbiome of the sample. The application of NGS is still in infancy when it comes to clinical mycology. However, giant strides are being made in mycology research that may soon translate into its application to routine diagnostic mycology.

D. Srinivas (✉)
Department of Neurosurgery, National Institute of Mental Health and Neurosciences (NIMHANS), Bangalore, India

H. Deora
National Institute of Mental Health and Neurosciences (NIMHANS), Bangalore, India

M. Turgut et al. (eds.), *Fungal Infections of the Central Nervous System*,
https://doi.org/10.1007/978-3-030-06088-6_39

39.3 Clinical Mycology

In addition to data obtained from population-scale projects such as HNP and MetaHIT, Bittinger et al. has demonstrated that the relative proportion of bacteria and mycobiota in the lung can be used to differentiate infection from colonization (Bittinger et al. 2014). However, fungal species constitute only 0.1–1% of the human microbiome and even less so in the CNS. This would imply that a level of 10^{12}–10^{14} nucleotides per sequencing run per sample is required to even detect subspecies of the fungi. This means that current available sequencers such as Illumina Miseq, Ion Torrent PGM, and HiSeq are far from the desired sensitivity required to diagnose fungal infections.

Using mycobiomes obtained by sequencing only amplicons of internal transcribed spacer (ITS) of the fungal ribosomal genes, using platforms like Illumina NextSeq, it may be possible to extract information in clinical samples. This would provide a relative composition of the microbiological flora and thus provide an opportunity for application to clinical mycology. Especially in the CNS, the relative proportion of fungi would also give an indication of the severity of the fungal infection. Salzberg et al. in a prospective pilot study applied NGS in combination with computational analysis to detect the presence of pathogenic microbes in brain and spinal cord biopsies from ten patients with findings suggestive of infection but clinical and microbiological studies yielding inconclusive results (Salzberg et al. 2016). They were able to detect infectious processes in eight of the ten cases, thus providing evidence that NGS can dramatically improve our ability to detect or rule out a wide range of CNS pathogens. This is especially applicable to cases where conventional microbiology has been negative or takes too much time to be clinically viable (Salzberg et al. 2016).

39.4 Research Mycology

NGS has been used frequently for research purposes. Options include single-nucleotide polymorphisms (SNPs), microsatellite analysis, amplicon sequencing of ribosomal ITS, and whole genome sequencing. While microsatellite analysis and SNPs are commonly used, ribosomal ITS and whole genome sequencing are the most sensitive in distinguishing various fungal pathogens (Araujo 2014; Dannemiller et al. 2014). Decker et al. showed that a NGS-based diagnostic approach was the best in patients with septic shock. They also demonstrated that invasiveness mycoses could be distinguished from colonization, thus indicating the need for antifungal therapy (Decker et al. 2017). Alonso et al. suggested that amyotrophic lateral sclerosis (ALS) may be a fungal disease and demonstrated a variety of fungal species in each case of ALS with the help of NGS. They even suggest that severity and evolution of the disease may vary from patient to patient in accordance with the fungal species (Alonso et al. 2017).

Azole resistance has been demonstrated in fungal infections including itraconazole, voriconazole, posaconazole, and isavuconazole, especially after long antifungal azole treatment (Bueid et al. 2010; Lockhart et al. 2011; Howard et al. 2009; Snelders et al. 2008; Verweij et al. 2009a). Mechanisms include efflux pumps, which reduce intracellular drug concentration, increased azole target enzyme production, and adaptation of target site of demethylases active in sterol synthetic pathways. Forward and reverse genetic approaches have demonstrated genes involved in *Cryptococcus neoformans* life cycle. Ianiri and Idnurm evaluated 35 genes required for viability in ascomycetes and drug resistance, demonstrating genes involved in ergosterol biosynthetic pathway (Ianiri and Idnurm 2015). Similarly, *Candida* isolates resistant to azoles have shown mutations in genes involved in formation of demethylases and efflux pumps (Garnaud et al. 2015).

Aspergillus fumigatus is an opportunistic fungus causing a variety of diseases in immunocompromised hosts, including invasive aspergillosis. Azole resistance is widespread in this species with resistant species being isolated form the environment (Snelders et al. 2009; Verweij et al. 2009b). Insight into the methods of azole resistance in this group has been investigated with the help of whole genome sequencing on isolated strains of *Aspergillus* from patients with long-term azole resistance. Elucidated mechanism points to mutations in Cyp51 A protein.

Cyp51 A protein is a demethylase involved in ergosterol synthesis which is a component of the fungal cellular wall and the main substrate for demethylase inhibitors like azoles (Latgé 1999). Mutations like amino acid substitution including G54A, P216L, M220V, Y121F, and duplication of 34 and 46 bp nucleotides in the promoter region of CYP51A gene have been found to be responsible for azole resistance. While former mutations are just a marker for azole resistance, duplication in the promoter region leads to increase in Cyp51 A protein synthesis.

Other more obscure mechanisms have been reported. Camps et al. reported four *Aspergillus fumigatus* isolates in which two species developed azole resistance after prolonged therapy and could not be explained by Cyp51 A protein mutations (Camps et al. 2012). They followed these changes with Whole genome sequencing of the isogenic *Aspergillus fumigatus* species and revealed several non-synonymous mutations. To correlate mutations with phenotypes, sexual crossing experiments were done on the progeny of azole resistance phenotype. These revealed that azole resistance was associated with a P88L amino acid substitution in the CCAAT-binding transcription factor complex subunit HapE. Also, the HapE P88L mutation caused an increased CYP51A gene expression thus causing resistance.

Similar study done by Fraczek et al. in *Aspergillus fumigatus* species lacking Cyp51 A mutation revealed 20 potential azole transporter genes (Fraczek et al. 2013). In one, CYP51A expression was increased 500 times in the presence of azoles. Others demonstrated an increase in CDR1B efflux transporter gene and in one out of five isolates, a P216L amino acid substitution was found in Cyp51A in conjunction with several other non- synonymous mutations and deletions of clusters of genes (Hagiwara et al. 2014). These authors thus concluded that the cdr1B efflux transporter is associated with Cyp51A-independent azole resistance.

While whole genome sequencing has offered us insight into the mechanisms of azole resistance, other NGS tools have demonstrated changes in genetic expression due to environmental changes. Gene expression changes with stress and is regulated with epigenetic mechanisms like DNA hydroxylation-methylation. Cytosine methylation or hydroxylation can be studied by the chemical conversion using bisulfate of cytosine into uracil.

Computational analysis along with NGS is powerful tool to study/diagnose fungal infections. Transcriptome analysis studies gene expression by growing fungal cells after messenger RNA are extracted from cells and sequenced after conversion to complementary DNA. Thus, the relative abundance of messenger RNA grown after and before exposure to azoles provides evidence to the change in gene expression because of these compounds.

Thus, while whole genome sequencing overcomes much of the limitations of currently available sequencers like Illumina NextSeq and HiSeq and provides insight into mechanisms of azole resistance, transcriptome analysis and DNA methylation provide proof of gene expression changes with azole exposure. These are the tools currently available for research in mycology.

39.5 Conclusion

Accuracy, speed, and sensitivity are the USP of NGS. It is especially valuable in fungal infections as these are notoriously difficult to grow in culture and thus offer "culture-independent" mechanisms of diagnosis. In addition, these offer similar if not better information considering the application of NGS to detect azole resistance, distinguishing infection and colonization and guiding treatment. Thus, "next" generation needs to be incorporated to current diagnostic methodologies.

References

Alonso R, Pisa D, Fernandez-fernandez AM, Rabano A, Carrasco L. Fungal infection in neural tissue of patients with amyotrophic lateral sclerosis. Neurobiol Dis. 2017;108:249–60.

Araujo R. Towards the genotyping of fungi: methods, benefits and challenges. Curr Fungal Infect Rep. 2014;8:203–10.

Bittinger K, Charlson ES, Loy E, Shirley DJ, Haas AR, Laughlin A, et al. Improved characterization of medically relevant fungi in the human respiratory tract using next-generation sequencing. Genome Biol. 2014;15:487.

Bueid A, Howard SJ, Moore CB, Richardson MD, Harrison E, et al. Azole antifungal resistance in Aspergillus fumigatus: 2008 and 2009. J Antimicrob Chemother. 2010;65:2116–8.

Camps SMT, Dutilh BE, Arendrup MC, Rijs AJMM, Snelders E, Huynen MA, et al. Discovery of a HapE mutation that causes azole resistance in Aspergillus fumigatus through whole genome sequencing and sexual crossing. PLoS One. 2012;7:e50034.

Dannemiller KC, Reeves D, Bibby K, Yamamoto N, Peccia J. Fungal high-throughput taxonomic identification tool for use with next-generation sequencing (FHiTINGS). J Basic Microbiol. 2014;54:315–21.

Decker SO, Sigl A, Grumaz C, et al. Immune-response patterns and next generation sequencing diagnostics for the detection of mycoses in patients with septic shock—results of a combined clinical and experimental investigation. Int J Mol Sci. 2017;18(8):1796. https://doi.org/10.3390/ijms18081796.

Fraczek MG, Bromley M, Buied A, Moore CB, Rajendran R, Rautemaa R, et al. The cdr1B efflux transporter is associated with non-cyp51a-mediated itraconazole resistance in Aspergillus fumigatus. J Antimicrob Chemother. 2013;68:1486–96.

Garnaud C, Botterel F, Sertour N, Bougnoux M, Dannaoui E, Larrat S, et al. Next-generation sequencing offers new insights into the resistance of Candida spp. to echinocandins and azoles. J Antimicrob Chemother. 2015;70:2556–65.

Glaser CA, Honarmand S, Anderson LJ, et al. Beyond viruses: clinical profiles and etiologies associated with encephalitis. Clin Infect Dis. 2006;43:1565–77.

Hagiwara D, Takahashi H, Watanabe A, Takahashi-Nakaguchi A, Kawamoto S, Kamei K, et al. Whole-genome comparison of Aspergillus fumigatus strains serially isolated from patients with Aspergillosis. J Clin Microbiol. 2014;52:4202–9.

Howard SJ, Cerar D, Anderson MJ, Albarrag A, Fisher MC, et al. Frequency and evolution of azole resistance in Aspergillus fumigatus associated with treatment failure. Emerg Infect Dis. 2009;15:1068–76.

Huttenhower C, Gevers D, Knight R, Abubucker S, Badger JH, Chinwalla AT, et al. Structure, function and diversity of the healthy human microbiome. Nature. 2012;486:207–14.

Ianiri G, Idnurm A. Essential gene discovery in the basidiomycete Cryptococcus neoformans for antifungal drug target prioritization. MBio. 2015;6(2):e02334–14.

Latgé JP. Aspergillus fumigatus and aspergillosis. Clin Microbiol Rev. 1999;12:310–50.

Lockhart SR, Frade JP, Etienne KA, Pfaller MA, Diekema DJ, et al. Azole resistance in Aspergillus fumigatus isolates from the ARTEMIS global surveillance is primarily due to the TR/L98H mutation in the cyp51A gene. Antimicrob Agents Chemother. 2011;55:4465–8.

Salzberg SL, Breitwieser FP, Kumar A, Hao H, Burger P, Rodriguez FJ, et al. Next-generation sequencing in neuropathologic diagnosis of infections of the nervous system. Neurol Neuroimmunol Neuroinflamm. 2016;3:e251. https://doi.org/10.1212/NXI.0000000000000251.

Snelders E, van der Lee HA, Kuijpers J, Rijs AJ, Varga J, et al. Emergence of azole resistance in Aspergillus fumigatus and spread of a single resistance mechanism. PLoS Med. 2008;5:e219.

Snelders E, Huis In 't Veld RA, Rijs AJ, Kema GH, Melchers WJ, Verweij PE. Possible environmental origin of resistance of Aspergillus fumigatus to medical triazoles. Appl Environ Microbiol. 2009;75(12):4053–7.

The NIH HMP Working Group, Peterson J, Garges S, Giovanni M, McInnes P, Wang L, et al. The NIH human microbiome project. Genome Res. 2009;19:2317–23.

Verweij PE, Howard SJ, Melchers WJ, Denning DW. Azole- resistance in Aspergillus: proposed nomenclature and breakpoints. Drug Resist Updat. 2009a;12:141–7.

Verweij PE, Snelders E, Kema GH, Mellado E, Melchers WJ. Azole resistance in Aspergillus fumigatus: a side-effect of environmental fungicide use? Lancet Infect Dis. 2009b;9:789–95.

Wylie KM, Weinstock GM, Storch GA. Virome genomics: a tool for defining the human virome. Curr Opin Microbiol. 2013;16:479–84.

Zoll J, Snelders E, Verweij PE, Melchers WJG. Next-generation sequencing in the mycology lab. Curr Fungal Infect Rep. 2016;10:37–42. https://doi.org/10.1007/s12281-016-0253-6.

Current Innovations and Future Trends

40

Neeraj Kumar, Ravindra Kumar Garg, and Hardeep Singh Malhotra

Abbreviations

CNS	Central nervous system
CSF	Cerebrospinal fluid
CSTET	Cryo-scanning transmission electron tomography
FIB-SEM	Focused ion beam scanning electron microscopy
LAMP	Loop-mediated isothermal amplification
MALDI-TOF	Matrix-assited laser desorption/ionization time of flight
MRI	Magnetic resonance imaging
PCR	Polymerase chain reaction

A dream will not become an innovation if there is no futuristic vision.

40.1 Introduction

Central nervous system (CNS) infection is a common entity in most part of the world. Prompt diagnosis and treatment is the key in saving life of a patient. Viral, bacterial, and mycobacterial agents are high in suspicion index in CNS infections. Fungal infections are mostly considered in immunocompromised state. In cases with no or poor response to treatment, fungal infection is suspected. The diagnosis of fungal infection is difficult and often delayed due to paucity of diagnostic methods.

40.2 Current Innovations in Diagnosis and Future Trends

Diagnosis of any infectious etiology depends upon either isolation of causative organism or demonstration of histopathological/serological changes.

40.2.1 Microscopy and Culture

The age-old method of microscopy is still relevant in early detection of fungal elements, but identification of actual fungal species may not be always possible.

The old saying "*A picture is worth a thousand words*" is very much relevant in microscopy of fungal infection. India ink stain and optical brighteners like calcofluor white helps in microscopic identification. The composition and structure of

N. Kumar · R. K. Garg (✉) · H. S. Malhotra
Department of Neurology, King George's Medical University, Lucknow, Uttar Pradesh, India
e-mail: rkgarg@kgmcindia.edu

M. Turgut et al. (eds.), *Fungal Infections of the Central Nervous System*,
https://doi.org/10.1007/978-3-030-06088-6_40

fungal agents are different, and newer stains are required to identify the actual fungal species.

Advances in the field of adaptive optics in scanning will be helpful (Lagree et al. 2018). New imaging modalities like cryo-scanning transmission electron tomography (CSTET), focused ion beam scanning electron microscopy (FIB-SEM), and soft X-ray tomography will be the future in diagnostics. Super resolution fluorescence microscopy helps in structural and functional delineation of cellular and subcellular structures. Combination of CSTET with fluorescent light microscopy will be an additional boon (Briegel and Uphoff 2018). Culture requires special media and takes a long time. The incubation period may range from 1 to 4 weeks. Augmented culture and new culture media is the need of the hour. Combination of fluorescence tagging with media substrate may expedite diagnosis.

40.2.2 Serology

Serological measurement of mannan antigen and antimannan antibodies is approved in Europe for diagnosis in fungal infections. The sensitivity and specificity is more than 80% in combined analysis (Ostrosky-Zeichner and Al-Obaidi 2017). Testing of 1,3-β-D-glucan levels in serum and cerebrospinal fluid (CSF) is also a sensitive marker of fungal infection. In abdominal candidiasis, it has been found to be better than culture and polymerase chain reaction (PCR) testing (Colombo et al. 2017). More biomarkers in CSF and serum are required to be discovered and tested for clinical efficacy.

40.2.3 Polymerase Chain Reaction-Based Assay

PCR-based assay is an excellent testing method for diagnosis. More and more information regarding genetics of fungi and resistant genome is being identified. The sensitivity (80–100%) and specificity (70–100%) varies but is high (Ostrosky-Zeichner and Al-Obaidi 2017). Fluorescent-based real-time PCR helps in early detection and diagnosis. Manual DNA extraction is having risk of contamination as compared to fully automated DNA extraction. Utilizing automated DNA extraction and real-time PCR will provide result in few hours.

Multiplex PCR is helpful in distinguishing various types of fungi, thus guiding appropriate treatment. Many commercial PCR-based panels are available. Two USFDA (United States Food and Drug Adminstration) approved panels are being used: (1) T2Candida Panel (2) SeptiFast (Ostrosky-Zeichner and Al-Obaidi 2017).

Quantitative PCR methodology requires evaluation for its utility in monitoring treatment response and virulence. Fungal ribosomal gene identification can also help in identification of different species. Luminex xMAP is a new DNA-based identification method using color-coded microspheres to detect specific gene sequence (Kozel and Wickes 2014). Increasingly, non-rDNA loci are being identified to recognize the particular fungal species. Future innovation requires techniques to detect and identify different species with more sensitivity and specificity.

40.2.4 Loop-Mediated Isothermal Amplification

Loop-mediated isothermal amplification (LAMP) is a newer technique that amplifies target DNA rapidly, efficiently, and specifically (Malhotra et al. 2014).

40.2.5 Fingerprinting/Proteomic Profiling

A newer non-nucleic acid-based diagnostic method is matrix-assisted laser desorption/ionization time of flight (MALDI-TOF). This technique utilizes spectra-based identification of different species. Commercial production is provided as MALDI Biotyper, AXIMA@SARAMIS, and ANDROMAS (Kozel and Wickes 2014).

The biggest challenge in future is to develop a diagnostic test that is simple, cost effective, available widely at point of patient care, and specific in all situations.

40.2.6 Radiology

Medical advances owe heavily to innovations in imaging technology. X-ray, computerized tomography, and magnetic resonance imaging (MRI) are widely available and help in diagnosis. Though some imaging features are characteristic in identifying the fungal organism type, many a times the radiological picture is inconclusive.

Positron emission tomography is now increasingly being advocated in fungal diseases too. It has been shown to be able to detect fungal involvement in the lung, bone, and other organs. Additionally, it shows promise in deciding the treatment completion end point. More research is required to fully utilize this technique in identifying different type of fungal organism.

Magnetic resonance spectroscopy can be improvised to detect various chemical differences in imaging signal, thus assisting in species identification.

In future, improved imaging modalities will be increasingly required. Higher Tesla machines with greater resolution will eventually be as good as microscopy. Innovations in software and linking with MRI machine will lead to species identification and characterization in a noninvasive manner.

40.3 Current Innovations in Treatment and Future Trends

40.3.1 Antifungals

Initiation of antifungals is usually delayed due to diagnostic difficulties and certainty. Many times, empirical treatment is started in a nonresponsive patient. Various antifungal groups like polyene, azoles, allylamines, and echinocandins are available. Resistance is now increasingly being identified (Revie et al. 2018). Albaconazole, CD101(biafungin), MK-3118(enfumafungin), VL-2397, and many other drugs are in phase 1 and phase 2 trial.

Newer drugs acting at various metabolic and enzymatic steps need to be discovered. Higher CNS penetration is also a requisite for better prognosis.

40.3.2 Adjuvants

Drug adjuvants like iron chelators have been shown good action as a synergist. A study by Lai et al. showed increased efficacy of amphotericin when combined with iron chelators (Lai et al. 2016). In the future, more such adjuvants are required to be discovered and tested.

40.4 Current Innovations in Vaccines and Future Trends

Aging population, industrialization, and increased antibiotics use are causing resurgence of fungal infections. Vaccination may be helpful in preventing such infections. Research in this area is at its naïve stage and requires a major thrust. Combined bacterial and fungal vaccine may be a reality in future.

40.5 Conclusion

Advancement in research is leading to new diagnostic and therapeutic tools, such as FIB-SEM, LAMP, etc. in the field of fungal infections of the CNS. Newer innovation in diagnosis will greatly reduce diagnostic time and specificity. Also, some new promising drugs are being tested. We hope that an upcoming vaccine may be a reality in the future.

References

Briegel A, Uphoff S. Editorial overview: the new microscopy. Curr Opin Microbiol. 2018;43:208–11. https://doi.org/10.1016/j.mib.2018.04.003.

Colombo AL, de Almeida Júnior JN, Slavin MA, Chen SC, Sorrell TC. Candida and invasive mould diseases in non-neutropenic critically ill patients and patients with haematological cancer. Lancet Infect Dis. 2017;17(11):e344–56. https://doi.org/10.1016/S1473-3099(17)30304-3.

Kozel TR, Wickes B. Fungal diagnostics. Cold Spring Harb Perspect Med. 2014;4(4):a019299.

Lagree K, Desai JV, Finkel JS, Lanni F. Microscopy of fungal biofilms. Curr Opin Microbiol. 2018;43:100–7.

Lai YW, Campbell LT, Wilkins MR, Pang CN, Chen S, Carter DA. Synergy and antagonism between iron chelators and antifungal drugs in Cryptococcus. Int J Antimicrob Agents. 2016;48(4):388–94.

Malhotra S, Sharma S, Bhatia NJ, Kumar P, Bhatia NK, Patil V, Hans C. Recent diagnostic techniques in mycology. J Med Microbiol Diagn. 2014;3(3):1.

Ostrosky-Zeichner L, Al-Obaidi M. Invasive fungal infections in the intensive care unit. Infect Dis Clin N Am. 2017;31(3):475–87.

Revie NM, Iyer KR, Robbins N, Cowen LE. Antifungal drug resistance: evolution, mechanisms and impact. Curr Opin Microbiol. 2018;45:70–6.

Conclusion

Although the most common causes of neuroinfections are bacteria and viruses, the role of fungi should not be ignored especially since these potentially devastating infections are encountered world wide. Fungal infections of the central nervous system (CNS) have a large spectrum of presenting features, and though most patients are immunocompromised hosts, immunocompetent subjects can also be affected. Unfortunately, the diagnosis is often delayed or not considered in routine clinical practice.

Diagnosis and management of CNS infections due to fungi is a true challenge because they often occur in a clinical context that is neither specific nor alarming. Neuroimaging data may be indicative but are not specific. However, pathology plays an important role for confirming the definitive diagnosis, especially if clinical findings, laboratory studies, and diagnostic imaging investigations are not conclusive. Systemic antifungal medications remain the cornerstone of management. However, in many patients diagnosis remains uncertain, or medical treatments are not effective, and severe complications needing surgical intervention may occur.

With these in mind, the main purpose of this richly illustrated book is to provide the reader with a frame of symptoms and signs of this particular infectious disease in an effort to suspect and confirm the diagnosis of CNS fungal infections at and early stage and therefore prevent damage to the brain parenchyma and meninges.

Education and training of medical personnel to recognize the disease early forms the pedestal of successful management along with careful infection control practices. Also, concomitant research to understand the pathogenesis of the disease, genetic risk factors for invasive fungal infections in humans, and the advance in diagnostic tools in addition to new therapeutic modalities can improve outcomes in the future.

Aydın, Turkey — Mehmet Turgut
Hyderabad, India — Sundaram Challa
Marrakech, Morocco — Ali Akhaddar

M. Turgut et al. (eds.), *Fungal Infections of the Central Nervous System*,
https://doi.org/10.1007/978-3-030-06088-6

Printed by Printforce, the Netherlands